Atlas of Neurotologic and Lateral Skull Base Surgery

John S. Oghalai • Colin L.W. Driscoll

Atlas of Neurotologic and Lateral Skull Base Surgery

Springer

John S. Oghalai, MD
Department of Otolaryngology – Head and Neck Surgery
Stanford University
Stanford, CA
USA

Colin L.W. Driscoll, MD
Department of Otorhinolaryngology
Mayo Medical School
Rochester, MN
USA

ISBN 978-3-662-46693-3 ISBN 978-3-662-46694-0 (eBook)
DOI 10.1007/978-3-662-46694-0

Library of Congress Control Number: 2015946111

Springer Heidelberg New York Dordrecht London

Illustrations by Scott A. Weldon, MA, CMI, Houston, TX, USA

Printed on acid-free paper

Springer-Verlag GmbH Berlin Heidelberg is part of Springer Science+Business Media (www.springer.com)

To my wife, Tracy, and my children, Kevin and Tom, for their support.

To my trainees for their inspiration. To my patients for their faith.

John S. Oghalai, MD

To my patients for their trust.

To my family, Sheri, Abigail and Avery for their support.

Colin L.W. Driscoll, MD

Acknowledgements

No one learns surgery in a vacuum. Most of the techniques we describe within this text are based upon techniques we learned during training. Since both of us were clinical fellows at the University of California, San Francisco, we certainly must acknowledge our fellowship director and mentor, Robert Jackler, MD. His training, leadership, and enthusiasm for scholarship helped build the foundation for our careers in academic medicine. Dr. Jackler's textbooks, lectures, and writings are wonderful models of educational materials. We hope this text will serve to honor and enhance his legacy.

Additional acknowledgments must go out to the other neurotologists that also trained us. This list is extensive, but includes Bobby Alford, MD, Herman Jenkins, MD, Newton Coker, MD, Anil Lalwani, MD, Steve Cheung, MD, and Steve Harner, MD. Of course, we have also learned from the neurosurgeons we have worked with, including Larry Pitts, MD, Mike McDermott, MD, Mitch Berger, MD, Dan Yoshor, MD, Youssef Comair, MD, David Baskin, MD, Gordon Li, MD, Larry Shuer, MD, Robert Dodd, MD, Gary Steinberg, MD, PhD, Mike Ebersold, MD, and Mike Link, MD.

Of course, we are indebted to Scott Weldon. His skill as a medical illustrator is of the highest level. Besides his incredible talent as an artist, Scott is an easy-going person and a great collaborator. We feel lucky to have been able to work with him on this large project.

Finally, we must express gratitude to the multitude of faculty, fellows, residents, medical students, and visitors that we have had the opportunity to work with, train, and learn from over the years. We find it is this spirit of collegiality, teamwork, learning, and optimism, all while striving to care for our patients with empathy, that makes us feel lucky to have careers as academic skull base surgeons.

John S. Oghalai, MD
Colin L.W. Driscoll, MD

Contents

1 Introduction 1

2 General Principles 3
Room Layout 3
Use of the Mayfield Head Holder 4
Computer-Guided Stereotactic Navigation 8
Cranial Nerve Monitoring 9
CSF Management. 10
Instrumentation 14

3 Middle Fossa Approaches 19
Approach to the Internal Auditory Canal. 19
Kawase's Triangle Approach 33
Orbitocraniozygomatic Approach 37

4 Posterior Fossa Approaches 51
Translabyrinthine Approach 51
Transcochlear Approach 72
Retrosigmoid Approach. 83
Far Lateral Approach. 104

5 Combined Approach to the Middle and Posterior Fossa 115

6 Infratemporal Fossa Approaches 131
Postauricular Approach to the Infratemporal Fossa 131
Preauricular Approach to the Infratemporal Fossa 162
Pre- and Postauricular Approach to the Infratemporal Fossa 181

7 Temporal Bone Surgery for Infectious Disease. 193
Simple Mastoidectomy for Acute Mastoiditis. 193
Retrolabyrinthine Craniotomy for Intracranial Complications of Acute Mastoiditis 196
Subtotal (Circumferential) Petrosectomy for Acute Petrositis or Skull Base Osteomyelitis. 214

8 Temporal Bone Surgery for Encephaloceles, Superior Semicircular Canal Dehiscence, Neoplasia, and Lesions of the Petrous Apex 221
Repair of Temporal Lobe Encephalocele 221
Repair of Superior Semicircular Canal Dehiscence. 235
Temporal Bone Resection 238
Drainage of Petrous Apex Lesions. 254

9 Facial Nerve Surgery 263

10 Cochlear Implantation. 281

11 Surgery for Vertigo 303
Endolymphatic Shunt 303
Vestibular Nerve Section 307
Labyrinthectomy 308

12 Complications and Additional Thoughts 311

Index 319

1 Introduction

Neurotology and skull base surgery is a wonderful career path. We highly recommend it! Patients range in age from the very young to the elderly and range in health from being completely normal to having multiple severe comorbidities. The pathologies are variable, spanning the spectrum from uncomplicated benign lesions to highly complex life-threatening lesions. Operating in and around the skull base is complex because of the detailed anatomy, large vascular structures, and the presence of cranial nerves. As you become an expert in this anatomy, you will be able to resect formidable-appearing tumors with superb survival rates and limited morbidity. Most patients will return to active and productive lives.

The importance of having a dedicated skull base surgical team cannot be overstated. There is a synergistic effect when the group works as a coordinated team in the management of these complex tumors and pathologies. A dedicated neurotologist, neurosurgeon, neuroradiologist, radiation oncologist, intraoperative monitoring technician, proficient surgical scrub, and experienced ICU staff are all critical to success. A high case volume is required to generate the necessary expertise.

The increasing use of stereotactic radiotherapy and observation strategies to treat vestibular schwannoma has led to a decline in surgical volume. However, these strategies have added options that increase patient choice and have improved outcomes for many patients. Since benign skull base tumors often have minimal presenting symptoms, surgical treatment and associated cranial neuropathies may make a patient feel worse after treatment than before treatment. Involving the patient in the selection of treatment planning, in our opinion, makes them much more satisfied when living with side effects after the chosen treatment strategy. Thus, you should embrace the consideration of these and any other future treatment strategies and always discuss these options.

This atlas contains both illustrations and case examples. The illustrations show the anatomy and the key steps in the surgical approaches. The case examples highlight unique features relevant to the approach. For example, pre- and postoperative radiographic images are included to demonstrate representative pathologies and the expected results. Similarly, intraoperative photos demonstrate specific features of the procedure that are often quite subtle but, when followed, can help to achieve ideal results. Most importantly, we have found that the careful review of case examples is an excellent way to teach residents and fellows the process of surgical decision-making. When you have a challenging case, we hope that by scanning the cases in this book, you will be able to find a similar case that can help guide your treatment planning.

Each chapter in this atlas covers approaches to different regions of the skull base. However, the head and neck are not easily divided up as many structures involve multiple regions. Also, many tumors involve more than one region. Thus, many of the approaches overlap. For example, a temporal bone tumor invading into the parotid gland and posterior fossa may be best treated with a transcochlear approach (Chap. 4) combined with a temporal bone resection (Chap. 8). Do not feel limited by the nomenclature of each approach, which is based upon CPT coding. Instead, treat each patient as an individual by considering the physical exam and radiographic imaging findings when deciding what structures need to be removed and what can be preserved. This thought process will help you to figure out which approach or combination of approaches will best allow you to perform the procedure you wish to perform. Many tumors call for creativity, an exciting aspect of the specialty.

J.S. Oghalai, C.L.W. Driscoll, *Atlas of Neurotologic and Lateral Skull Base Surgery*,
DOI 10.1007/978-3-662-46694-0_1, © Springer-Verlag Berlin Heidelberg 2016

General Principles

2

Room Layout

1. Room layout for an approach on the right side. The bed should be turned 180° from the anesthesiologist to allow maximum room around the patient's head. Having the microscope base at the head of the bed allows the assistant to sit under the boom arm and observe through the side arm. The scrub nurse sits across the patient from the surgeon to facilitate the handing of instruments. He/she can have a Mayo stand near the patient's head to hold the commonly used instruments, cottonoid patties, Surgicel, and Gelfoam. All of the rest of the less frequently used instruments can be kept on the back table.

The neurophysiologist can realistically be placed anywhere in the room. However, he/she should be close enough so that the surgeon can communicate with the neurophysiologist and be able to hear the speaker from their machine.

Your anesthesia colleagues may initially not be enthusiastic about being away from the head of the bed but will adapt. The sooner after induction of anesthesia that the table can be turned, the sooner the case can be started. An experienced team should be ready to make an incision 45 min after the patient enters the OR. Once the OR table is turned, multiple people can work simultaneously to place an arterial line, Foley catheter, or EMG monitoring electrodes and to work on patient positioning.

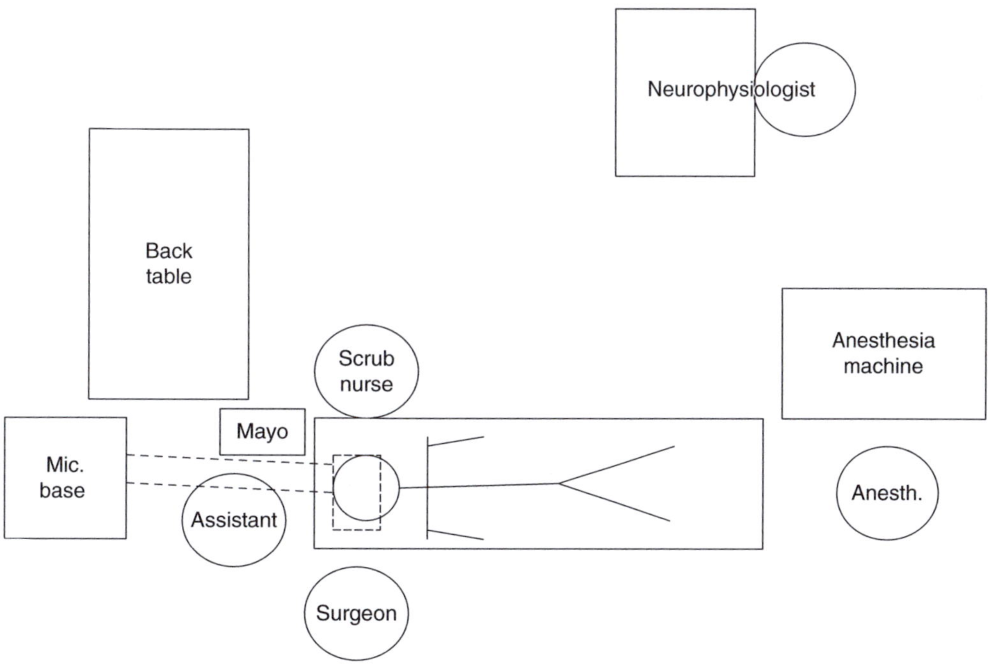

J.S. Oghalai, C.L.W. Driscoll, *Atlas of Neurotologic and Lateral Skull Base Surgery*,
DOI 10.1007/978-3-662-46694-0_2, © Springer-Verlag Berlin Heidelberg 2016

Use of the Mayfield Head Holder

2. A Mayfield head holder serves two important purposes. First, it rigidly fixates the head so it will not move relative to the operating table. Second, it allows for the attachment of adjustable retractors. We typically use the Greenberg retractor system or the Budde Halo system. By rigidly connecting the table, the head, and the retractor, there is less opportunity for unexpected movements to occur during the surgery. While not every skull base surgery needs the use of the Mayfield, it is often helpful in long cases or those where careful brain retraction is expected.

   The Mayfield has three pins. To securely clamp the head, the two pins are typically placed near the back of the head and must be seated above the nuchal line (the horizontal ridge of bone in the back of the head where the posterior paraspinal muscles attach). Ideally, pinning is performed so that one of these two pins is placed under the head to reduce the risk of gravity pulling the patient's head out of the pins during the long surgery. After first making sure the two pins are firmly in contact with the head, the side with the single pin is then clamped down near the front of the head. Before pinning the patient, bacitracin ointment is applied to the three pins. Also, the anesthesiologist should be warned. The stimulation associated with pinning can often require additional sedation.

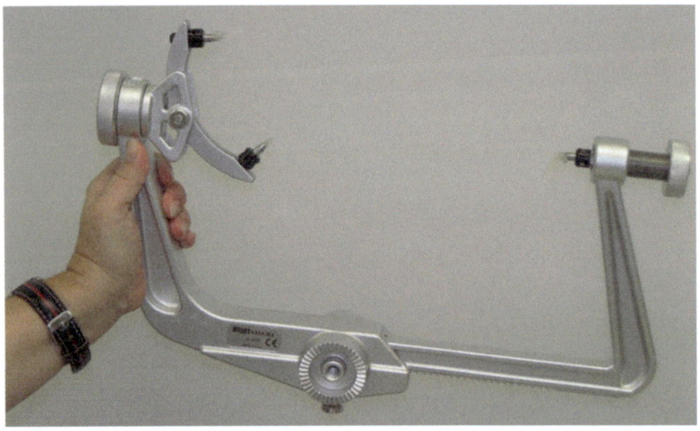

3. Pinning must be performed carefully so as not to traumatize the patient's neck or brachial plexus with overstretching. In this example, the patient was pinned for a retrosigmoid approach for vestibular schwannoma resection. Note the large café au lait spot consistent with this patient's diagnosis of neurofibromatosis type II. A shoulder bump was placed to help rotate the torso slightly.

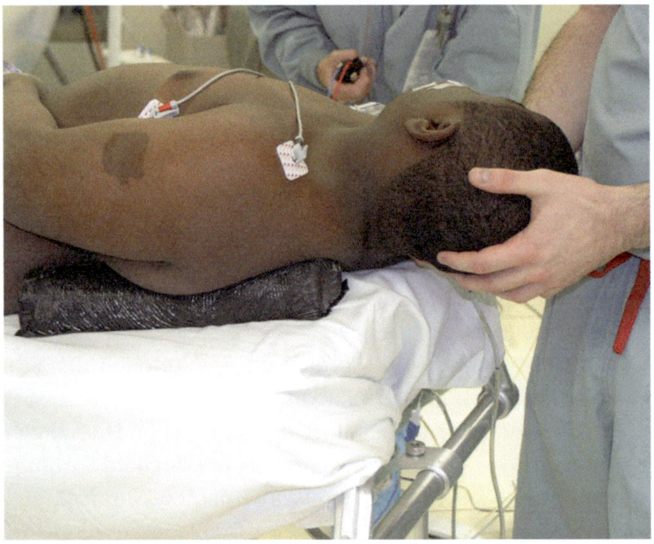

4. The posterior two pins are seated first to ensure that they both make firm contact with the skull above the nuchal line. During this process, the person applying the pins must be sure not to accidentally poke the hand of the person holding the patient's head. Note the glob of bacitracin ointment on the anterior pin.

5. Next, the single pin is brought in. With lateral skull base surgery, this pin often needs to be placed in the forehead. While this is not ideal because of the postoperative pigmentation that can occur in that spot, it is not worth the risk of trying to move the pin to a hair-bearing area. It will not hold the head tightly, and the head may slide out of the pins during the long surgery.

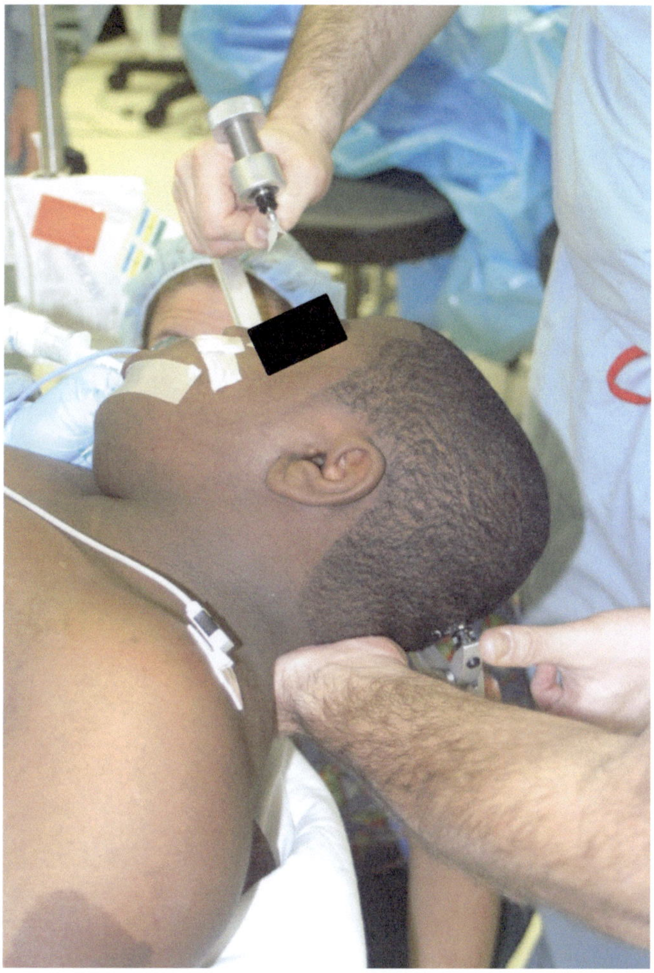

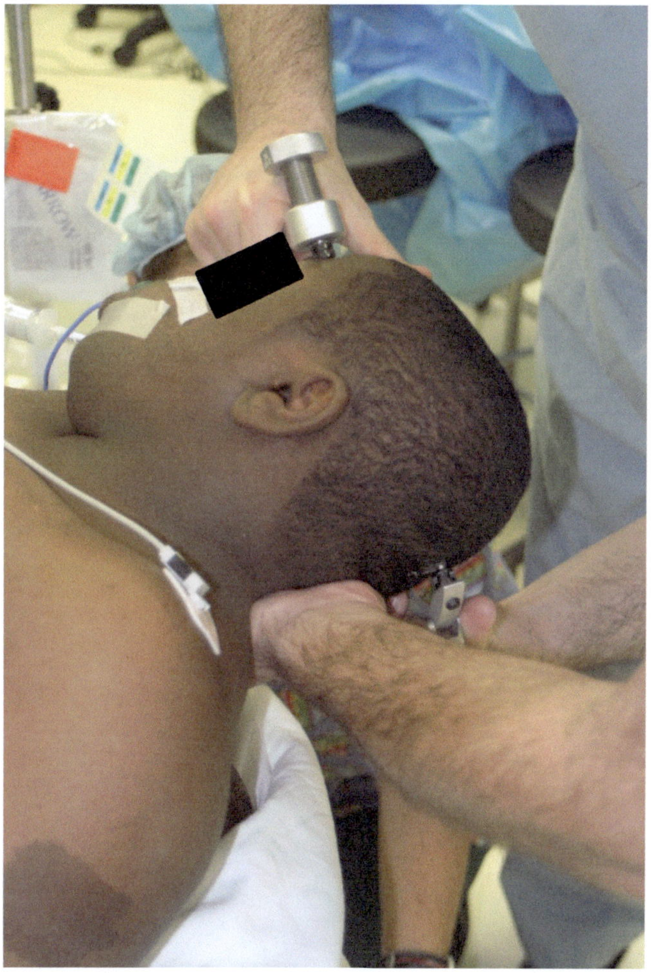

6. The screw is turned to tighten the pins.

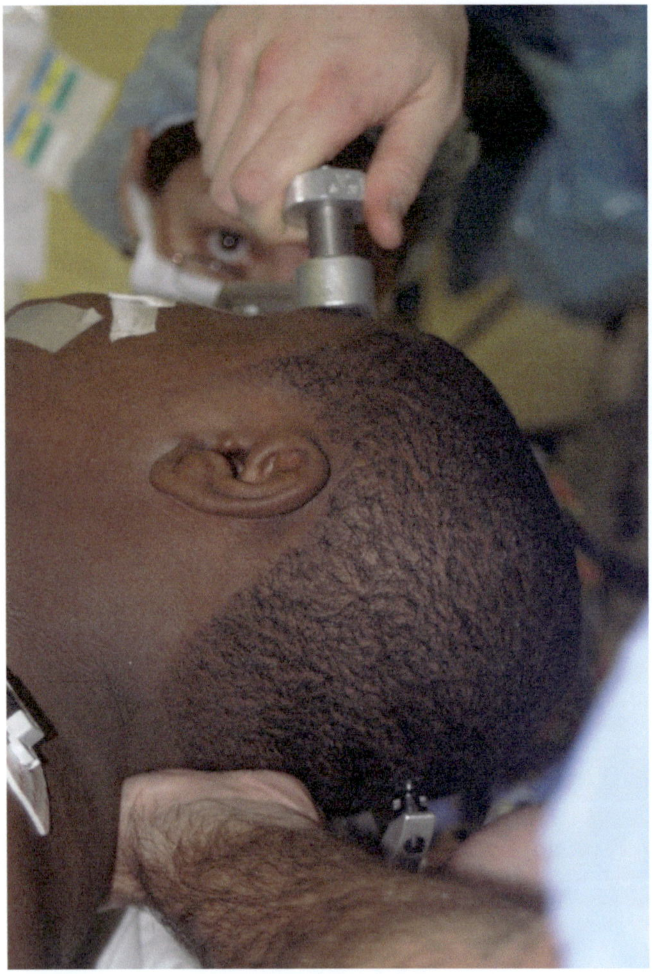

7. For adults, the screw should be tightened until the third line is reached (60 lbs pressure). When pinning children, shorter pins are used, and the pressure is lowered to prevent a skull fracture.

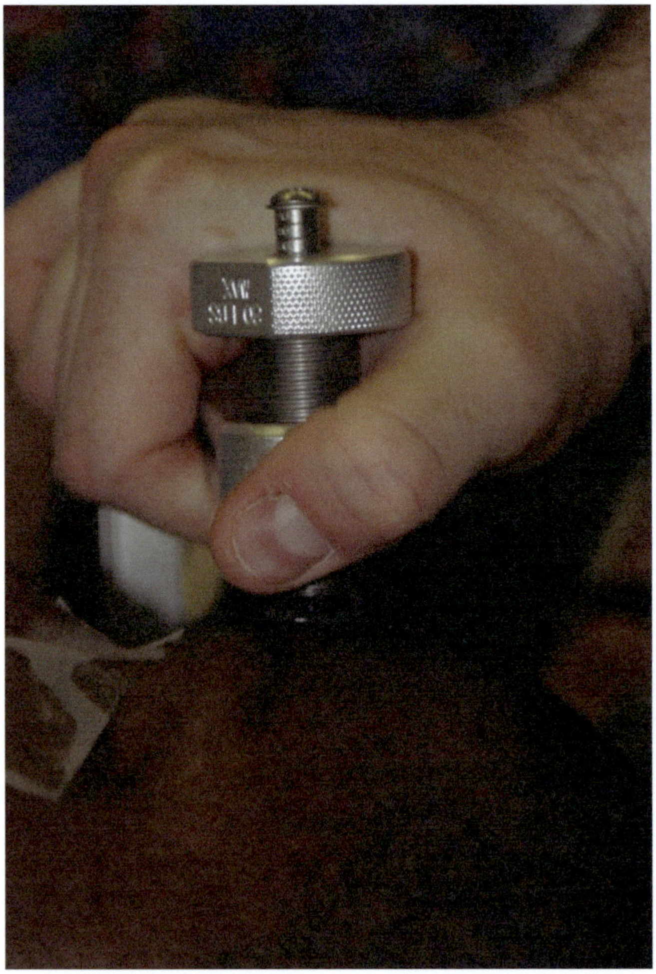

8. Finally, the head is placed in the proper position. The surgeon must think about what view he/she wants during surgery before finalizing the head position. Typically, we like to have the head flat and tilted forward slightly to keep the operative field as far away from the shoulder as possible. However, care should be taken to make sure that a hand can fit between the patient's chin and shoulder. If space is not left here, a brachial plexus stretch injury can occur. Head and neck positioning is important when using the Mayfield head frame. Although the OR table can be tilted, every effort should be made to properly position the patient to minimize the need to tilt the bed. There is increased risk of a compressive neuropathy or of falling off the bed when it is tilted, particularly for prolonged procedures.

   The screws are tightened at each joint, working from the top down. Before releasing the head, verify the integrity of the Mayfield head holder by trying to jiggle the head slightly. It should not move at all.

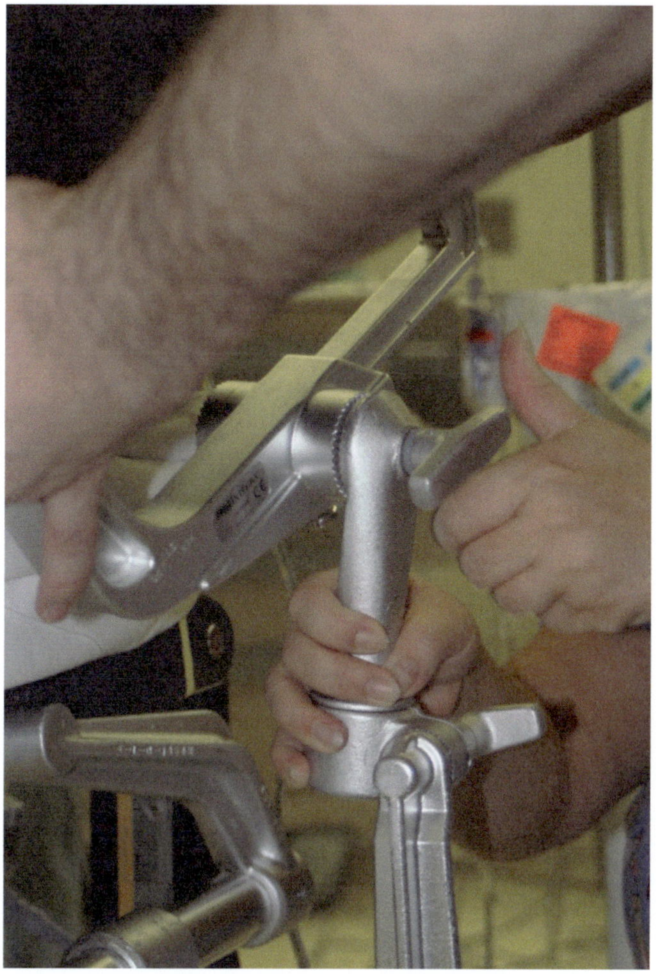

9. The final view of the patient after placing the Mayfield head holder.

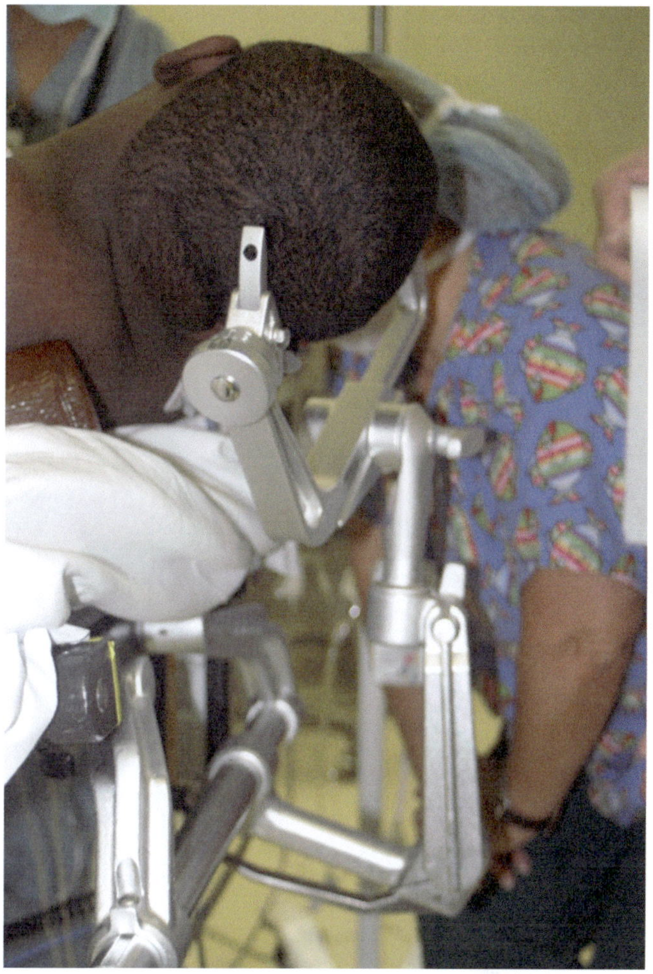

Computer-Guided Stereotactic Navigation

10. A typical setup for a Stealth navigation system is shown here. The patient has already had an MRI and/or CT scan with the fiducials in place. The Mayfield head holder is placed. Then, each fiducial is located using the computer software. After this has been done, the fiducials can be removed.

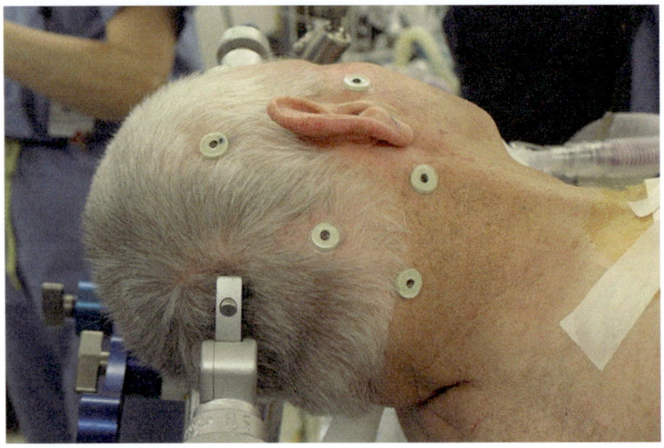

11. During surgery, the Stealth probe is used to identify the anatomic position of structures noted intraoperatively. This is particularly helpful when assessing structures fixed to the skull as they do not shift position as do structures within or attached to the brain. One minor problem with the Stealth system is that the microscope must sometimes be moved out of the way to fit the probe into the wound. Finding an appropriate position for the viewing screen and other stereotactic navigation equipment can be challenging in smaller ORs.

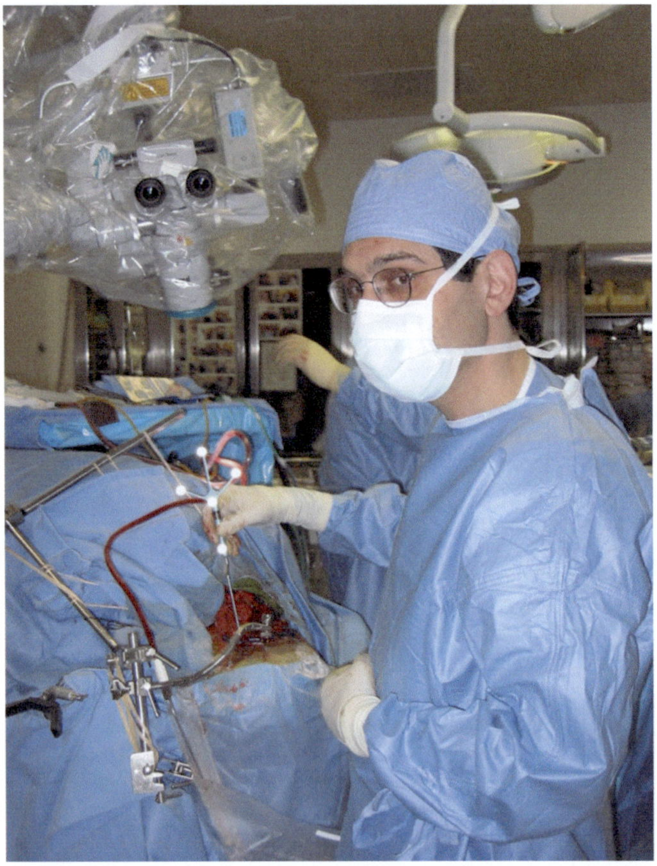

Cranial Nerve Monitoring

12. A typical setup for facial nerve monitoring is shown here. This is what we use for routine ear surgery and cochlear implant. The automated facial nerve monitoring machine is used instead of a dedicated neurophysiologist. The paired electrodes (red and blue) are placed at the corner of the eye and mouth. They are placed in a subdermal position, meaning that they do not penetrate deep, just parallel to the skin. There is no significance to whether the red or blue paired electrode is placed at either the corner of the eyes or the corner of the mouth. In either case, activation of the orbicularis oculus and orbicularis oris muscles will be detected. The ground for the recording electrode (green) and the ground for the stimulating electrode (white) are placed anywhere on the chest.

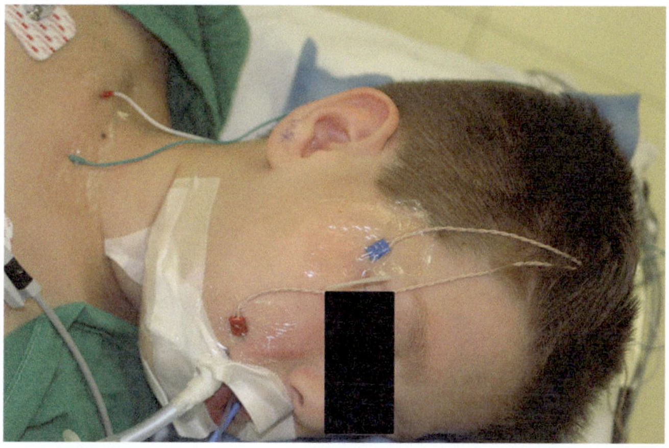

13. When skull base surgery is to be performed, we always use a neurophysiologist. At a minimum, we measure cranial nerves V, VII, and XI. In this example, where we were doing a hearing preservation middle fossa approach, we also measured ABRs. The facial nerve electrodes were placed at the corner of the eye and mouth. Also, the electrodes for the masseter muscle (CN V) are visible in the midcheek region. Lastly, the electrode for the ABR was placed in the earlobe.

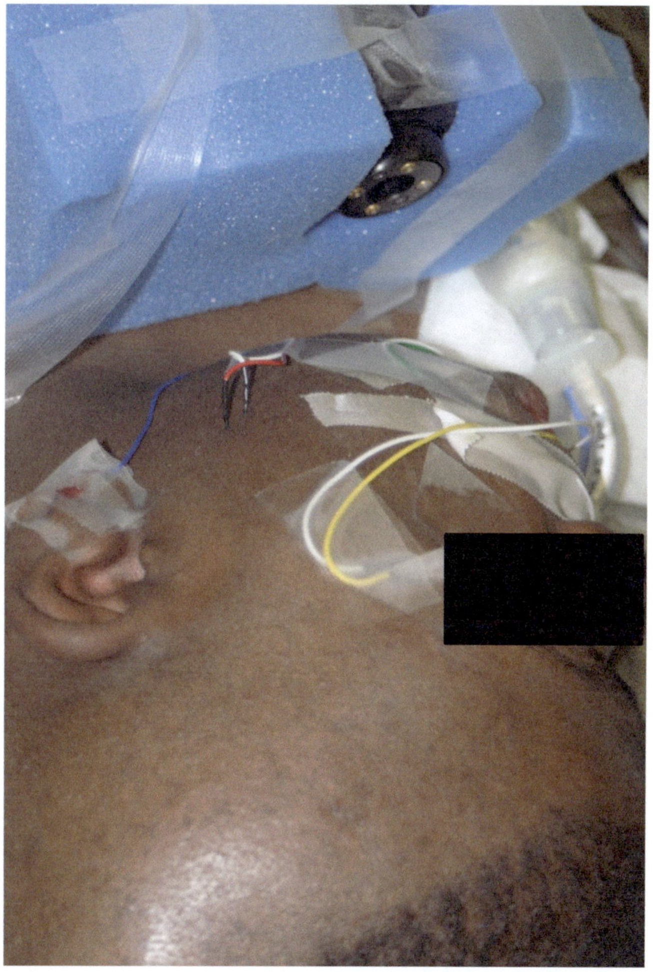

14. Next, the earphone was placed in the ear canal. Sound travels through the blue tube, and care needs to be taken that the tubing will not become kinked during the case. After applying Mastisol, a sticky drape was applied around the ear to keep the ear canal dry. This is important because if blood or fluid gets into the ear canal, it can cause a conductive hearing loss and abolish the ABR tracing.

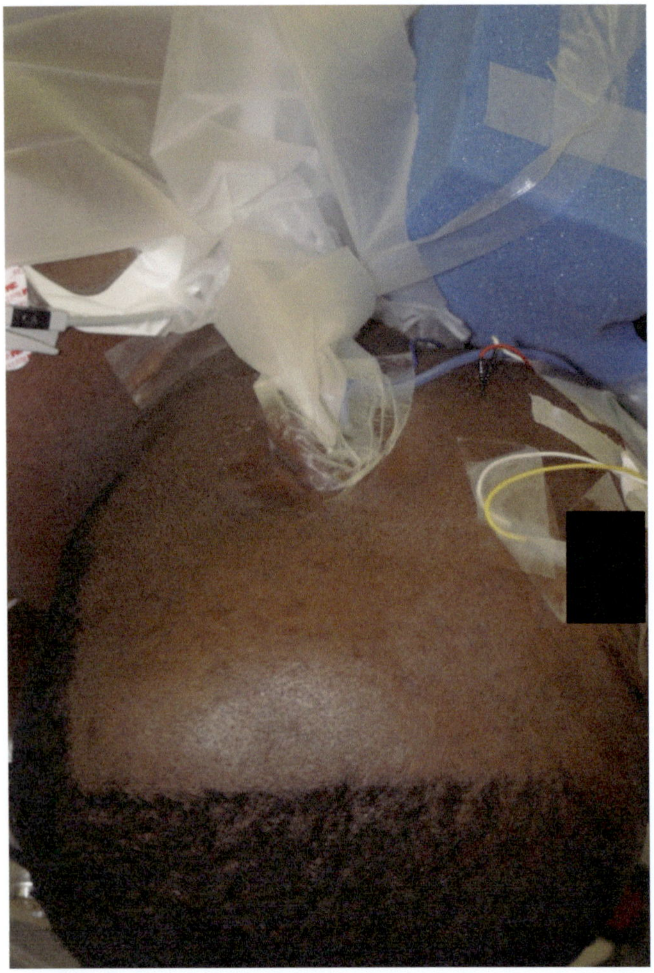

CSF Management

15. After skull base surgery, patients can have CSF rhinorrhea. This occurs when the dura is not closed in a watertight fashion (as is common after skull base procedures). CSF can percolate through the air cell tracts in the temporal bone and reach the middle ear space. It will then drain down the Eustachian tube and enter the nasopharynx. When the patient is lying back in bed, he/she may notice a salty-tasting drainage, but most often, they won't appreciate this. By having them lean forward, the presence of CSF rhinorrhea can be diagnosed by visually seeing the CSF drip out of the nose. In this representative patient, the CSF trickled down his mustache (*arrow*) before dropping to the floor. To treat this, a lumbar subarachnoid drain (LSAD) can be placed.

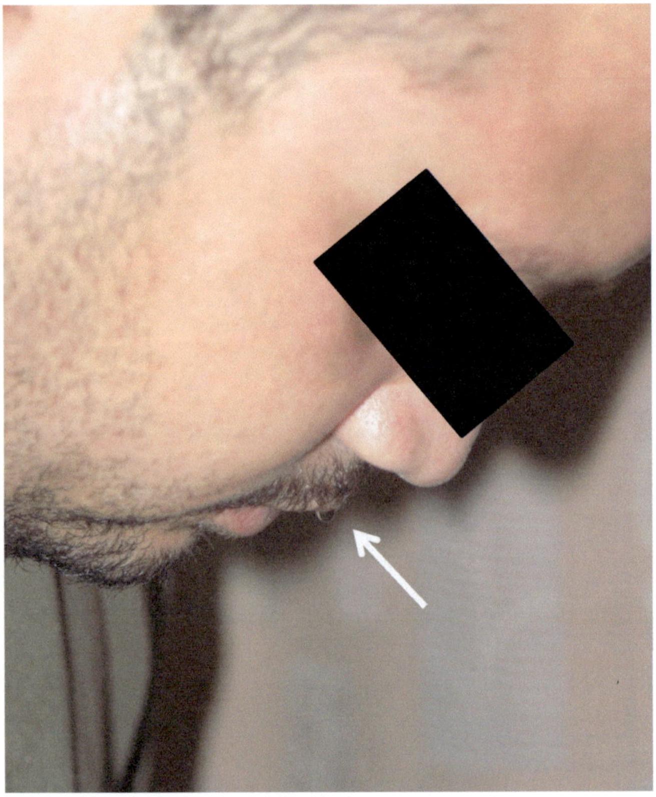

16. In this example, a postoperative CSF leak was expected because the patient had a very large tumor, and so a LSAD was placed in the operating room before the surgery was started. It was used during the postoperative period to help prevent a CSF leak from developing. First, the patient is turned on his side, and the iliac crest is palpated as a landmark.

17. The area is prepped in a sterile fashion, and the space between L3 and L4 is found. The trocar from the LSAD kit is inserted into the interspace at a slight superior angle of approach. The bevel of the trocar is oriented vertically to minimize trauma to the dura when it is penetrated.

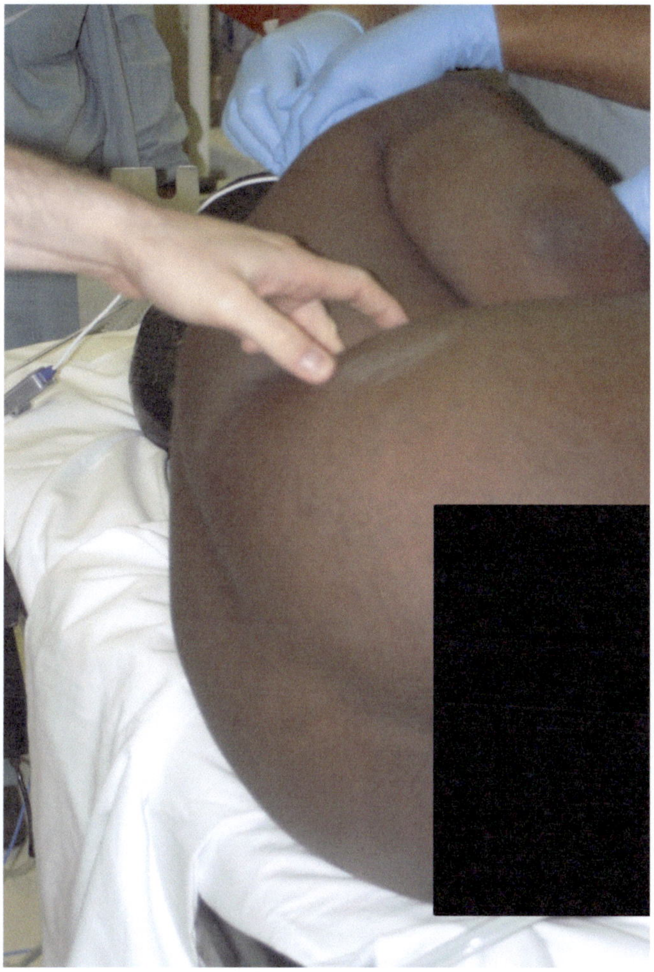

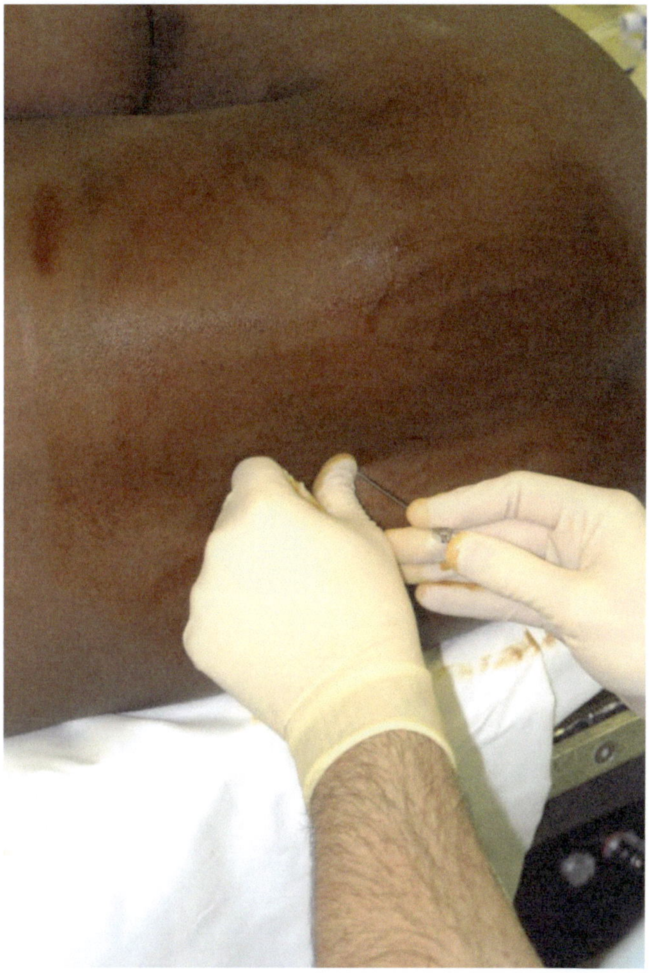

18. Periodically, the inner cannula is removed to see if CSF is flowing. If it is not, the cannula is reinserted, and the trocar is advanced further. Sometimes but not always, a very slight "give" is felt when entering the intradural space.

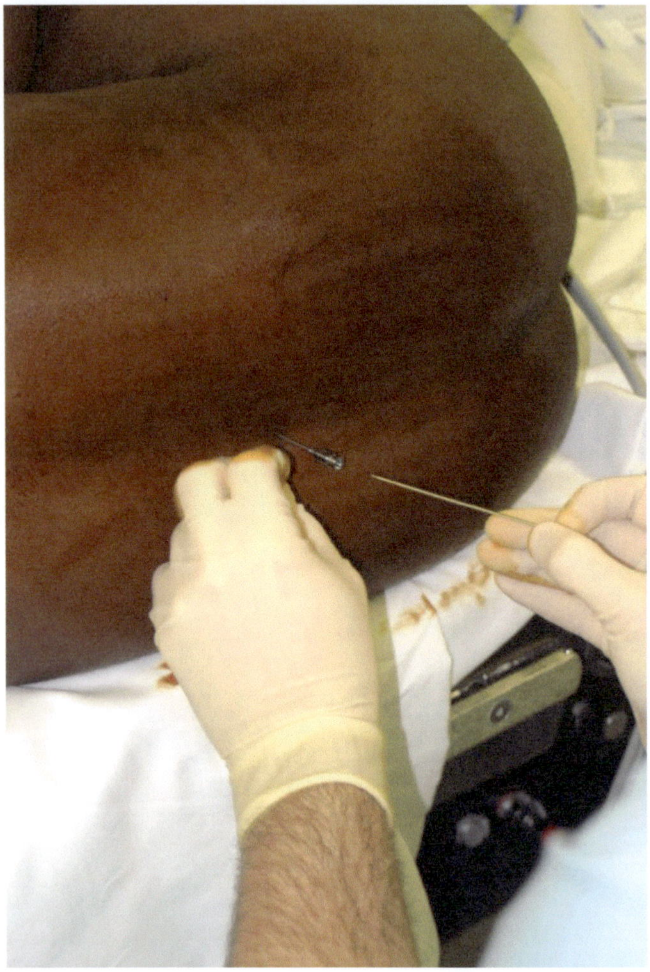

19. When CSF flows, the trocar is turned 90° so that its bevel is oriented superiorly (cephalad).

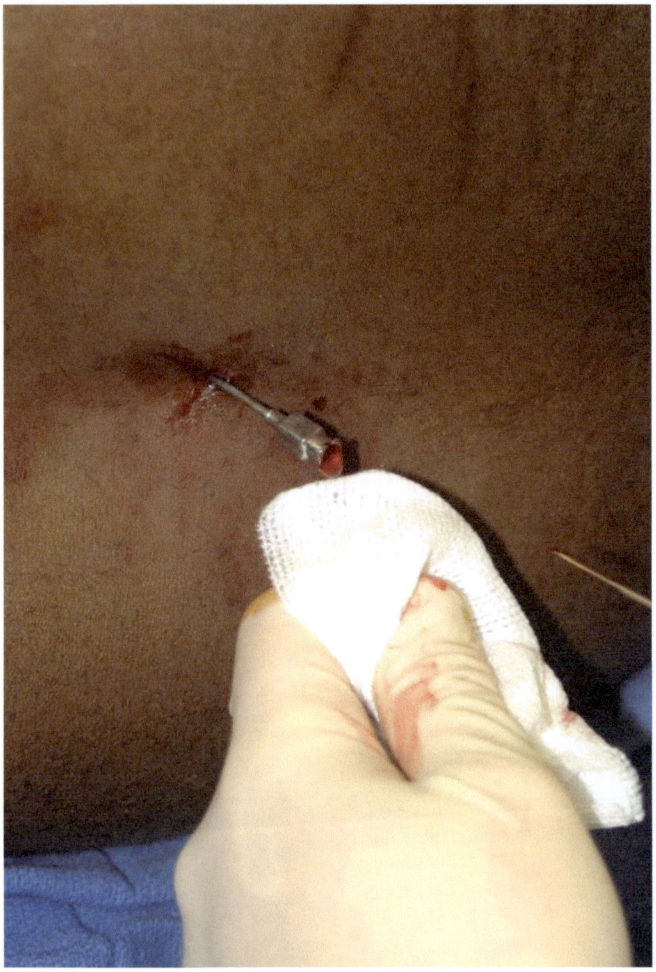

20. The catheter is then gently inserted and advanced at least 10 cm beyond the tip of the trocar.

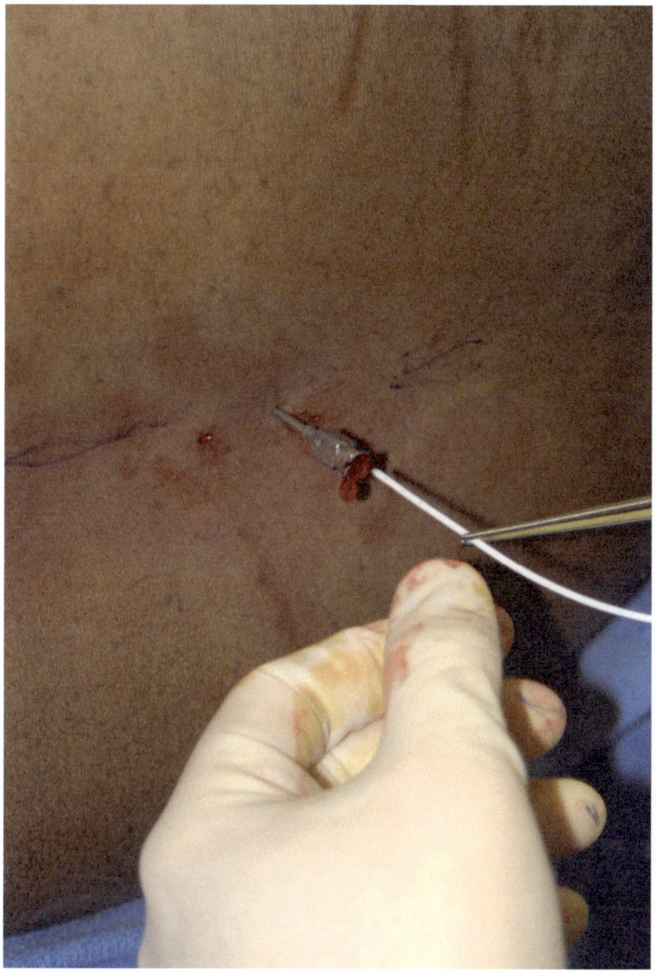

21. The trocar is then carefully removed, and flow of CSF through the catheter is verified. If it is working, the catheter is sutured to the back in two different locations. A sterile dressing is applied. For extra safety, the catheter is also coiled twice and secured to the skin next to the entry point with a large Tegaderm.

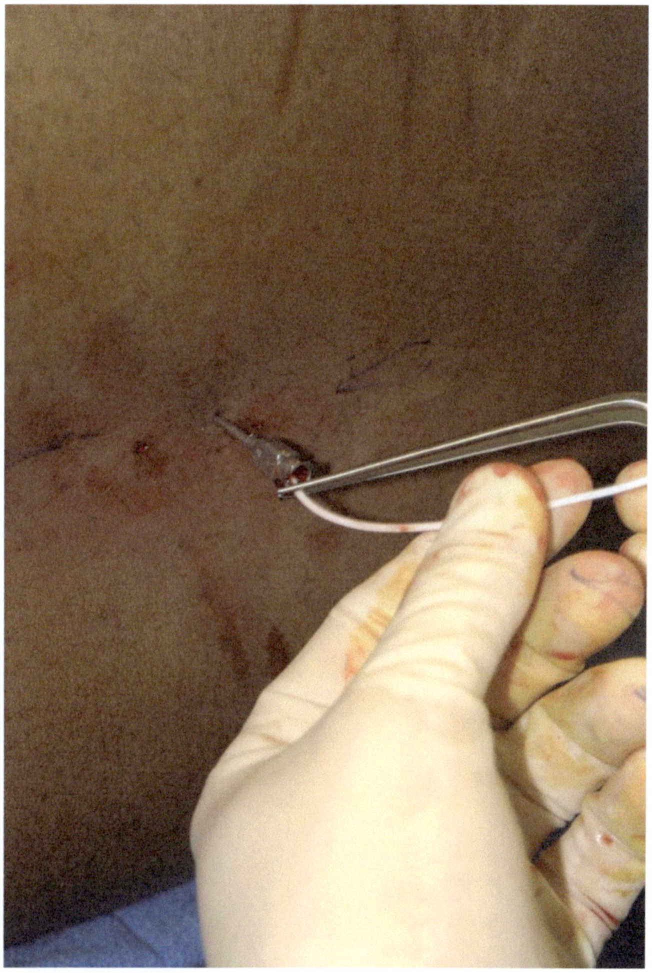

Instrumentation

22. Skull base surgery requires a standard craniotomy set, a neurotology set, and a fat graft set. Some of the specialized microdissectors in the neurotology set are shown in the picture. The purpose of the microdissectors is mainly to allow careful dissection of tumors off the cranial nerves and out of the internal auditory canal. (1) Angled scissors. (2–3) Microcurettes allow removal of residual tumor that rests under a lip of bone, typically the lateral aspect of the internal auditory canal. (4–5) Angled knives allow the dura of the internal auditory canal to be opened in a careful and precise manner without disturbing the tumor or nerves that may lie directly underneath. (6–8) Smaller microcurettes at various angles allow probing of the fundus of the internal auditory canal to verify that all the tumor has been removed.

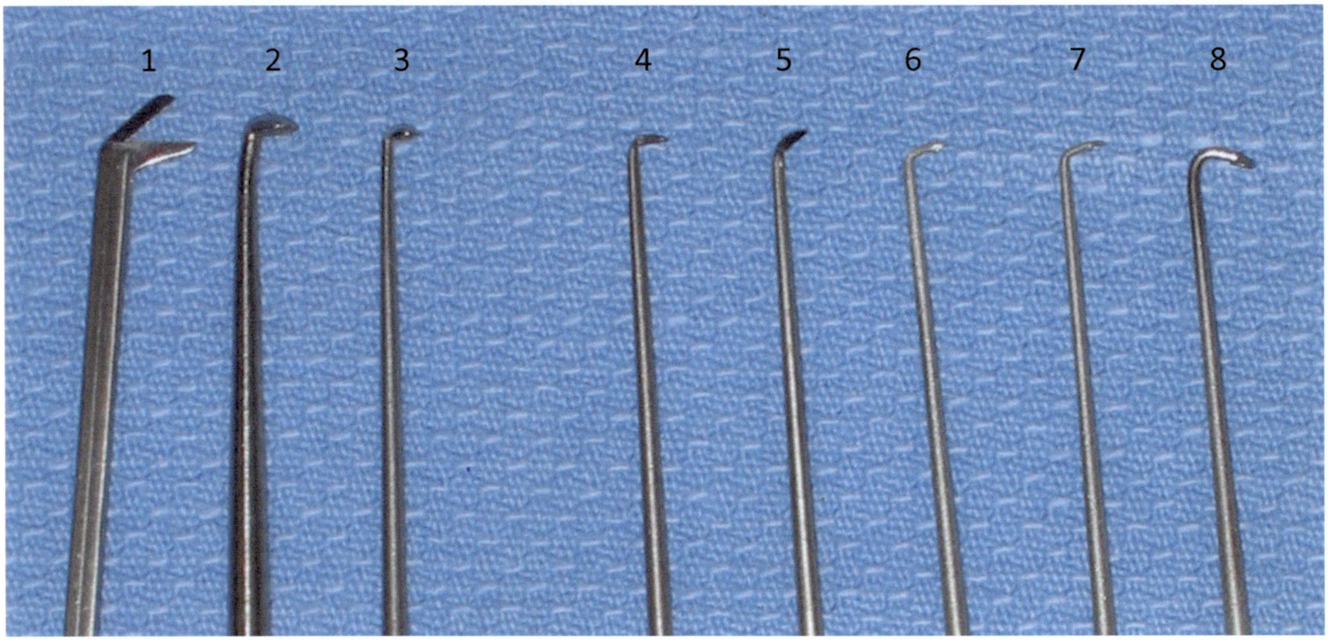

23. Three views of a custom-modified version of the House-Urban and Fisch retractors. Such a device can be used instead of malleable retractors and the Greenberg retractor set for middle fossa approaches if desired.

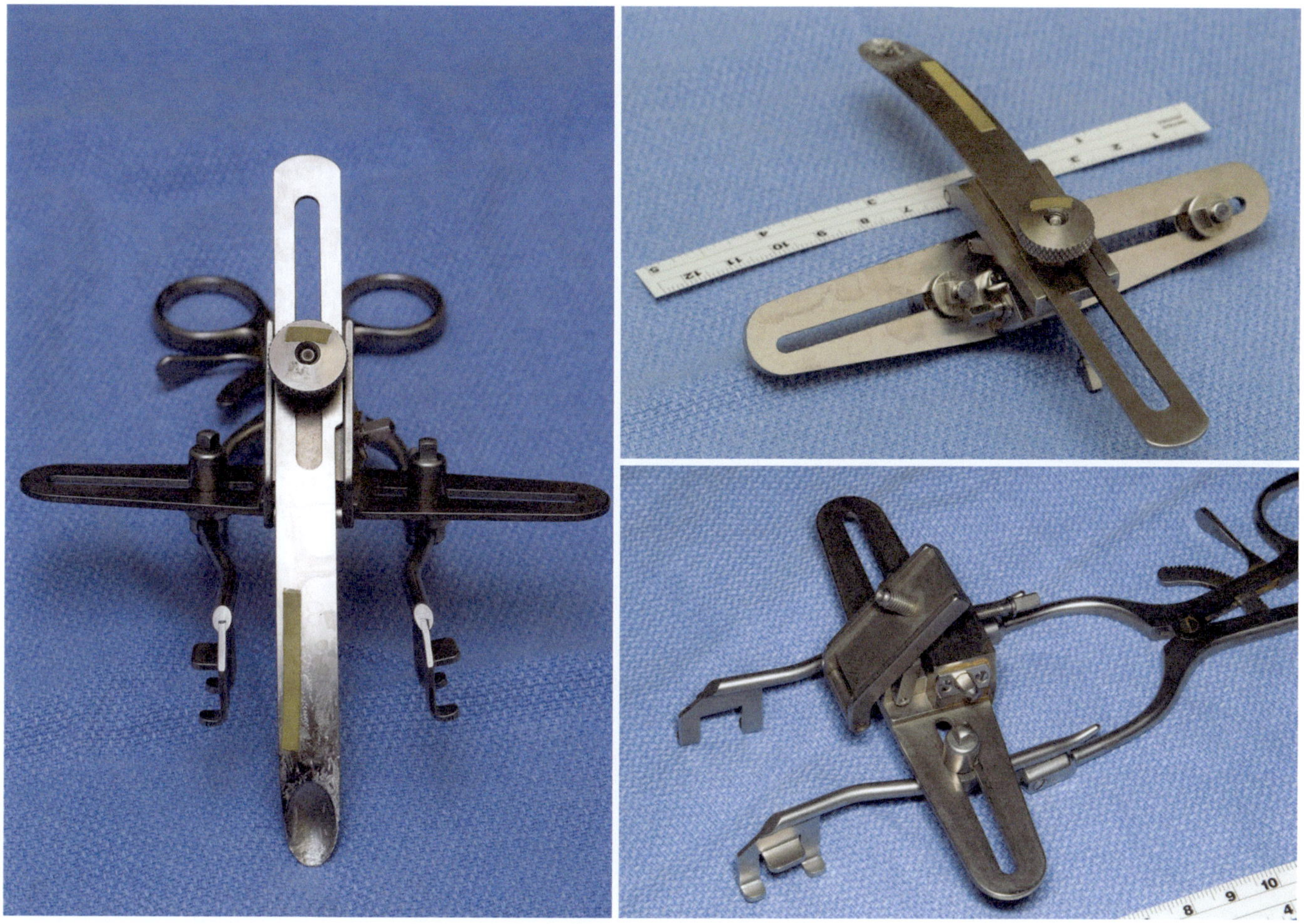

A list of the contents of our instrument sets are given below in the following tables:

Craniotomy set

Manuf	Prod Num	Inst/Cmt	Qty
Codman	50-1194	Retractor Weitlaner Small Sharp 3×4 5 1/8″	2
Codman	50-1020	Retractor Vein Large 13 mm	2
Vmueller	NL1020	Retractor Cushing	1
Vmueller	NL1302	Spatula Brain Silver 3/4″×7″	1
Integra	NL8700208	Spatula Brain Teflon 5/8″×8″	1
Integra	NL8700210	Spatula Brain Teflon 1/2″×8″	1
Codman	59-1085	Spatula Brain 1″×7″	1
Codman	59-1082	Spatula Brain 1/2″×8″	1
Codman	50-1181	Retractor Adson Cerebellar	2
Pilling	34-3550	Ruler 6″	1
Weck	588200	Adson Rongeur	1
MedtrSof	9560565	Micropituitary 2 mm	1
Vmueller	AU6780	Rongeur Ruskin Double Action 5 mm Jaws	1
Codman	65-1116	Elevator Langenbeck	1
Codman	53-1224	Wilde Takahashi Medium	1
Codman	23-1042	Curette Straight #00	1
Vmueller	SU1403-001	Handle Knife #3	1
Pilling	35-2957	Handle Knife #7	1
Codman	53-4005	Forceps Alligator Micro Cup Straight	1
Vmueller	NL4251-81 T	Kerrison 1 mm UpBiting 40°	1
Vmueller	NL4251-82 T	Kerrison 40° Upbiting 2 mm (Gold & Black Handle)	1
Vmueller	NL4251-83 T	Kerrison 40° Upbiting 3 mm (Gold & Black Handle)	1
Codman	36-2016	Needleholder Mayo Hegar Diamond Jaw 6″	4
Codman	36-3014	Needleholder Ryder 6″	2
Codman	36-5051	Scissors Mayo Classic Plus Straight 6 3/4″	1
Codman	36-5016	Scissors Metzenbaum 7″ Curved	1
Codman	54-5566	Scissors Metzenbaum 5″	1
Weck	520130	Scissors Wire	1
Codman	32-4001	Clamp Mosquito Curved 5″	10
Codman	32-4021	Clamp Kelly Curved 5.5″	2
Codman	32-7000	Clamp Allis 6″	12
Vmueller	SU2800	Clamp Kocher Straight 6″	2
Codman	30-4291	Clamp Schnidt 8″ Curved	2
Codman	20-5115	Applier Raney Clip	3
EthicEnd	LX107	Applier Clip Short Small Blue Handled 7.25″	2
Codman	32-5015	Clamp Edna Towel	4
Codman	32-5000	Clip Towel Small	2
Codman	80-2901	Forceps Bipolar Irrigating Insulated Bayonette-Blue Coated 7.75	1
Vmueller	SU-2332	Forceps Tissue 5 3/4″	1
Codman	30-1172	Forceps Dura Fine Toothed	1
Weck	468220	Forceps Cushing 7″ w/ Teeth	2
Vmueller	NL3138	Forceps Gerald Bayonet	2
Codman	65-1015	Dissector Penfield Broad Curved #1	2
Codman	65-1016	Dissector Penfield Curved #2	2
Codman	65-1017	Dissector Penfield Full Curved #3	2
Codman	65-1018	Dissector Penfield Slight Curved #4	2
Vmueller	NL1902	Suction Tip Frazier 10fr #3 w/ Stylet	1
Vmueller	NL1903	Suction Tip Frazier 12fr w/ Stylet	1
Storz	SP7-57488	Suction Tip Brackmann Short #5	2
Storz	SP7-35326	Suction Tip Brackmann Medium #5	2
Storz	SP7-57780	Suction Tip Brackmann Short #7	2
Storz	SP7-35326A	Suction Tip Brackmann Medium #7	2

Manuf	Prod Num	Inst/Cmt	Qty
Storz	N4725	Skin Hook Double Prong Medium Wide	2
Jarit	277-241	Hook Nerve Sharp Small	1
Jarit	277-235	Hook Krayenbuehl Nerve Fine Dull 7 1/4″	1
Codman	38-1042	Hook Dura	1
Codman	54-1041	Scissors Dandy	1
Codman	30-1186	Forceps Adson w/ Teeth 4″	2
Fukash		Hook Scalp	4

Neurotology set

Manuf	Prod Num	Inst/Cmt	Qty
		Rongeurs	
Codman	53-4000	Rongeur Decker Alligator Action Straight 2 mm × 6 mm	1
Codman	53-4002	Rongeur Decker Alligator Action Curved Left 2 mm × 6 mm	1
Codman	53-1235	Love Gruenwald Straight 3 mm × 10 mm	1
		Scissors	
Vmueller	NL3799	Scissors Kurze Dissecting straight	1
Vmueller	NL3800	Scissors Kurze Dissection Curved left	1
Vmueller	NL3801	Scissors Kurze Dissecting Curved right	1
Vmueller	NL4003	Scissors Yasargil bayonet shaped straight 12.5 mm	1
Vmueller	NL4004	Scissors Yasargil bayonet shaped Curved up 12 mm	1
Instrume	s.50.411.13	Scissors Special Sinus 130 mm Long Shaft Straight	1
Instrume	s.50.420.13	Scissors Special Sinus 130 mm Long Shaft Left	1
Instrume	s.50.421.13	Scissors Special Sinus 130 mm Long Shaft Right	1
Vmueller	RH1680	Scissors Foman Upper Lateral Fully Curved 5 1/4″	1
Codman	80-1524	Scissors Bayonet Titanium Straight Fine Tip	1
Codman	80-1525	Scissors Bayonet Titanium Curved	1
		Forceps	
Codman	53-4006	Forceps Rhoton Micro Cup Curved Right 1 mm × 6″	1
Codman	53-4007	Forceps Rhoton Micro Cup Curved Left 1 mm × 6″	1
Codman	53-4005	Forceps Alligator Micro Cup Straight	1
		Bipolar forceps	
Kirwan	10-1603NS	Cautery Irrigating Bipolar regular 1.5 mm	1
Kirwan	12-1600NS	Cautery Irrigating Bipolar Micro 0.7 mm	1
		Suctions	
Storz	SP7-57718	Suction Brackmann 5fr Long (Custom – fenestrated)	2
Storz	SP7-57607	Suction Brackmann 7fr. Long (Custom – fenestrated)	2
Storz	SP7-54918	Suction Brackmann 9 Fr.	1
Storz	N0607-5	Suction Brackmann Irrigating 4 × 5fr	2
Storz	N0607-7A	Suction Brackmann Irrigating 5 × 7fr	2
Storz	N1705-76A5	Suction Irrigating House 5 × 7fr	2
Storz	N1705-77A	Suction Irrigator House 7 × 10fr	2
Storz	N1705-77B	Suciton Irrigator House 8 × 12Fr.	2
Vmueller	58-6313	Rhoton atraumatic suction, straight tip, angled tube, 4" 3 Fr	2
Vmueller	58-6315	Rhoton atraumatic suction, straight tip, angled tube, 4" 5 Fr	2
Vmueller	58-6317	Rhoton atraumatic suction, straight tip, angled tube, 4" 7 Fr	2
		Retractors and elevators	
Codman	50-1520	Retractor Cerebellar w/ 9.5 cm Flexible Arm (2 Pieces Each)	2
Codman	50-1511	Retractor Greenberg 6.5 cm flexible secondary arm	1
Codman	0308 N	Retractor Malleable Blades Right/Left/Midline 2 Each	6
Codman	SP01031	Retractor Blade Old Style 1/2″ × 4″	2
Codman	SPO1031-3	Retractor Blade Old Style 5/8″ × 4″	2
Storz	N1705-71	Retractor Middle Fossa Dura Custom	1
Codman	50-1186	1 Curved Weitlaner Custom Made	1
W Lorenz	26-0028	Retactor Adson Cerebellar	1
Vmueller	NL1305-3	Retractor Davis Malleable 1/2″	2

Manuf	Prod Num	Inst/Cmt	Qty
Aesculap	OL153R	Elevator Cottle	1
Storz	N1124	Elevator Lempert 7 mm	1
Storz	N4610	Elevator Joseph 4 mm	1
Codman	65-1075	Elevator Cushing Periosteal sharp 16 mm	1
		Rhoton Rack	
Boss	71-5101	Dissector Round 1 mm Angled Blade	1
Boss	71-5101	Dissector Round 1 mm Custom Straight Blade	1
Boss	71-5102	Dissector Round 2 mm Angled Blade	1
Boss	71-5102	Dissector Round 2 mm Custom Straight Blade	1
Boss	71-5103	Dissector Round 3 mm Angled Blade	1
Boss	71-5103	Dissector Round 3 mm Custom Straight Blade	1
Codman	80-1683	Elevator General Purpose Small #4	1
Codman	80-1684	Elevator General Purpose Large #5	1
Codman	80-1685	Dissector/Spatula Rhoton Small #6	1
Codman	80-1688	Hook Nerve Fine Semi Sharp 90° #9 Blue	1
Codman	80-1689	Hook Nerve Blunt 90° #10	1
Codman	80-1690	Hook Semi Sharp 45° #11	1
Codman	80-1692	Curette Micro Straight #13	1
Codman	80-1693	Curette Micro Angled #14	1
Codman	80-1696	Dissector Rhoton Teardrop 90° 3 mm #16	1
		Rack #2	
Mizuho	07-821-12	Knife McEleen 90′	1
Storz	N1690-7	Knife Rosen Canal Large	1
GyrusACM	13-0562	Knife Lancet #2 2 mm	1
Mizuho	07-821-01	CP-1 Sickle Style Knife	1
Mizuho	07-821-02	Knife 2.5 mm Tumor Microbayonet	1
Mizuho	07-821-03	CP-3 Tumor Knife Blunt Tip	1
Mizuho	07-821-04	Knife 2.5 mm Tumor sharp tip 80′ angled up Microbayonet	1
Mizuho	07-821-08	CP-8 1.2 mm Tumor Ring Curr. 60°	1
Mizuho	07-821-09	CP-9 1.55 m Tumor Ring Curr. 45°	1
Mizuho	07-821-10	Curette Cup 1 × 1.5 mm angled up Microbayonet	1
Mizuho	07-821-11	Curette Cup 1.5 × 2.0 mm angled up Microbayonet	1
Vmueller	NL2400	Hook Adson Dural 5 mm tip	1
Storz	NI705-HM	Knife Sickle	1

Fat graft set

Manuf	Prod Num	Inst/Cmt	Qty
Vmueller	SU1403-001	Handle Knife #3	1
Codman	36-5032	Scissor Metzembaun 7″	1
Jarit	099-210	Scissors Mayo 6 – 3/4″ Straight	1
Jarit	130-265	Forceps Brown 6″	1
Jarit	129-234	Forceps Adson W/Teeth	1
Jarit	107-102	Clamp Mosquito Curved	4
Jarit	136-100	Clamp Allis 6″ 4 × 5 Teeth	4
Jarit	120-135	Needle Holder Mayo-Hegar 6″	1
Codman	50-1197	Retractor Weitlaner Dull Medium 6 1/2″	1
Codman	70-6560	Suction Tip Andrews Pynchon (Andrews)	1

Special cochlear implant instruments

Manuf	Prod Num	Inst/Cmt	Qty
Cochlear Corp	Z60770	AOS Forceps – to insert the electrode	1
Richards	13-0577	House Pick 90°, 0.5 mm– to open the round window membrane	1

Middle Fossa Approaches

3

Approach to the Internal Auditory Canal

- *Concept*
  - Retract the temporal lobe in an extradural fashion, and drill through the petrous apex to reach the posterior cranial fossa and internal auditory canal
- *Conditions treated*
  - Small vestibular schwannoma (intracanalicular lesions and those with a diameter in the cerebellopontine angle <1.0 cm)
  - Facial nerve decompression or repair
- *Risks*
  - Retraction injuries to the temporal lobe can cause contusion, edema, or stroke.
  - Temporal lobe seizure.
  - Anomic aphasia.
  - Hearing loss if the labyrinth is violated or auditory nerve involved with the tumor.
  - Facial nerve injury, particularly if the geniculate ganglion is dehiscent and not recognized.
  - Carotid artery injury along the horizontal segment.
  - Dry eye if the GSPN is transected.
  - CSF leak.
- *Benefits*
  - Best approach for hearing preservation when removing a vestibular schwannoma that extends to the fundus
  - Only way to access the labyrinthine course of the facial nerve while preserving hearing

J.S. Oghalai, C.L.W. Driscoll, *Atlas of Neurotologic and Lateral Skull Base Surgery*,
DOI 10.1007/978-3-662-46694-0_3, © Springer-Verlag Berlin Heidelberg 2016

1. Coronal view of the temporal bone. An intracanalicular vestibular schwannoma is shown. The facial nerve lies superior to the tumor.

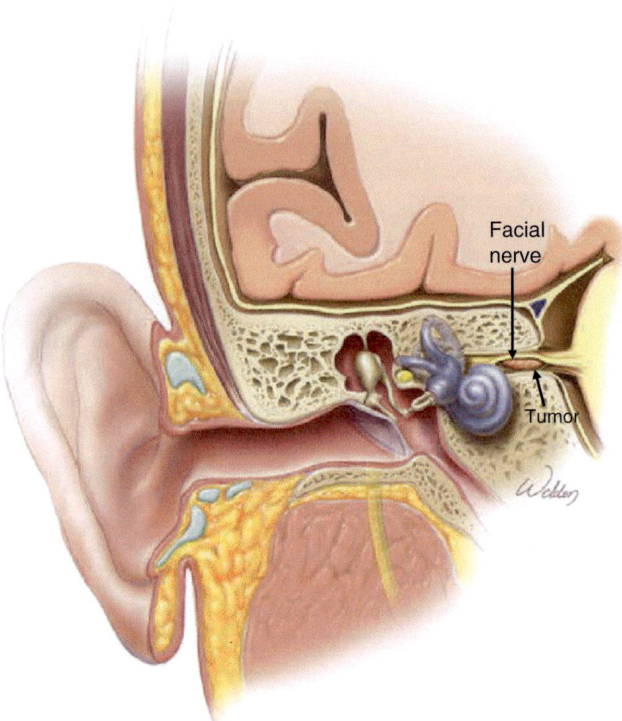

2. Theory of the middle fossa approach to the internal auditory canal. Elevation of the middle fossa dura is performed, followed by drilling out the petrous apex to expose the posterior fossa dura and the dura of the internal auditory canal. These are then opened to expose the tumor.

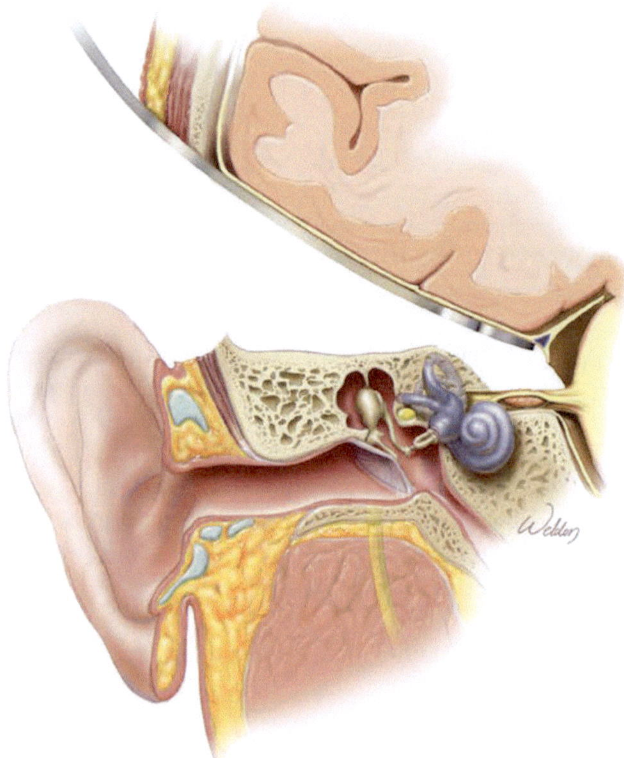

3. Overview of the bone to be removed (*gray*).

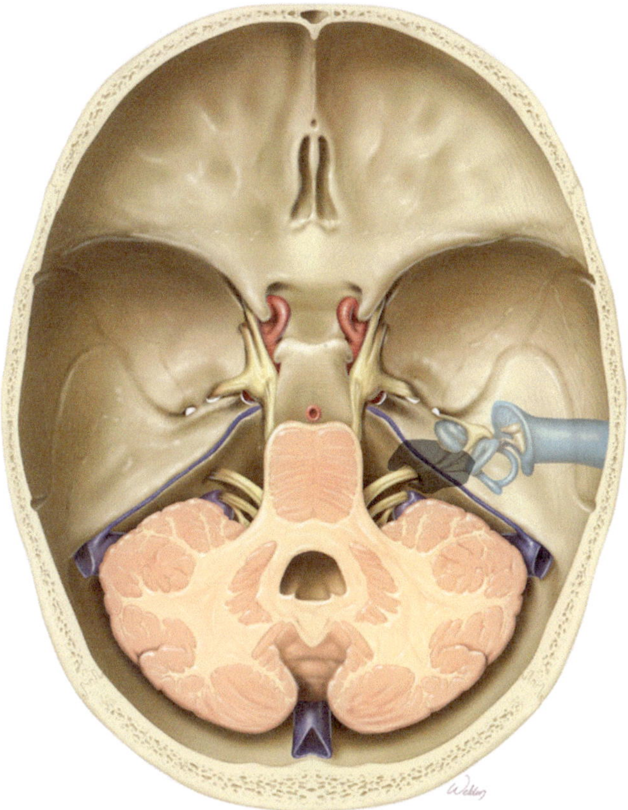

4. To start the procedure, an inferiorly based U-flap provides excellent exposure. The important point is to start the anterior limb down at the root of the zygoma. This is necessary to provide enough anterior–inferior exposure and provides the required line of sight to the internal auditory canal. An inadequate opening may seriously impair the ability to expose and remove the tumor. It is a critical step in the operation.

   This incision can be shortened if desired. It still needs to start at the root of the zygoma, but the posterior limb may be reduced in length as long as adequate retraction is possible. Although it is possible to not clip any hair, we do remove some just along the incision line to facilitate closure. Cosmetically, this is camouflaged by the surrounding hair.

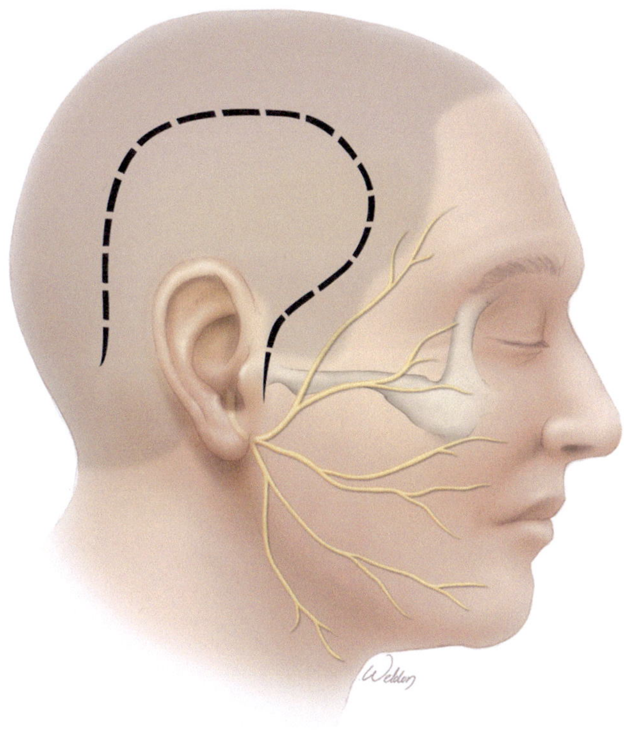

5. An alternate incision is vertical, which splits the fibers of the temporalis muscle. Although the ultimate opening is a little smaller than the U-flap, there is often less post-operative atrophy of the temporalis muscle. The incision choice should be influenced by the patient's scalp and temporalis muscle thickness. This incision can be limiting, particularly in the anterior inferior corner in patients with thick scalps and a big temporalis muscle.

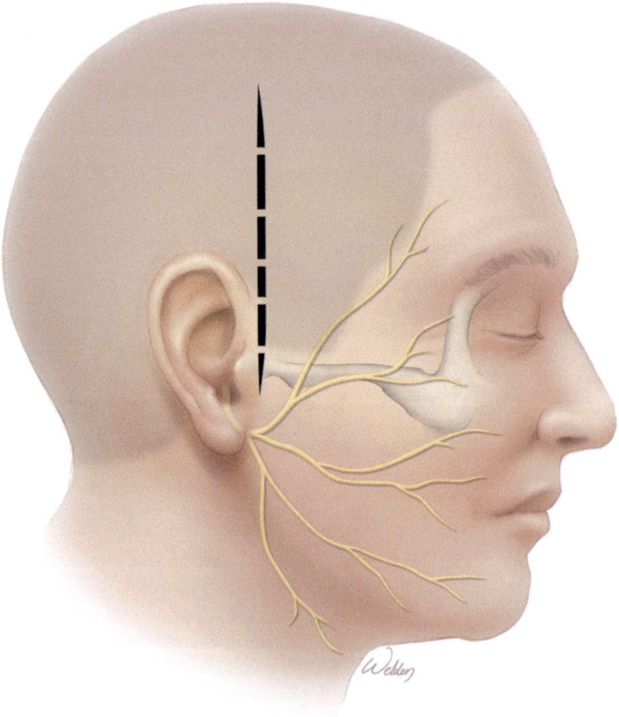

6. The skin, temporoparietal fascia, temporalis muscle, and periosteum are elevated off the skull. These tissues can be elevated as a single, thick flap rather than dissecting between each layer. This reduces the risk of a postoperative hematoma forming between the layers and is more efficient.

   A burr hole (*BH*) is first placed just anterosuperior to the root of the zygoma. The next two burr holes are drilled about 4 cm superiorly and are centered over the external auditory canal (*EAC*). While a posterior–inferior burr hole can also be made, it is not necessary.

   The dura is separated from the underside of the bone flap using an elevator. Care is taken to minimize this dissection in regions outside the bone flap as this raises the risk of a post-op epidural hematoma.

   Finally, a craniotome is used to turn the bone flap. The flap is placed in moist gauze or soaked in Bacitracin solution and saved on the back table until closing at the end of the procedure.

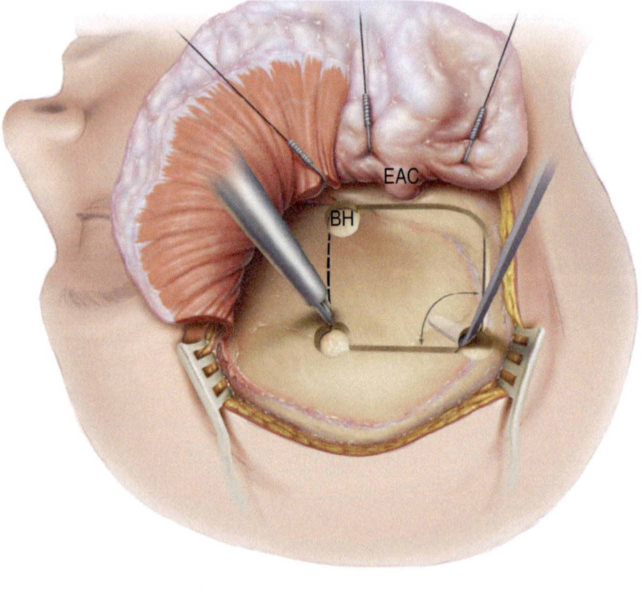

7. The dura is elevated off the temporal floor. This can be done with a Freer elevator, although we prefer the Joseph (narrow mastoid) elevator as it is stiffer. A key part of this portion of the procedure is to identify the greater superficial petrosal nerve (*GSPN*) as it leaves the temporal bone. It is often quite adherent to the overlying dura. Its fibrous adhesions to the dura can be separated with the elevator or an 11 blade scalpel. Dissection from posterior to anterior decreases the risk of injuring an exposed geniculate ganglion and dissecting under the GSPN nerve fibers.

   In most cases, it is not necessary to distinguish the foramen spinosum containing the middle meningeal artery (*MMA*) from the foramen ovale (*FO*). All of this tissue contains thin-walled veins, and the more they are dissected, the more they bleed. However, for larger tumors or if a wider opening is needed, division of the MMA artery does permit more exposure of the posterior fossa. In any case, expect dissection in this area to bleed.

   Once the dura can no longer be elevated anteriorly any further because of the foramen ovale, the bleeding should be controlled with hemostatic agents (such as Flowseal and Surgicel). A cottonoid should then be placed on top of it and left in place for the remainder of the case. By the time surgery is done, the cottonoid can be removed, and there is usually no further bleeding.

   The elevation of the dura needs to continue medially all the way to the petrous ridge, where the superior petrosal sinus (*SPS*) runs. It is often easiest to identify this structure posteriorly near the junction of the transverse sinus and sigmoid sinus. This area also tends to bleed and can be controlled with hemostatic agents and a cottonoid. The SPS can then be followed as it courses anteriorly and medially. This is helpful in identifying the true posterior/medial edge of the petrous bone as there are often misleading false ridges.

   The arcuate eminence (*AE*) is a bulge that approximates the location of the superior semicircular canal.

   Dural elevation begins posteriorly, and the petrous ridge and superior petrosal sinus are identified first.

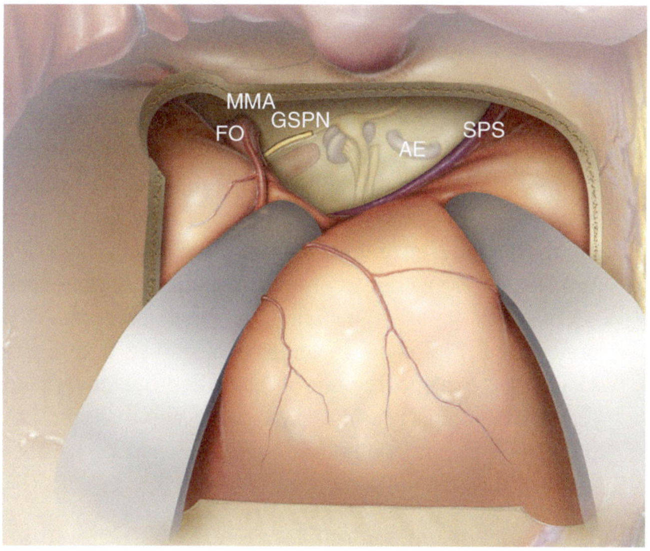

   Dissecting medially and anteriorly will then permit identification of the GSPN as described. These two landmarks (the petrous ridge and the GSPN) should give you sufficient orientation to anticipate the location of all other structures. There is a tendency to not dissect far enough medially along the petrous apex, and it is also important to be certain your retractor fits over the true posterior ridge of the petrous bone.

   A modified version of the House-Urban and Fisch middle fossa retractors can be used instead of malleable retractors held by the Mayfield head holder if desired. The main benefit of these middle fossa retractors is that a Mayfield head holder is not needed as it is securely fixed to the edges of the craniotomy. Furthermore, the modified version has the benefit of a wider base to accommodate larger craniotomies while still lowering the profile of the blade by curving it. Both of these retractors permit the generation of significant pressure to hold the dura. The downside of these retractors is that they are finicky and take a lot of time to orient and reorient it as the dissection progresses. They don't offer as much adjustability and retraction ability as the malleable retractors either.

8. To reach the internal auditory canal and posterior fossa, the petrous bone needs to be drilled away. The retractors are positioned so that their tips are held securely in place at the petrous ridge. Care is taken to bend the retractors (*bend*) so that the lateral temporal lobe is not overly compressed. The dark dotted line highlights the area of bone to be removed deeply, and the light dotted line highlights the area of bone to be removed in a more shallow fashion so as not to injure the geniculate ganglion, cochlea, or superior semicircular canal. Nevertheless, bone in this region does need to be removed in order to visualize the deeper regions of the drilled-out cavity, and fear of damaging hearing or the facial nerve should not prevent one from obtaining enough exposure to adequately perform the procedure.

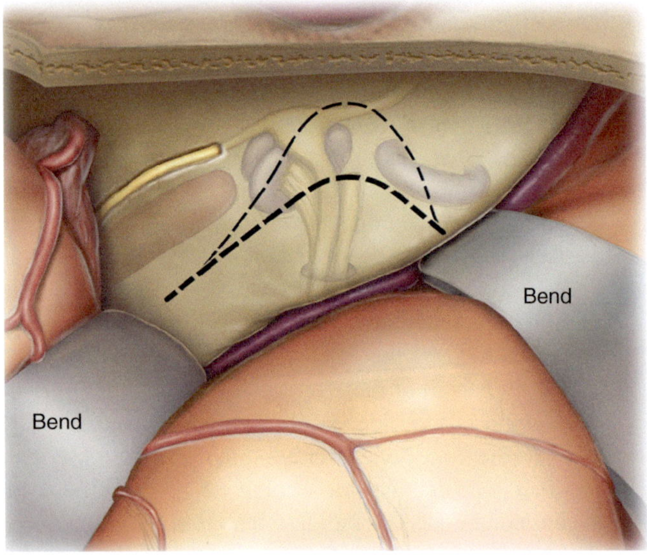

9. After removal of the petrous bone deep to the superior petrosal sinus (SPS), the posterior fossa dura is visible (*asterisks*), and the internal auditory canal has been skeletonized. Note the >180° exposure of the internal auditory canal.

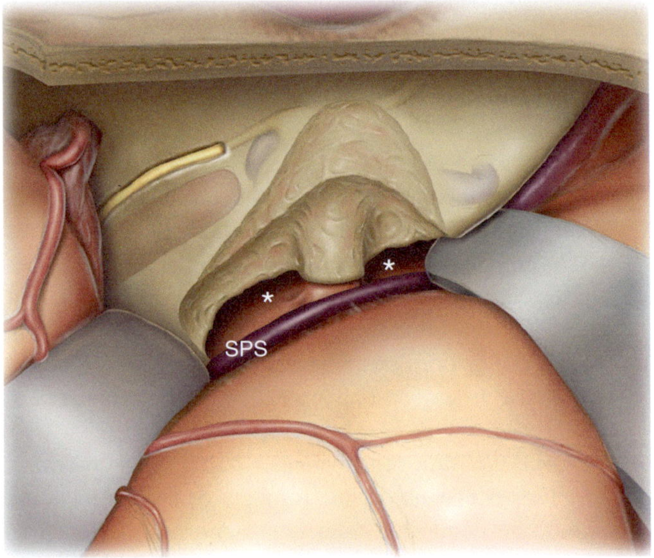

10. The complete view depicted in the illustrations is not obtainable in surgery without rotating the microscope to the three different angles depicted. The retractors do not need to be adjusted, just the microscope.

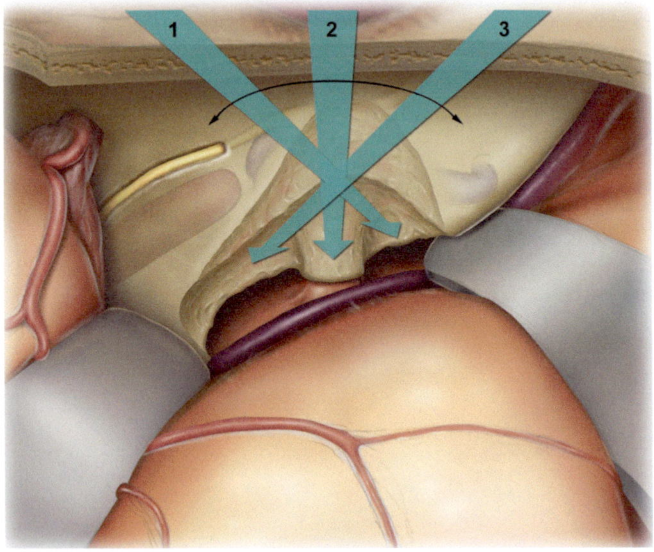

11. Appropriate decompression of the internal auditory canal is essential for a good outcome. The two most difficult and important areas to be dissected are the lateral end of the canal and the bone posterior to the internal auditory canal and medial to the superior semicircular canal. The dissection should continue laterally until the labyrinthine segment of the facial nerve is decompressed and the first millimeter or so of the superior vestibular nerve exposed. The superior semicircular canal should be positively identified so that bone can be removed up to it for decompression of the posterior aspect of the internal auditory canal. This space that is created provides room to push the tumor into as it is dissected medially and anteriorly.

    The inset depicts the layout of the nerves of the internal auditory canal: facial nerve (*F*), cochlear nerve (*C*), superior vestibular nerve (*SV*), and inferior vestibular nerve (*IV*). The degree of drilling necessary along the internal auditory canal varies. Deeper troughs are needed medially at the porus acusticus (*inset, bottom panel*) than medially (*inset, middle panel*). Along the labyrinthine portion of the facial nerve, only a very shallow exposure is performed (*inset, top panel*). The cochlea is less than 1 mm away. Watch carefully when drilling at the fundus and along the labyrinthine facial nerve. The cochlea can be "blue lined" much like the superior canal without causing injury. If it is accidentally opened, do not suction out the intracochlear fluids. Gently, seal the opening with bone wax.

    The dotted line indicates the dural opening. This is performed along the posterior fossa dura with an 11 blade scalpel or microscissors. Then, the nerve stimulator is used to identify the rough location of the facial nerve within the internal auditory canal by stimulating through the dura. An angled sickle knife is then used to open the dura of the internal auditory canal from lateral to medial in an area away from the nerve. The dura becomes flimsy at the fundus and easily tears open.

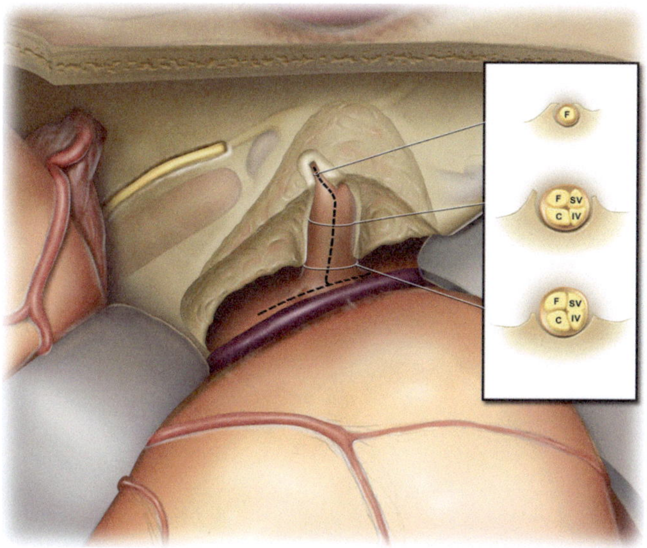

12. After opening the dura, the facial nerve is typically found on top of the tumor. In this case, the tumor is depicted as an inferior vestibular nerve tumor. The facial nerve is usually splayed somewhat and covers part of the tumor. It is important to zoom in with the microscope and visually identify the posterior edge of the facial nerve (*arrows*). The nerve stimulator should also be used to confirm this critical landmark. This plane can be developed sharply with a #1 or #2 Rhoton dissector or similar preferred instrument.

    Then, a window can be cut into the tumor using microscissors (*dotted lines*). This should not be directly adjacent to the facial nerve but a little bit posterior to its edge. This is so that the interface between the facial nerve and the tumor capsule is not lost.

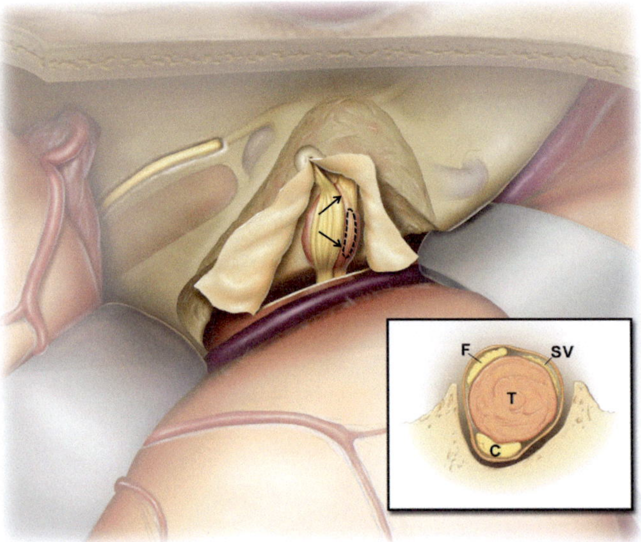

13. For a tumor extending into the cerebellopontine angle, a similar procedure is performed, but the window can be larger. The core of the tumor is then debulked with a small cup forceps and microscissors through the window (not shown). This releases the tension from the facial nerve, reduces its splaying, and makes the nerve even easier to visualize.

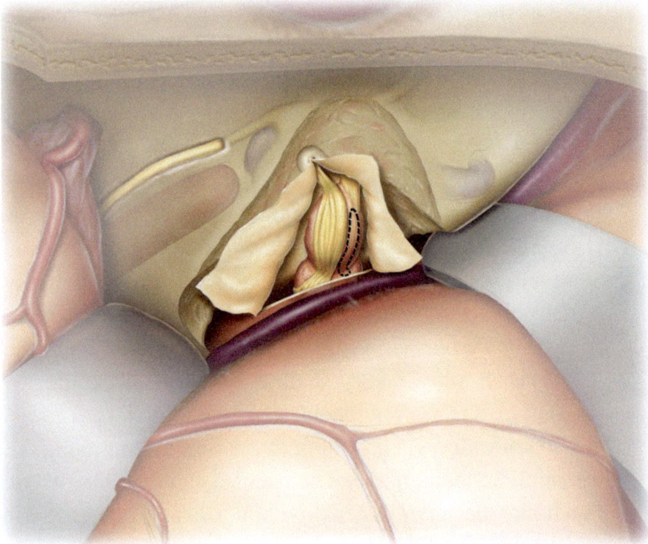

14. The proximal vestibular nerve (*V*) is transected with a microscissors. This includes both the inferior vestibular (*IV*) and superior vestibular (*SV*) nerves. Careful microdissection is then performed to separate the tumor (*T*) off the facial nerve (*F*). Sharp dissection is often helpful for this process. Dissecting medially to laterally, when possible, is helpful as it reduces tension on the facial nerve as it enters the temporal bone.

    The auditory nerve (also known as the cochlear nerve, *C*) is under the tumor and difficult to see until this point. If the tumor is not infiltrating into the auditory nerve, there is typically a plane between the tumor and the auditory nerve which clearly presents itself. This allows the surgeon to lift the tumor off the auditory nerve in order to spare hearing. The labyrinthine artery may also be noted (not shown) but is difficult to spare if adherent to the tumor.

    If they are to occur, changes in the ABR usually occur during this point in the process. Changes may occur even if the auditory nerve is spared. This indicates that there was trauma to the labyrinthine artery (spasm or division) or to the auditory nerve (edema or division). In any case, there is little the surgeon can do to restore the ABR once it is lost. Similarly, if the tumor infiltrates the auditory nerve or labyrinthine artery, there is no way to preserve hearing. These issues reflect properties of the patient's tumor, not the surgeon's technical skills. Tumors that extend fully to the fundus (and particularly if they extend under the transverse crest and into the base of the modiolus) are much more difficult to remove completely with hearing preservation. Soft tumors will fragment and small residuals may be left behind; removal of firm tumors may result in stretch injury to the nerve fibers or artery as the tumor is pulled away.

    Finally, the distal superior and inferior vestibular nerves are transected and the tumor removed (not shown).

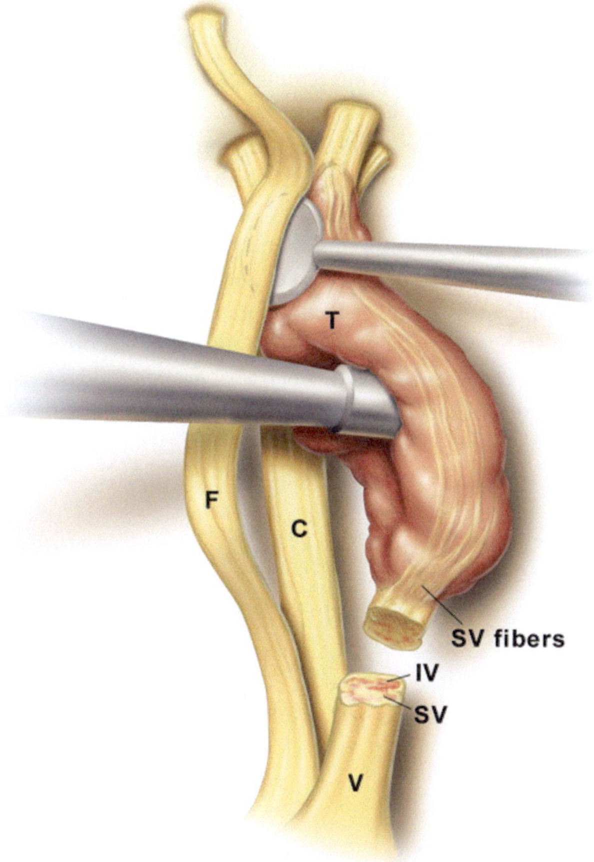

15. Exposed air cells within the area of petrous bone drilling are plugged with bone wax (not shown). Often, this works best by applying a round piece of bone wax stuck to the back of a thin elevator or dissector. A bipolar forceps is then used to push a cottonoid into the bone wax, compressing the wax into the air cells.

    Finally, a piece of abdominal fat is placed into the bony defect. While a muscle plug can be used, it tends to become highly vascularized and enhance with gadolinium within a few months. This can make it difficult to distinguish between the muscle plug and tumor recurrence by MRI. On the other hand, when a fat graft is used, fat saturation MRI techniques can eliminate this potential for artifacts.

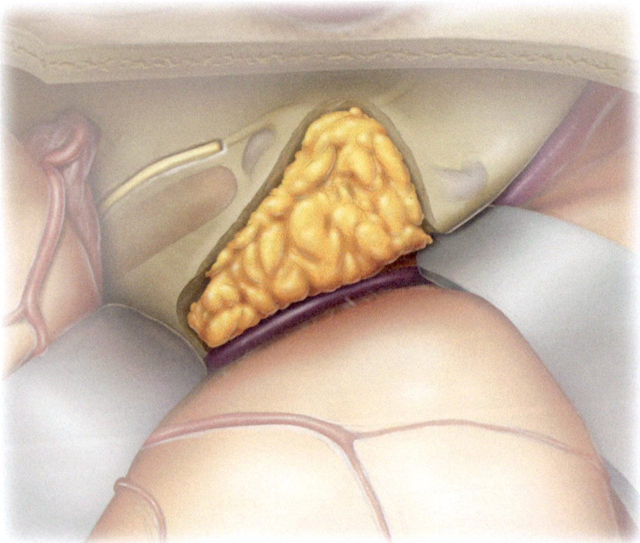

16. Case 1: Gadolinium-enhanced T1 MRI axial section of an intracanalicular left vestibular schwannoma (*arrow*). This tumor would be ideal for removal by the middle fossa approach.

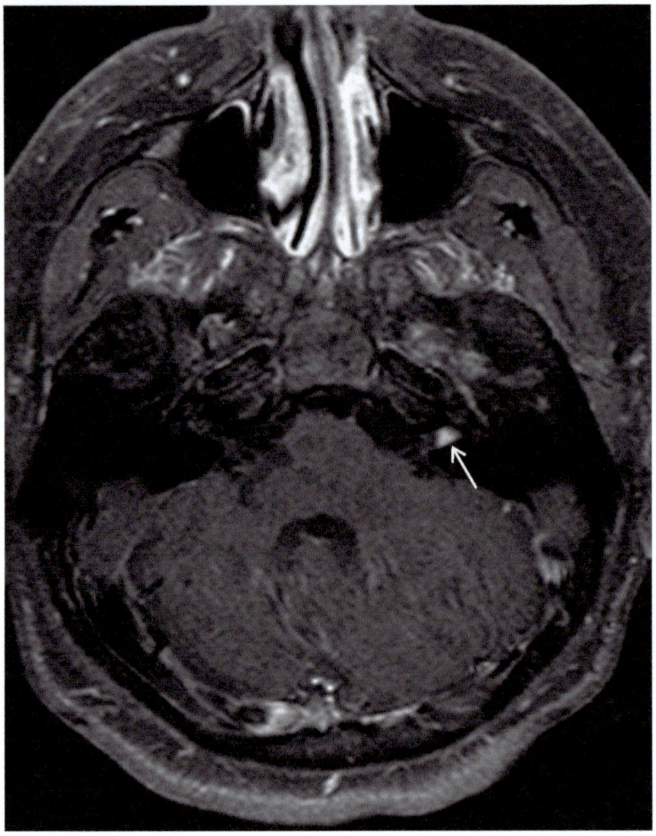

17. FIESTA T2-weighted sequence of the same tumor. The CSF space lateral to the tumor (between the tumor and the fundus) increases the chances of hearing preservation.

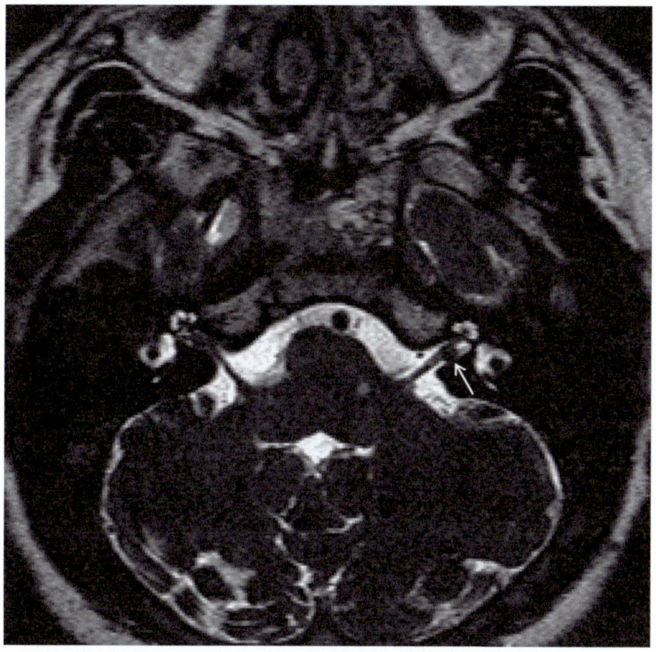

18. Case 2: A right intracanalicular vestibular schwannoma appropriate for the middle fossa approach.

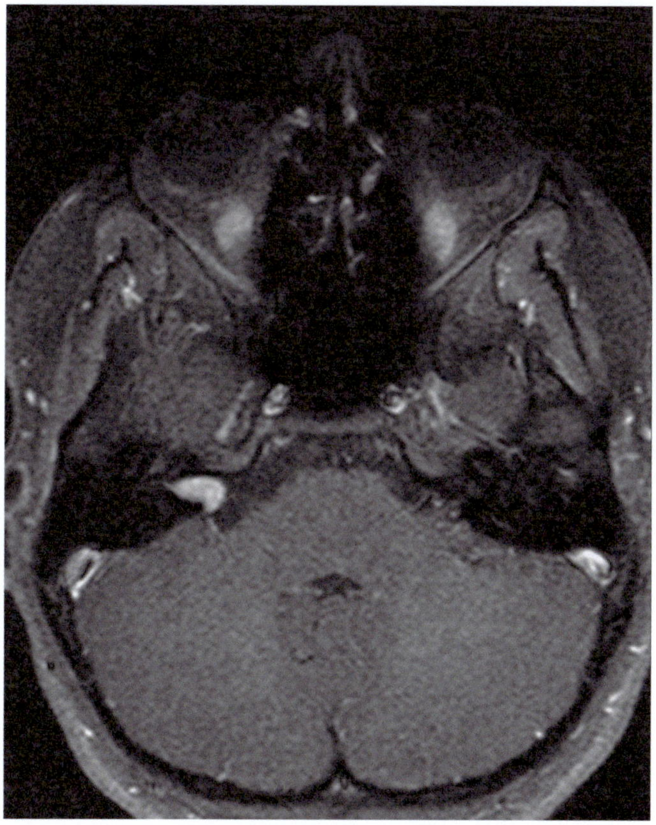

19. Intraoperative view during elevation of the temporal lobe dura in this patient. The instruments are directly over the epitympanum.

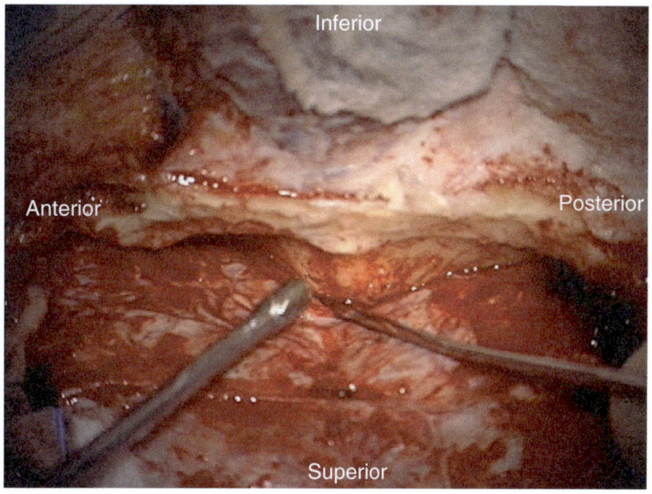

20. Dissection of the greater superficial petrosal nerve (*GSPN*). Note that a 1/2 in. square cottonoid kite (*kite*) is on top of the bleeding veins from around the foramen ovale and foramen spinosum. The Joseph elevator is between the GSPN and the dura. By sliding it anteriorly, the GSPN can be released from the dura, allowing more medial dissection to take place easily.

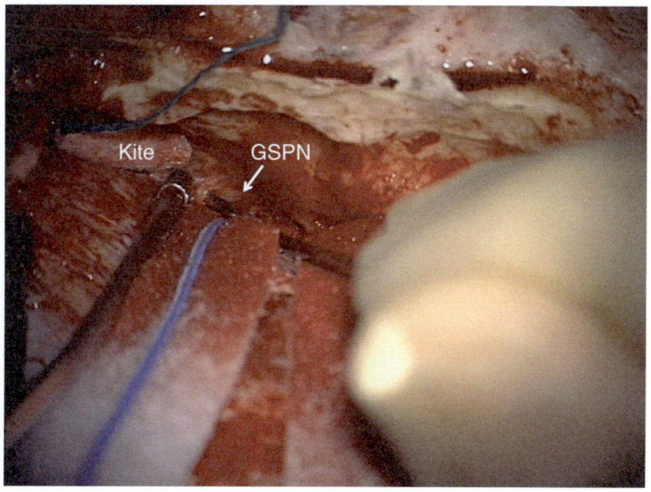

21. Drilling of the petrous bone commences. Note that there is very little space until some bone is removed. We prefer to begin drilling in the petrous apex anterior to the internal auditory canal. This is a safe area to begin identifying important landmarks. The superior petrosal sinus and GSPN are highly reliable and allow for accurate estimation of the location of other structures. As bone in the apex is removed, the posterior fossa dura is identified, followed by the porous acusticus. The internal auditory canal can then be followed out laterally. Depending on the structure of the floor of the middle cranial fossa, it is often necessary to remove bone around the geniculate ganglion and lateral to the internal auditory canal over the epitympanum. As the internal auditory canal is gradually identified, the location of the superior semicircular canal can be better predicted and subsequently "blue lined." The remainder of the bone removal can then be completed.

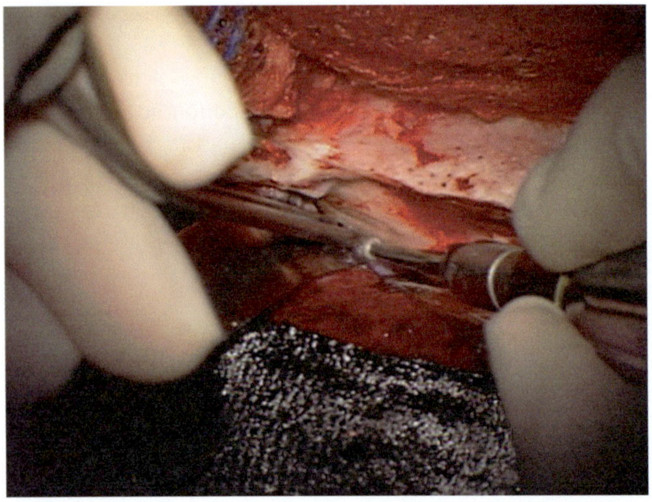

22. After drilling away the petrous ridge, the internal auditory canal (*IAC*) has been skeletonized but is still covered in bone. The posterior fossa dura, both anterior and posterior to the internal auditory canal, is visible.

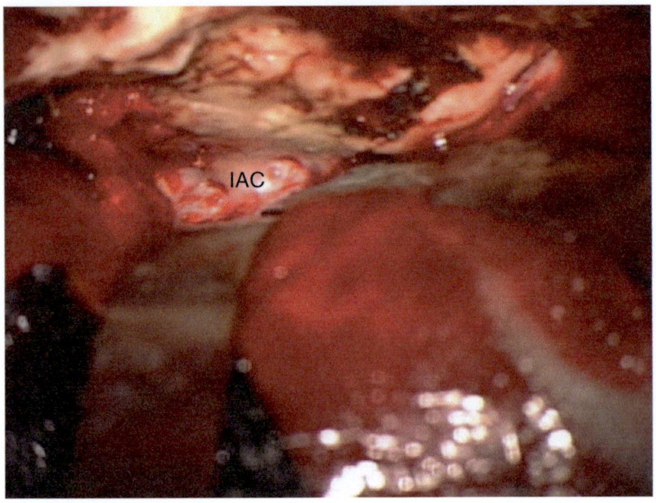

23. The dura of the internal auditory canal is now visible after removing the overlying bone. Note that cerebrospinal fluid has been released, likely from a small tear in the posterior fossa dura.

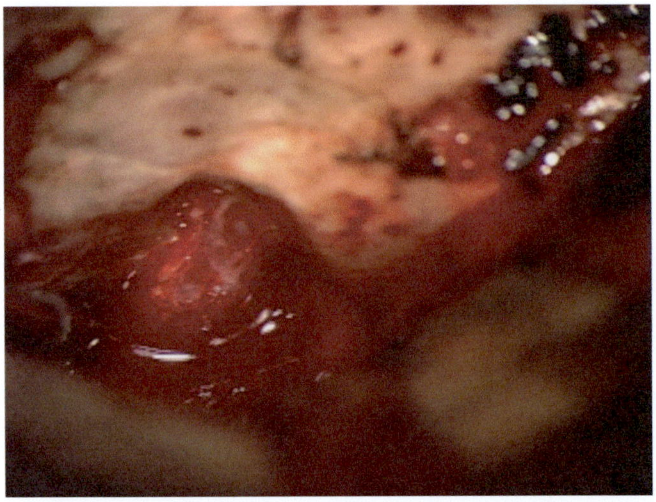

24. Blood vessels in the posterior fossa dura have been cauterized using the bipolar to prevent bleeding when opening it. Note the superior petrosal sinus (*SPS*) is under the tip of the retractor. The posterior fossa dura (*PF*) and middle fossa dura (*MF*) are identified.

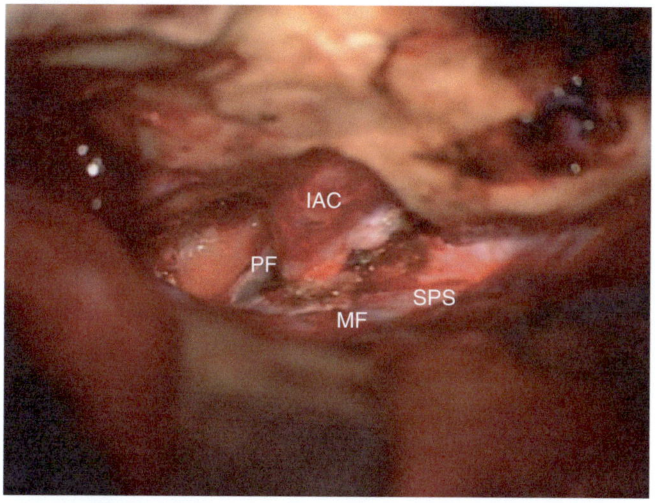

25. The dura of the posterior fossa and internal auditory canal has been opened. The facial nerve is just barely visible on top of the tumor (*F*). The posterior edge of the facial nerve is highlighted (*arrows*).

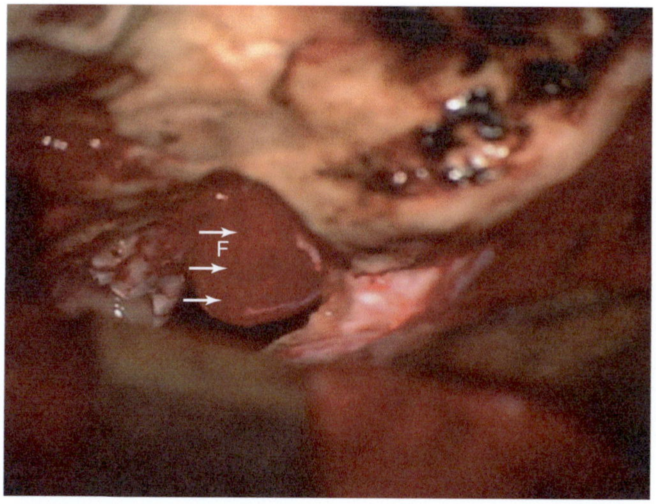

26. After removing the tumor and waxing any open air cells, a plug of fat is placed into the drilled-out cavity.

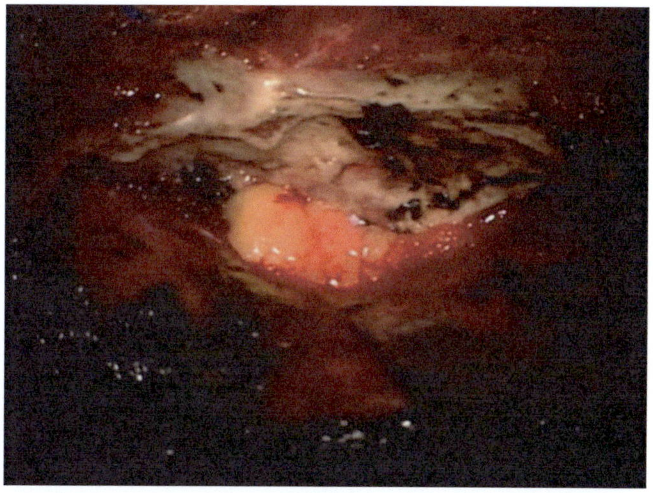

27. MRI taken on post-op day 1, demonstrating complete tumor removal, with normal postoperative inflammatory changes within the dura of the anterior internal auditory canal and clivus.

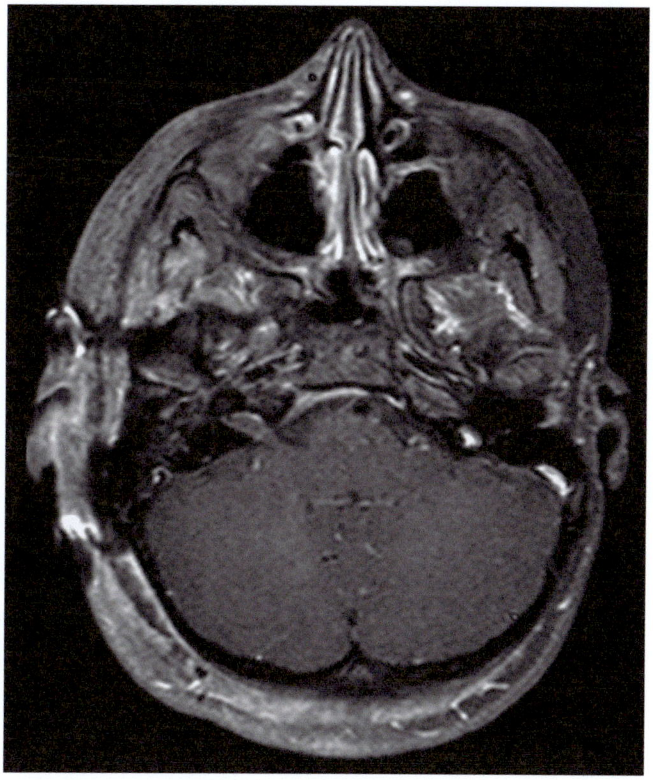

28. A pre-op CT of this patient that had been taken as an initial evaluation for headaches. The diameter of the internal auditory canal is perhaps slightly larger than normal but is not obviously dilated.

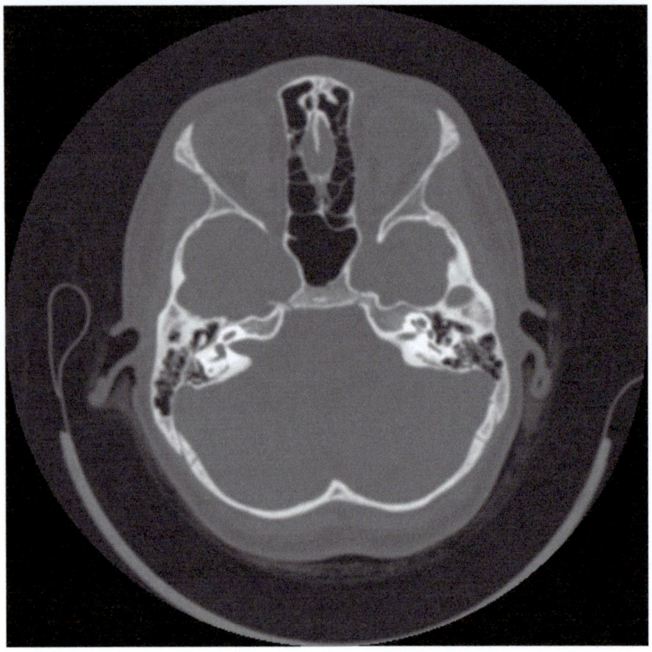

29. A post-op CT of this patient that was taken because of concern for bleeding the first night after surgery. While there was no bleed, the image nicely shows the amount of petrous apex bone that had been removed (*arrow*).

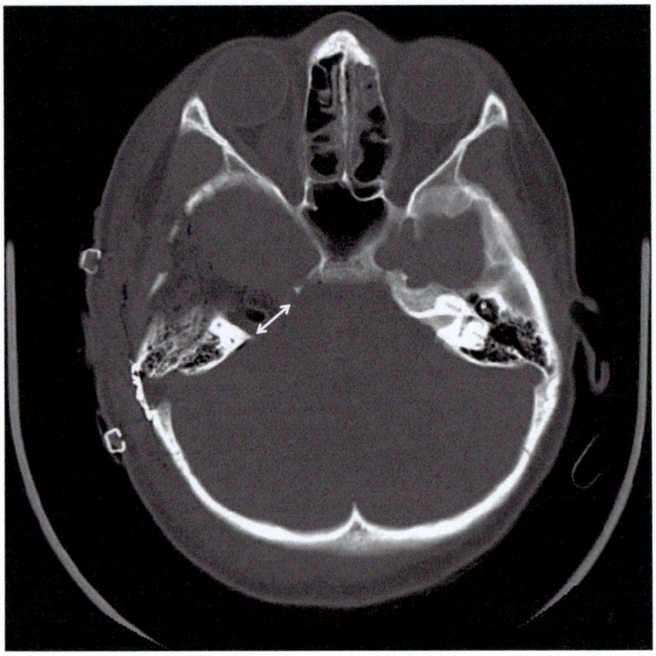

Kawase's Triangle Approach

- *Concept*
  - Retract the temporal lobe in an extradural fashion, and drill through the petrous apex anterior to the internal auditory canal to reach the posterior cranial fossa, ventral brainstem, and upper clivus.
- *Conditions treated*
  - Small posterior fossa meningiomas anterior to the internal auditory canal
  - Posterior fossa epidermoids anterior to the internal auditory canal
  - Basilar artery aneurysms
  - Trigeminal nerve schwannomas primarily based within the middle fossa that extends into the posterior fossa
- *Risks*
  - Retraction injuries to the temporal lobe can cause contusion, edema, or stroke.
  - Temporal lobe seizure.
  - Anomic aphasia.
  - Hearing loss and/or vertigo if the labyrinth is violated.
  - Facial nerve injury, typically if the geniculate ganglion is dehiscent and not recognized.
  - Carotid artery injury along the horizontal segment.
  - Dry eye if the GSPN is transected.
  - CSF leak.
- *Benefits*
  - Better than the posterior fossa approaches when approaching tumors anterior to the internal auditory canal because cranial nerves VII and VIII are not between the surgeon and the tumor. Thus, there is a lower risk of hearing loss and facial nerve weakness.
  - Drilling away the underlying petrous apex bone removes most of the blood supply to meningiomas prior to tumor dissection, facilitating tumor removal.
  - Allows simultaneous access to the middle fossa and posterior fossa.

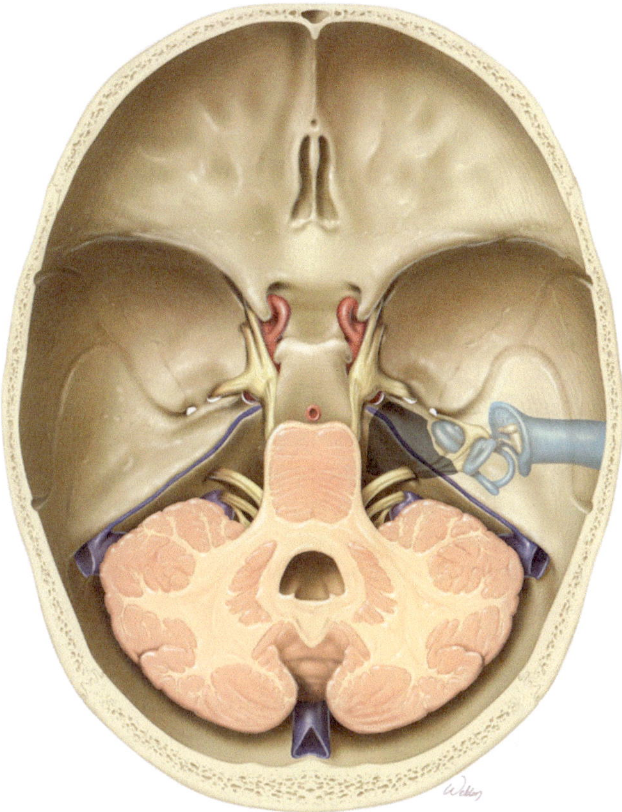

30. Overview of the bone to be removed (*gray*). Less bone posterior to the internal auditory canal needs to be removed compared to the approach for resection of a vestibular schwannoma. The anterior limit is the cavernous sinus, which partially covers the trigeminal ganglion.

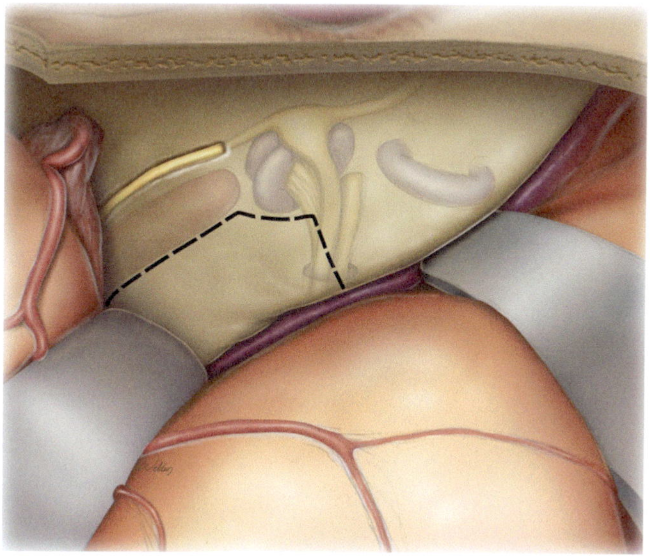

31. The procedure starts exactly as described in Figs. 4, 5, 6, and 7. The area of petrous apex bone to remove for a Kawase's triangle approach is highlighted. It is not really a triangle. The basic concept is to remove as much of the petrous apex bone anterior to the internal auditory canal as possible.

32. The posterior fossa dura is exposed and then opened. The anterior limit of exposure is the cavernous sinus. One recognizes this because it begins to bleed. The bleeding can be voluminous. However, since it is under low pressure, it can be controlled with Surgicel and a cottonoid held in place by the malleable retractor.

    The inferior limit of exposure is the inferior petrosal sinus (*IPS*), the posterior limit is the internal auditory canal (*IAC*), the lateral limit is the carotid artery (*CA*), and the medial limit is the superior petrosal sinus (*SPS*). Additional access can be obtained by decompressing the internal auditory canal as is done in a middle fossa approach for a vestibular schwannoma. The dissection does not need to be carried aggressively to the fundus, but as is true with most approaches, the more thorough the bone removal, the better the access and visibility. This improved access needs to be balanced with the increased risk to regional structures. The visible structures include CN V and VI, the ventral pons, and the basilar artery (*BA*).

    The access to the posterior fossa is fairly limited, and tumors with larger posterior fossa components should be assessed carefully before considering this approach. A trigeminal nerve schwannoma will likely be much easier to remove compared to a meningioma with extensive dural involvement. The course of the cranial nerves may be discernable on preoperative imaging. If the nerves are pushed anteriorly, a posterior fossa approach may be best. If they are pushed posteriorly, this approach may be preferred. Most concerning with this approach is the potential inability to manage a vascular injury. Vessels may fall back into the posterior fossa and be difficult to visualize and reach.

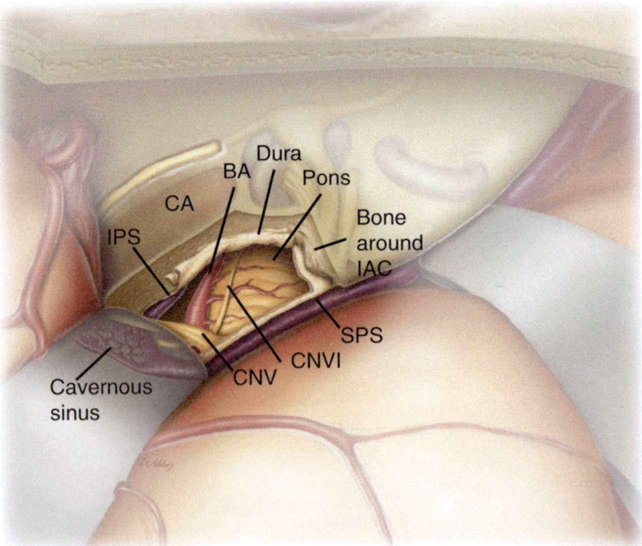

33. Case 1: Postoperative CT scan showing the amount of bone removal after a Kawase's triangle approach (*arrow*). The entire anterior petrous apex and part of the clivus have been removed.

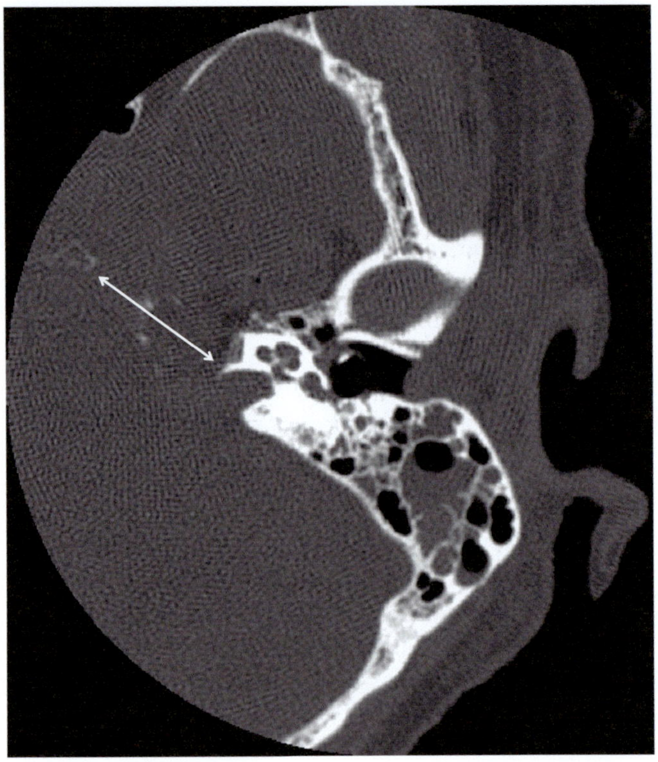

34. The unoperated contralateral side.

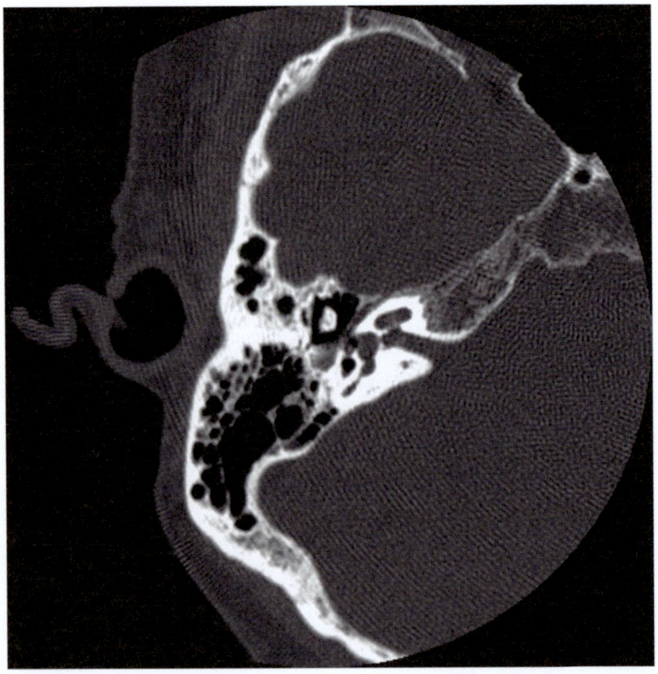

35. Case 2: Preoperative CT demonstrating an erosive arachnoid cyst (meningocele) involving the right petrous apex (*arrow*). This patient presented with trigeminal neuralgia.

This approach is what we generally use to approach chondrosarcomas, epidermoids, and cholesterol granulomas of the petrous apex. The entire procedure is extradural in these cases. For a cholesterol granuloma, we may combine this with a transmastoid retrofacial dissection to create a drainage pathway. In the setting of larger tumors and when widely exposing the carotid artery, the ultrasonic bone aspirators can be easier to use and safer than a high-speed drill.

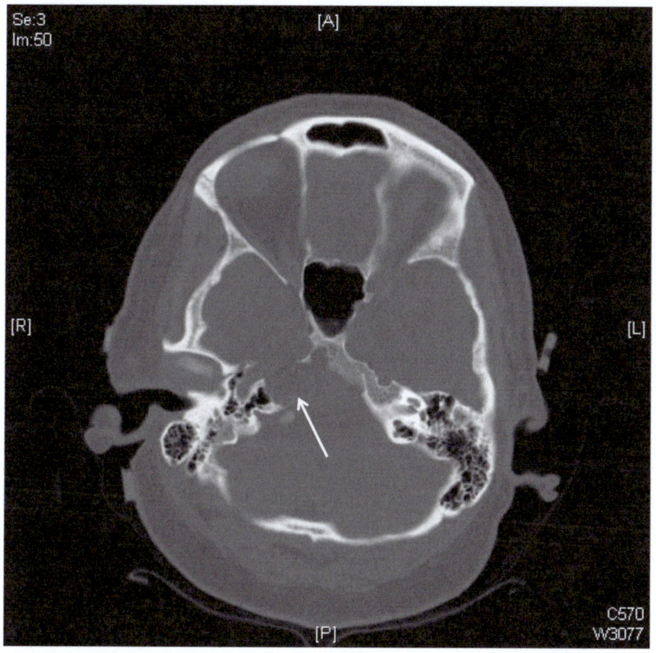

36. Postoperative T1-weighted MRI after Kawase's triangle approach with packing of the defect with a fat graft.

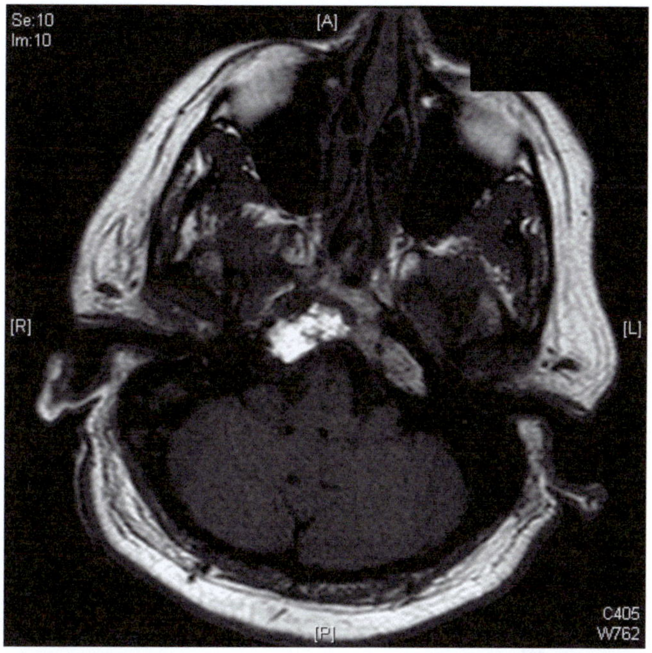

37. Postoperative T1-weighted MRI with gadolinium and fat saturation demonstrates that the bright signal on the previous figure was the fat graft.

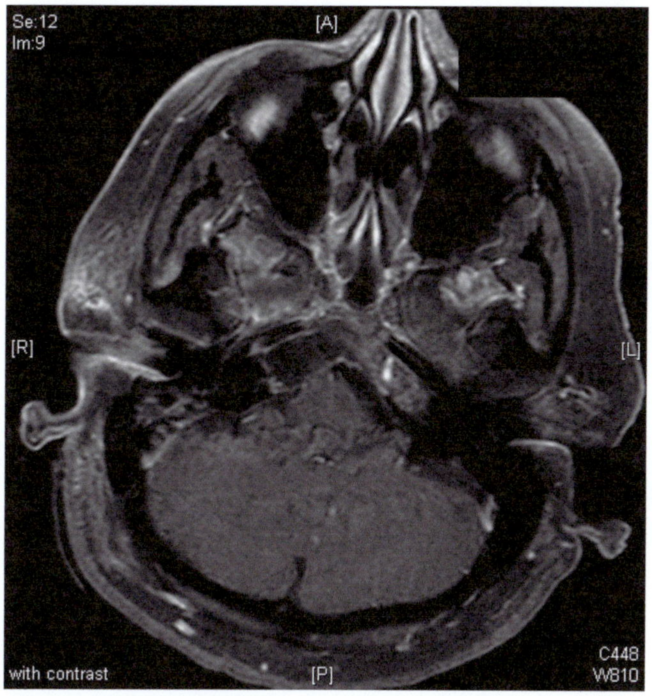

38. Postoperative T2-weighted MRI with the gray fat graft visible in the drilled-out defect in the petrous apex and clivus.

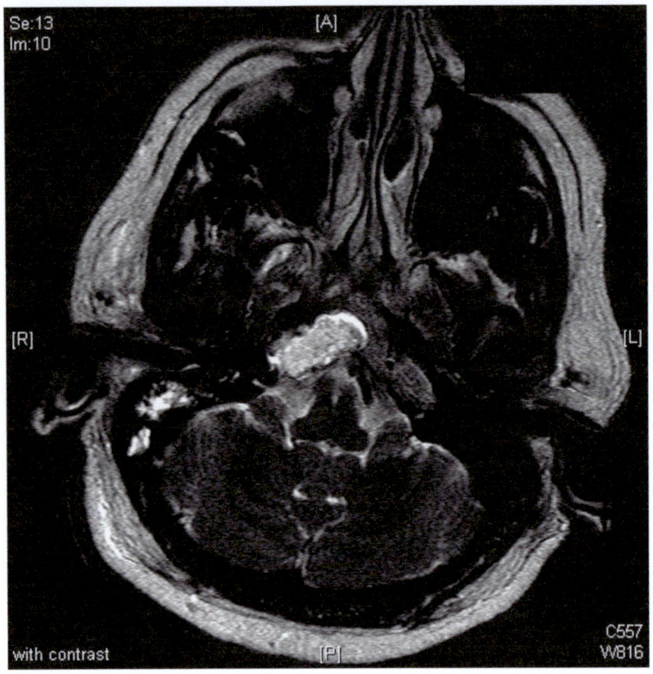

39. Case 3: Preoperative T1-weighted MRI with gadolinium showing a small posterior fossa meningioma based along the anterior petrous apex. This tumor can be resected quite nicely with the Kawase's triangle approach.

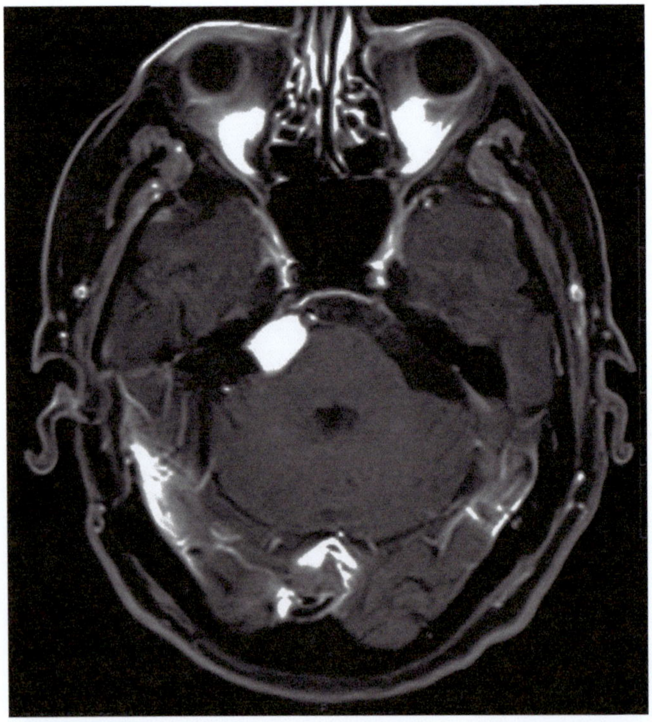

40. Coronal view of the same patient. The tumor is anterior and superior to the internal auditory canal, pushing the nerves posteriorly and inferiorly. This makes an anterior approach like this more attractive than a posterior approach (such as a retrosigmoid craniotomy).

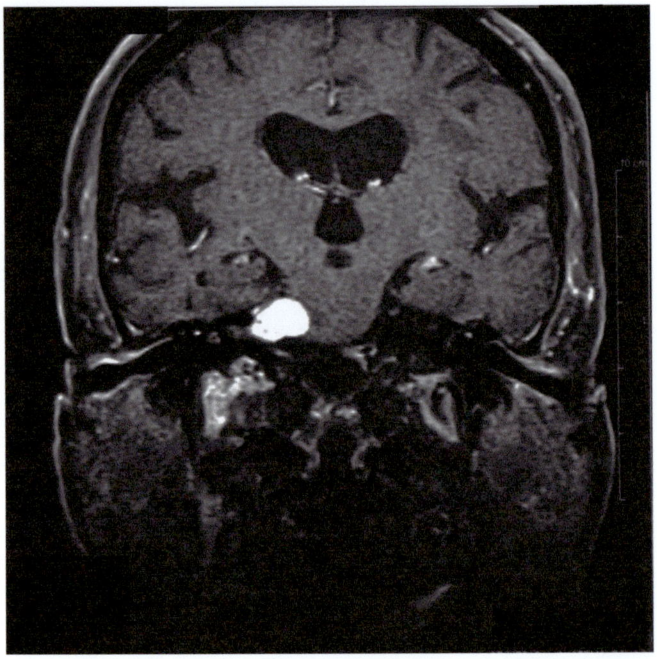

Orbitocraniozygomatic Approach

- *Concept*
  - Retract the anterior temporal lobe and the anterior cranial fossa contents in an extradural fashion to reach the foramen ovale, the foramen rotundum, the optic canal, and the cavernous sinus
  - This approach can be tailored to meet the unique needs of each specific case. Thus, the specific tumor characteristics and extent and preexisting deficits need to be carefully assessed to determine the best way to tailor this more generalized surgical approach.
- *Conditions treated*
  - Chordoma
  - Chondrosarcoma
  - Decompression of the optic nerve for traumatic optic neuropathy
  - Sphenoid wing meningioma
  - Trigeminal schwannoma
  - Juvenile nasopharyngeal angiofibroma with intracranial extension
  - Other tumors of the nasopharynx, pterygopalatine fossa, or infratemporal fossa that extend intracranially to the cavernous sinus
- *Risks*
  - Brain contusion, edema, or stroke
  - Seizure
  - Anomic aphasia
  - Visual loss, partial or complete
  - Diplopia. This can be transient from postoperative edema within the orbit or permanent if cranial nerves III, IV, or VI are injured.
  - Enophthalmos
  - Facial numbness in any or all divisions of trigeminal nerve
  - Facial nerve injury, typically if the geniculate ganglion is dehiscent and not recognized
  - Carotid artery injury
  - Dry eye if the GSPN is transected
  - CSF leak
  - Temporal hollowing from atrophy of the temporalis muscle
  - Scar at incision site on forehead
- *Benefits*
  - Wide exposure of the middle cranial fossa, cavernous sinus, and lateral orbit
  - Allows the surgeon to safely separate the cavernous sinus from tumors that originated within the face or parapharyngeal space and which have extended intracranially

41. Overview of the bone to be removed (*gray*). This can be tailored based upon the extent of the disease.

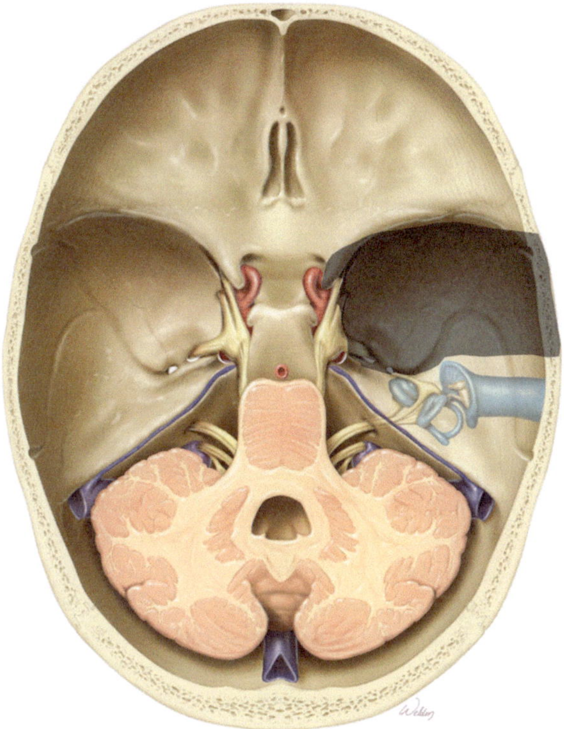

42. The incision for the orbitocraniozygomatic approach. The tip of the incision often needs to extend down into the forehead a little bit to obtain adequate exposure. This may leave a noticeable scar. If this is unacceptable, a bicoronal approach could also be used.

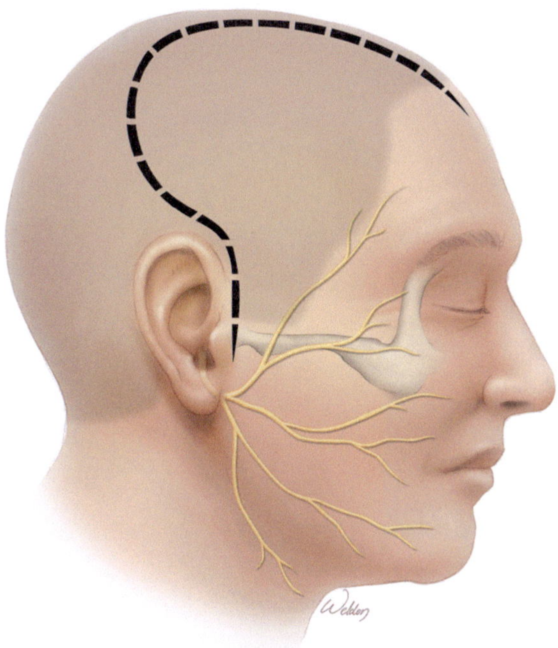

43. The skin, subcutaneous tissues, and periosteum are lifted off the skull, while the temporalis muscle is left in place. Care must be taken when elevating over the zygoma not to damage the frontal branch of the facial nerve. This nerve is preserved by lifting this plane deep to the superficial temporalis fascia prior to the midpoint of the zygoma and elevating posteriorly. This avoids injury to the temporal branch of the facial nerve as it transitions from deep to superficial in this area.

    Next, the periosteum along the underside of the superior edge of the zygoma is incised. A Freer elevator is then used to carefully elevate the periosteum off the zygoma until reaching the insertion of the masseter muscle. The periorbita is released along the lateral and superior orbit, with care taken to preserve the supraorbital nerve (*arrow*).

    The dotted lines show where the cuts should be made to remove the zygoma. We like to use the reciprocating saw because its kerf is thin, preserving as much bone as possible. The strategy of creating a V at the anterior segment is helpful when plating the zygoma back at the end of the procedure because it helps to align the bone properly. Alternatively, prior to making the cuts, the plates can be bent, the holes drilled, and the screws put in and taken out again. This process takes longer, however. The zygoma is placed in a bacitracin solution on the back table.

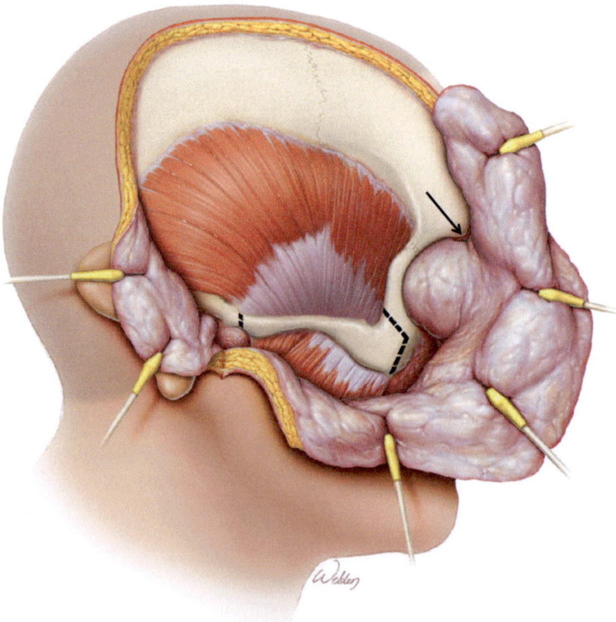

44. The temporalis muscle is elevated in a subperiosteal fashion. It is reflected inferiorly but left attached to the coronoid process of the mandible.

    The keyhole (*arrow*) is then exposed with an otologic drill and a large bit. This is the point where the dura of the middle cranial fossa, the dura of the anterior cranial fossa, and the periorbita meet.

    Three more burr holes are then made as shown and a craniotome used along the dotted lines to open the bone flap. The bone cuts over the orbit can course across the lateral and superior aspects of the orbital rim so that the lateral orbital bone and rim comes out as a separate piece (as shown here). This provides the greatest exposure of the orbit. Alternatively, the inferior cut can be brought up directly to the keyhole if the lateral orbital bone doesn't need to be removed this low. This is what we typically do for intracranial pathology as surgery within the orbit is seldom necessary.

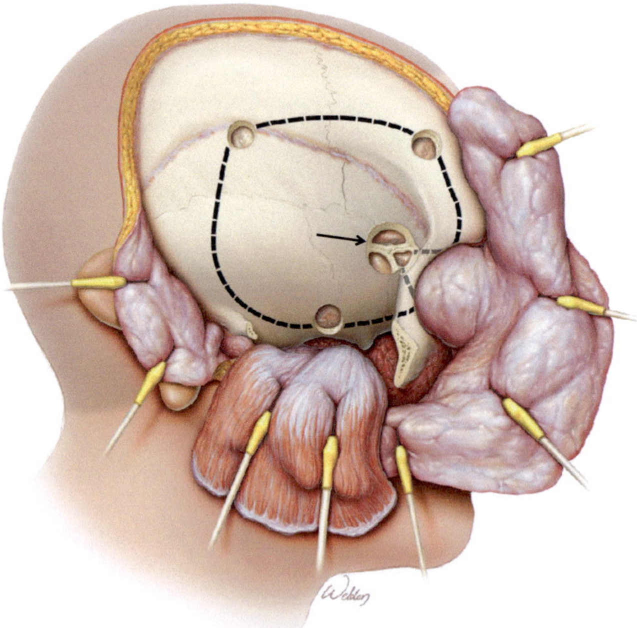

45. After removing the bone flap, malleable retractors are used to carefully elevate the contents of the anterior cranial fossa and retract the temporal horn. All dissection is done in an extradural fashion if the pathology allows.

The gasserian ganglion, cranial nerve V3 (entering the foramen ovale), and cranial nerve V2 (entering the foramen rotundum) are easily visible after this process. Bleeding from around them comes from the cavernous sinus and can be controlled with gentle packing and pressure.

Depending upon the tumor to be removed, cranial nerves V1 and V2 can be divided here and the dissection carried along the skull medially another centimeter or so. As many parapharyngeal space and nasopharyngeal tumors extend intracranially through the foramen ovale and the foramen rotundum, this maneuver allows the surgeon to separate the main tumor mass from its blood supply coming from the cavernous sinus. This makes removal of the lower portion of the tumor much simpler and safer.

The internal carotid artery (ICA), oculomotor nerve, trochlear nerve, abducens nerve, and cranial nerve V1 run inside the cavernous sinus. Therefore, they are not visible unless the cavernous sinus dura is opened. If this is performed, the bleeding is persistent, and while it can still be controlled with packing and gentle pressure, one needs to be concerned about the total amount of accumulated blood loss. An attentive anesthesiologist who is keeping up with blood products is invaluable.

Also, the surgeon should be worried about damaging the cranial nerves that run within the cavernous sinus unexpectedly because of the poor visualization. These types of postoperative neuropathies, together with the difficulty in removing all residual tumor within the cavernous sinus, is why removing tumor from within the cavernous sinus is not a fulfilling endeavor. Therefore, we typically plan ahead to leave behind tumor that has invaded the cavernous sinus. Residual tumor within the dura of the cavernous sinus can be cauterized intraoperatively, followed with serial imaging, and treated with stereotactic radiation as needed.

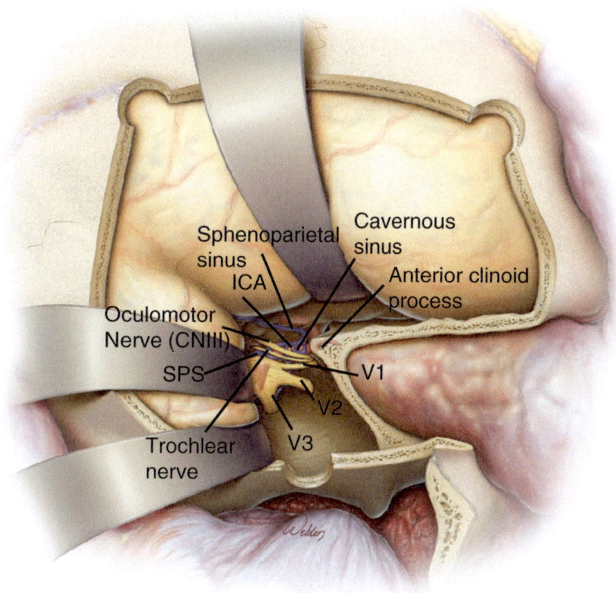

46. The anterior clinoid process can be drilled away if necessary to decompress the optic nerve.

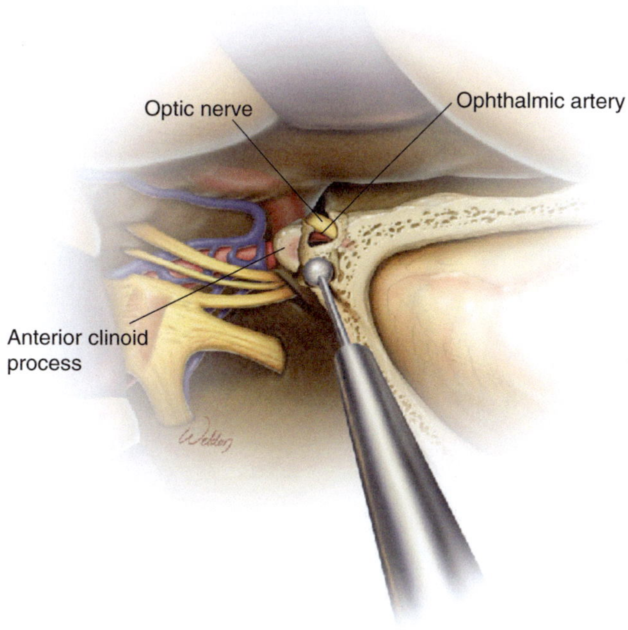

47. Case 1: Axial MRI of a teenager with a large juvenile nasopharyngeal angiofibroma.

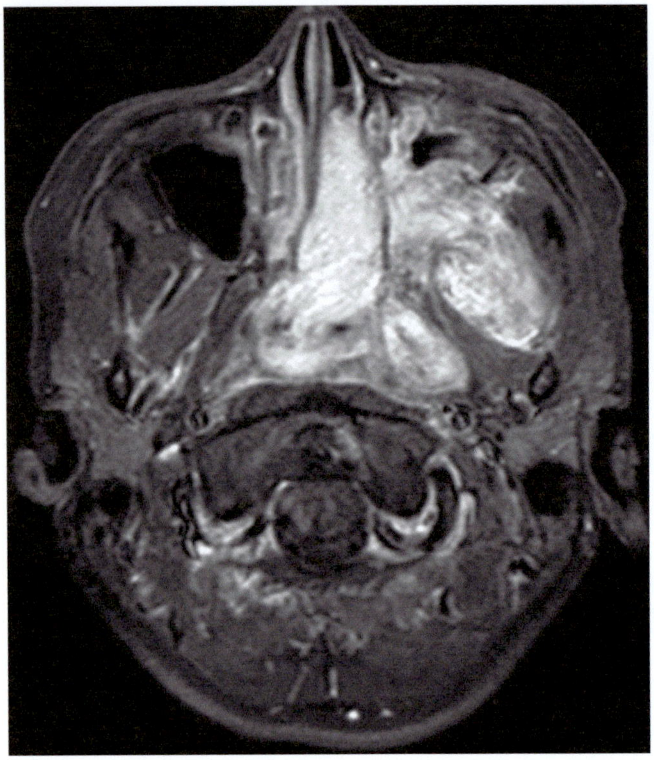

48. Coronal MRI demonstrates intracranial extension of the tumor through the foramen ovale to involve the cavernous sinus (*arrow*).

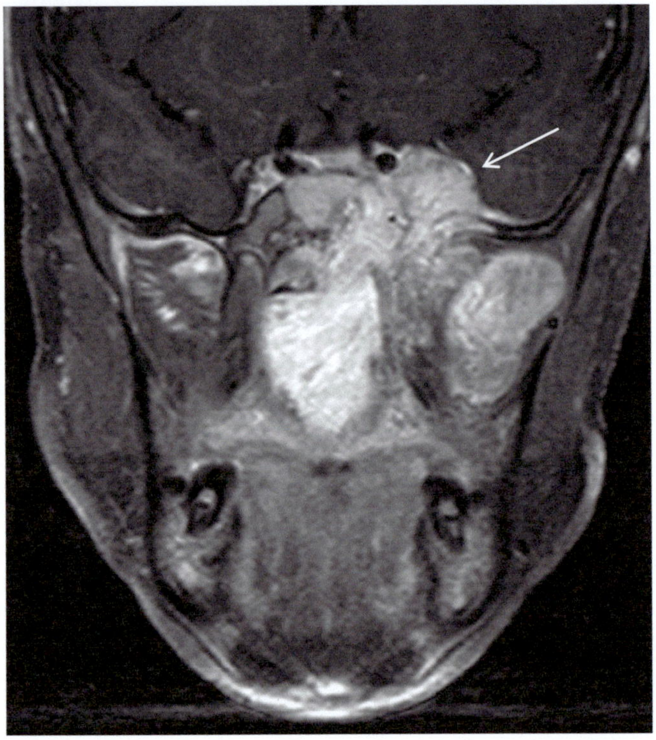

49. There is also significant lateral extension into the parapharyngeal space (*arrow*).

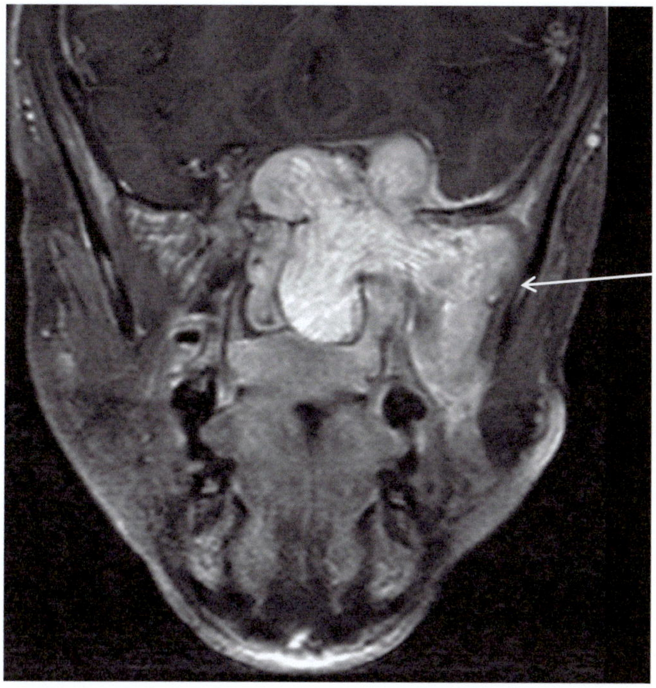

50. Coronal CT revealing significant bony destruction of the skull base.

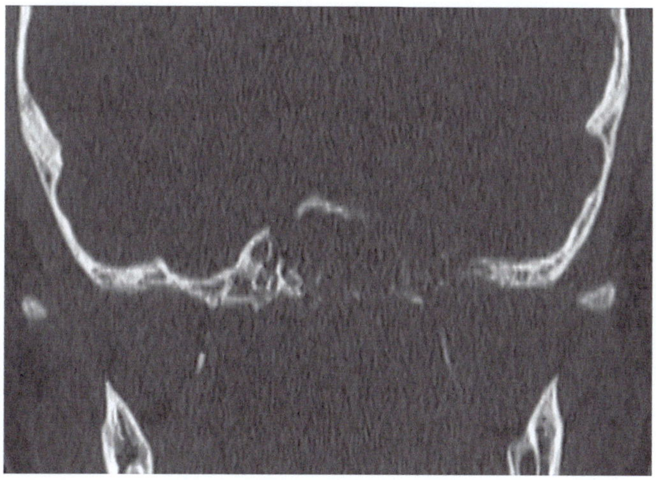

51. The day before surgery, embolization of the extracranial vascular feeding vessels was performed. Embolization of feeding vessels coming from the dura around the cavernous sinus is not possible. Tumors like this need to be separated from the intracranial vascular supply prior to transfacial resection of the tumor to prevent potentially life-threatening bleeding throughout the surgery. Thus, a bicoronal incison was planned for the orbitocraniozygomatic approach. At the time we performed this surgery, the front of the head was prepared with a significant shave. Currently, we simply shave a strip across the top of the head, leaving hair in front and behind the incision site.

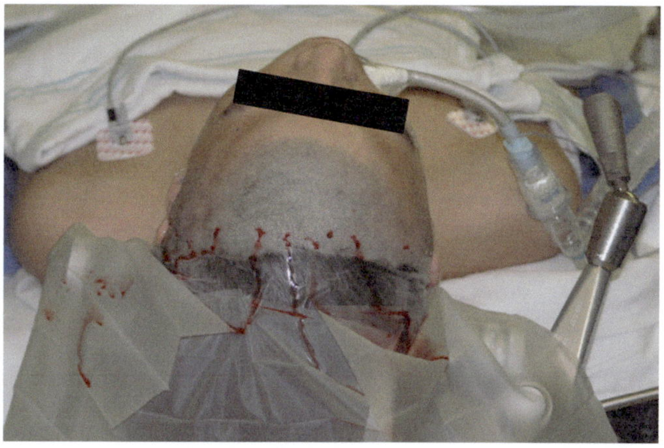

52. The periosteum and superficial layer of the deep temporal fascia was elevated, leaving the temporalis muscle down.

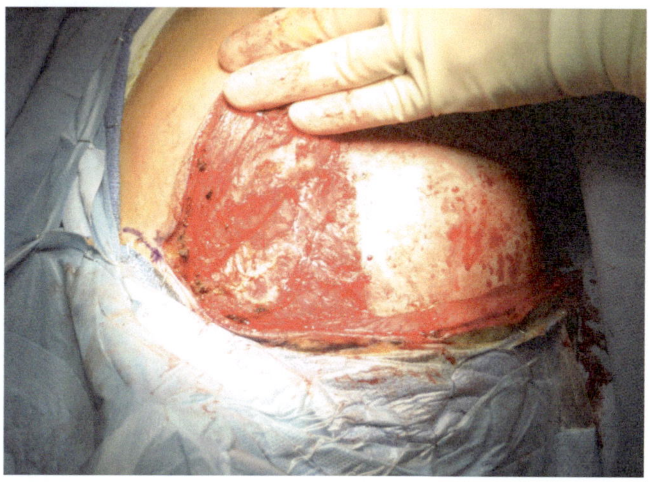

53. The zygoma was then removed and the temporalis muscle elevated. It was covered by a moist sponge and retracted inferiorly by the yellow fishhook. Burr holes were drilled and connected with the craniotome. Note the keyhole (*arrow*). We used a more minimalistic bone flap, preserving the lateral orbital rim while removing the superior orbital rim.

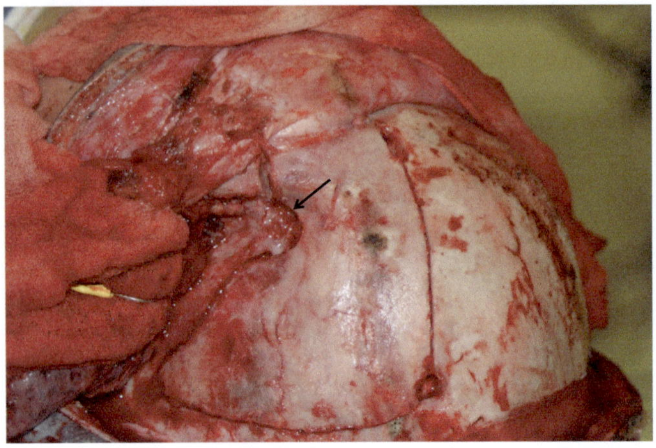

54. Removing the bone flap reveals the dura of the anterior cranial fossa (*AF*), the dura of the middle cranial fossa (*MF*), and the lateral periorbita (*P*). The medial skull base bone that leads superiorly to the anterior clinoid process and inferiorly to the foramen rotundum and ovale is visible (*bone*). This bone will be removed to obtain deeper access to the central skull base.

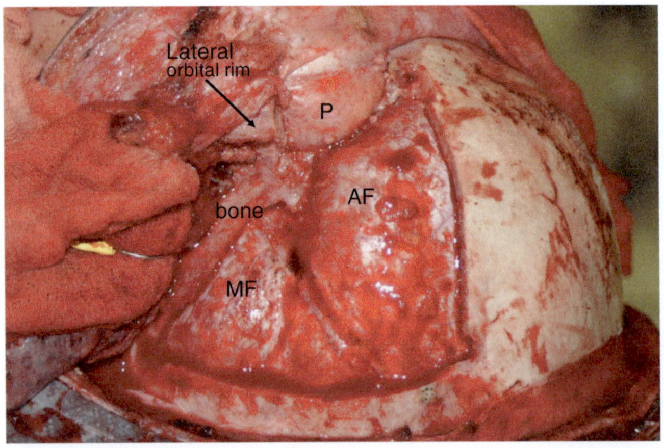

55. The bone flap after plating an additional piece of the superior orbital bone that was removed for exposure. The keyhole (*arrow*) is visible.

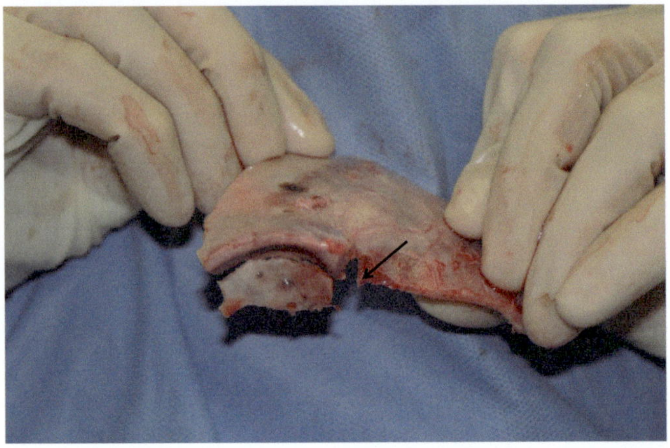

56. To drill away the medial skull base bone, cottonoids and retractors were placed to protect the periorbita and dura.

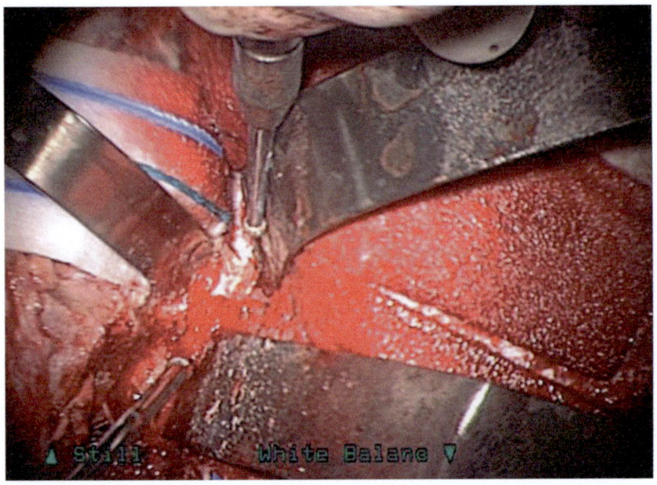

57. Extradural drilling was continued medially and inferiorly. CN V2 was divided, and the distal stump can be seen as it is held up by the suction. The nasopharyngeal tumor was separated from the dura using a bipolar. Surgicel (*S*) was placed on top of the tumor within the pterygopalatine fossa after it was separated from the middle fossa dura to control bleeding inferiorly. The tip of the malleable retractor is tenting up the lateral side of the cavernous sinus. This structure limits the extent of resection that can be performed.

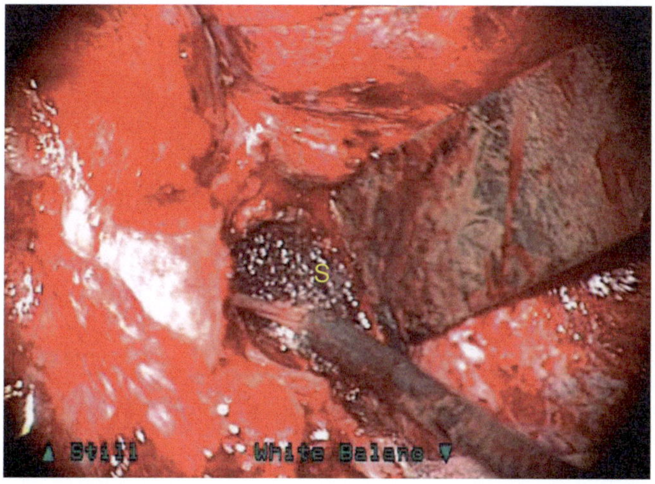

58. Once the tumor was separated from the dura around the cavernous sinus, its vascular supply became based solely upon its extracranial vessels (which had already been partially embolized). A standard transfacial approach to resect the tumor was then feasible and safe. In this case, a lateral rhinotomy incision was used to perform a medial maxillectomy. All of the tumor could be safely removed.

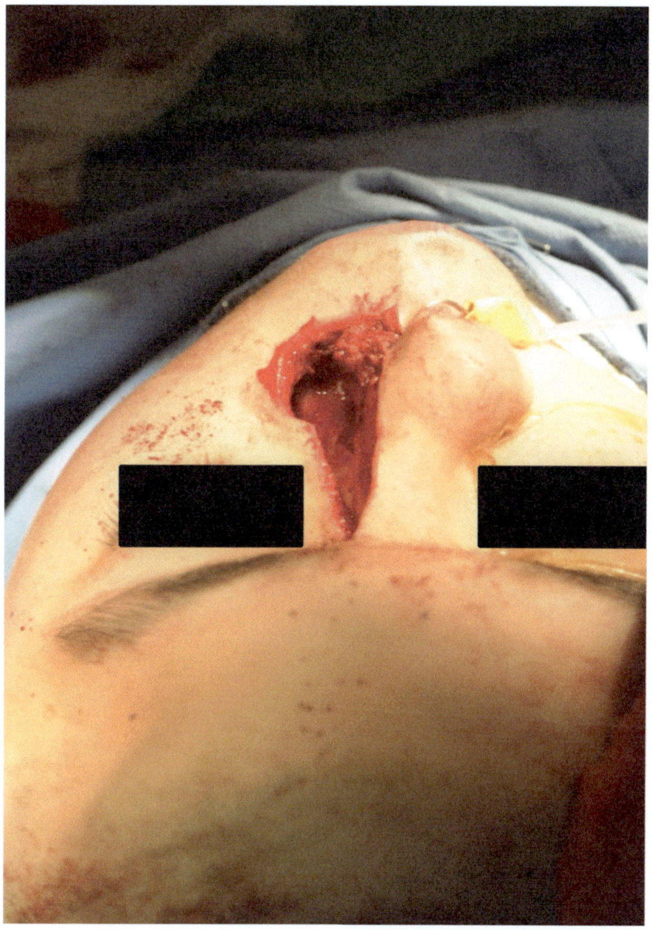

59. Finally, the bone flap was plated back into position, and a fat graft harvested from the abdomen was used to fill in the skull base defect under the temporal lobe where the bone had been drilled away. This separated the dura from the nasopharynx and parapharyngeal space.

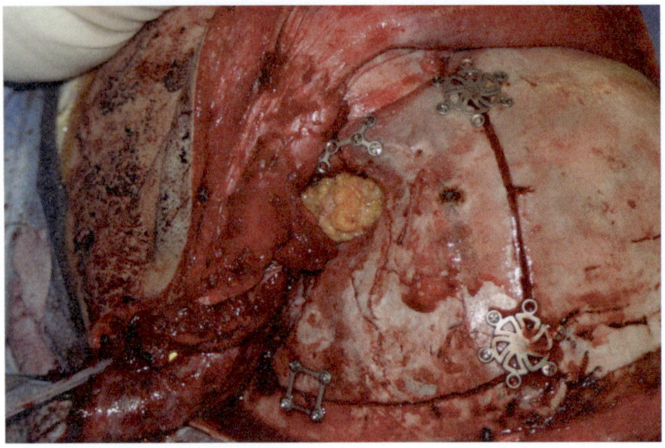

60. A coronal MRI taken 3 months postoperatively revealed excellent tumor resection.

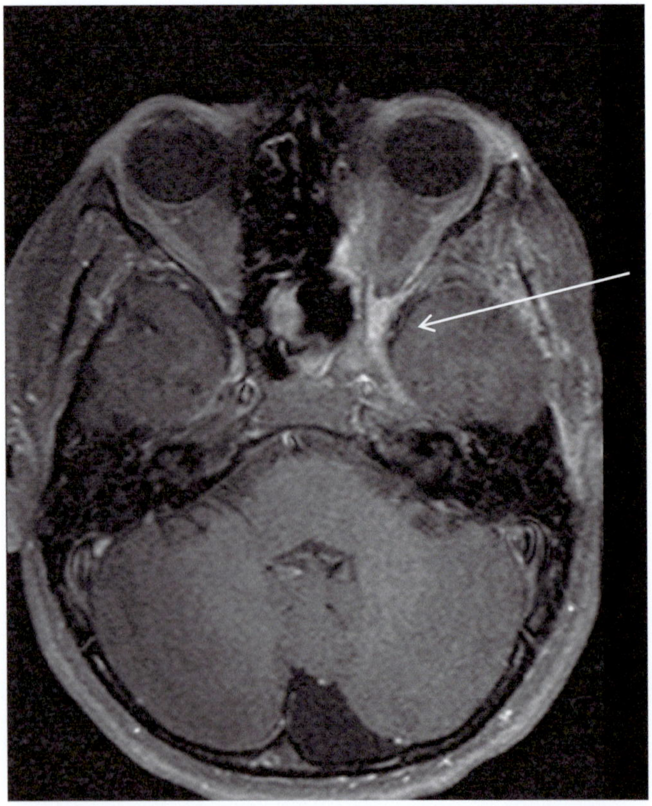

61. Axial MRI reveals inflammatory changes in the area of the keyhole where the fat was placed (*arrow*) but no evidence of tumor or enophthalmos.

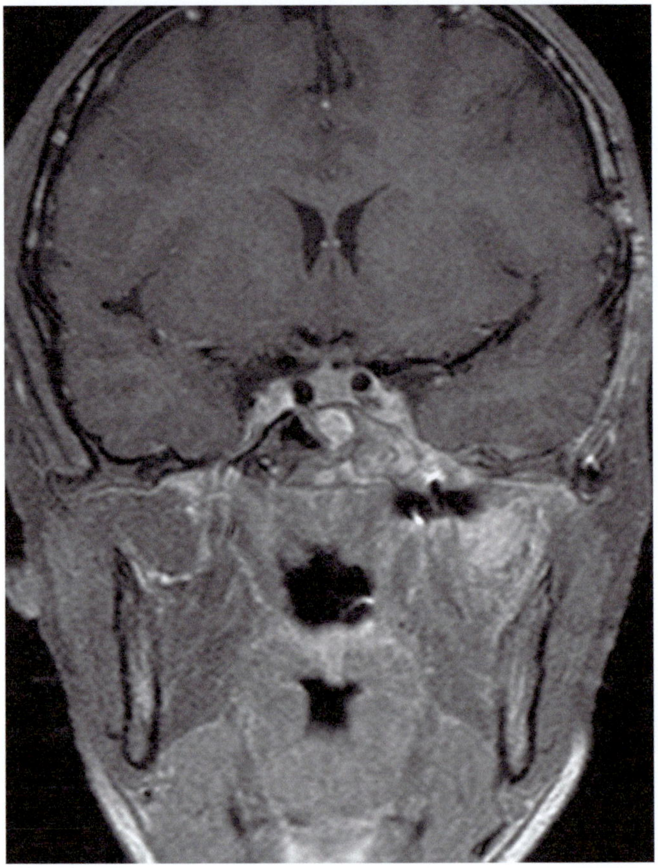

62. The lateral rhinotomy incision healed quite nicely as well.

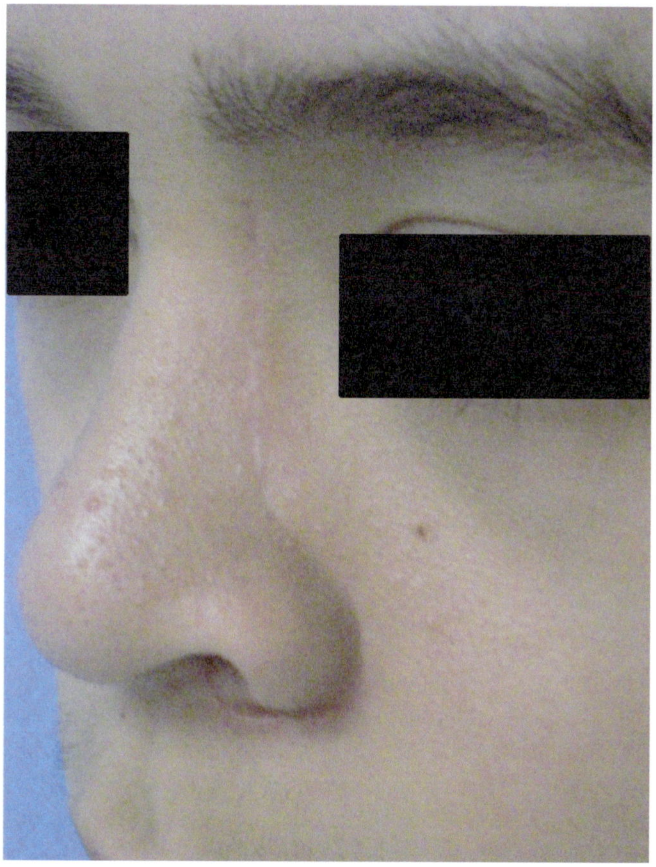

63. Case 2: A large cavernous sinus meningioma. This patient had no cranial nerve deficits, with the exception of facial numbness in the V2 and V3 distribution.

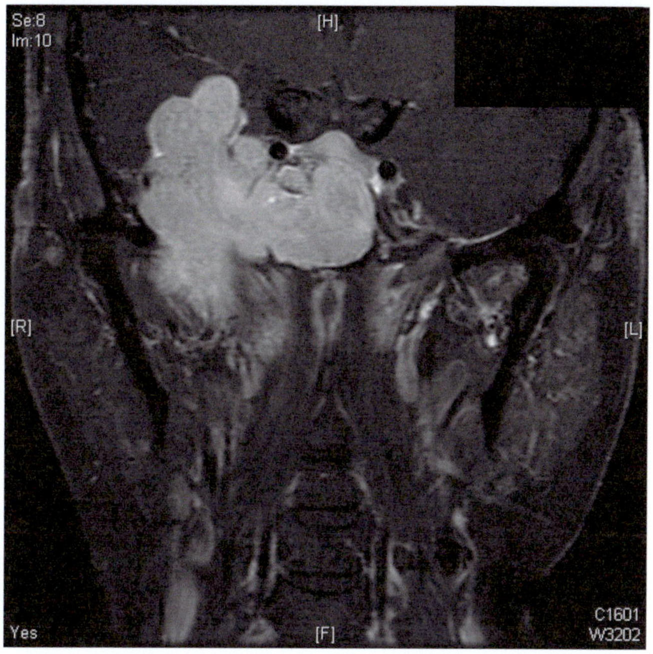

64. It extended into the sphenoid sinus, nasopharynx, and infratemporal fossa.

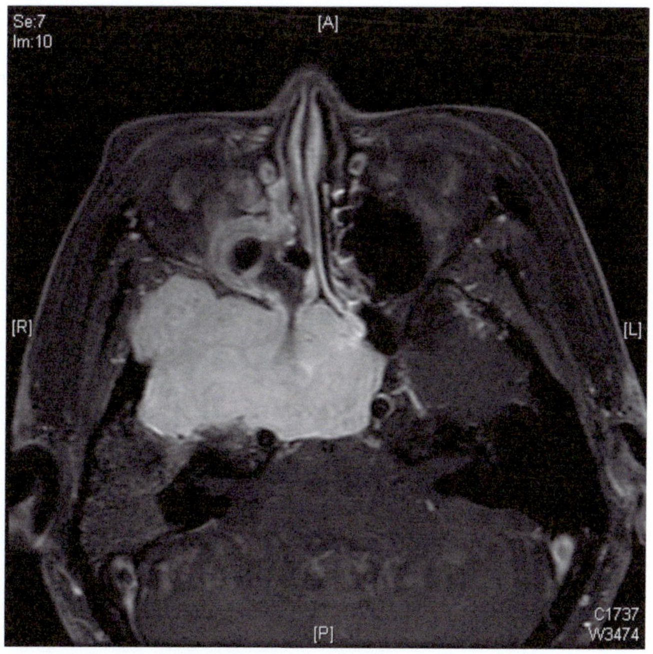

65. Coronal CT scan demonstrating the expansion of the bony margins of the tumor.

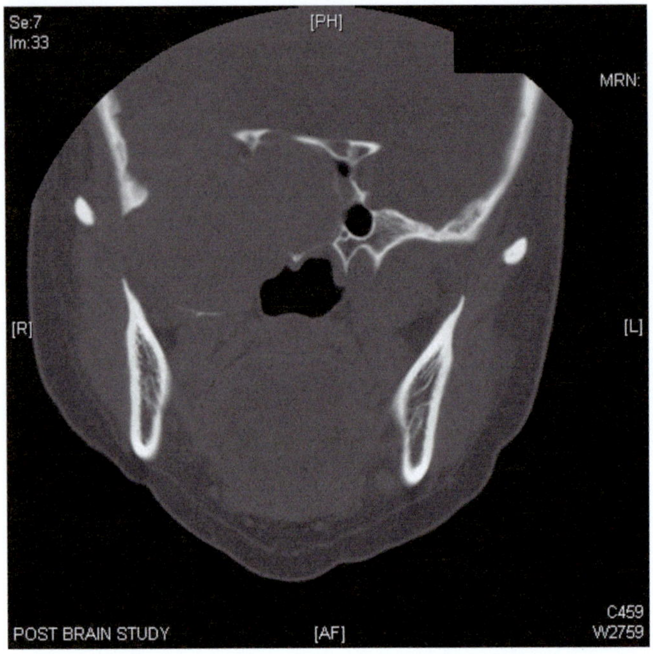

66. Axial CT demonstrating erosion of the clivus and displacement of the right internal carotid artery compared to the left (*arrows*).

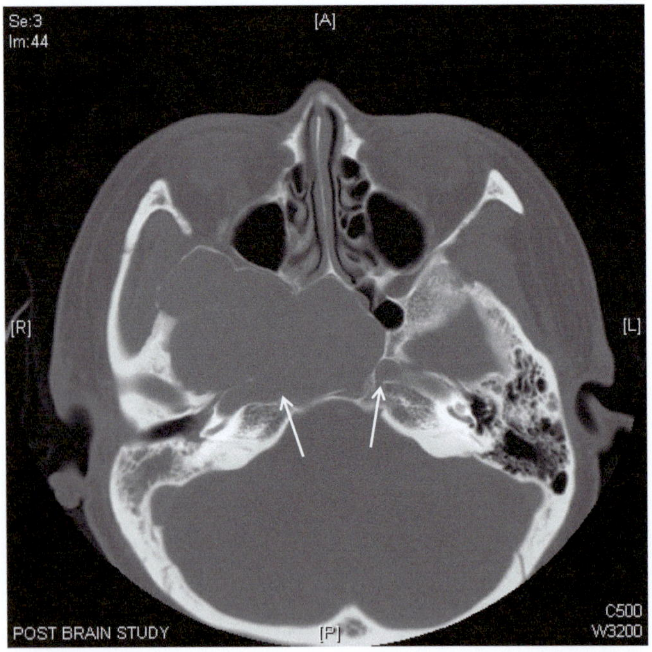

67. A bicoronal incision was used for this approach. For personal reasons, this patient requested a complete shave of the head rather than a strip as we more commonly do at this time.

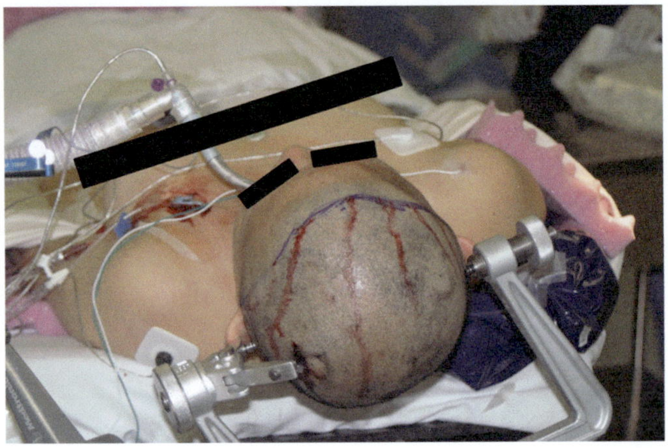

68. The temporalis muscle (T) was left down, but the periosteum was elevated off the zygoma (*Z*) and the frontal bone (*F*) in order to preserve the temporal branch of the facial nerve. Note that the lateral periorbita (*P*) has been violated, exposing the orbital fat. Ideally, the periorbita would have been left intact as this procedure does not include intraorbital dissection.

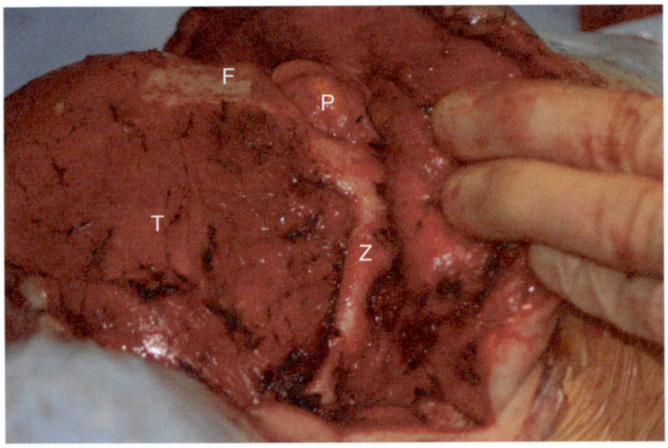

69. The zygomatic arch after removal. Note that the anterior cut (top) was performed in a V-shape.

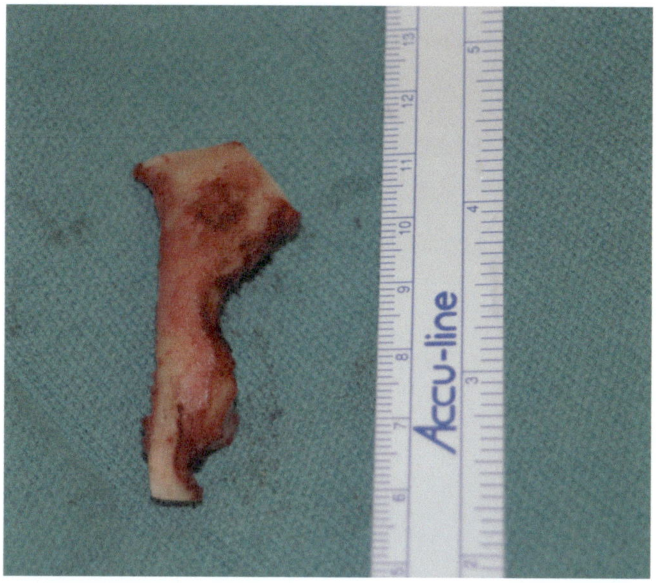

70. The temporalis muscle was then reflected inferiorly off the skull in a subperiosteal plane. The Bovie indicates where the tumor has eroded through the skull.

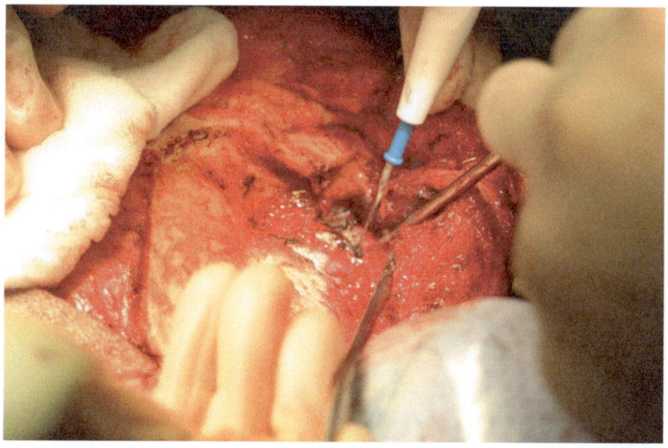

71. A view after removing easily accessible extracranial tumor through the region of bone erosion. Note that we really like the use of the yellow fishhook retractors (sometimes called "Lone-Stars") to hold the overlying soft tissues out of the way during skull base procedures. They are easy to reposition and do not require an assistant to reach into the operative field under the microscope to hold a retractor.

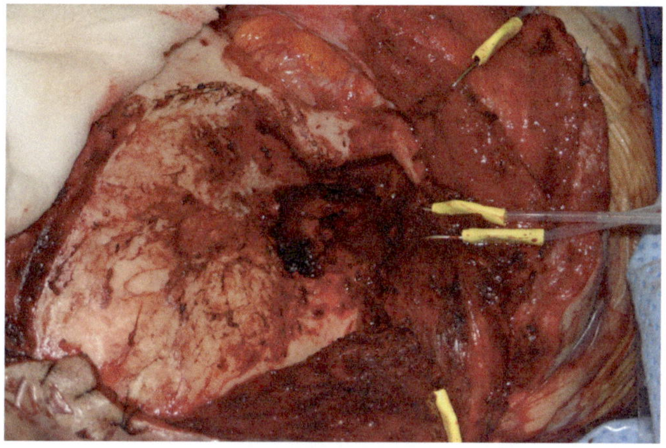

72. Because the tumor was large, debulking some of the tumor provided improved access to the rest of the tumor. Thus, we did not need to remove the lateral orbital rim as the tumor impinging upon the posterior orbit could be accessed directly. Also, the tumor in the sphenoid sinus could be removed. Thus, the periorbita (*P*) and the sphenoid sinus mucosa (*SS*) are visible in this image. However, we did remove a bone flap over the temporal lobe in order to remove the intracranial portion of the tumor. We resected the dura at the base of the meningioma. While some of the dura could be closed primarily (*stitches*), there was exposed brain medially (*brain*) near the lateral edge of the cavernous sinus (*CS*).

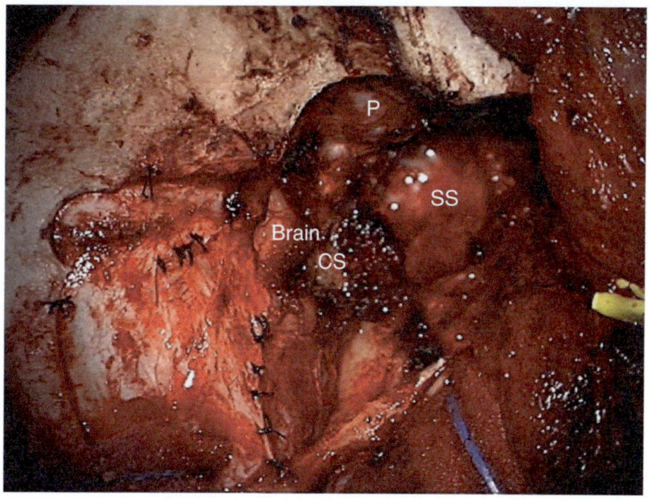

73. Artificial dura (DuraGen) was used to cover the residual defect, and it was made watertight with a sealent (DuraSeal, the blue material). A vascularized muscular free flap was then used to fill the defect and the zygoma plated back in place. Almost any type of free flap can be used in this area with excellent results, although the degree of bulk needs to be matched to the defect.

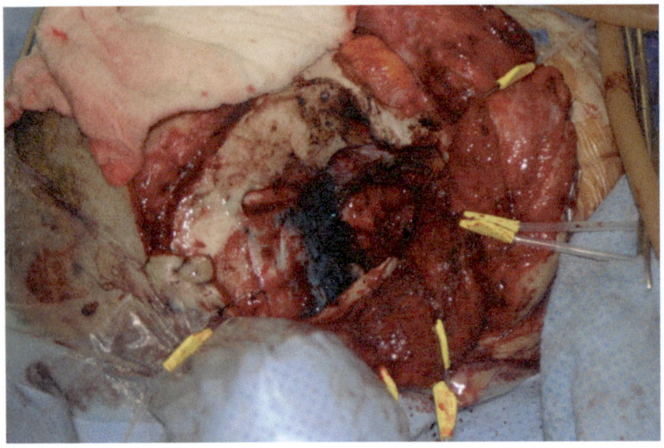

74. Postoperative coronal view demonstrating excellent resection, although there is residual tumor within the cavernous sinus (*arrow*). It is impossible to completely remove tumor in this area without sacrificing the cranial nerves within it. This patient had no new cranial nerve deficits after surgery. In particular, the extraocular muscles functioned normally.

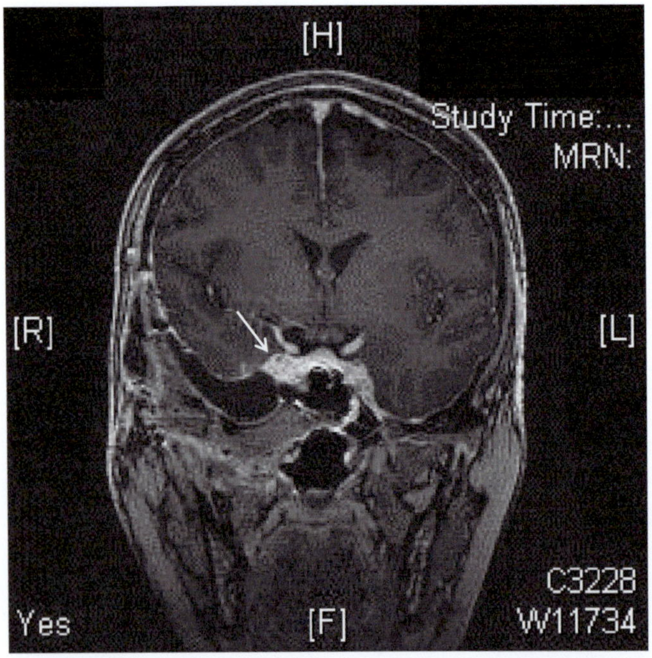

75. Postoperative axial view demonstrating the extent of the free flap. It crossed the midline and filled the entire sphenoid sinus.

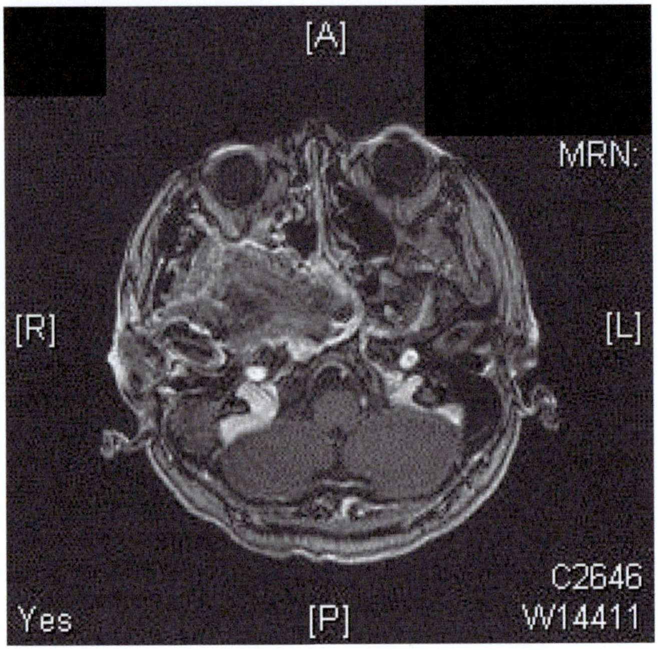

76. Case 3: A cavernous sinus meningioma with extracranial extension inferiorly though the skull base.

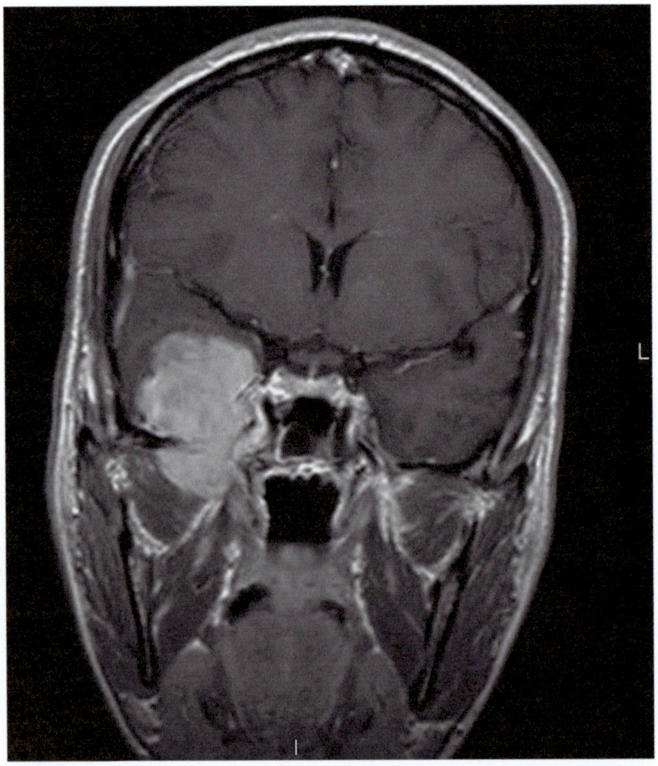

77. The axial view demonstrated that the tumor extended medially into the sphenoid sinus.

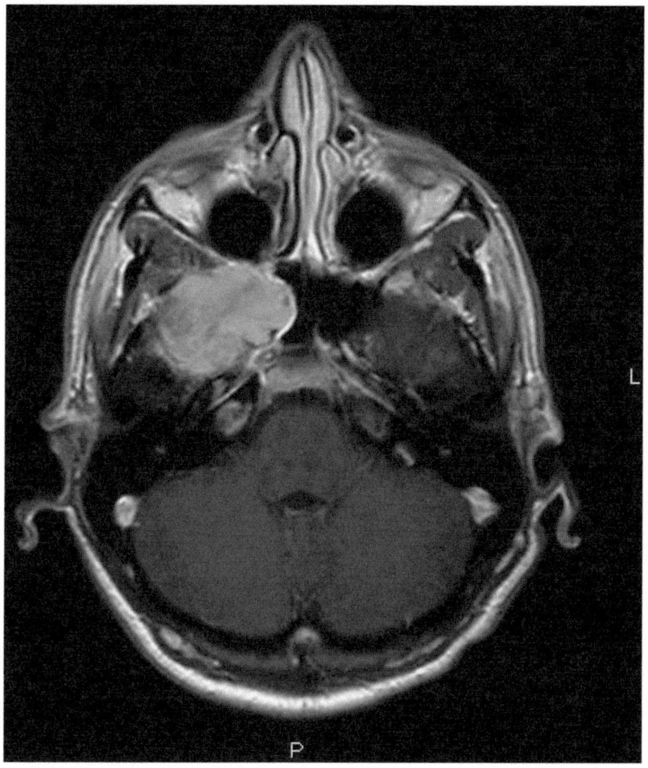

78. After resection via an orbitocraniozygomatic approach, reconstruction was performed by rotating a pedicled temporalis muscle flap (*T*). It was pulled into the sphenoid sinus and tacked in place. The goal was to interpose this pedicled flap between the brain and the nose to prevent CSF rhinorrhea. An abdominal fat graft (*arrow*) was used to prevent temporal hollowing. A free flap was not needed.

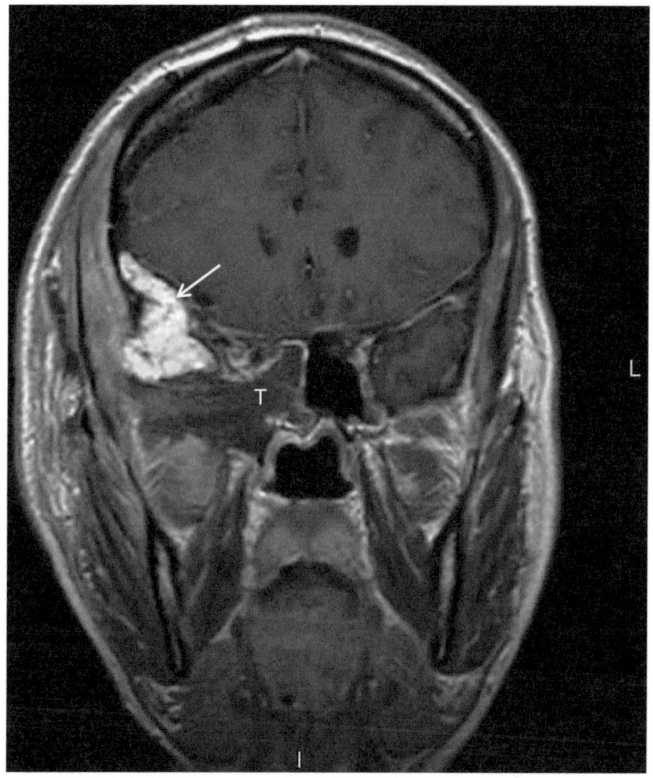

79. Postoperative axial view demonstrating no evidence of residual tumor.

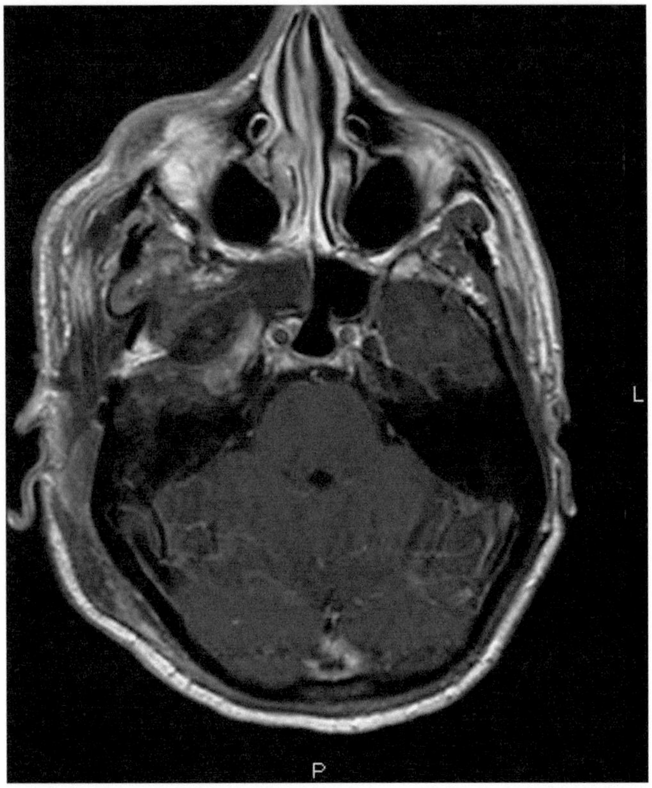

4 Posterior Fossa Approaches

Translabyrinthine Approach

- *Concept*
  - Drill through the mastoid and semicircular canals to reach the posterior cranial fossa and internal auditory canal. The approach is anterior to the sigmoid sinus.
- *Conditions treated*
  - Vestibular schwannomas
  - Other cranial nerve schwannomas within the posterior cranial fossa
  - Meningiomas within the posterior cranial fossa
  - Temporal bone tumors that involve the posterior fossa dura or have posterior fossa extension
  - Facial nerve decompression or repair in a non-hearing ear
- *Risks*
  - Complete hearing loss in the operated ear and the potential for persistent tinnitus
  - Complete vestibular loss with disequilibrium that should improve with time, assuming there is normal vestibular function in the other ear and appropriate compensation occurs
  - Facial nerve injury
  - CSF leak
  - Necrosis or infection of the abdominal fat graft in the ensuing weeks after the surgery
  - Meningitis
  - Dysmetria if there is direct injury or vascular compromise to the cerebellar peduncle or brainstem
- *Benefits*
  - This approach for resection of a vestibular schwannoma requires less brain retraction than the other approaches.
  - It provides a direct view of the entire course of the facial nerve.
  - The facial nerve is anterior to the vestibular schwannoma, making it less likely to be injured during drilling of the internal auditory canal or tumor removal as compared to the middle fossa approach.
  - Less headache, neck pain, and stiffness compared to the retrosigmoid approach
- *Additional notes*
  - This approach is an excellent procedure for training residents and fellows in how to do mastoid and temporal bone surgery. However, it should be noted that the approach is not the key part of the procedure; tumor removal is. If too much time is spent appreciating the anatomy of the temporal bone during the approach, it may be late in the day when the careful and meticulous microdissection needed to remove the tumor is begun.

J.S. Oghalai, C.L.W. Driscoll, *Atlas of Neurotologic and Lateral Skull Base Surgery*,
DOI 10.1007/978-3-662-46694-0_4,

1. The concept of the translabyrinthine approach to access a vestibular schwannoma. Note that the opening in the skull is anterior to the sigmoid sinus. The cochlea is intact, but the semicircular canals have been removed. A malleable retractor is between the tumor and the cerebellar peduncle in this example. However, much of the surgery can be performed without the use of retraction. Retractors can create a more stable open field and allow visualization of the most medial tumor extent. Retractors may also be helpful when drilling to provide a solid barrier between the sigmoid sinus and dura to limit the risk of injury. However, retractors do not help with visualization of the lateral tumor, and in many patients with smaller tumors, no retraction is needed at all. Thus, retractors can be removed from the field when they are not necessary. This decreases the risk of retraction injury to the brain and thrombosis of the sigmoid sinus.

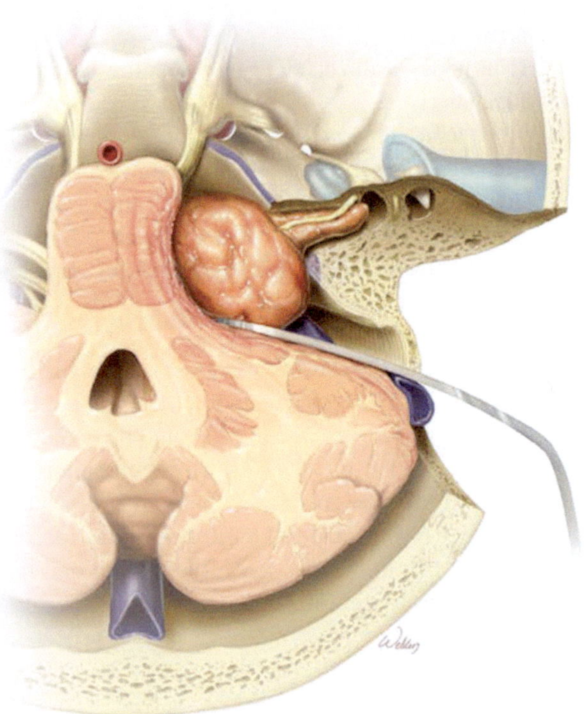

2. Overview of the bone to be removed (*gray*).

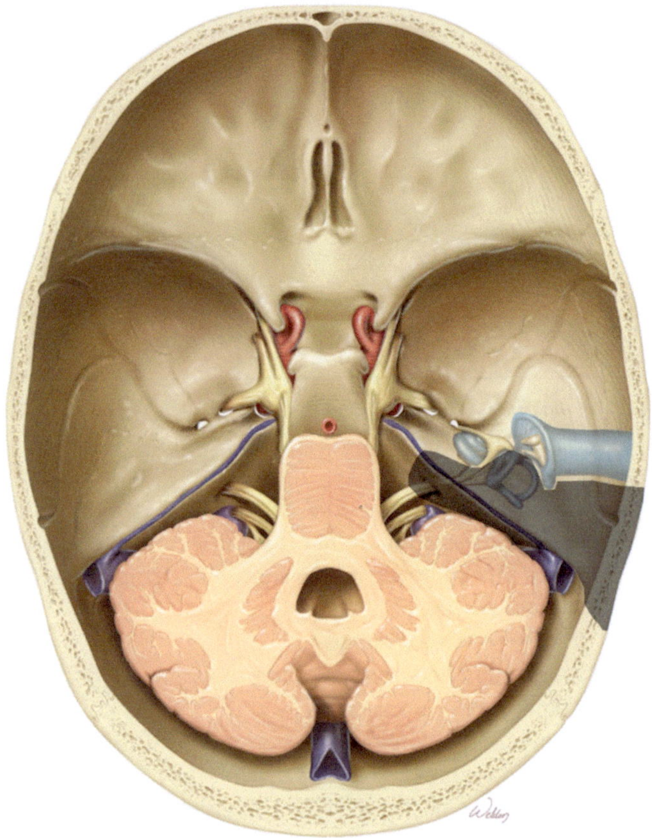

3. The incision is ~2–3 cm behind the postauricular sulcus. It is further back than what is typically used for otologic surgery to permit removal of enough bone for adequate visualization.

   Although it is possible to use the same standard approach in all cases, there is value in considering each case individually and adapting your surgery to the particular challenges and opportunities presented. As a useful exercise, pause at the end of each operation and review the exposure and consider how it could be improved. Using a standard approach for all tumors will mean you are doing too much surgery for some tumors and you will also be less creative when you need to tackle the unusual tumors. For example, an intracanalicular tumor can be removed with a smaller incision and does not require decompression of the middle fossa dura or sacrifice of the emissary vein. These simple variations save time and decrease risk. There are several factors to consider when planning your approach. Tumor size and location are most important, but the course of sigmoid sinus, location and size of the jugular bulb, and scalp thickness (particularly in the posterior–inferior area) also can influence the plan. Be a thoughtful surgeon; have a reason for all you do.

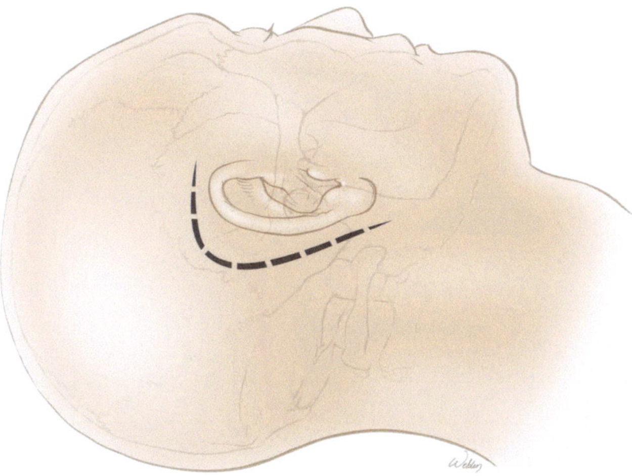

4. The mastoid cortex is exposed. It is unnecessary to dissect down the ear canal, and doing so simply increases the risk of creating a hole in the ear canal skin, which would connect the nonsterile ear canal to the sterile craniotomy wound. It is most efficient to create a full-thickness scalp flap with a single incision down to bone superiorly and posteriorly. As you extend inferiorly, the sternocleidomastoid muscle (SCM) is initially left attached to the bone and the scalp flap elevated to the anterior mastoid tip. The SCM is then taken down off the mastoid with cautery. For larger tumors, the digastric muscle is also taken out of its groove.

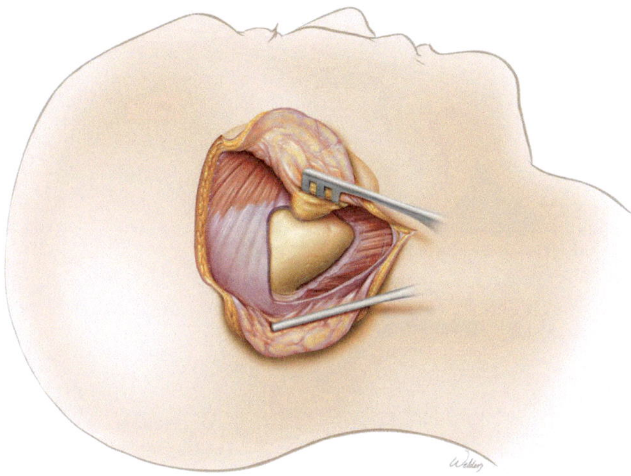

5. A simple mastoidectomy is performed with identification of the sigmoid sinus, the tegmen, the mastoid antrum, and the lateral semicircular canal. Only the antrum should be opened. The aditus ad antrum will need to be sealed with fascia at the conclusion of the procedure to prevent CSF leak, and it is easier to do this when the opening is small.

   Another option for this portion of the procedure is to remove the incus and open the superior part of the facial recess. This allows direct packing of the Eustachian tube orifice at the end of the procedure which may reduce the incidence of postoperative CSF leak.

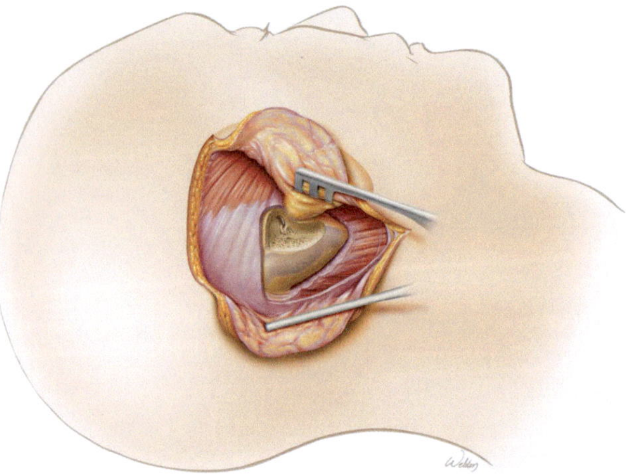

6. The retrosigmoid dura is identified and the overlying bone thinned with a large cutting burr. It is then "egg-shelled" into fragments with a large diamond burr. The bone fragments are then dissected off the dura with a Joseph or Freer elevator. Removing the bone allows the sigmoid sinus to be retracted posteriorly, permitting wider exposure. This is particularly critical for tumors >2 cm, but it is helpful for nearly all tumors.

   During this process, the mastoid emissary vein is often sacrificed. Carefully decompressing this structure and coagulating with bipolar cautery at least a few millimeters from the sigmoid sinus will prevent getting a larger hole in the sidewall of the sinus. If the sigmoid sinus is more posterior or the tumor is small (so less retraction is anticipated to be necessary), the emissary vein can often be preserved.

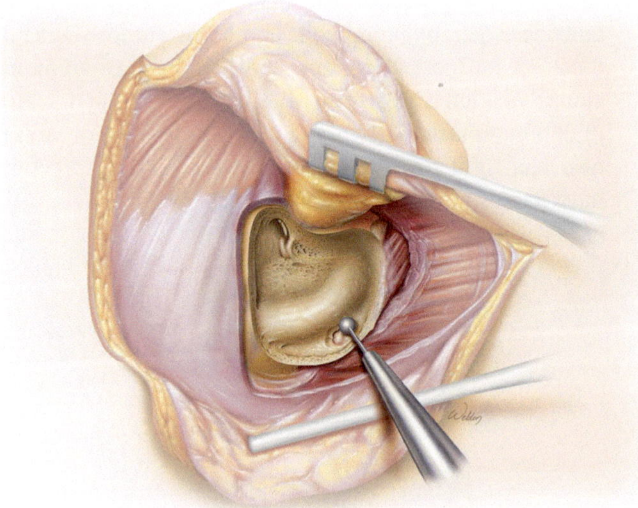

7. The bone over the sigmoid sinus is then thinned and "egg-shelled" in a similar fashion. The bone fragments can be removed or loosened as necessary to reach the lip of bone anterior to the sigmoid sinus. It is easier and safer to remove smaller bone islands rather than one large piece. If the sinus tears while elevating a bone island, stop and leave that fragment in place. Prior to removing the bone over the sinus, it is important to have removed the retrosigmoid bone as shown in the previous illustration. This is because if the sinus is accidentally opened, it can be easily compressed with Surgicel and a cottonoid to control the bleeding.

   Great care should be employed to avoid entering the sinus as this increases risk of thrombosis, venous congestion with the potential for increased intracranial pressure, and devastating venous infarction. It is most vulnerable as it turns medially toward the jugular bulb. If the sigmoid sinus is inadvertently entered, Surgicel and gelfoam can be placed, and gentle pressure with a cottonoid can be used to control the bleeding. This usually does not completely obstruct the blood flow within the sinus.

   This is a part of the operation where it is important to mentally shift from an aggressive drilling mindset to a careful microdissection mode. Careful management of the sigmoid not only limits the risk of serious complications but also saves time and allows for more flexibility in retractor placement. Bleeding from the sinus is easily controlled but requires extra care in that area for the remainder of the case.

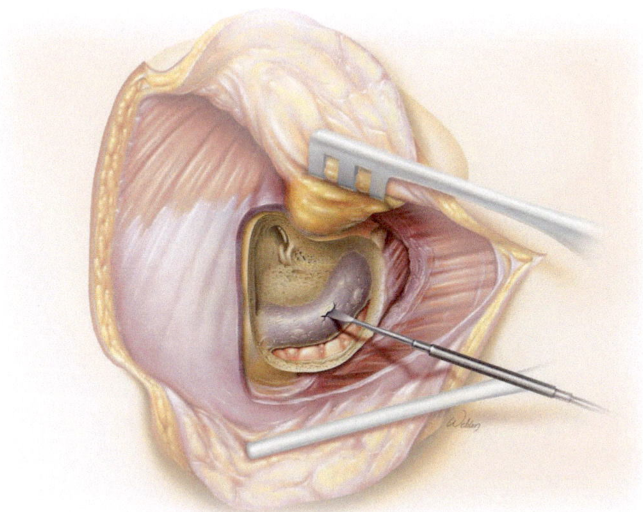

8. Malleable retractors are then positioned between the posterior and middle cranial fossa dura and their bony plates. This bone can then be quickly removed with a rongeur or a drill down to the level of the labyrinth without risk of tearing the dura.

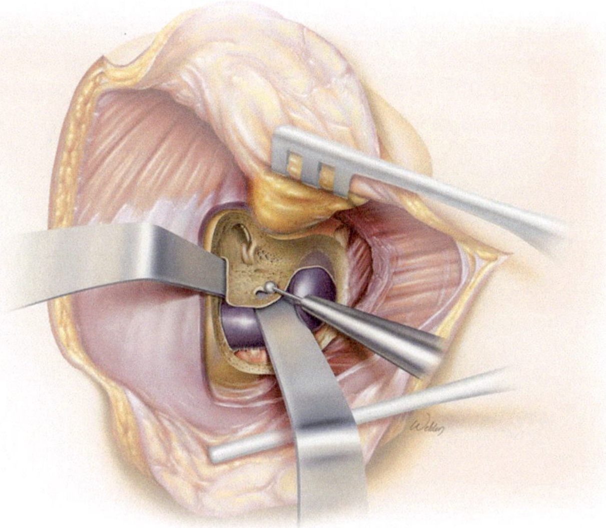

9. After removal of the mastoid, the middle and posterior fossa dura are exposed. Bleeding from the superior petrosal sinus (*arrow*) can be managed with bipolar cautery. If cautery is ineffective, a piece of Surgicel can be inserted through the opening intraluminally both proximally and distally to plug the sinus. Elevating the sinus out of the bony groove will limit the risk of injuring the sinus.

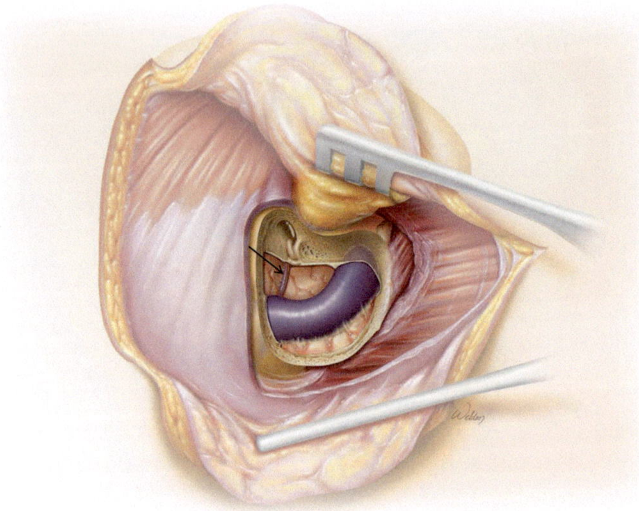

10. Next, identify the course of the vertical segment of the facial nerve just distal to the second genu. It should be left within its bony sheath but traced out inferiorly. This will allow safe exposure of the sigmoid sinus as it courses medially to the facial nerve and forms the jugular bulb. This maneuver is particularly helpful for tumors >2 cm in the cerebellopontine angle where a larger opening is needed to dissect the tumor off the cerebellum and the cerebellar peduncle.

    The endolymphatic duct can be noted as a tether between the posterior face of the temporal bone and the posterior fossa dura (*arrow*). It should be transected with an 11 blade scalpel where it enters the bone. Once this is performed, the malleable retractor in the posterior fossa can be advanced all the way to the porus acusticus.

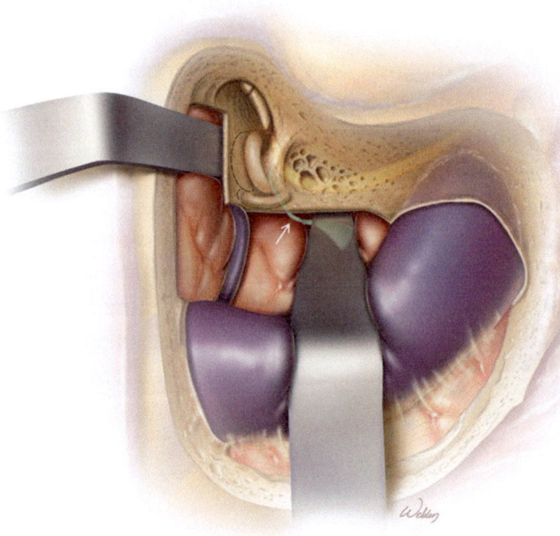

11. The labyrinthectomy is performed by drilling parallel to the middle and posterior fossa dura (*arrows*). We typically do not trace out the canals during this process. Doing so expends time that could be better used later in the procedure when dissecting out the tumor. Care should be taken not to drill anterior to the ampullate ends of the lateral and superior semicircular canals (*arrowhead*) as the facial nerve might be damaged within the labyrinthine segment or geniculate ganglion.

    The duct of the lateral semicircular canal is parallel to and directly superior to the horizontal segment of the facial nerve. By drilling through the lateral semicircular canal from superior to inferior, the facial nerve can be safely identified proximal to the second genu.

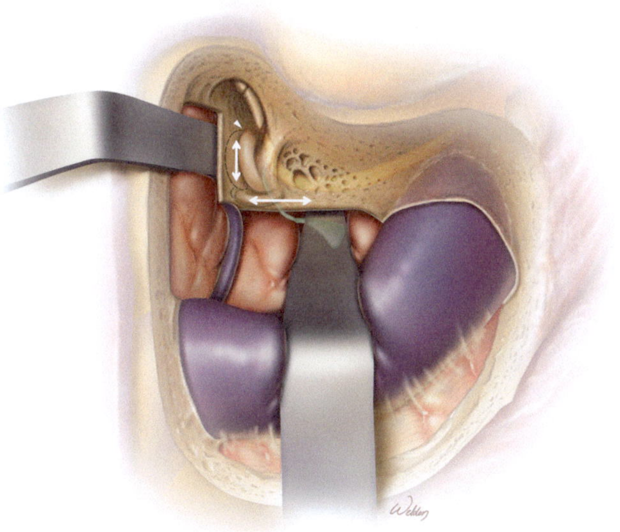

12. The ampullated ends of the lateral and superior semicircular canals open into the anterior vestibule (*arrowhead*). The vestibule is directly medial to the horizontal facial nerve. A diamond bit is used to extend the opening of the vestibule posteriorly toward the ampulla of the posterior semicircular canal (*arrow*). Note that the horizontal and vertical segments of the facial nerve should be traced out all the way from the anterior edge of the vestibule to the sigmoid sinus. A thin layer of bony fallopian canal should be left covering it for safety, but this exposure is critical to achieve ideal visualization of the cerebellar peduncle during tumor dissection.

    Remember that the vestibular nerve innervates the utricle and saccule within the vestibule as well as the ampullae of the semicircular canals. Therefore, the vestibule marks the location of the fundus of the internal auditory canal. Completing the approach now requires finding the porus acusticus and tracing the internal auditory canal (*dotted lines*) out to the vestibule.

    The porus acusticus is much deeper than the fundus. However, by simply drilling the temporal bone parallel to the posterior fossa dura as was done during the labyrinthectomy, you will eventually find it. Drilling through this bone can be frustrating because it is very dense. However, if you get concerned that you are not drilling in the proper location, you can also palpate within the intracranial space between the dura and the bone to find the porus acusticus. This will give you confidence that you are aiming in the proper direction and give you a clue about how much further you need to drill to get there.

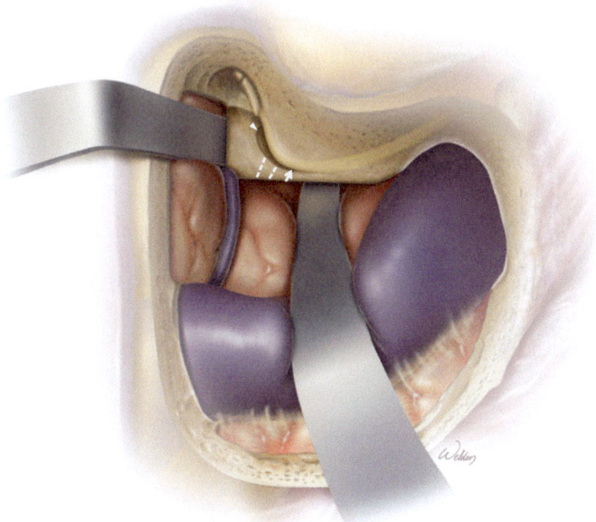

13. Once the porus acusticus (*PA*) is identified, drill troughs superior and inferior to the internal auditory canal, and trace it out to the vestibule. Since the facial nerve may take a course over the superior aspect of the tumor, the dura absolutely needs to remain intact while drilling the superior trough. This is best achieved by leaving a thin layer of bone over the dura to protect its contents during drilling. This is perhaps not quite as critical when drilling the inferior trough, and a small dural tear is acceptable.

    The cross-sections show the normal layout of the nerves of the internal auditory canal (*lower inset*) and what they look like with an inferior vestibular nerve tumor (*IVT*) present (*upper inset*). Facial nerve (*F*), cochlear nerve (*C*), superior vestibular nerve (*SV*), and inferior vestibular nerve (*IV*).

    When drilling out laterally near the fundus, care should be taken near the labyrinthine portion of the facial nerve (*arrow*). This segment of the nerve is quite thin and not enveloped with a thick epineurial covering yet. Also, it is very close to the vestibule at the edge of the superior trough. Thus, the superior troughs can be drilled deeper medially but should be kept shallower laterally.

    Initially, the bone is thinned all along the internal auditory canal, and then the remaining thin layer is removed around the edges of the dissection, and the cap of bone can be removed. It is safest to remove bone down to the dura inferiorly along the internal auditory canal first and then across the transverse crest and lastly along the superior internal auditory canal in the region of the facial nerve. The dissection of the bone can be blind around the superior internal auditory canal, but as it is thinned, the bone covering the internal auditory canal will become mobile. Thus, the last very thin eggshell can be fractured rather than drilled, offering more protection to the underlying facial nerve.

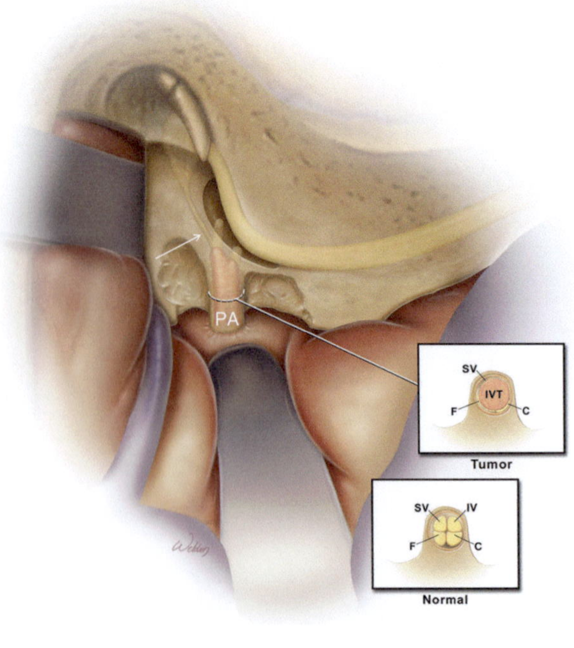

14. Drill the troughs deeper to expose the dura anterior to the porus acusticus. Also, the jugular bulb (*JB*) should be skeletonized. The superior aspect of the JB is the inferior limit of drilling and easily identified. It is also critical to remove the bone along the posterior aspect of the JB to obtain adequate room to expose the tumor. At this point in the operation, there is a tendency to feel like you have removed enough bone and you want to get on with tumor removal. Removing a few more millimeters of bone deep in the troughs can pay big dividends later in the case when following the facial nerve. Tumors are centered on the internal auditory canal so half the tumor volume is anterior to the internal auditory canal. Having good exposure to this part of the tumor is important.

    The dotted lines show the area of dural opening. The posterior limit is the sigmoid sinus, and the superior limit is the superior petrosal sinus. The square of dura between the sigmoid sinus and the internal auditory canal can be removed and discarded or left attached in the presigmoid area. While fancy dural flaps can be developed, in practicality it is impossible to close them in a watertight fashion at the end of the case, and it is not worth the effort.

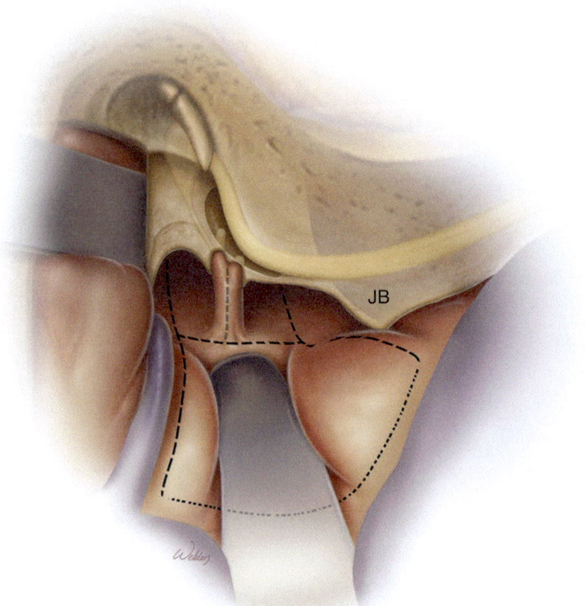

15. Initially, only the posterior fossa dura is opened. The dura of the internal auditory canal is not immediately opened because it helps to support the tumor during the dissection process, thereby reducing traction on the facial nerve.

A moist Telfa pledget is used between the malleable and the exposed cerebellum. This distributes the retraction pressure and minimizes trauma.

Cerebrospinal fluid can be released by gently opening the arachnoid membranes inferior to the tumor (*arrow*). We prefer to perform this maneuver using a blunt broad instrument, like a Penrose #2.

A bridging (or Dandy's) vein (*arrowhead*), which drains blood from the cerebellum into the superior petrosal sinus, is often not in the way for smaller tumors and can be left alone. For larger tumors, more retraction of the cerebellum may be needed, and this vein will need to be divided. While there is significant collateral circulation in the cerebellum, venous infarction is an unpredictable and potentially devastating event, so veins should be preserved where possible.

The posterior face of the tumor is tested with the nerve stimulator to make sure the facial nerve is not draped across it. This would be highly unusual as the facial nerve is almost always anterior to the tumor, but it is critical to check. We use a high current or voltage for this maneuver as we expect the results to be negative. When we think we should be probing the facial nerve, we use a low-level stimulus to best identify the border of the nerve.

A window is then made in the tumor with a scalpel or scissors (*dotted lines*) and the core of the tumor debulked.

16. After debulking, the tumor capsule can be microdissected off the surrounding tissues and collapsed inward. The capsule is removed in pieces during this process. The nerve stimulator should be used repeatedly during this process to verify that the facial nerve is not draped over the section of capsule to be removed.

An important goal is to dissect directly within the tumor–arachnoid interface. If one begins leaving arachnoid on the tumor, there are many more blood vessels to contend with, and the dissection plane is not obvious. If you get out of the correct plane, go back to a place where you are sure you are in the correct place and start again. This is why it is good to leave an edge of tumor visible when making a window (*arrowheads*)

The eighth cranial nerve is divided proximally to the tumor (*VIII*). Just deep to this is the root entry zone of the facial nerve (*VII*). It should be identified using the facial nerve stimulator before sectioning the eighth cranial nerve. Also, there is typically a small artery between the root entry zones of cranial nerve *VII* and *VIII*. This artery is a branch of the anterior inferior cerebellar artery that feeds the brainstem. Every effort should be made to preserve all arteries.

Larger tumors often are adjacent to the trigeminal nerve (*V*). Most of the bulk of the trigeminal nerve is sensory, and only a small bundle consists of motor fibers (*arrow*). Thus, it should not be surprising to be unable to stimulate the fifth cranial nerve with the nerve stimulator until you move the probe superiorly to reach the motor division.

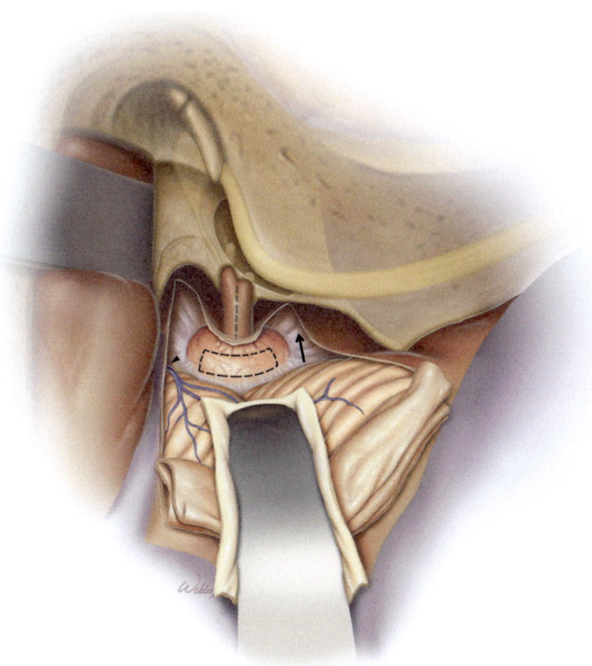

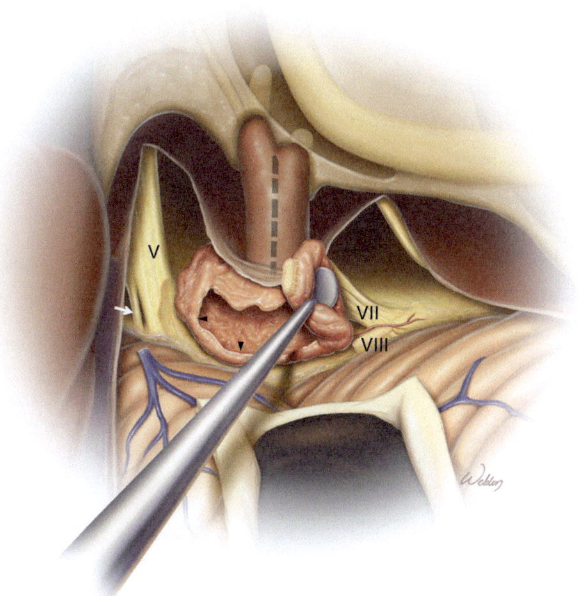

17. After the majority of the tumor within the cerebellopontine angle has been debulked and the facial nerve has been identified at the brainstem, the internal auditory canal can be dissected.

    Left panel: The dura of the internal auditory canal is opened after verifying with the nerve stimulator that the facial nerve is not directly underneath the planned incision. A microscissors or an angled sickle knife works well to make this opening.

    Middle panel: The superior pole of the tumor is carefully separated from the internal auditory canal dura near the fundus until the facial nerve is identified. If the tumor has dilated the internal auditory canal and there is a lot of bulk, the posterior aspect of the tumor can be removed before doing this maneuver. This makes it easier to rotate the tumor and minimizes traction on the facial nerve.

    Right panel: The superior vestibular nerve (*SV*) and inferior vestibular nerve (*IV*) are divided at the fundus (or simply teased out of the fundus) and the plane between the cochlear nerve (*C*) and the facial nerve (*F*) identified. If possible, the cochlear nerve is left in place to minimize dissection trauma to the facial nerve. If the cochlear nerve is infiltrated with tumor, it is also separated at the fundus and sharp dissection used to carefully separate the tumor from the facial nerve. Identifying the correct plane is critical, or tumor adherent to the facial nerve will be left behind.

    It is beneficial to be flexible in how you go about removing the tumor. There should not be a sense of urgency when finding the facial nerve or other landmarks. All of the important structures will eventually be delineated. Each patient and tumor provides challenges and opportunities. Take advantage of what is most accessible and easy.

    Do not dissect the internal auditory canal until the tumor in the cerebellopontine angle has been debulked to limit the risk of stretching the facial nerve. A significant debulking of the internal mass of the tumor with an ultrasonic aspirator (i.e., the CUSA) is extremely helpful as it allows for the capsule to be able to be teased away from the surrounding normal structures. It is preferable to retract tumor from nerves and blood vessels rather than push these structures off the tumor surface. When possible, force should be directed to the tumor and not the nerves. In general, less manipulation equates with less risk of injury and better function.

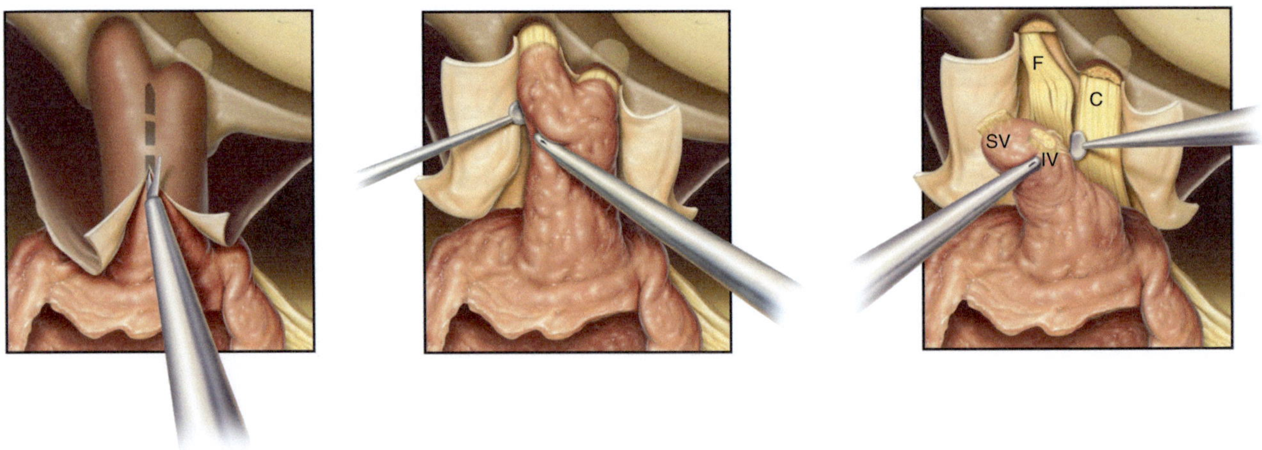

18. As the tumor removal progresses and the dissection is carried down to the portion most adherent to the facial nerve along its course in the midcerebellopontine angle, it is easy to create too much traction on the nerve. The tumor remnant can be supported in the posterior fossa with gelfoam. Also, rather than working from either proximal or distal along the nerve, the tumor can be rolled inferiorly or superiorly and the facial nerve plane followed without pulling.

    Also, this is the time of the operation that the decision to perform a total, near-total, or subtotal tumor removal is made. If the tumor is highly adherent to the facial nerve, it is typically better to leave a small and thin remnant attached to the facial nerve rather than to damage the facial nerve in a heroic attempt to remove all tumors. The remnant is unlikely to grow, and if it does, it can be treated with stereotactic radiotherapy. In contrast, aggressive dissection of the facial nerve is guaranteed to produce facial nerve weakness.

    For smaller tumors, the cochlear nerve may be able to be preserved and thus offer the possibility of cochlear implantation (which should be considered for patients with NF II). For most tumors, over 1.5 cm becomes quite difficult to preserve a satisfactory cochlear nerve.

19. To close the craniotomy, start by removing all Telfa strips and cottonoids. Counts must be correct. Surgicel on the sigmoid sinus can be left in place. The wound is irrigated, and any bleeding is controlled. If there are large air cells in the petrous apex, these should be occluded with bone wax to prevent CSF leak.

    A piece of temporalis fascia or a dural substitute (like Duragen) is then laid over the aditus ad antrum. Tisseal can be used around it to obtain a watertight seal. Finally, two or three pieces of abdominal fat are placed into the defect to fill it. We typically dumbbell a little bit of fat through the defect in the posterior fossa dura to help plug it. Care is taken not to stretch the facial nerve when placing the fat and to not fill up the cerebellopontine angle with fat.

    Another closure technique advocated by some surgeons (not shown) is to open the facial recess, separate the incudal–stapedial joint, remove the incus, and drill away the incudal buttress. The middle ear and Eustachian tube are then packed with an abdominal adipose graft at the time of closure. This works well and may reduce the risk of CSF leak.

    If desired, a titanium or resorbable mesh plate can be placed over the fat graft to help keep the appropriate pressure. This also makes soft tissue closure easier and may result in improved cosmesis.

    The wound is then closed in three layers (periosteum, subcutaneous tissues, and skin). A pressure dressing is applied for 1 day if the plate was used or 4 days if no plate was used.

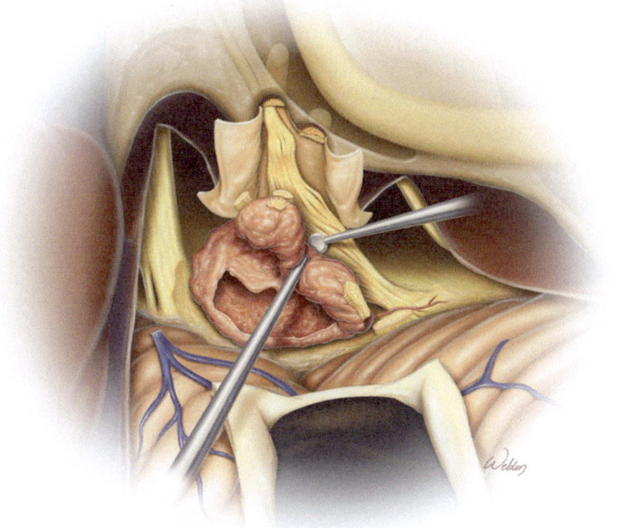

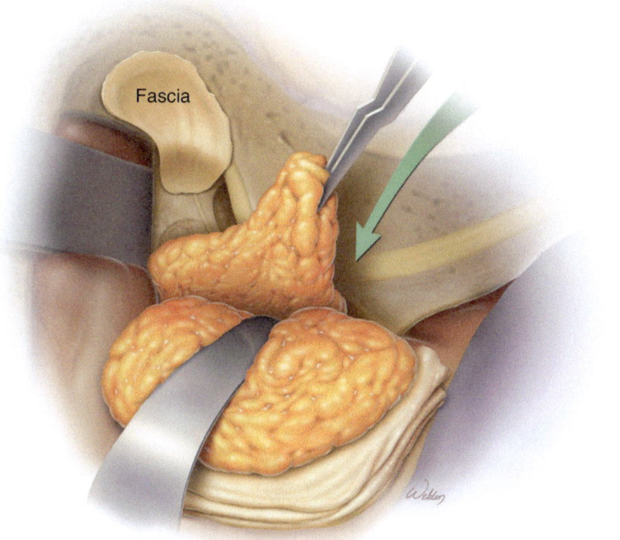

20. Case 1. Axial T1 MRI with gadolinium of a patient with a 3.4 cm left vestibular schwannoma. The dimension is taken from the largest dimension in the cerebellopontine angle, excluding the tumor within the internal auditory canal (*arrow*). There is significant compression of the brainstem, cerebellar peduncle, and cerebellum. A small arachnoid cyst is visible posterior to the tumor. This is not a cyst within the tumor because the margin between the cyst and the cerebellum does not enhance (*arrowheads*).

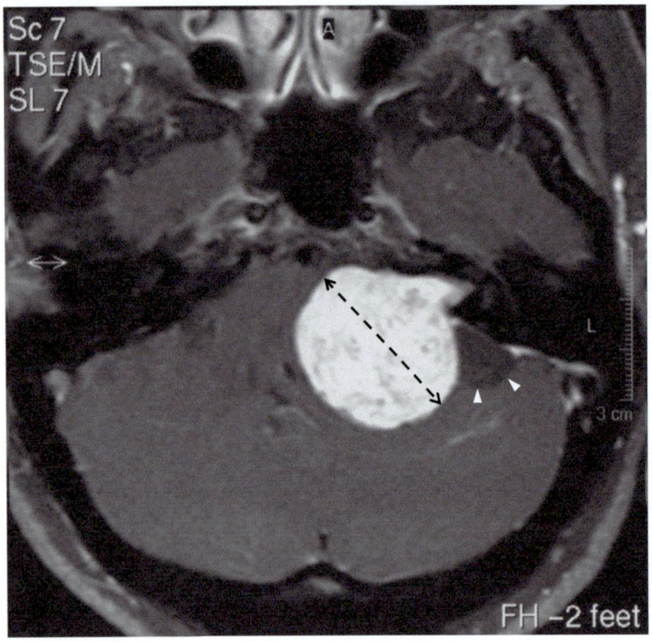

21. Axial FIESTA T2-weighted image of the same tumor. The tumor is solid, and there is CSF within the arachnoid cyst. There is a slight amount of CSF between the distal end of the tumor and the fundus of the internal auditory canal (*arrow*). There is compression and distortion of the fourth ventricle, but it remains patent (*arrowhead*).

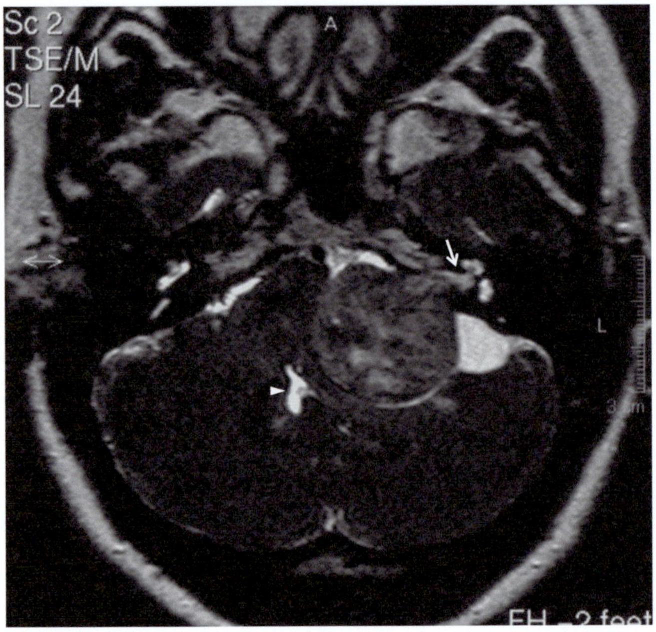

22. A translabyrinthine approach was used to remove the tumor. Here, we only demonstrate specific features of the bony drilling and tumor dissection process. A mastoidectomy was performed, the tegmen and sigmoid sinus were identified, and the retrosigmoid dura was exposed. The ear canal was left intact.

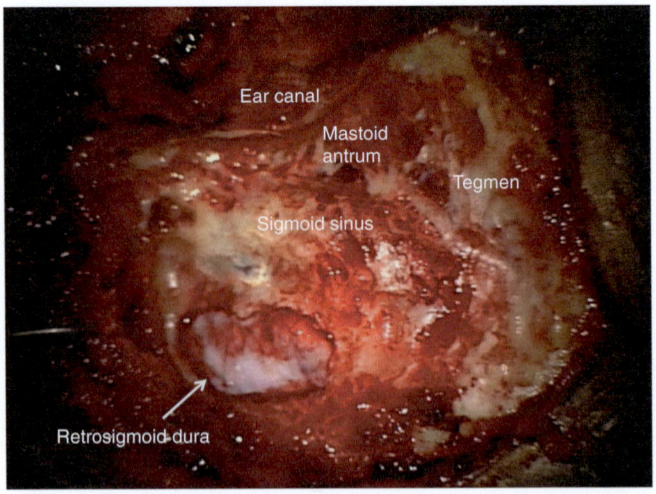

23. The bone over the sigmoid sinus was thinned to allow the sinus to be compressed. The bone covering the presigmoid posterior fossa dura and the dura of the floor of the middle cranial fossa was removed. The lateral, posterior, and superior semicircular canals are within the dense otic capsule bone (*L*, *P*, *S*).

Malleable retractors were placed between otic capsule bone and the dura to reduce the chance of damaging the dura in case the drill slips during the labyrinthectomy. A cottonoid was placed over the sigmoid sinus and compressed by the retractor. There was a piece of surgical under it, which covered a small area of bleeding from the sigmoid sinus.

The air cells over the facial nerve still needed to be removed (*arrowhead*). The fossa incudis (*arrow*) can also be seen. This is as far forward as it needs to be opened.

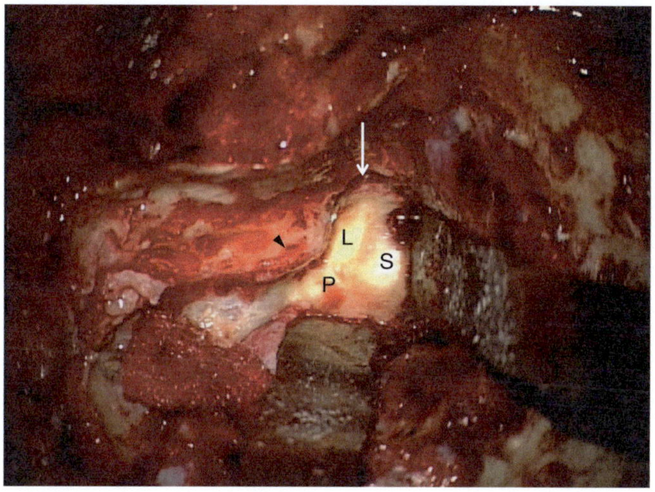

24. The rest of the approach was performed, and most of the tumor was removed (not shown). After debulking the mass of the tumor in the cerebellopontine angle, the dura of the internal auditory canal was opened and the tumor teased out of the fundus with division of the superior and inferior vestibular nerves. This image, taken after all of these steps were performed, demonstrates the transverse crest (*arrow*) and the facial nerve (*arrowhead*).

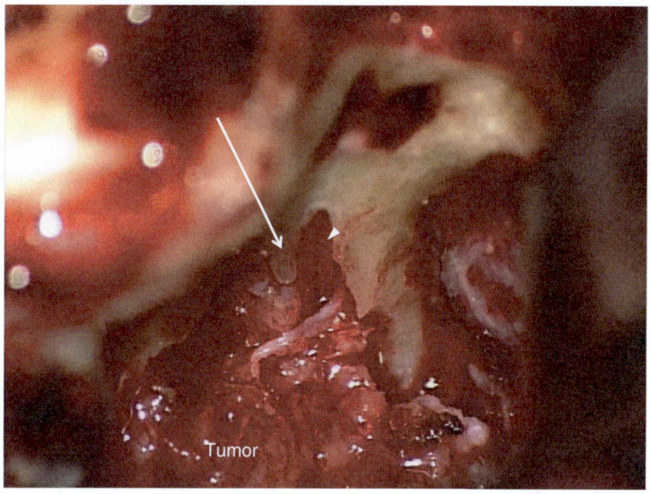

25. Continuing the dissection to the mid-cerebellopontine angle, the facial nerve (*arrow*) can be seen along the anterior aspect of the tumor capsule. Extreme care must be taken not to stretch the facial nerve during the process of separating the tumor from the nerve.

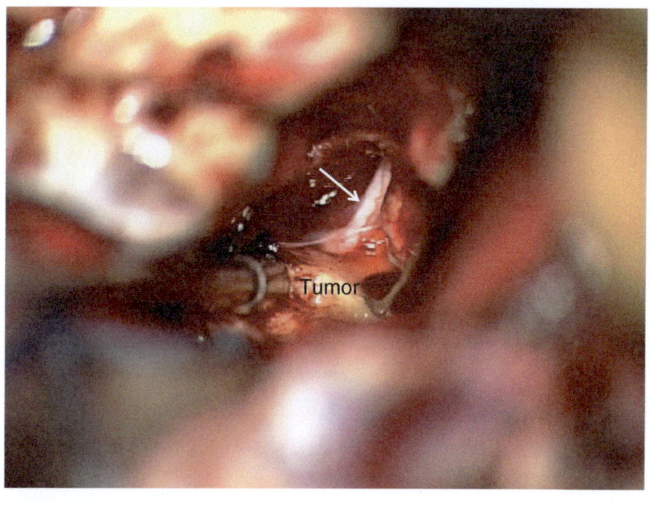

26. Immediate post-op axial T1 MRI with gadolinium and fat saturation demonstrated a total tumor resection. The slight amount of enhancement along the cerebellar peduncle represents inflammation, not tumor.

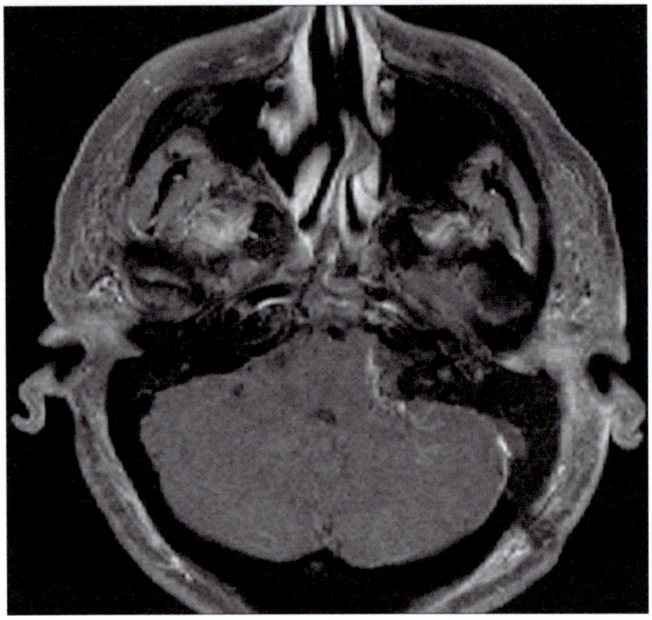

27. Precontrast T1 MRI without fat saturation demonstrated the extent of the fat graft placement. Also, the white discoloration to the cerebellar peduncle represents postoperative blood and should be expected after the resection of larger tumors.

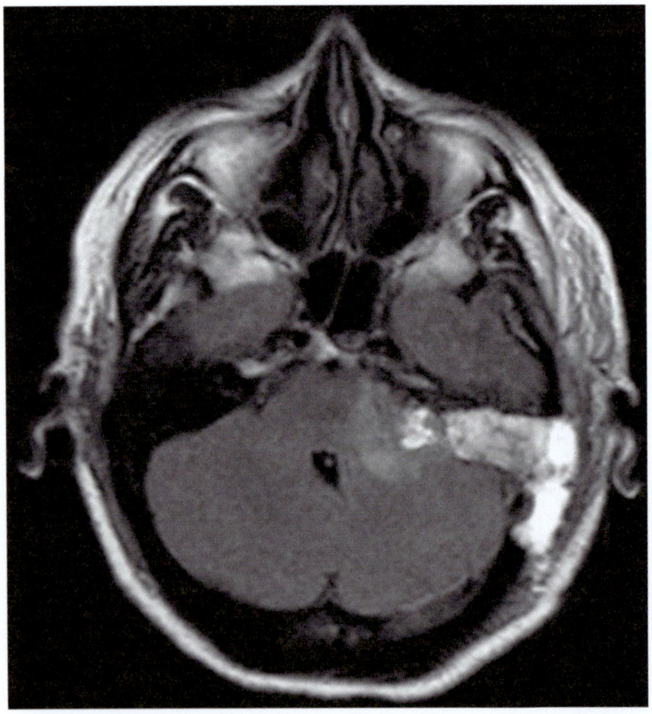

28. Case 2. A multicystic vestibular schwannoma.

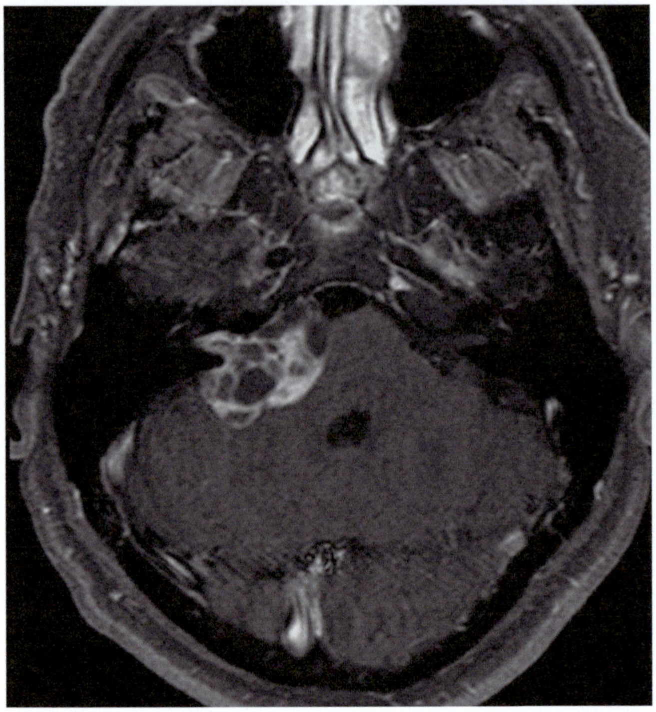

29. Postoperative image demonstrating a subtotal resection. A subtotal resection was selected for this patient based on his older age and comorbidities. With the availability of postoperative stereotactic XRT (i.e., Gamma knife, Cyberknife, Novalis, proton beam), this approach is becoming more commonplace. Typically, we only recommend post-op stereotactic XRT if the tumor remnant demonstrates growth on serial MRI. A small remnant like this usually will "ball up" into a well-circumscribed mass within 6–12 months. This makes it relatively straightforward to deliver an adequate radiation dose to the tumor remnant while minimizing unwanted exposure to the brainstem and inner ear.

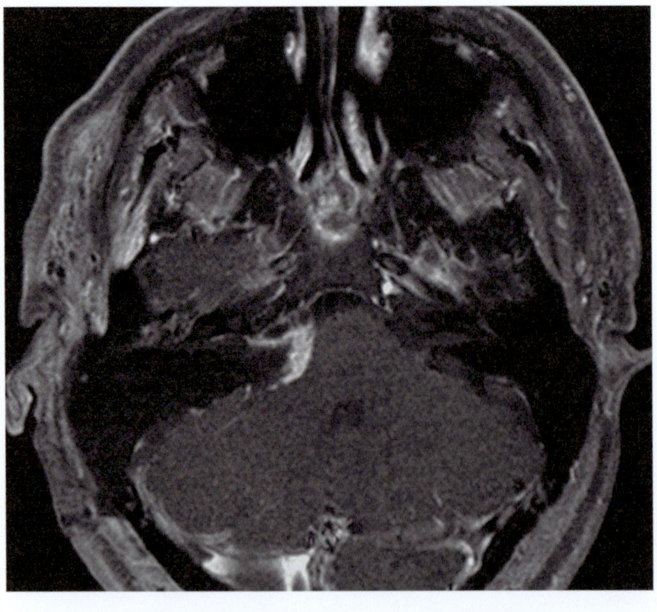

30. Case 3. Axial MRI with gadolinium of a patient with a medium-sized right vestibular schwannoma. The tumor extends to the fundus of the internal auditory canal. A subtotal dissection was planned for this patient according to his wishes to minimize the risk of any (even temporary) facial nerve dysfunction.

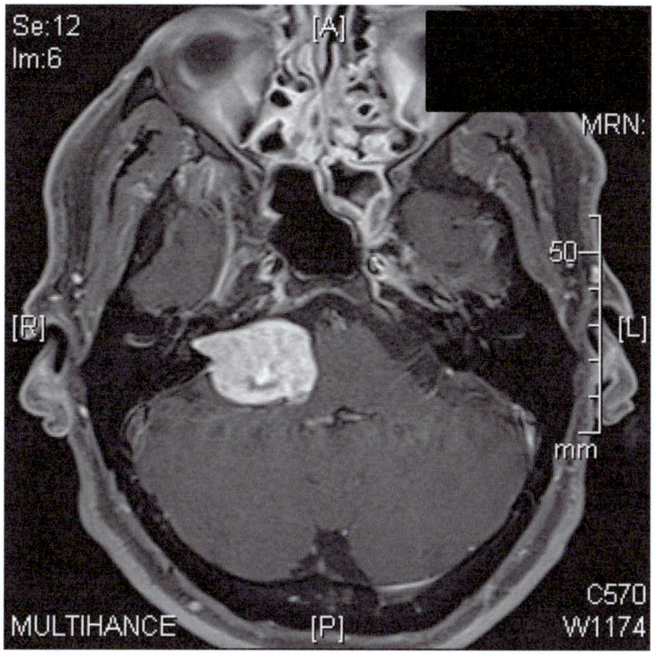

31. Coronal view of the tumor. The superior extent of the tumor is the tentorium (*arrowhead*).

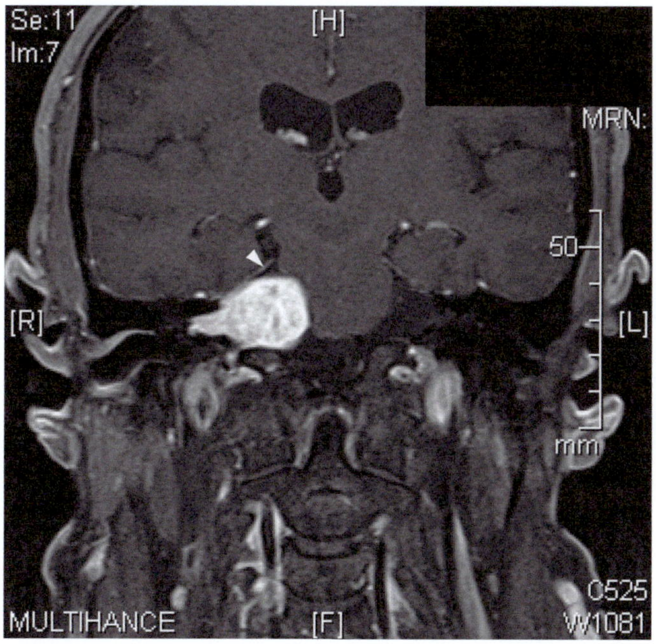

32. Fiesta T2-weighted MRI demonstrating that only a thin crevice of CSF is present within the distal internal auditory canal (*arrow*). Care must be taken during surgery to resect the lateral-most extent of the tumor.

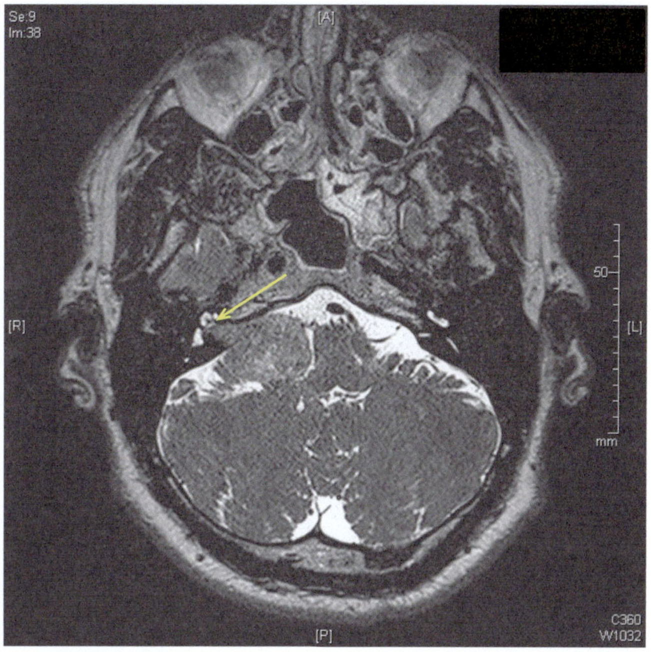

33. After opening the postauricular incision, drilling was performed to identify the sigmoid sinus and expose the retrosigmoid dura.

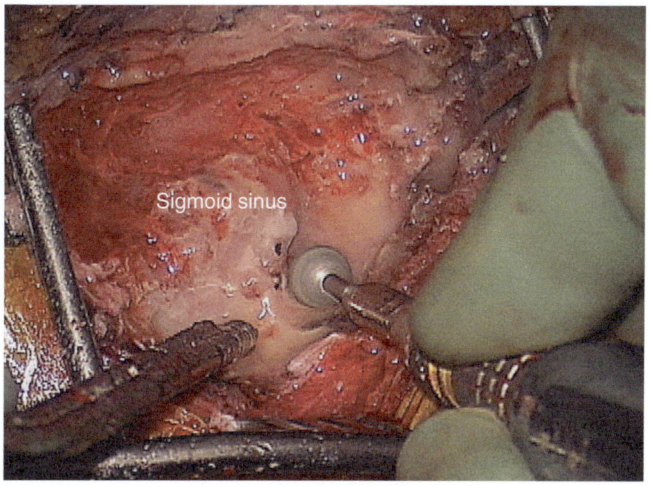

34. After thinning the bone over the sigmoid sinus, a malleable was placed between the posterior fossa dura and the bone.

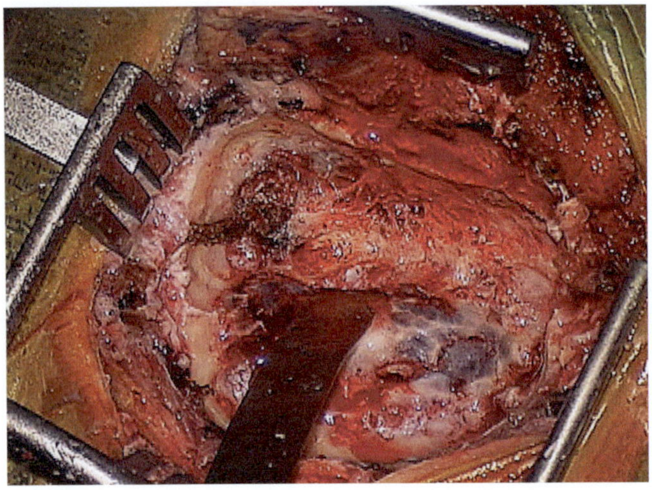

35. The mastoidectomy was completed and the tegmen removed, allowing the superior retractor to be placed between the middle fossa dura and the bone. The lateral semicircular canal (*LSSC*) can be seen.

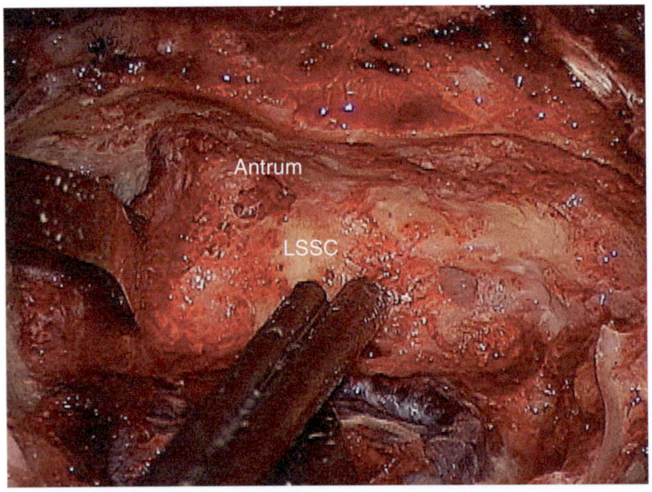

36. The labyrinthectomy was begun by using a 4 mm cutting burr to drill troughs that parallel the middle fossa and posterior fossa dura (*arrows*). This is not a "canal exploration," and so there is no need to nicely blue-line each canal. The goal is to get to the tumor quickly so that time can be spent on the tumor microdissection. This approach of drilling parallel to the dura quickly advances the dissection medially in a safe fashion. The jugular bulb (*JB*) is visible through the bone.

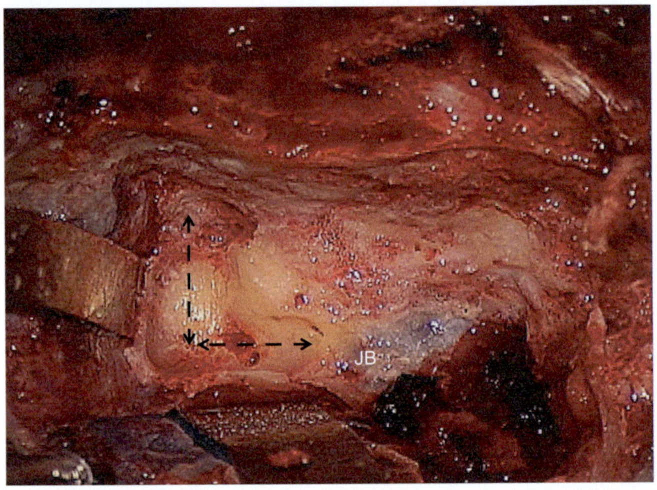

37. As the bone was removed, the endolymphatic duct (*arrow*) could be seen running from the endolymphatic sac in the dura to the posterior petrous bone. This was then divided with an 11 blade scalpel.

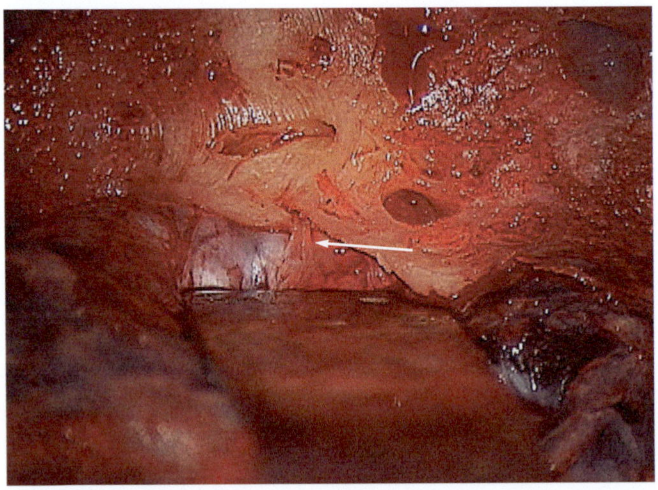

38. After completing the labyrinthectomy, the facial nerve was defined along its horizontal and vertical segments (*arrowheads*). Also, note how thin the ear canal bone is (*EAC*). These steps are critical to perform when resecting larger tumors as inadequate thinning of these structures will limit the ability to view the interface between the posterior face of the tumor and the cerebellar peduncle. For smaller tumors, it is not that important.

    The vestibule (*arrow*) was opened under the second genu. The jugular bulb (*JB*) was the inferior limit of exposure. In this case, it was higher than optimal, but there was still plenty of room for tumor removal. A bone covering was left over it to reduce the risk of accidentally puncturing it during tumor removal.

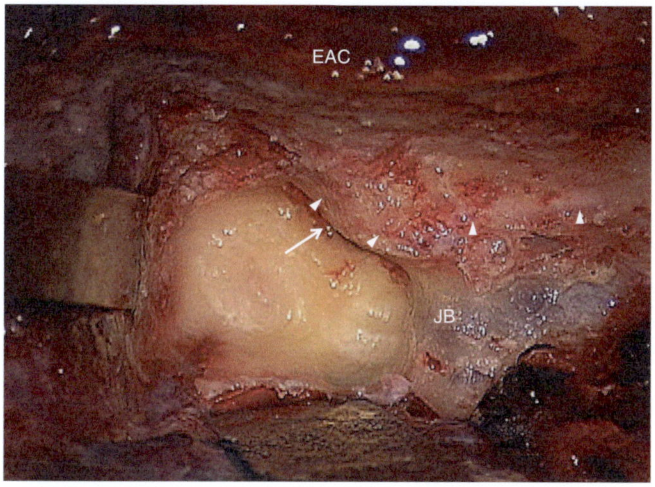

39. To find the internal auditory canal, the porus acusticus (*PA*) was first identified by drilling along the posterior fossa dura. Then, the length of the internal auditory canal (*IAC*) was delineated.

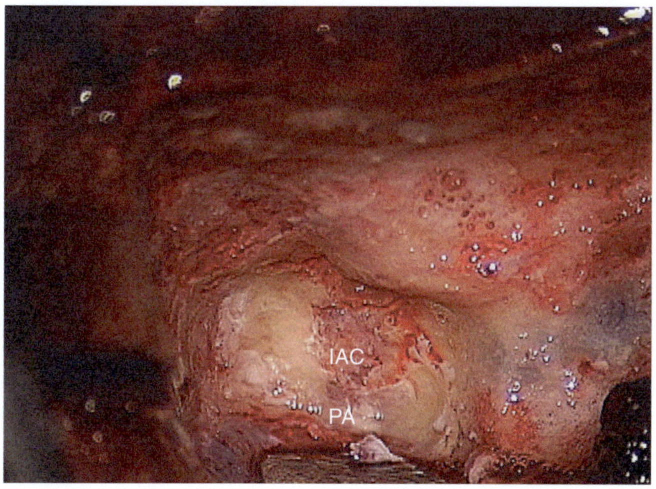

40. Troughs (*asterisks*) were drilled superior and inferior to the internal auditory canal (*IAC*). The superior trough was deeper than the inferior trough in this case because of the relatively high jugular bulb. Note the cottonoid pledget in the "crotch" of the sigmoid sinus. The sigmoid sinus often bleeds in this area because its dural lining is very thin.

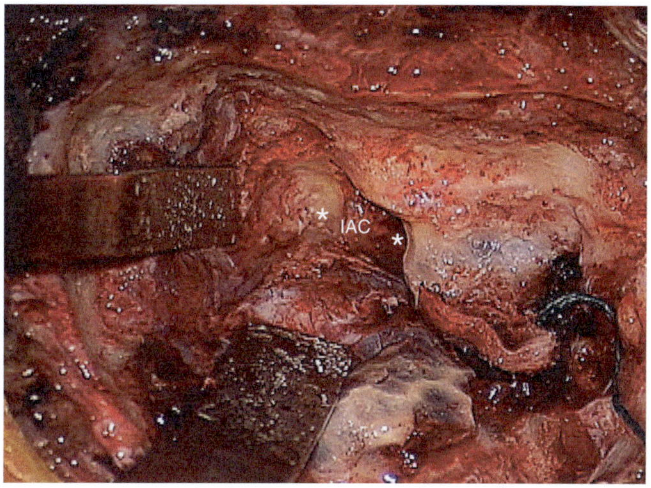

41. The posterior fossa dura was opened. A moist Telfa strip was placed on the cerebellum and the retractor positioned. A #2 Penfield retractor was placed under the tumor to gently open the arachnoid membranes and release cerebrospinal fluid. This maneuver is important because it lowers the intracranial pressure and allows the brain to relax, providing more space to perform the dissection.

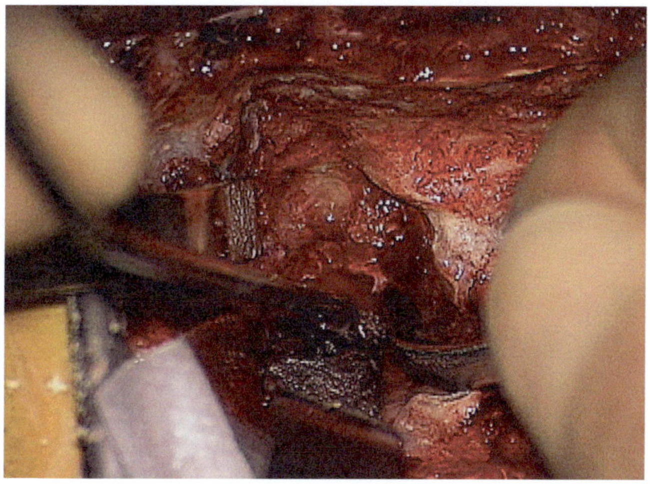

42. The cerebellum was under the retractor, and the posterior face of the tumor was exposed. Testing with the nerve stimulator was performed to verify that the facial nerve was not in this area.

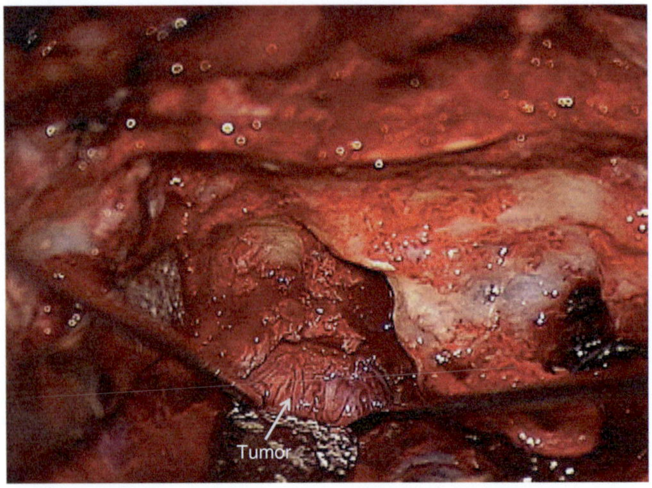

43. A square opening was made in the posterior face of the tumor (*dotted quadrangle*), and the internal portion of the tumor was debulked. An instrument can be used to palpate the inside of the tumor to appreciate the thickness of the residual capsule lining. Once it is thin enough to permit it to be collapsed in upon itself, dissection of the capsule can be started.

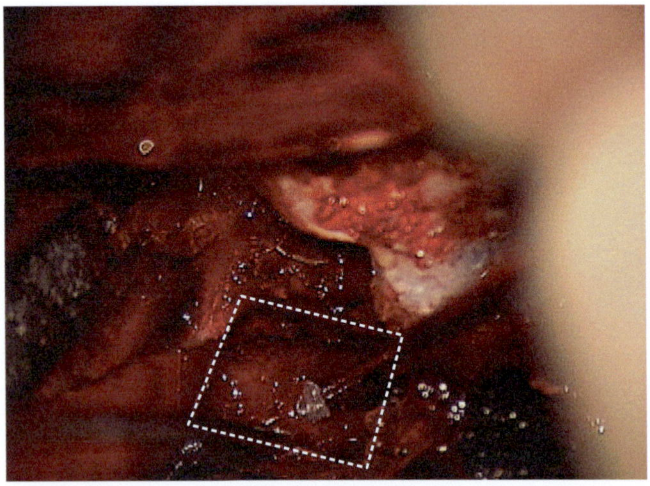

44. After removing the majority of the medial capsule, only the anterior capsule (*arrow*) was left. As the facial nerve is draped along its deep side (and not seen in this image), this part is saved until the end. A subtotal resection could stop here although the tumor within the internal auditory canal (*IAC*) is typically also removed. The blood supply to the tumor remnant in the cerebellopontine angle comes either from the brainstem or from the dura of the internal auditory canal. Removing tumor at both ends reduces the blood supply to the remnant and thus minimizes the chance of this residual tumor demonstrating growth.

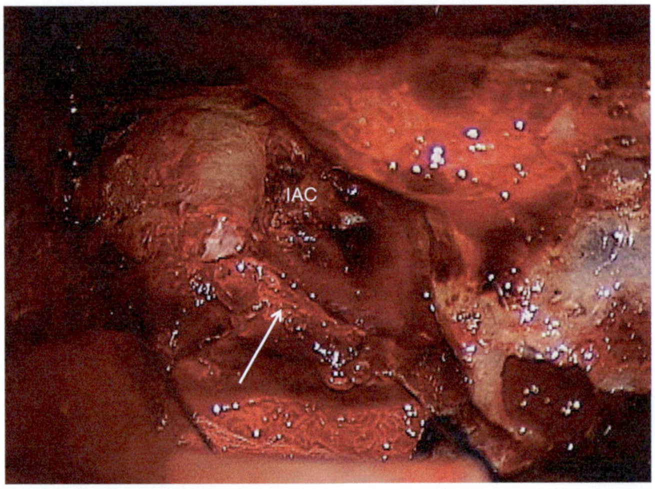

45. The edge of the facial nerve (*F*) was identified by meticulously freeing up the superior aspect of the tumor (*T*) from the fundus. Frequent use of the nerve stimulator is helpful during this process to identify the true edge of the facial nerve.

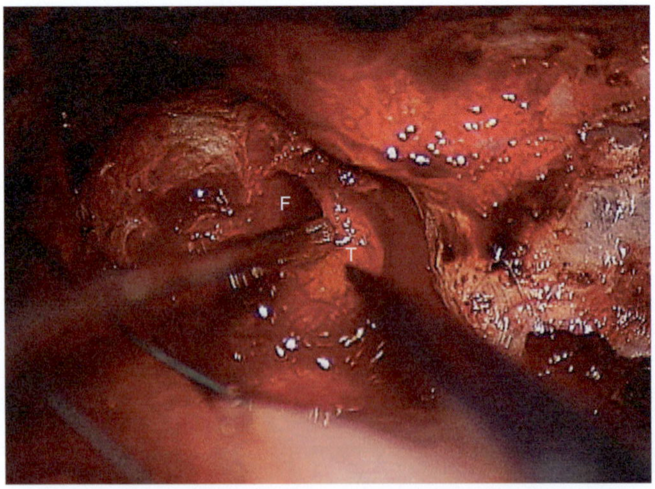

46. After removal of the tumor from the internal auditory canal with preservation of the facial nerve (*F*). While dissection could be continued further to take the tumor (*T*) within the cerebellopontine angle off the nerve, we stopped here according to the patient's wishes to have a subtotal resection.

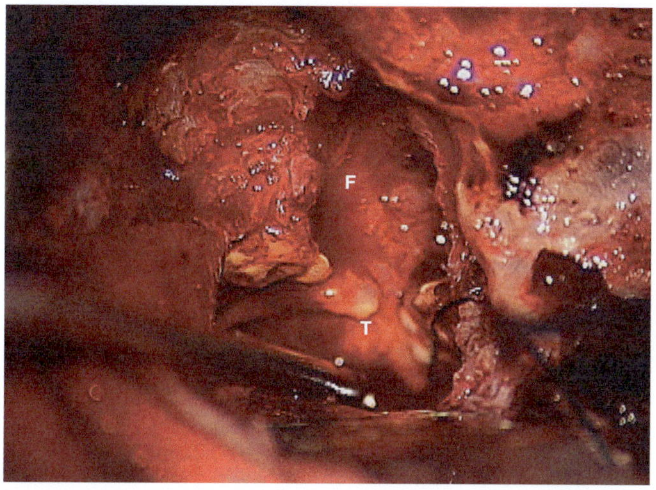

47. Following tumor removal, a piece of temporalis fascia was laid over the aditus ad antrum (*arrow*).

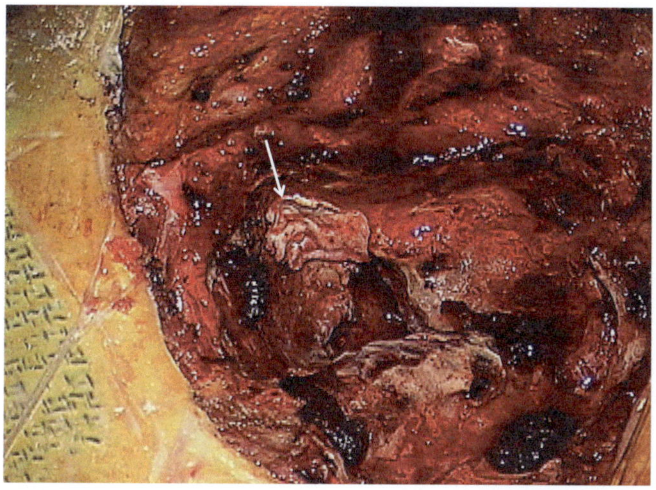

48. A fat graft harvested from the abdomen was then placed in. While it can be cut into multiple strips, one or two short, fat sausage-shaped pieces often work best because cerebrospinal fluid can trickle between the pieces of fat graft. It is preferable if the fat graft protrudes through the dural opening into the posterior fossa a little bit to help it cork well. However, one does not want the fat to compress the brainstem. Also, the neurophysiologist should carefully monitor the facial nerve during the process to verify that it does not protrude too deeply and stretch the nerve.

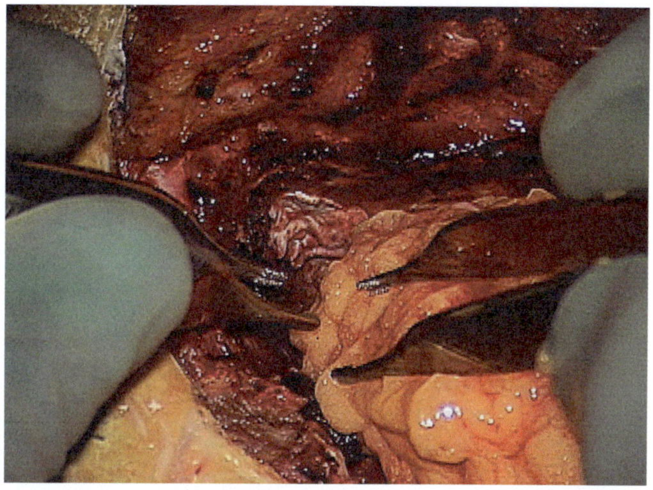

49. Completed fat graft placement. The wound was then closed in three layers. Particular attention should be paid to tightly close the lower end of the incision. If a cerebrospinal fluid leak through the skin is going to occur, it always leaks out through the inferior pole of the incision.

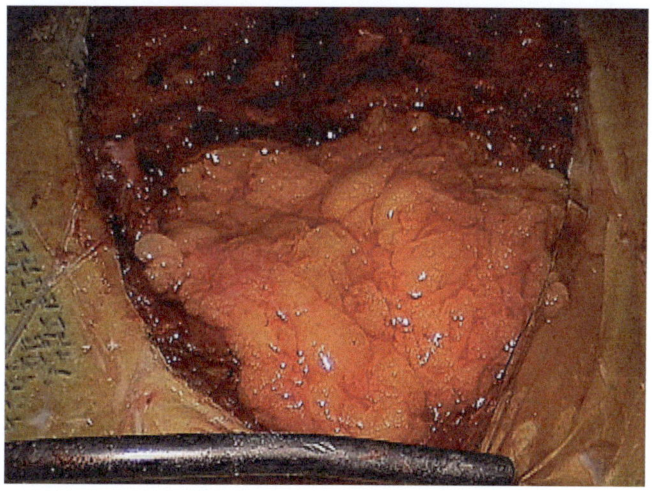

50. Immediate post-op MRI demonstrated the residual tumor within the cerebellopontine angle. This remnant was a little thicker than we typically would like. Nevertheless, the brainstem pressure was relieved, the internal auditory canal was clear, and the facial nerve function was normal.

It is common to underestimate the amount of residual tumor. If you cannot see the anterior aspect of the tumor, it is likely there is still considerable bulk remaining. Recall that 50 % of the tumor volume is anterior to the internal auditory canal. To avoid this, continue to remove tumor either along the superior or inferior edge depending on the facial nerve course. Separating the tumor from the dura around the porous acusticus and just proximal will allow the tumor to be rolled inferiorly or superiorly, and this will provide access to more tumor. If the bone removal in the troughs at the beginning of the case was inadequate, more bone can be removed at this point. There is a tendency to "cheat" on openings when performing a planned subtotal resection.

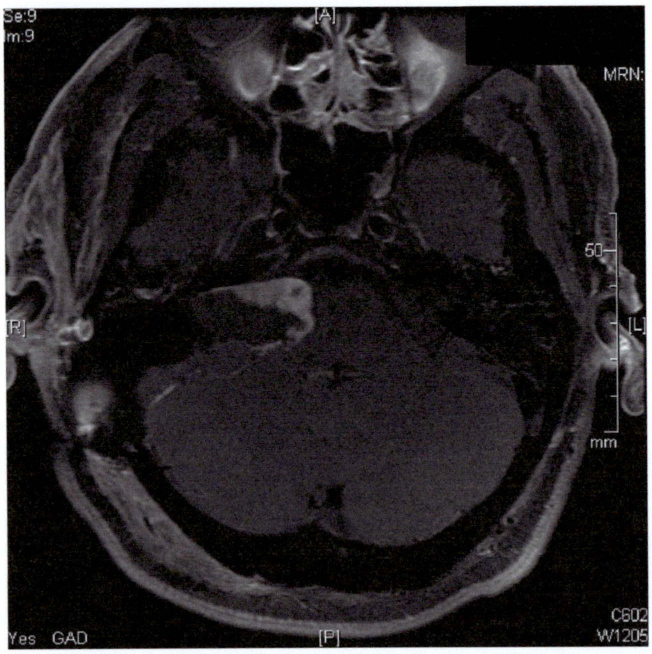

51. Post-op FIESTA T2-weighted image demonstrated the fat graft placement (*arrow shows the deep extent*). Note that it did not fill in the space where the tumor was. The goal is to cork the dural opening without recreating the brainstem compression the patient started with.

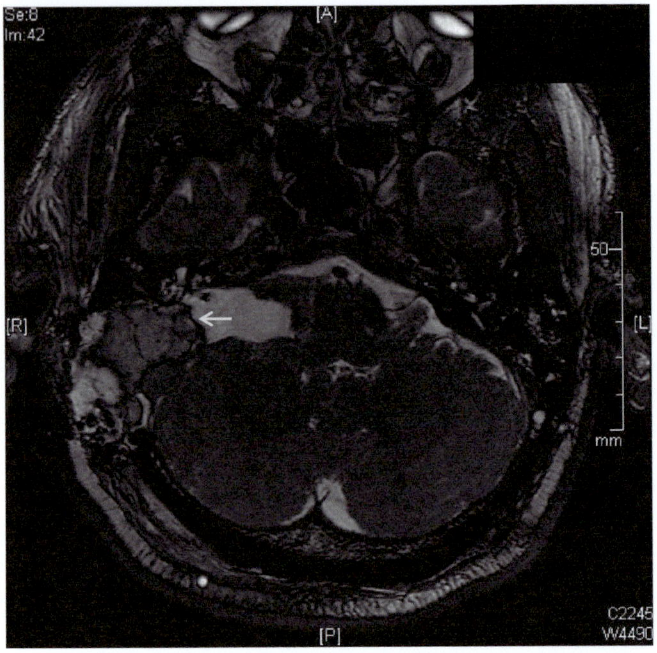

52. Case 4. A small left vestibular schwannoma with nonserviceable hearing. There was no extension into the fundus.

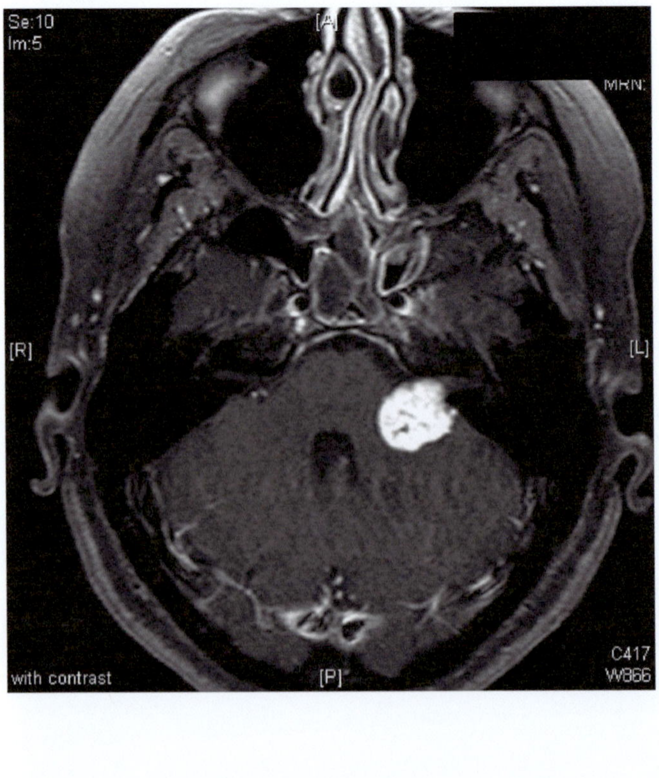

53. Post-op image after total resection via the translabyrinthine approach. If the patient had serviceable hearing preoperatively, a retrosigmoid approach would have been used in an attempt to preserve hearing.

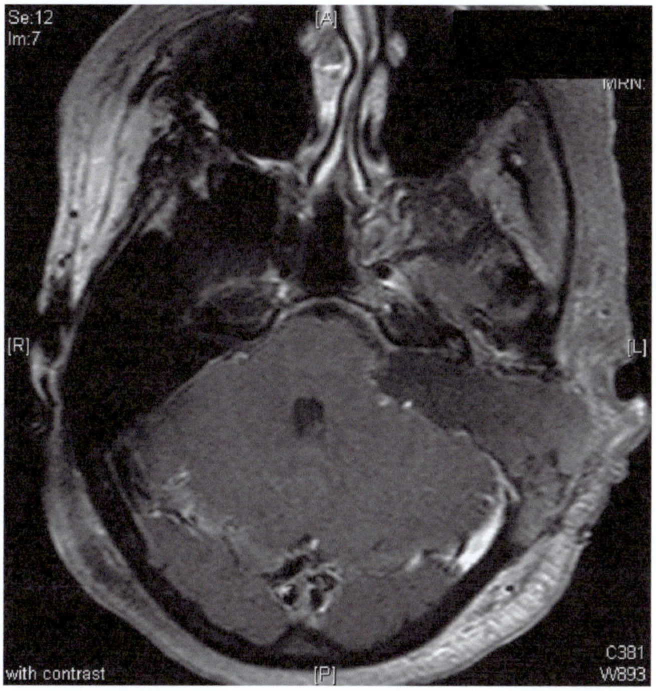

54. Case 5. This patient had a small left endolymphatic sac tumor. A translabyrinthine approach was performed. While these types of tumors are often very large, this patient had a tumor localized to the sac (see the bulge along the posterior fossa dura). Because of the small size of this tumor, the tegmen was left in place and only the posterior fossa dura exposed.

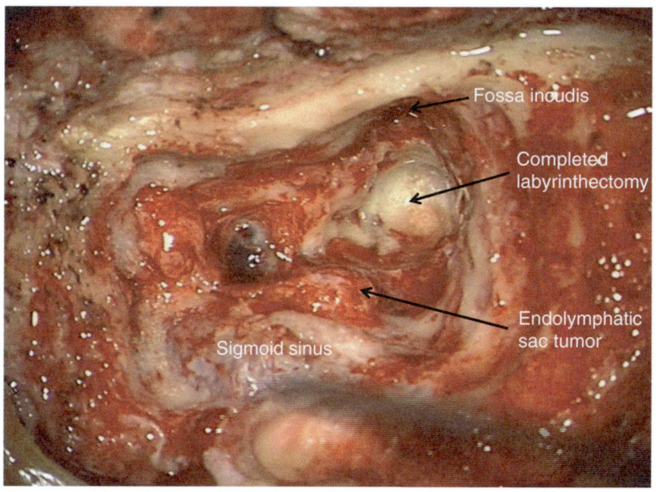

55. After resection of the tumor, much of the dura could be preserved. Closure was performed with an abdominal fat graft.

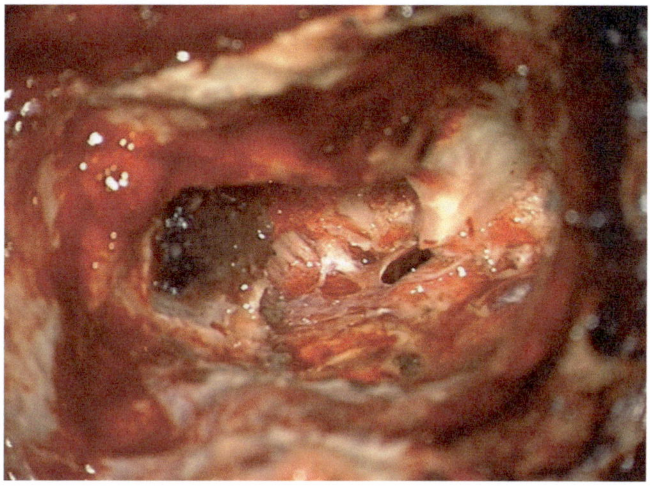

Transcochlear Approach

- *Concept*
  - This is essentially a total temporal bone resection. The translabyrinthine approach is extended to remove the cochlea and ear canal. The external auditory canal is oversewn.
  - If the tumor permits, the facial nerve is best managed by preserving the fallopian canal. This reduces the chance of facial nerve dysfunction.
  - If more exposure of the posterior fossa is required, the facial nerve can be mobilized from the first genu. This typically results in a complete palsy that recovers to a House–Brackmann grade III-IV function.
  - With malignant tumors of the temporal bone, facial nerve resection may be necessary to achieve oncologic control.
- *Conditions treated*
  - Large tumors within the posterior cranial fossa, particularly those ventral to the brainstem
  - Extensive endolymphatic sac tumors
  - Deeply invasive skin cancers or parotid gland carcinomas
  - Unusual temporal bone lesions with significant temporal bone and skull base involvement
- *Risks*
  - Complete hearing loss in the operated ear always occurs.
  - Disequilibrium that should resolve with time, assuming there is vestibular function in the other ear and appropriate compensation occurs.
  - Facial nerve weakness is common, but the risk is reduced if the nerve is not mobilized and when operating on benign lesions.
  - CSF leak.
  - Necrosis of the abdominal fat graft in the ensuing weeks after the surgery.
  - Meningitis.
  - Dysmetria if there is direct injury or vascular compromise to the cerebellar peduncle or brainstem.
- *Benefits*
  - Wide exposure of the lateral aspect of the posterior fossa.
  - Favorable line of sight to ventral brainstem and central skull base.
  - Limited brain retraction.
  - When operating on a tumor involving the temporal bone, most of the vascularized portion of the tumor is removed prior to opening the dura. This makes the intradural tumor dissection safer.
- *Additional notes*
  - The transcochlear approach can be helpful in managing a wide variety of complex benign and malignant skull base lesions as illustrated by the cases presented in this section. Careful consideration needs to be given to the goals of surgery and the potential morbidity of operative intervention. This approach necessitates the loss of hearing and vestibular function and potentially results in permanent facial nerve weakness. For benign tumors or unresectable tumors such as a diffusely infiltrative meningioma (which may require radiation to achieve long-term control), every effort should be made to preserve function. This may translate to working around the otic capsule through a combined middle and posterior fossa approach rather than a transcochlear approach. A patient with an extensive malignant tumor may benefit from aggressive tumor debulking, but surgical cure is often impossible. Leaving microscopic disease on a functioning facial nerve may provide the best outcome when considering life expectancy and quality of life. Be creative, but don't compromise the primary mission.

56. Overview of the amount of bone that can be removed with this approach (*gray*). The bone removal is tailored to the pathology. A cochlear schwannoma can be removed with limited bone removal, for example, modest widening of the external auditory canal alone may provide adequate access. A large chondrosarcoma may require removal of essentially all the temporal bone except the fallopian canal.

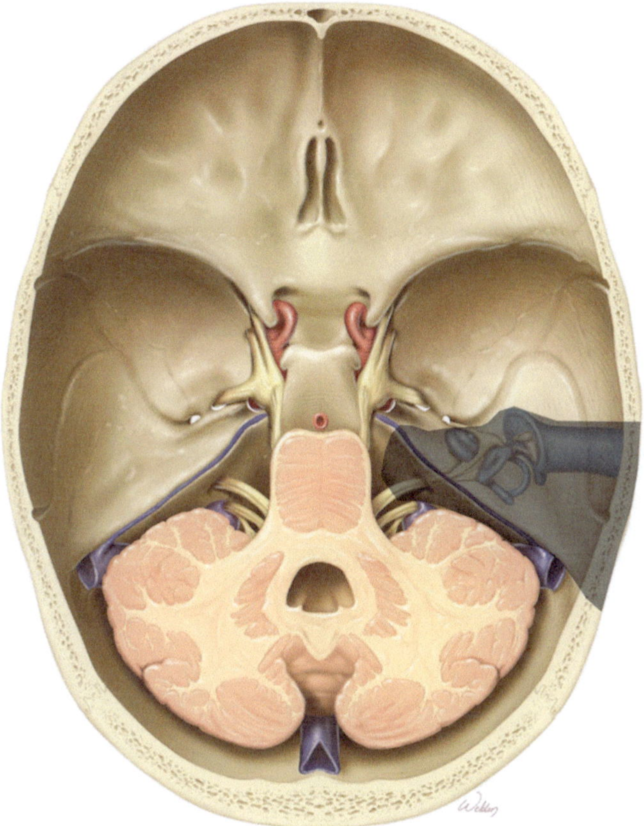

57. Case 1. CT of a boy with recurrent meningitis and profound left sensorineural hearing loss that was found to have multiple congenital meningoceles with erosive changes within the left temporal bone. Note the enlargement of the geniculate ganglion (*arrow*) and the internal auditory canal.

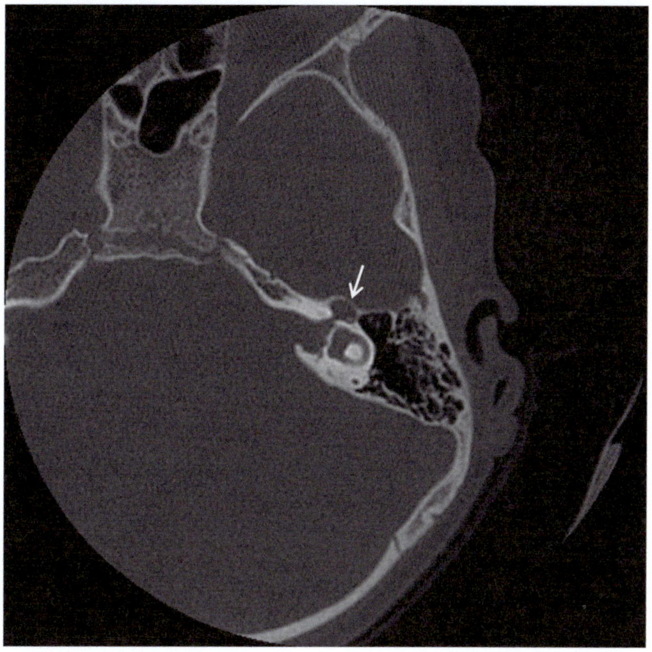

58. A lower cut demonstrates unusual cystic erosion of the internal auditory canal (*arrow*).

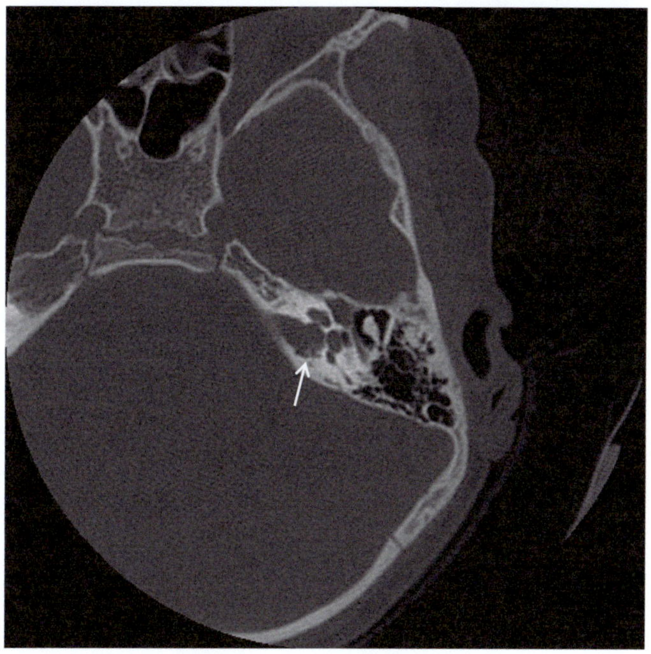

59. The lesions extended down to the jugular foramen (*arrow*). The dome of the jugular bulb (*asterisk*) can be seen posterior to the basal turn of the cochlea.

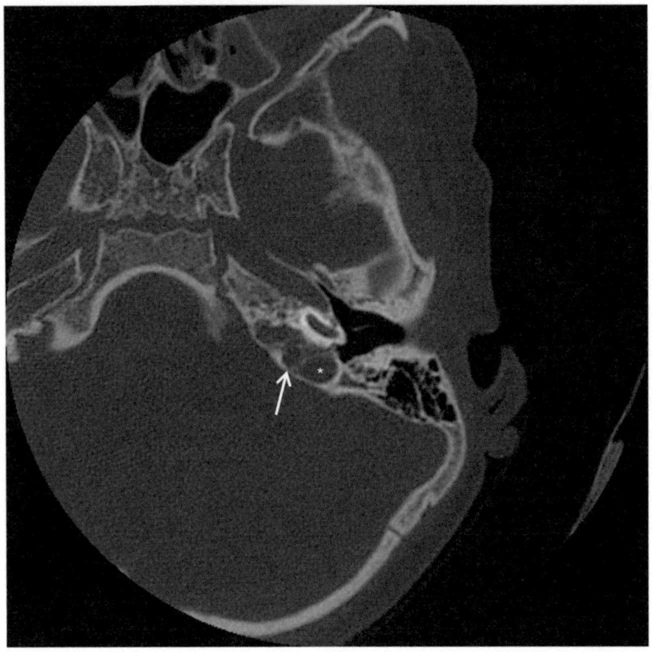

60. T2 MRI demonstrated that these lesions were filled with CSF (*arrow*).

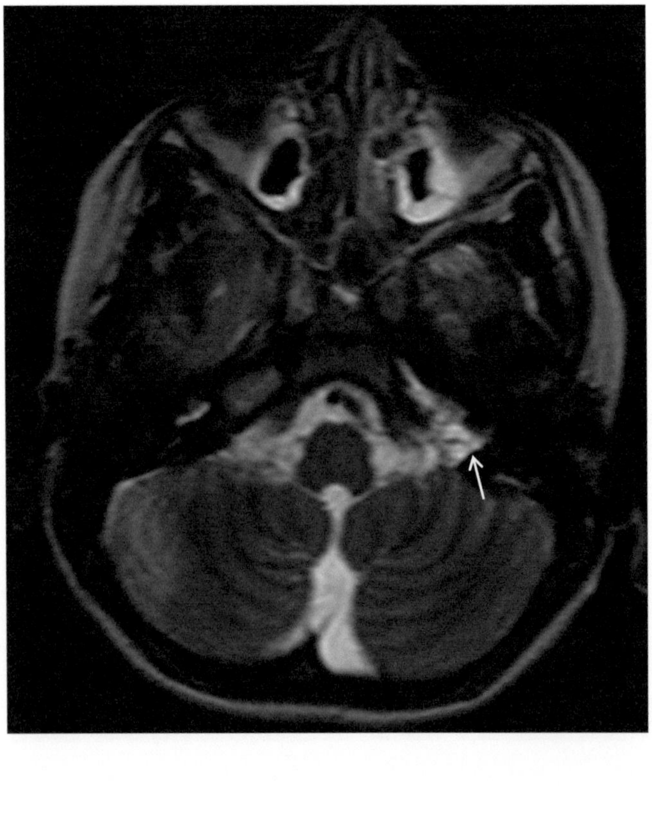

61. Coronal T2 MRI demonstrated that the meningoceles penetrated through the skull base into the upper neck (*arrow*). Based upon this imaging, his complete hearing loss in that ear, and history of recurrent meningitis with the associated risks of serious neurological injury, we elected to perform a definitive approach to treat this problem. We performed a transcochlear approach to expose and repair the multiple meningoceles combined with closing the Eustachian tube and packing the cavity off with fat. Thus, a definitive separation of the CSF from the upper aerodigestive tract could be achieved.

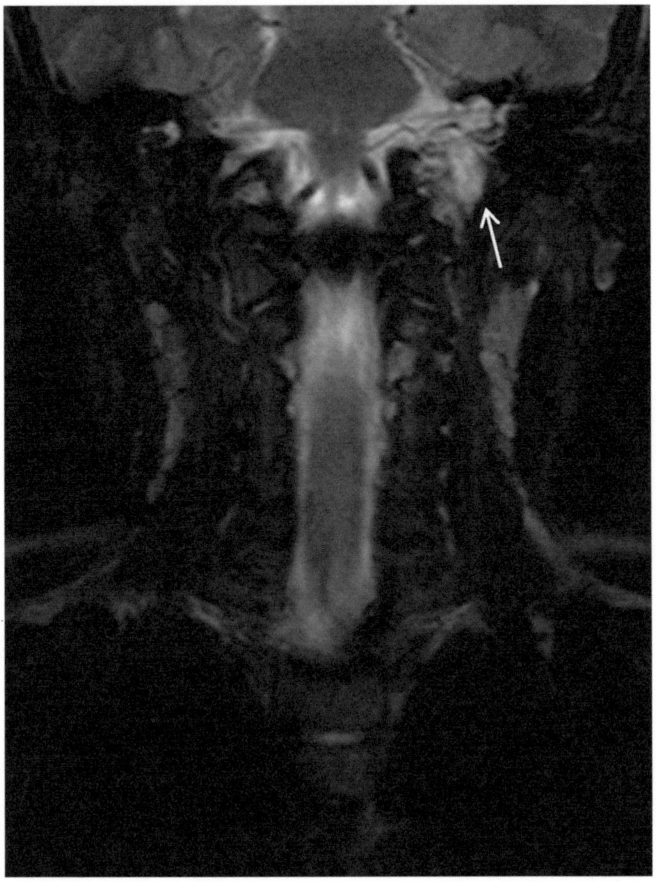

62. Initially, a canal wall down mastoidectomy was performed. During this procedure, the malleus and the incus were removed. Also, the skin of the ear canal was completely removed and the ear canal oversewn (explained in Chap. 8, temporal bone resection). The posterior fossa dura was exposed and a malleable used to retract it.

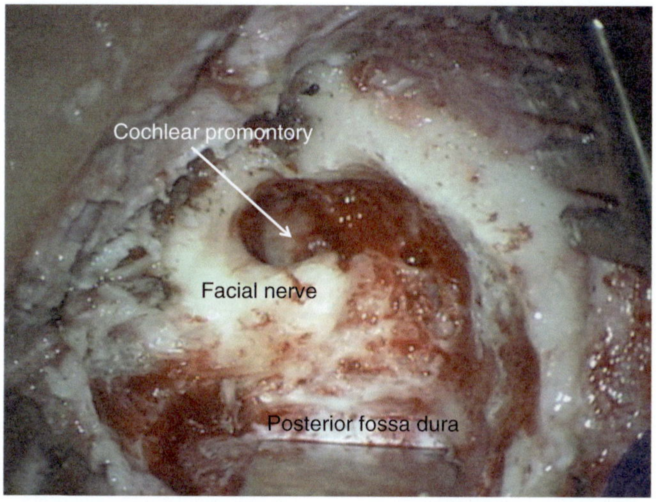

63. A labyrinthectomy was performed. The endolymphatic sac is the white tissue anterior to the retractor (*arrow*). The vestibule (*arrowhead*) was opened under the facial nerve.

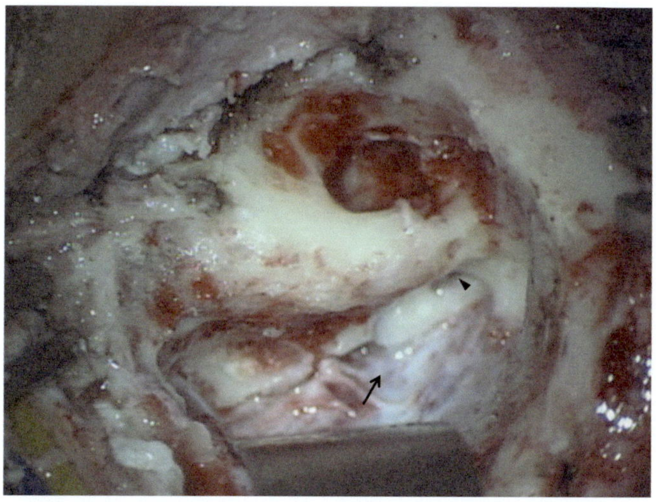

64. The internal auditory canal was opened (*arrowhead*). Note the well-circumscribed bony defects associated with the meningocele through which cranial nerves VII and VIII (*arrow*) were visible. The posterior aspect of the jugular bulb was also visible (*JB*).

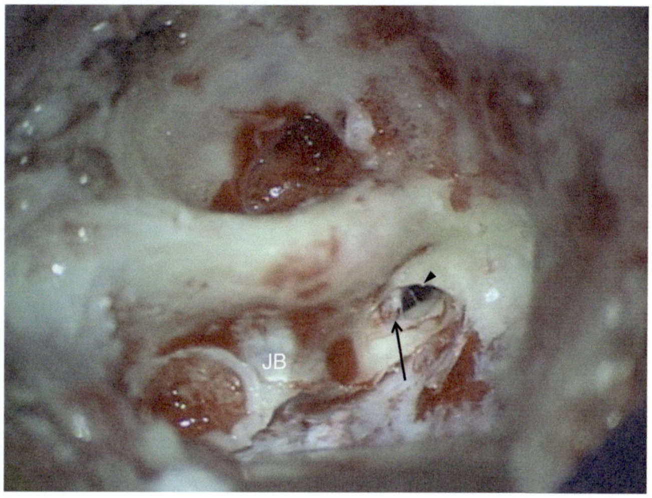

65. To remove the cochlea, the promontory was drilled away. Here, it is shown as partially resected (*arrow*). The jugular bulb (*JB*) and the carotid artery (*CA*) should be identified and preserved within the middle ear.

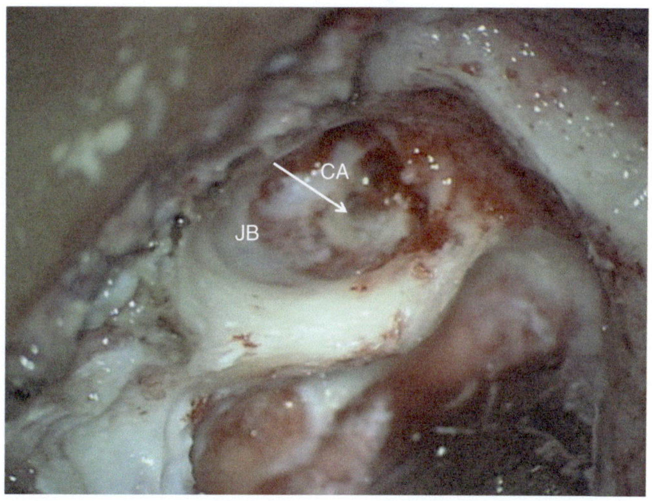

66. After completing the transcochlear approach, there was a wide connection under the horizontal facial nerve (*arrow*). The facial nerve was left intact within the fallopian canal so as to preserve its function.

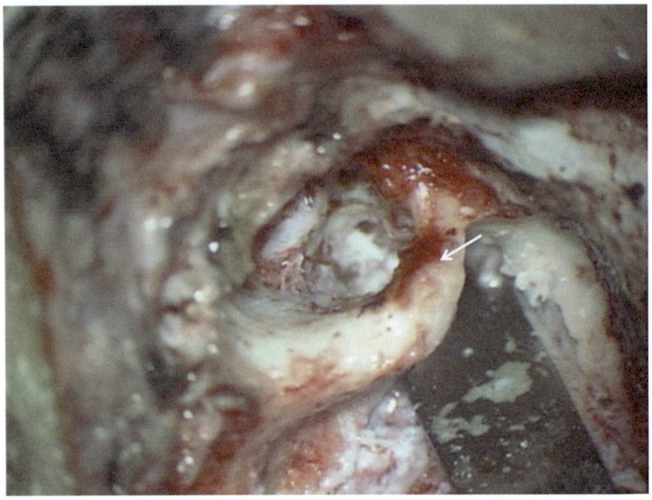

67. Post-op axial CT demonstrated the extent of resection. While more of the anterior petrous apex could certainly have been removed, it was not needed to accomplish the goal of this procedure. At this inferior cut, the dome of the jugular bulb separates the anterior and posterior spaces created by drilling out the cochlea and the vestibular system, respectively. Fat was filling the cavity.

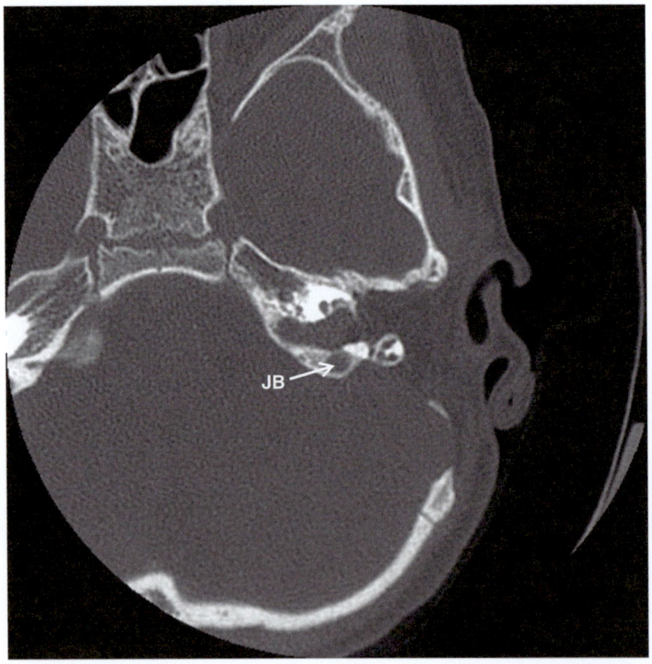

68. Post-op coronal CT demonstrated the "fallopian bridge" through which the horizontal facial nerve passes (*arrowhead*).

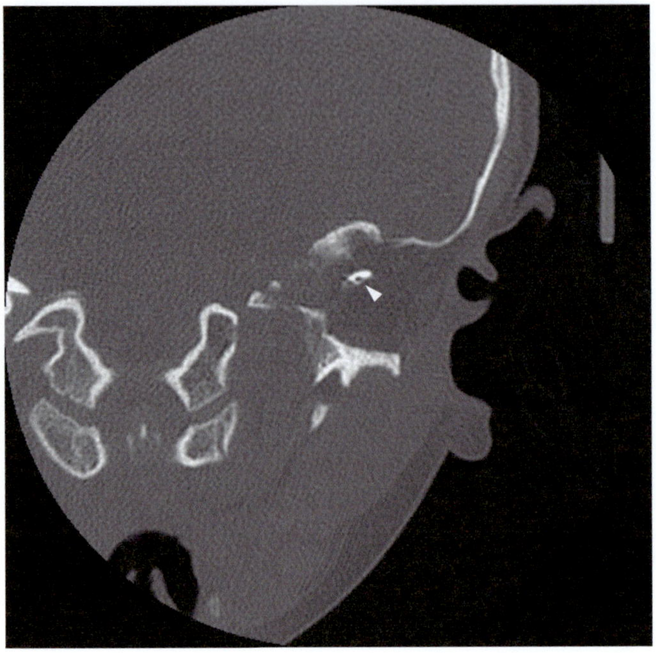

69. Post-op T2 MRI demonstrated that the residual meningocele was isolated from the middle ear cleft and Eustachian tube. Thus, this should prevent further episodes of meningitis.

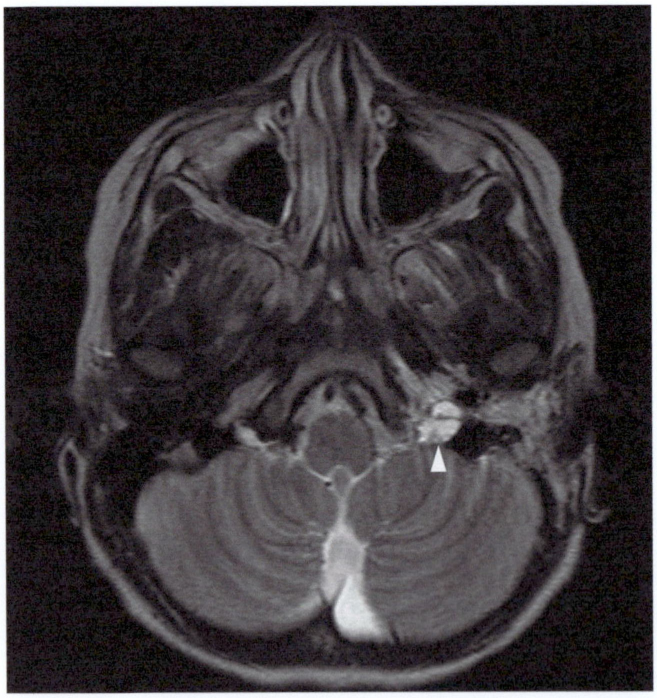

70. Case 2. A right endolymphatic sac tumor. In this gadolinium-enhanced MRI, it is clear that the entire temporal bone was involved with disease. The tumor also extended into the posterior fossa.

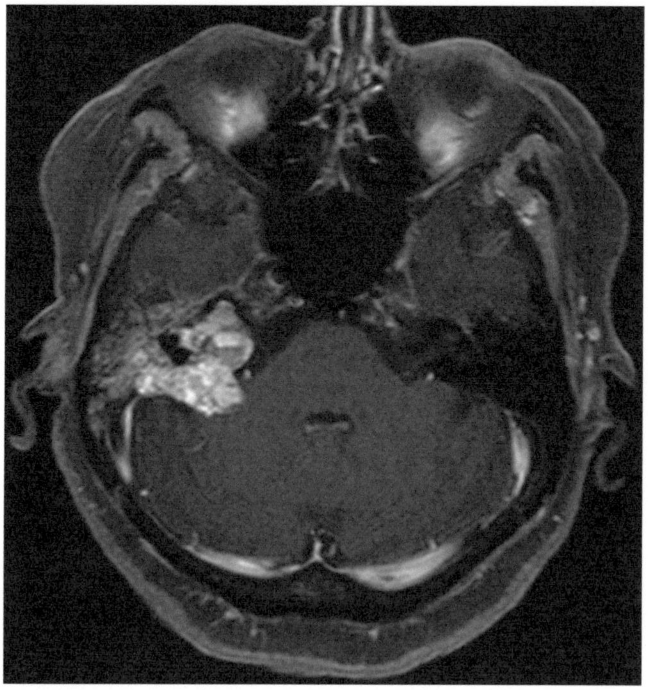

71. Coronal MRI demonstrated that the tumor involved the middle fossa dura.

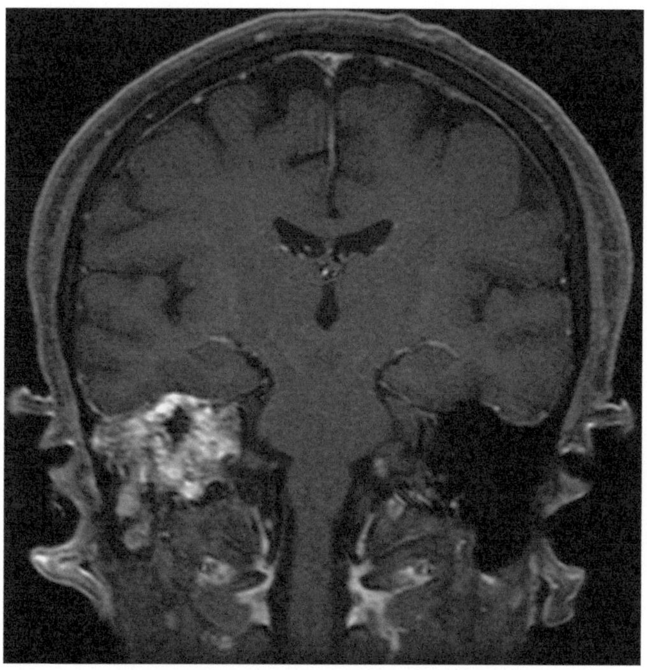

72. T2 MRI demonstrated that the tumor had some solid areas and some cystic areas. This is characteristic of endolymphatic sac tumors.

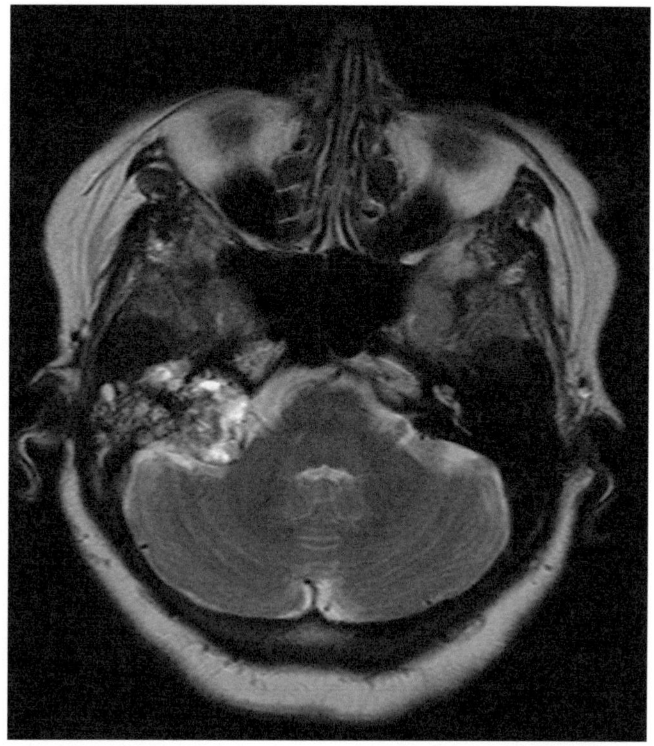

73. Pre-op CT demonstrated substantial erosion of the temporal bone.

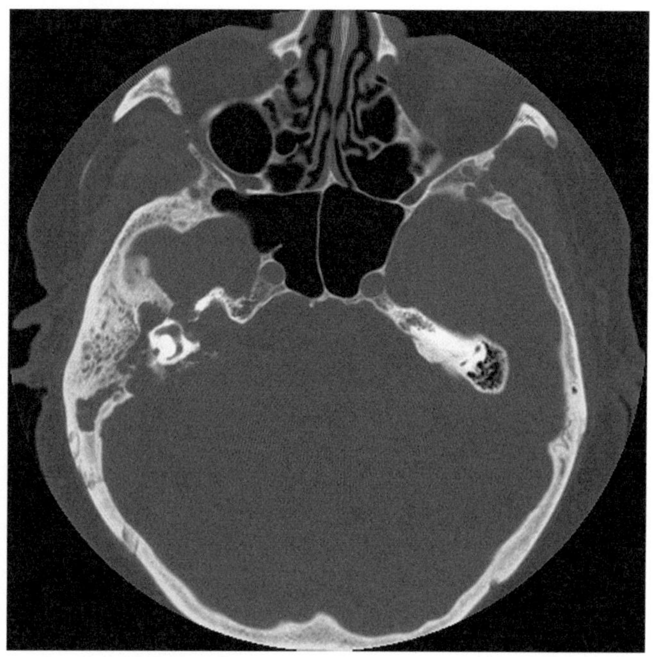

74. After completion of a transcochlear resection, an immediate post-op CT demonstrated the extent of resection. A complete resection was achieved, and a large fat graft was in place. In this case, because the facial nerve was paralyzed preoperatively, a facial nerve resection was performed.

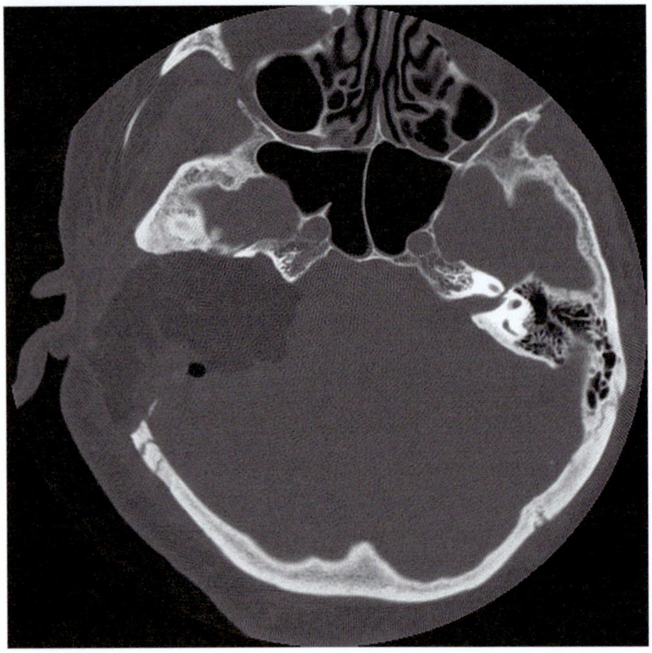

75. Post-op T1 MRI with gadolinium demonstrated that there was no residual tumor.

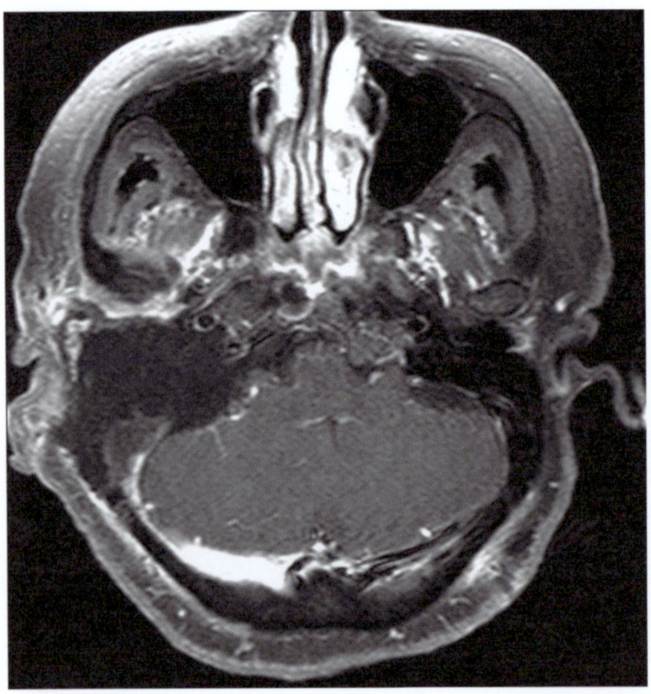

76. Post-op T2 MRI demonstrated the fat graft.

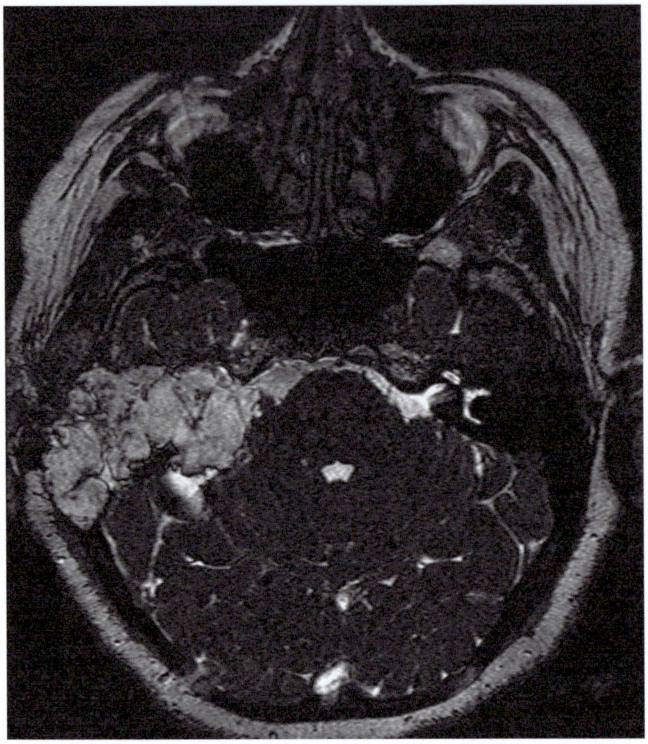

77. Case 3: An intracochlear schwannoma was found in a patient with asymmetric sensorineural hearing loss. Note the small area of enhancement within the basal turn of the right cochlea (*arrow*).

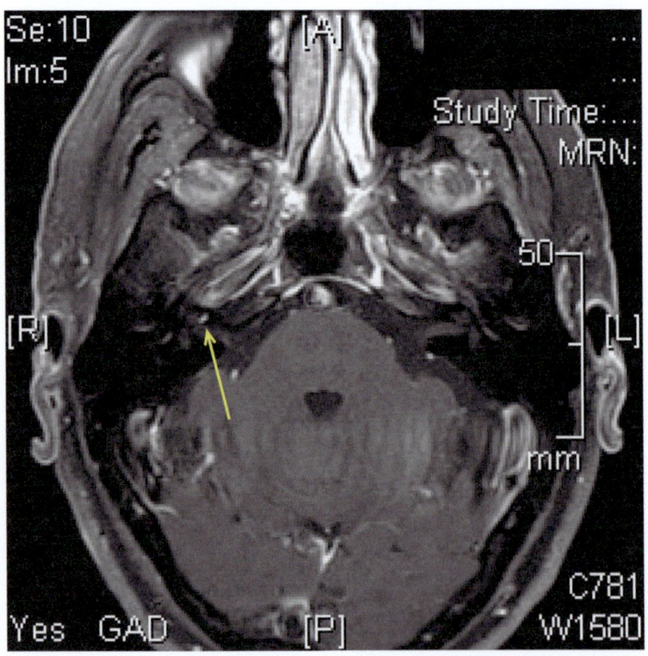

78. FIESTA T2 MRI demonstrated a filling defect within the basal turn of the cochlea corresponding to the area of enhancement. This was not present on the left side. The patient desired surgical removal due to hearing loss and vertigo.

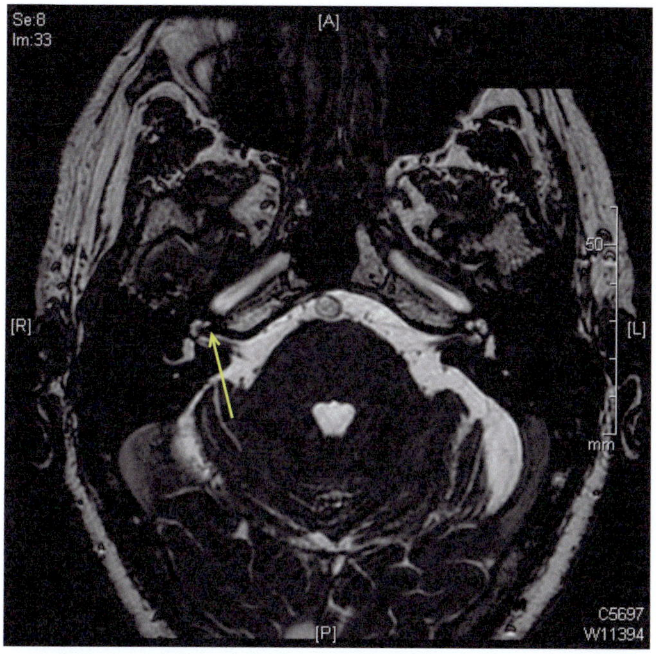

79. A transcochlear approach was performed and the cochlea opened. The tumor was first dissected out of the cochlea.

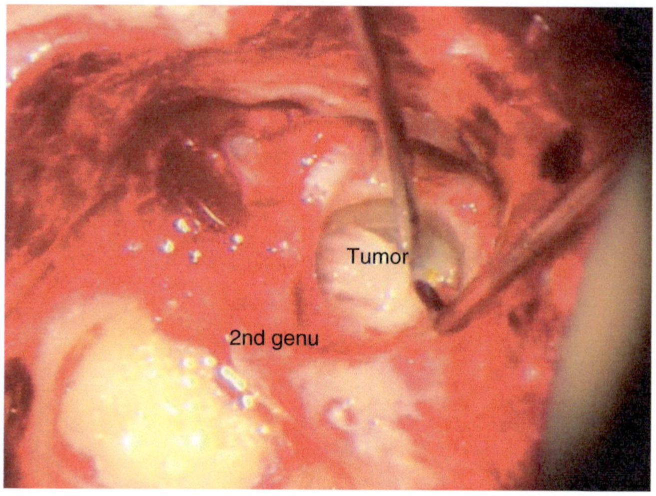

80. A tumor remnant was still present within the modiolus (*asterisk*), which then needed to be removed. Note how the suction could be passed under the second genu of the facial nerve during this dissection process because of the fallopian bridge of the horizontal facial nerve.

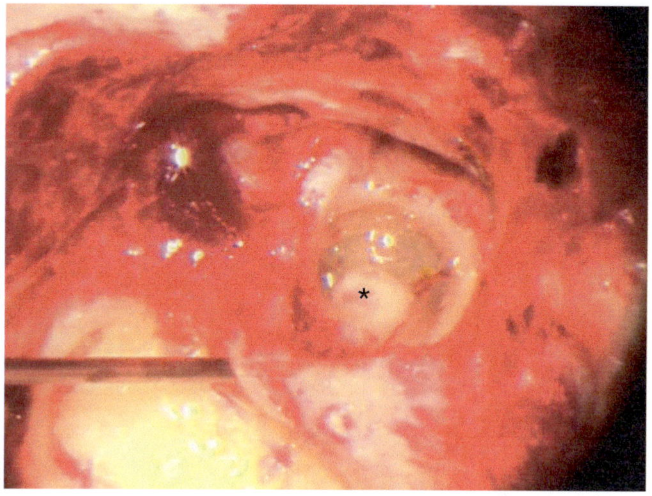

81. After removal, the fundus of the internal auditory canal was open.

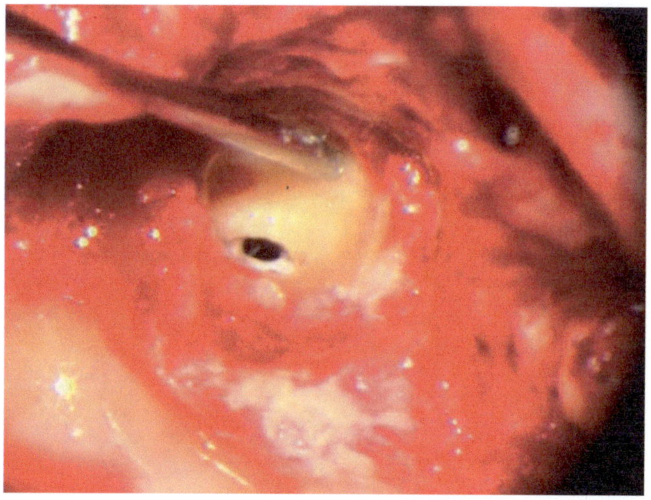

82. A small piece of fat was dumbbelled through the fundus to plug it. A larger piece of fat was used to fill the defect and the wound closed in layers.

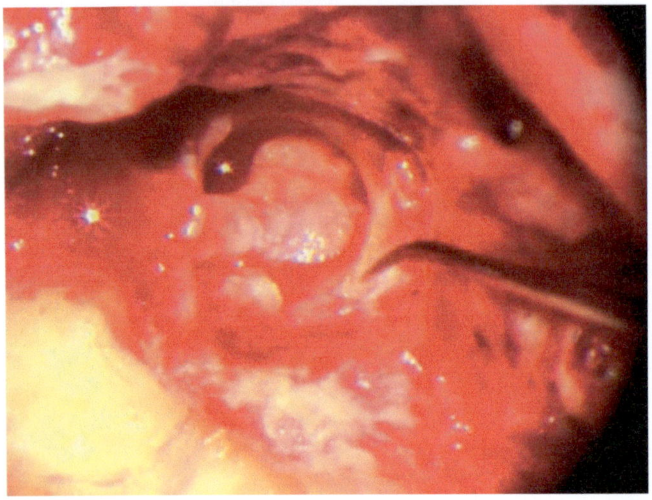

83. Post-op T2 MRI demonstrated the extent of resection with the fat graft in position.

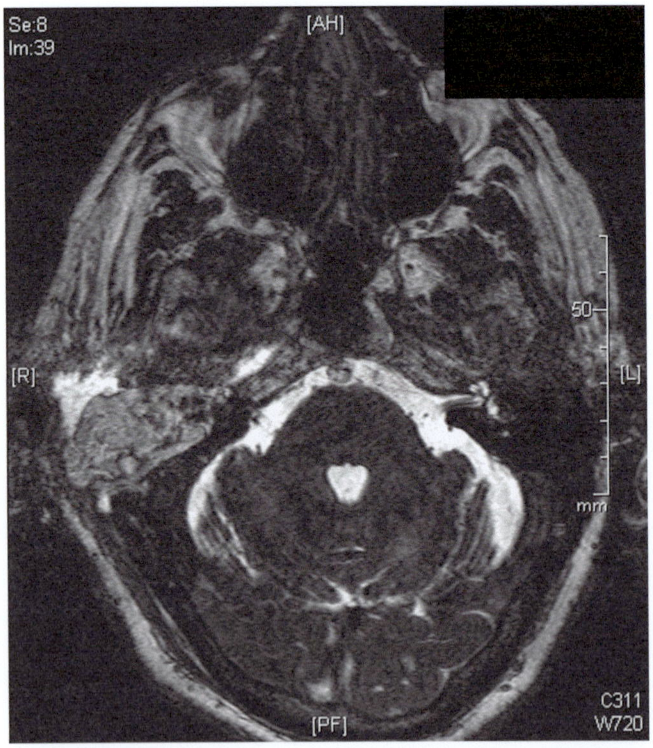

84. Case 4. A large recurrent glomus jugulare tumor. Note the large flow voids in the lesion. Previous surgeries included a Fisch type A approach used 11 years previously by one surgeon and a retrosigmoid approach used by another surgeon 6 years later.

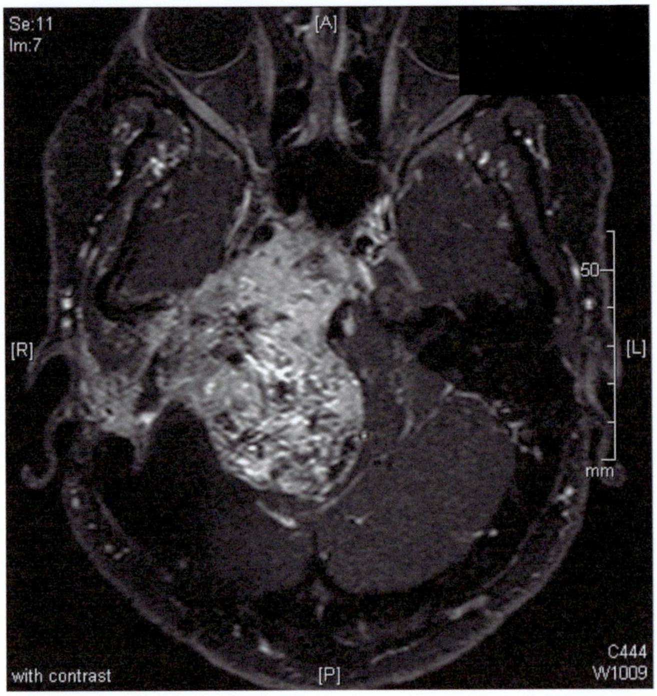

85. T2 MRI demonstrated substantial brain compression.

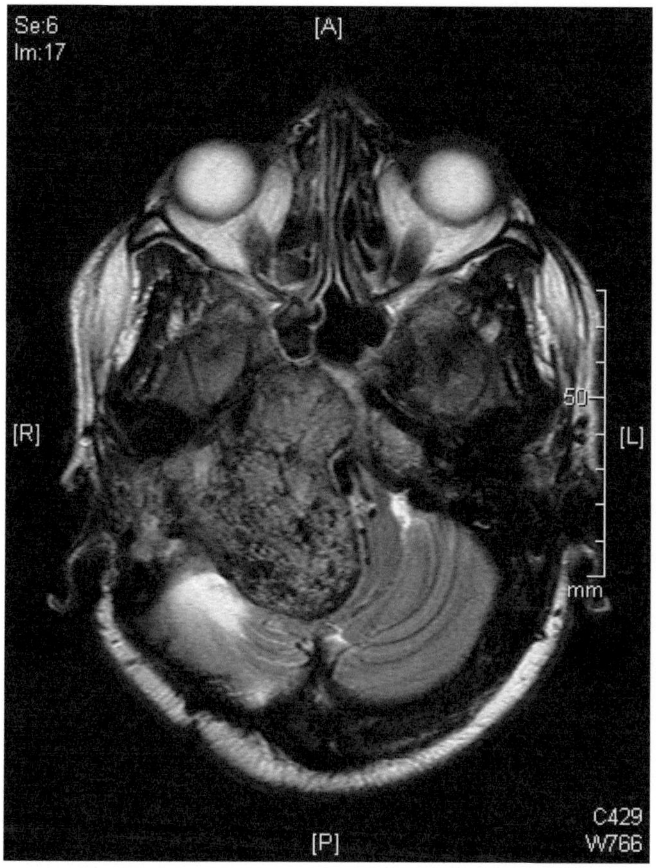

86. Preoperative CT scan demonstrated near-complete destruction of the petrous apex and tumor extension into the clivus. The mesh plate used for the retrosigmoid approach is visible.

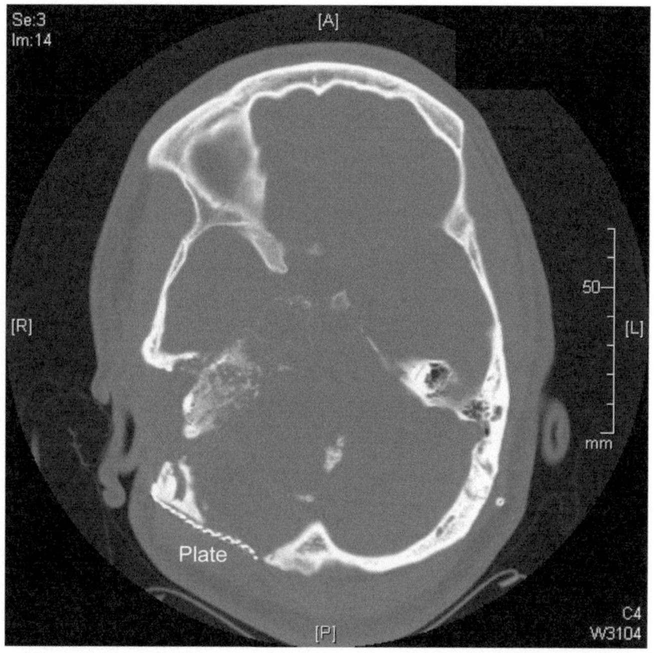

87. Preoperatively, the tumor was embolized with Onyx, which is highly visible by CT.

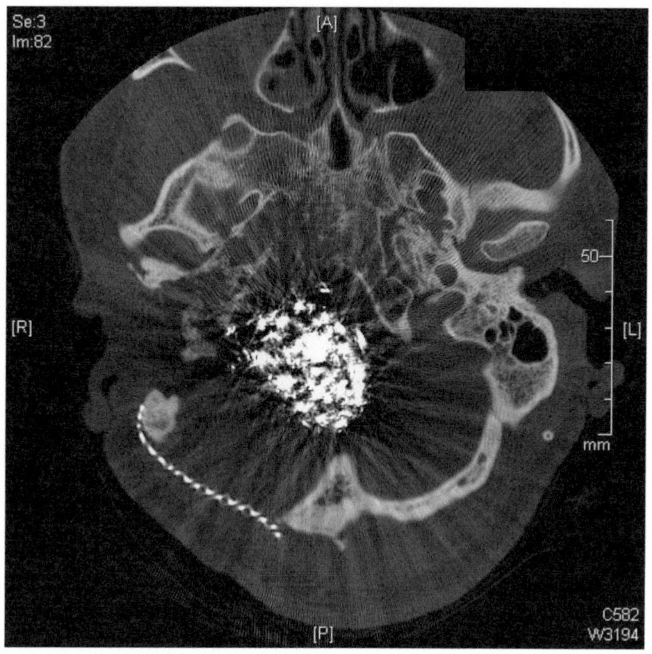

88. Post-op MRI. After transcochlear resection, the vast majority of the tumor had been removed, and the posterior fossa was decompressed. Due to the extent of bleeding, we elected to leave disease in the clivus. We resected the internal carotid artery together with the tumor. The patient had passed a balloon occlusion study preoperatively.

The patient developed a postoperative pseudomeningocele with CSF lateral to the fat graft (*asterisk*). This resolved after placement of a lumboperitoneal shunt.

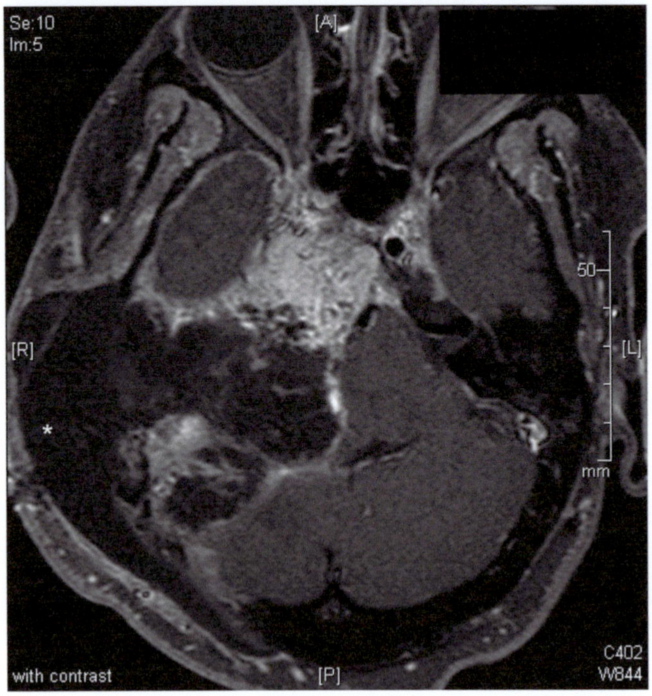

89. Post-op CT. Note the residual onyx within the tumor remnant in the clivus.

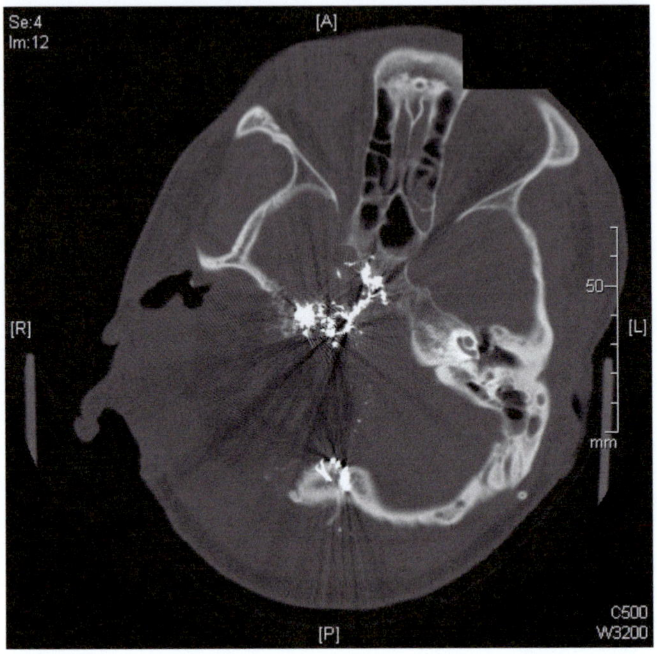

Retrosigmoid Approach

- *Concept*
  - The skull is opened posterior to the sigmoid sinus and the cerebellum retracted to visualize the cerebellopontine angle. The posterior face of the temporal bone is drilled away to expose the internal auditory canal.
- *Conditions treated*
  - Vestibular schwannomas of any size
  - Meningiomas and other posterior fossa tumors
  - Jugular foramen schwanommas and meningiomas that have minimal extracranial disease.
  - Posterior cranial fossa subdural or intraparenchymal abscess
- *Risks*
  - Hearing loss
  - Facial nerve injury
  - CSF leak
  - Brainstem injury producing dysmetria
  - Dysphagia, possibly with aspiration
  - Vocal cord paralysis
  - Shoulder weakness
- *Benefits*
  - This hearing preservation approach is preferred for larger vestibular schwannomas and small tumors that are medially located.
  - The opening is relatively quick compared to the translabyrinthine approach.
  - This approach provides tremendous exposure from the trigeminal nerve down to the jugular foramen.
- *Additional notes*
  - When using this approach to remove a vestibular schwannoma, it is important not to just remove the cerebellopontine angle component of the tumor. Drilling of the temporal bone should be performed to remove the intracanalicular component as well. The tumor receives blood supply from the dura of the internal auditory canal, and the risk of recurrence is high if not removed.
  - A subtotal tumor resection is indicated in some situations (e.g., an elderly patient with a large tumor,) and in these cases, it is enticing to not open the internal auditory canal. Doing so saves time and decreases the risk of CSF leak. However, if it is not done, there is a tendency to overestimate the amount of tumor that has been resected. Most tumors are centered on the internal auditory canal; therefore, 50 % of the tumor volume is anterior to the internal auditory canal. Debulking the internal auditory canal portion allows for better access to the remaining tumor, and often a substantial amount of additional tumor can be resected without risk to the facial nerve.
  - This approach is not typically used for primary temporal bone tumors (such as endolymphatic sac tumors or glomus jugular tumors) as the extracranial blood supply to the tumor is not controlled.

90. The retrosigmoid approach involves removing the bone posterior to the sigmoid sinus and retracting the cerebellum.

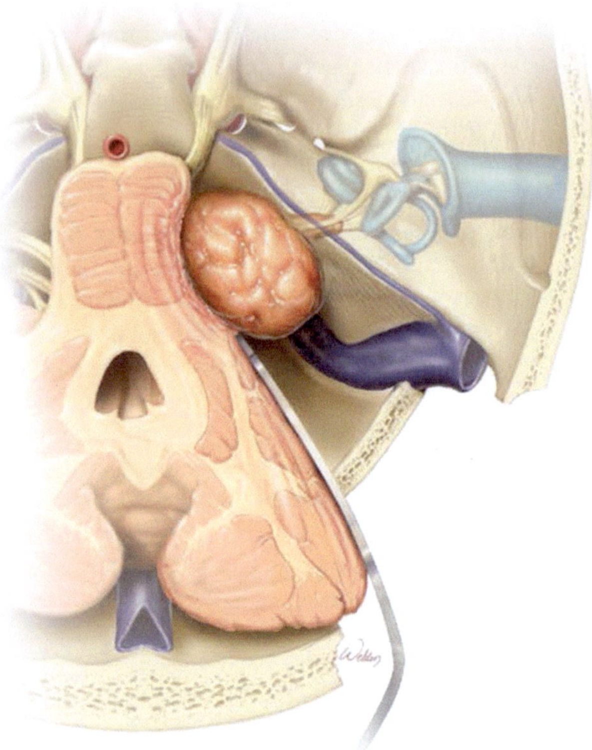

91. Overview of the bone to be removed (*gray*).

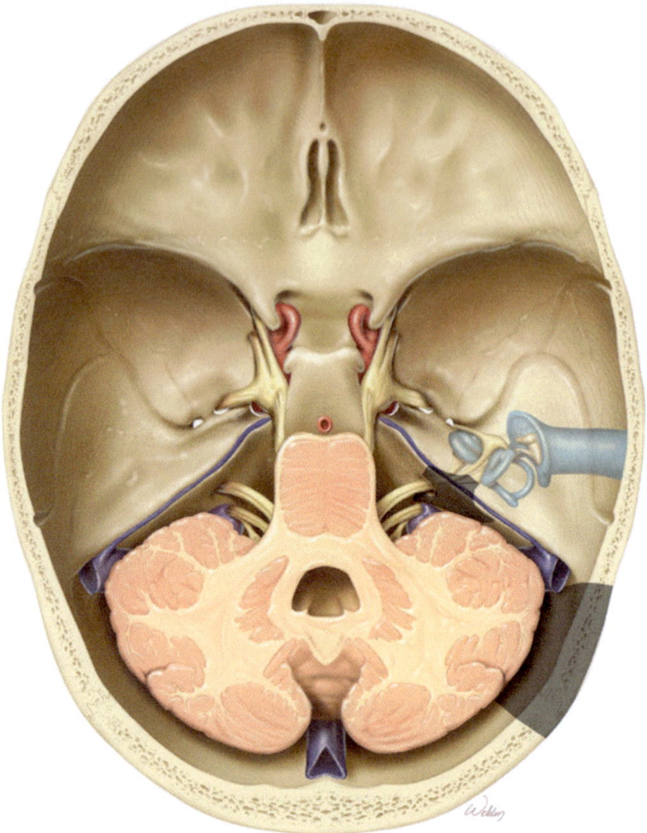

92. The incision for the retrosigmoid approach is ~3-4 cm behind the postauricular sulcus.

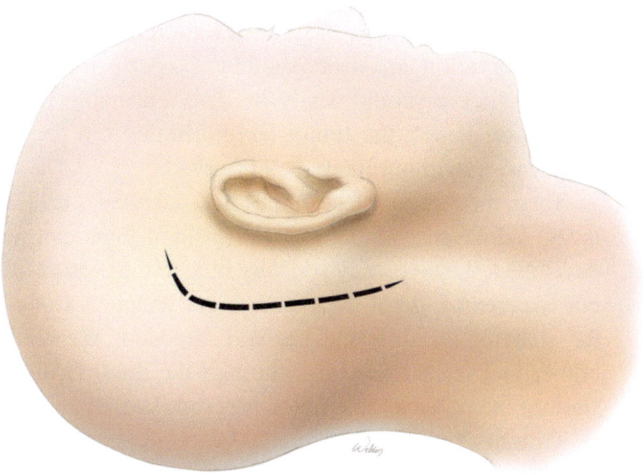

93. The periosteum is elevated off the skull and mastoid process. The muscles at the base of the skull are lifted off. Foramen magnum does not need to be identified, although some surgeons like to do this.

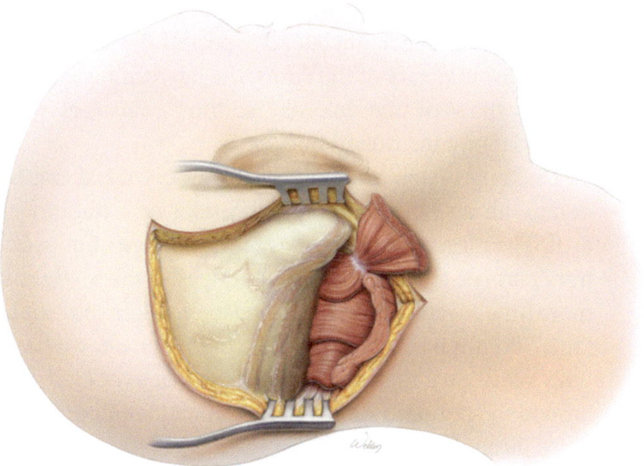

94. The sigmoid sinus (*SS*) and transverse sinus (*TS*) are identified using a drill. It is important to clearly see them and not just presume that you have found them in order to obtain adequate exposure. A bone flap can then be removed using a craniotome to expose the retrosigmoid dura. The skull is significantly thinner inferiorly compared to superiorly. Therefore, footplate of the craniotome needs to be angled appropriately while turning the flap to prevent tearing the dura inadvertently.

The dural opening is marked. It is important not to cut into the cerebellum accidentally when opening dura. We prefer to use a dural hook or Cushing forceps to elevate the dura while gently making an opening with a 15 blade scalpel. Once a small opening is made, scissors can be used to make the rest of the opening. Care should be taken that the dura is safely lifted away from the brain during this process.

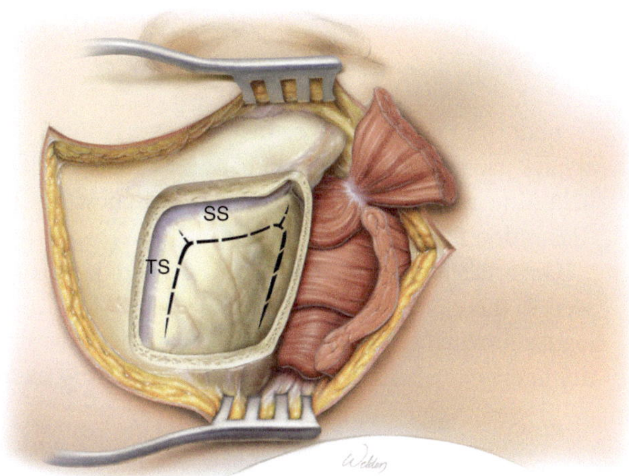

95. After opening the dura, the edges are sutured up. In particular, suturing the anterior and superior dural edges helps to prevent bleeding from the sigmoid and transverse sinuses.

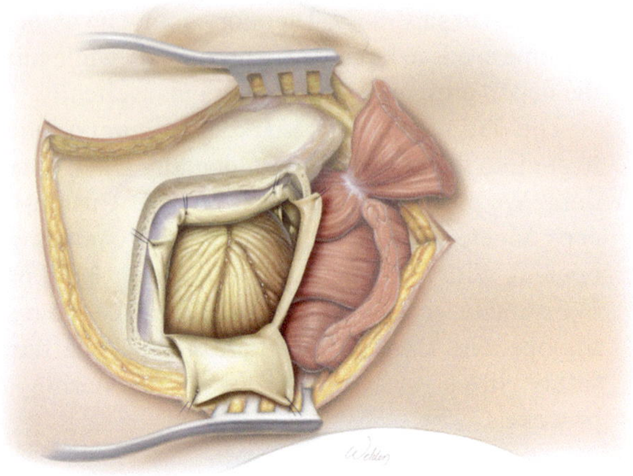

96. A malleable is used to retract the cerebellum. We always use a moist Telfa strip between it and the cerebellum to reduce trauma, but this is not shown in the illustration for simplicity.

Once the retractor is positioned, the tumor is easily seen. In this case, a vestibular scwhannoma is shown. The jugular foramen containing CN IX, X, and XI and the anterior inferior cerebellar artery (*AICA*) are also easily seen.

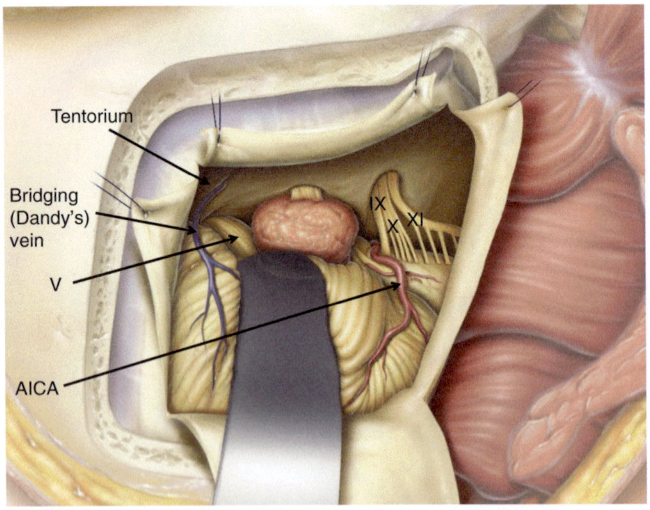

97. After verifying that the facial nerve is not in the way, a window is cut in the tumor and its core debulked.

The vestibular nerve medial to the tumor should be divided (as shown in the translabyrinthine approach) and the root entry zone of CN VII identified. If a hearing preservation approach is able to be performed, the cochlear nerve should easily be distinguishable from the tumor. If not, the tumor has infiltrated the nerve, and hearing will not likely be preserved.

Then, the posterior face of the temporal bone is drilled away. While all sorts of innovative dural flaps can be developed, they typically add very little to the closure. In our experience, dural flaps tend to get wrapped around the shaft of the drill and become shredded. We don't bother and instead just drill through the dura. Drilling starts at the porus acusticus and proceeds laterally.

Troughs (*arrows*) are created around the internal auditory canal just like with the translabyrinthine approach. The main risk is drilling into the posterior semicircular canal in a hearing preservation procedure, which can happen if drilling is continued too far laterally. Unfortunately, there are no great landmarks for determining this. Although theoretically the operculum and endolymphatic sac/duct can be identified and used to protect from entry into the labyrinth, it is often difficult to appreciate these structures through the dura. The MRI can be studied to estimate how much bone can be safely removed without entering the labyrinth. Typically, we just drill out the internal auditory canal so that we can reach the lateral aspect of the tumor, and in the vast majority of the cases, the labyrinth is spared.

The dura of the internal auditory canal is then opened along the dotted line.

Decompression of the internal auditory canal can be done with an ultrasonic bone aspirator or a traditional drill. The ultrasonic device has the advantage of no spinning parts or tendency to slip off edges. It takes slightly more time to remove the bone, and the existing ultrasonic "tips" do not provide the variety and precision we have with a drill. In either case, place large pieces of Gelfoam around the tumor to limit the dissemination of bone particles throughout the posterior fossa.

When we are attempting to preserve hearing, we focus on following the tumor capsule and leaving all vessels and nerve fibers behind (vestibular, cochlear, and of course facial). In contrast, if hearing is not an issue, we will resect all nerve fibers except the facial nerve. It is easier to precisely follow the facial nerve plane when the other fibers are not preserved. Debulking the tumor in the inferior part of the internal auditory canal will allow the remaining tumor to be rotated inferiorly away from the facial nerve. The tumor-nerve plane can be clearly seen and developed. Working in this direction prevents placing traction on the nerve.

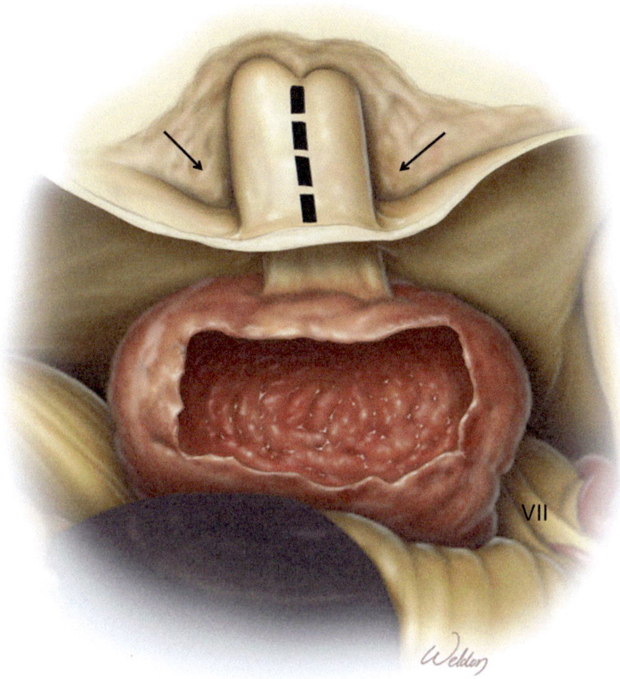

98. As with the translabyrinthine approach, the superior vestibular nerve (*SV*) and inferior vestibular nerve (*IV*) are divided and the lateral aspect of the tumor microdissected off the facial nerve (*F*) and cochlear nerve (*C*). Sharp dissection is often needed to stay in the proper plane between the facial nerve and the tumor. To do this, we typically use Rhoton 1, 2, and 3 dissectors.

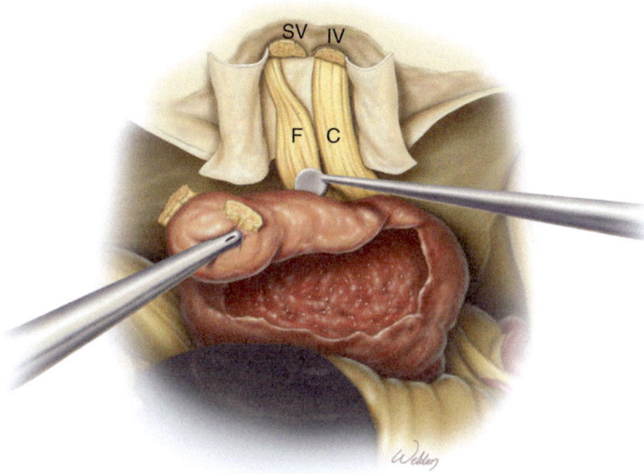

99. Occasionally, drilling of the internal auditory canal does not proceed far enough to visualize the lateral aspect of the tumor. Angled microcuretes are used to reach into the superior and vestibular nerve canals and scoop out residual tumor (*inset*). The fundus is easily palpable so you can tell when you have adequately cleaned out these areas. A mirror or endoscope is helpful in assessing for additional tumor that is not directly visible.

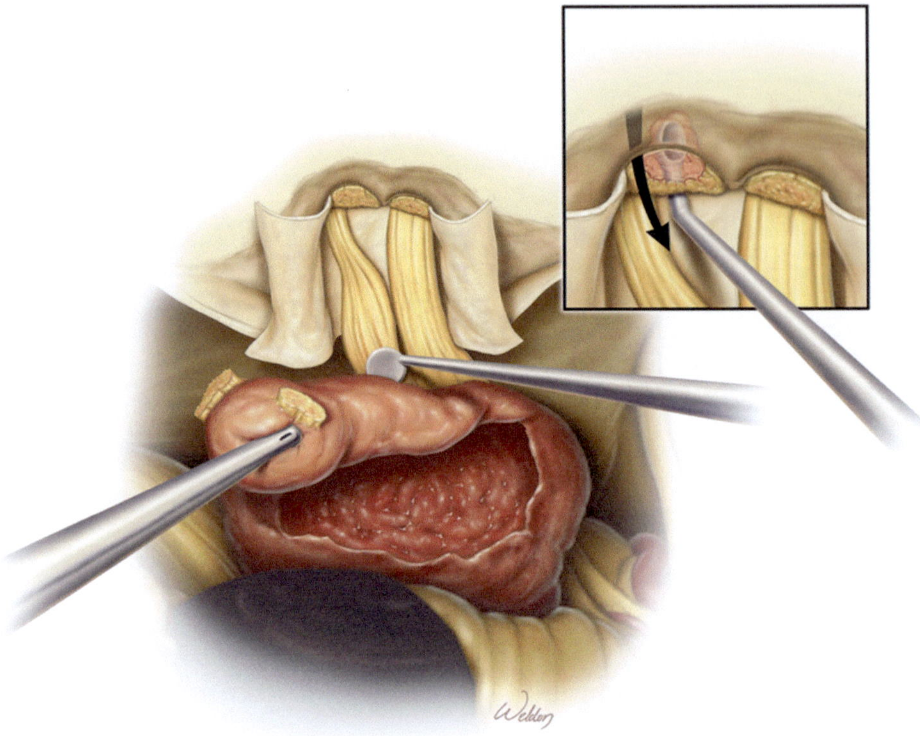

100. Case 1. Axial MRI with gadolinium demonstrated a small right posterior fossa tumor (*arrow*) in a patient with serviceable hearing. There was reduced enhancement within the anterior portion of the tumor. The dura of the posterior internal auditory canal demonstrated enhancement.

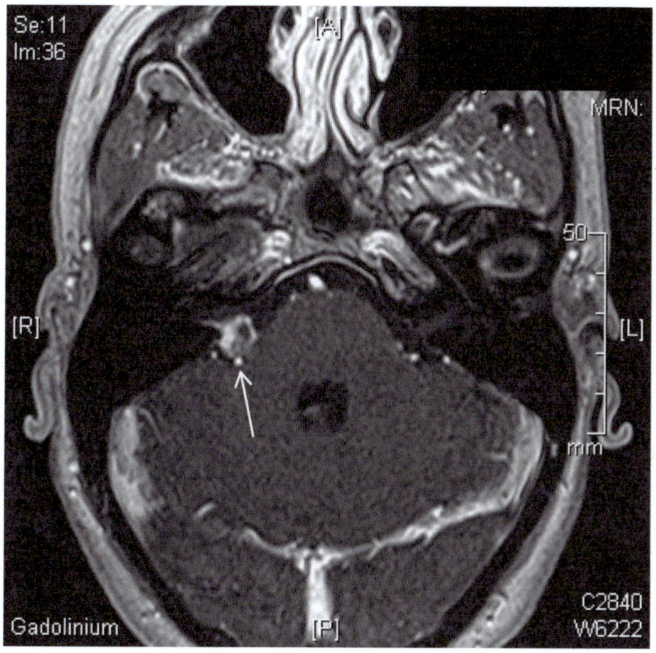

101. A lower cut revealed that most of the tumor did not enhance.

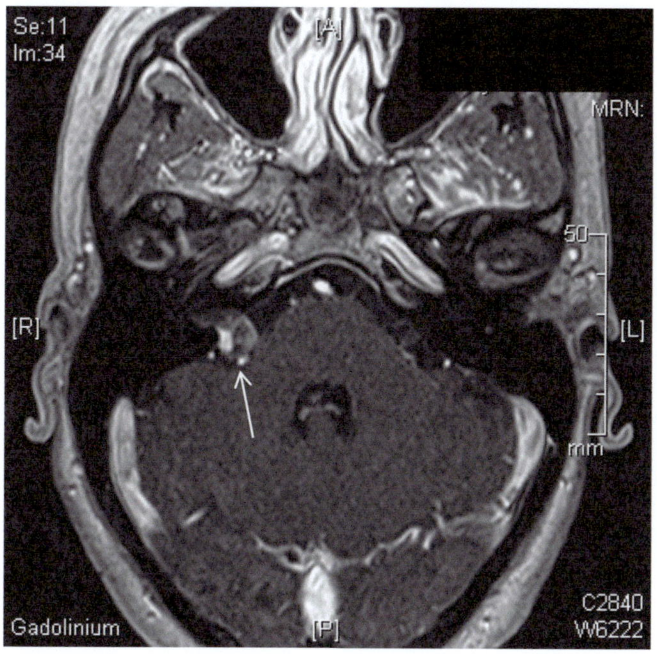

102. T2 MRI revealed that the tumor was solid, not cystic, and based over the posterior lip of the porus acusticus. It did not extend all the way to the fundus of the internal auditory canal. The differential diagnosis was vestibular schwannoma versus meningioma. Because of the good hearing and the lack of a significant internal auditory canal component, the retrosigmoid approach was chosen. In the end, the pathology demonstrated that this was a vestibular schwannoma.

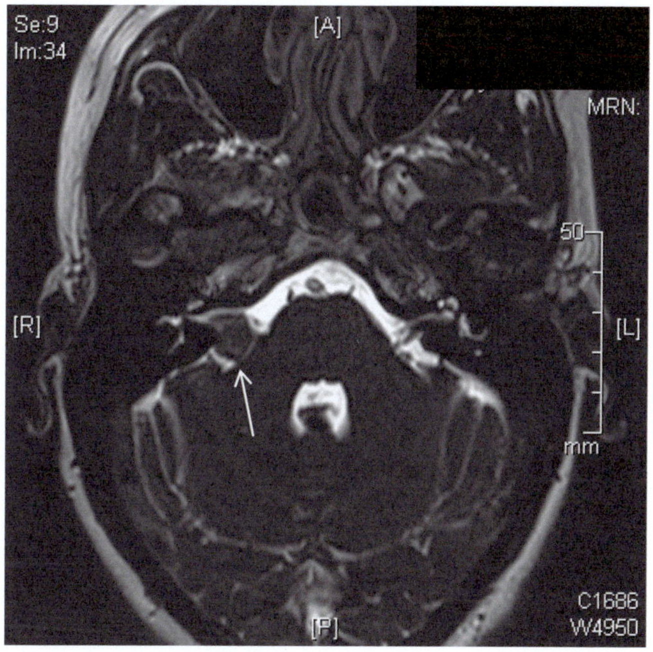

103. The right mastoid was exposed and the sigmoid sinus (*SS*) – transverse sinus (*TS*) junction identified.

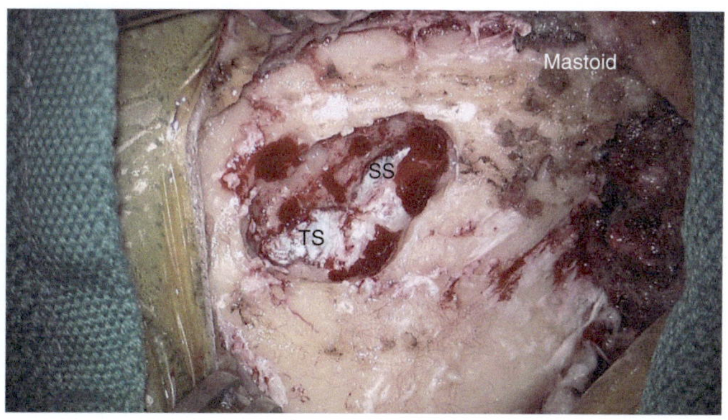

104. The outline of the bone flap to be removed is shown.

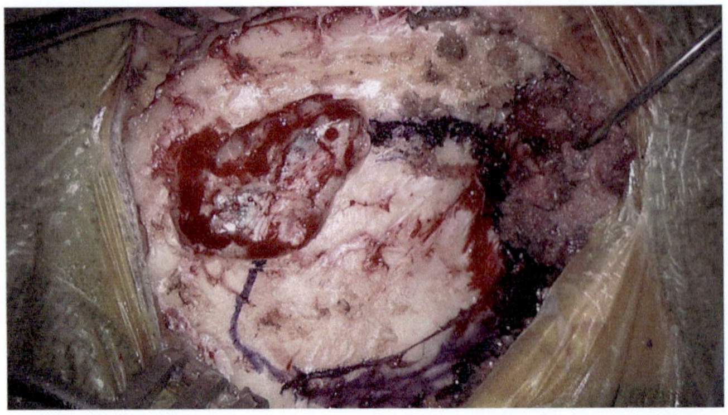

105. After removing the bone flap, the retrosigmoid dura was exposed. Note that the sigmoid sinus (*SS*) was left covered with bone. Transverse sinus (*TS*).

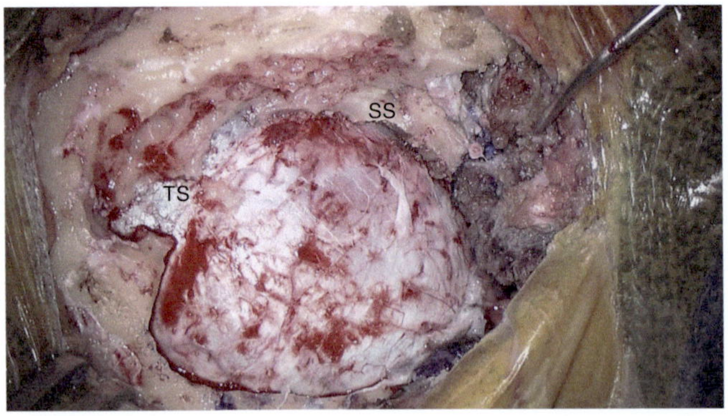

106. Bone wax was applied to the mastoid air cells. It is a good policy to wax on the way in and again on the way out in order to reduce the risk of cerebrospinal fluid leak.

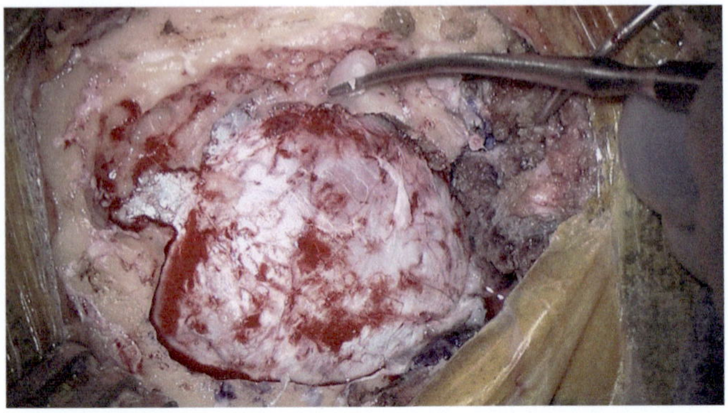

107. At the inferior aspect of the craniotomy, rongeurs were used to remove the thin bone in order to achieve an adequate exposure.

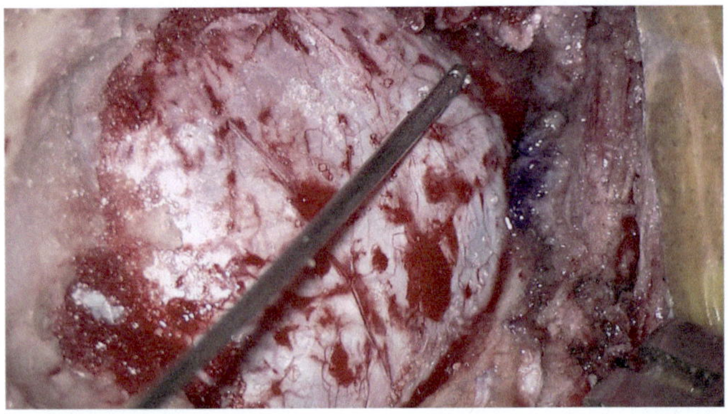

108. The dura was then opened posterior to the sigmoid sinus. In this example, a Y-shaped dural opening was performed. Note how the cerebellum was pushing out. This is typical and should be controlled by releasing CSF from cisterna magna, which lies inferior to the cerebellum.

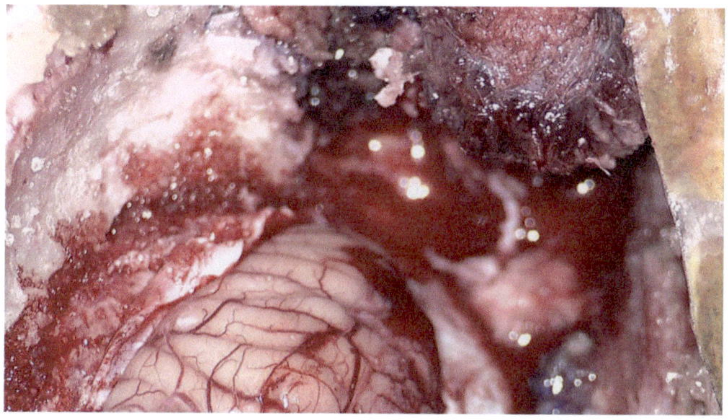

109. The first step in opening cisterna magna is to use a malleable to retract the lower pole of the cerebellum.

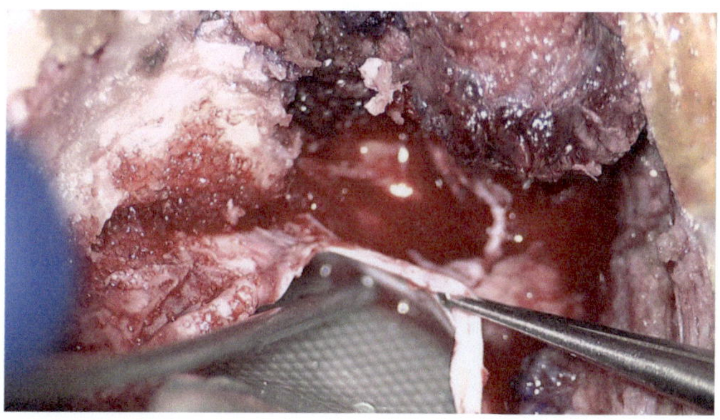

110. The arachnoid encompassing cisterna magna can then be visualized (*arrow*). By opening this up with a Rhoton or Penfield dissector, rapid release of cerebrospinal fluid was achieved.

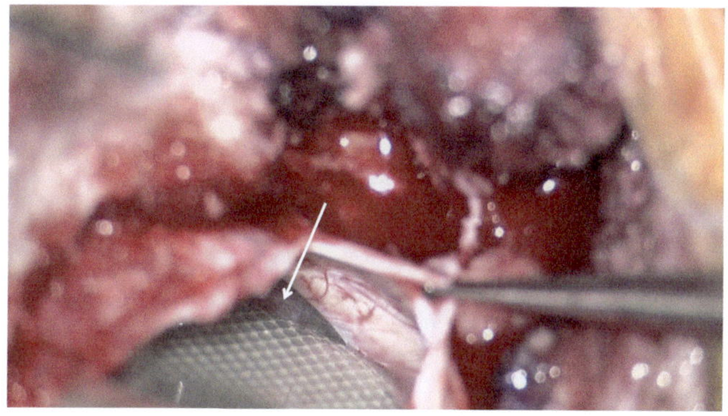

111. Once cerebrospinal fluid release was performed, the cerebellum no longer expanded out through the dural opening. Note that an Adaptic strip was used on the brain for protection. This works as well as a Telfa strip. The dural flaps were sutured up to expose the posterior fossa and to protect the sigmoid and transverse sinuses.

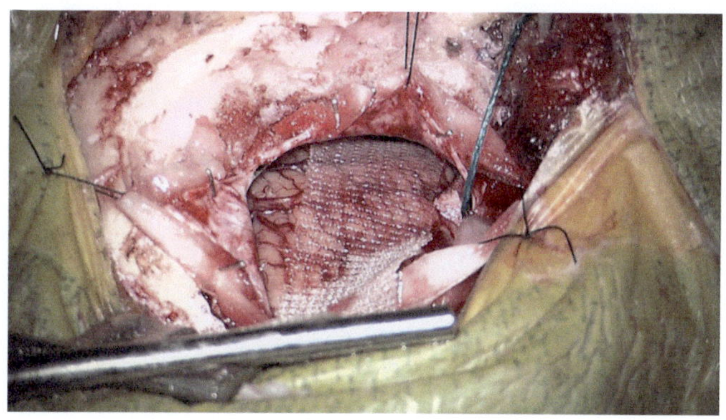

112. Gentle retraction of the cerebellum was then performed to follow the posterior face of the temporal bone and find the tumor at the porus acusticus.

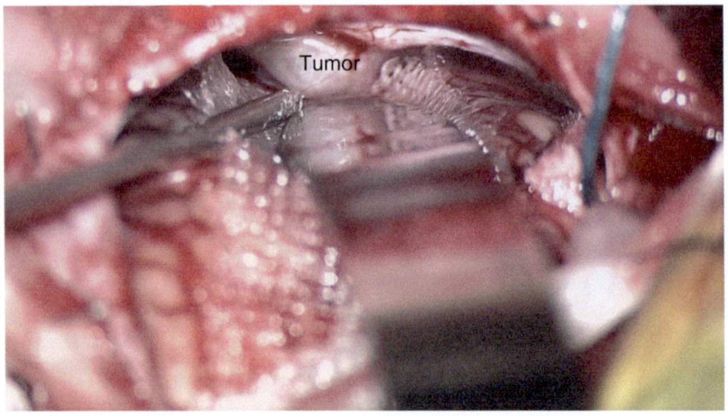

113. There was arachnoid mater bridging between the cerebellum and the tumor that needed to be divided. A large cerebellar vein was visible.

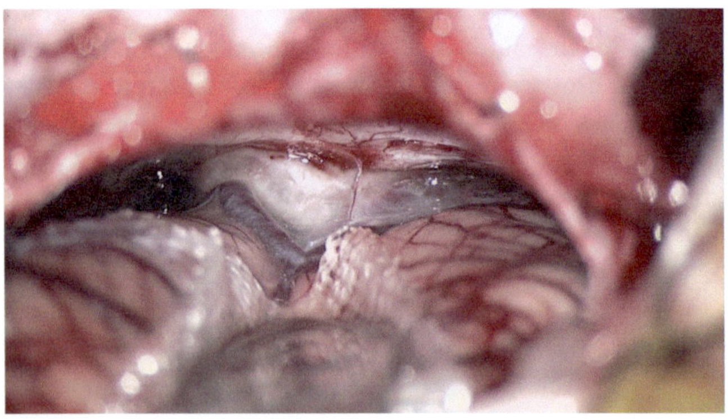

114. Dividing the arachnoid should be performed as closely to the tumor as possible in order to minimize the trauma to vessels feeding the brain. The importance of various small veins and branches of arteries is impossible to discern. Every effort should be made to meticulously dissect these free from the tumor surface. This starts with dissecting in the correct plane between the tumor capsule and arachnoid. Only coagulate and sharply divide vessels directly supplying the tumor.

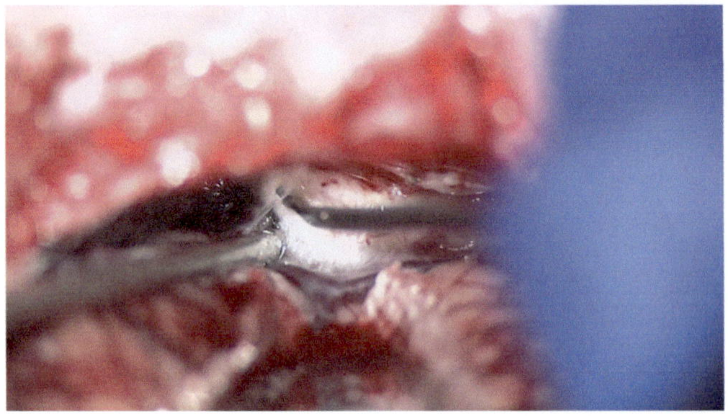

115. The superior pole of the tumor was partially dissected.

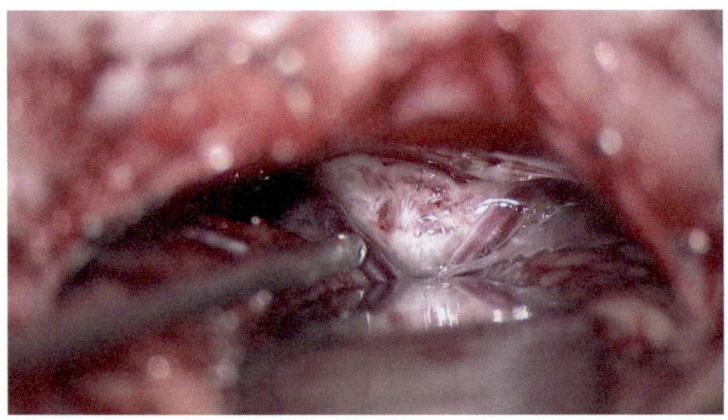

116. A nerve stimulator is used to probe the face of the tumor to see if the facial nerve is present. We typically use a Yingling stimulator probe because it has a flexible tip. This minimizes trauma to the facial nerve.

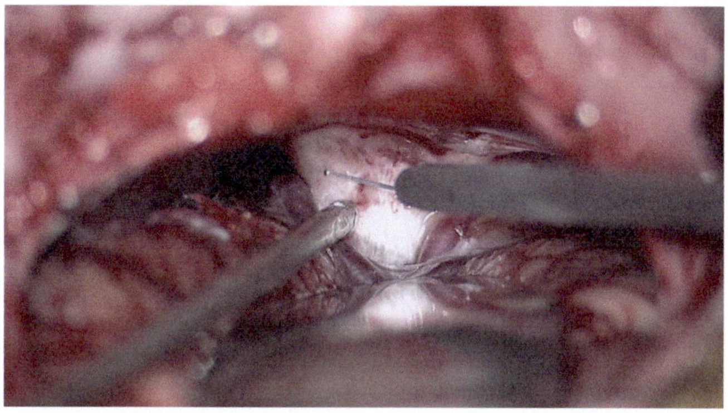

117. Continuing to dissect the arachnoid off the tumor. A Rhoton #6 dissector was being used for blunt dissection in this image, although sharp dissection with Rhoton #2 or #3 dissectors also works well.

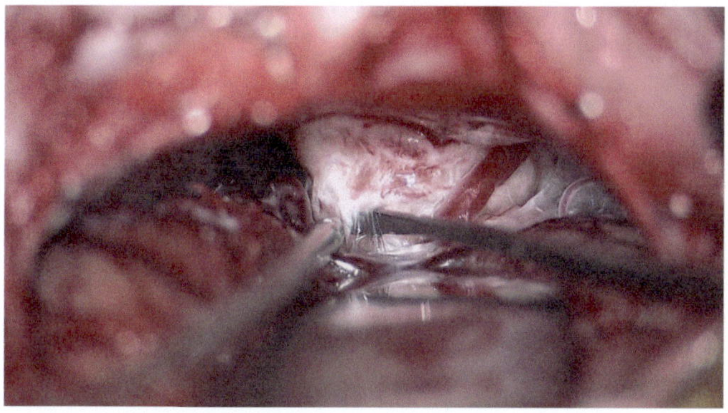

118. Vessels within the capsule of the tumor can be cauterized with the bipolar. An irrigating bipolar minimizes heat transfer to surrounding normal tissues.

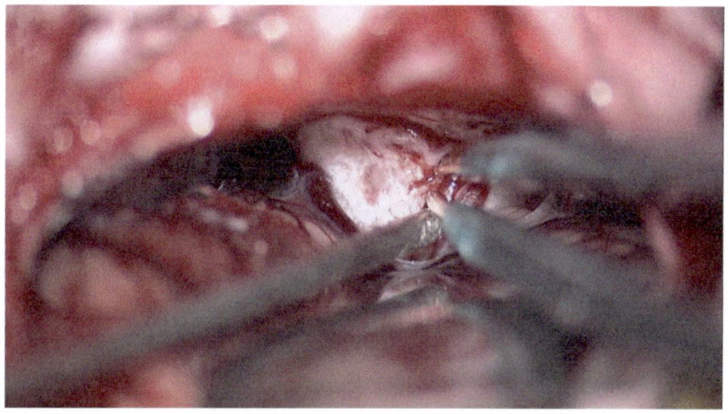

119. The posterior face of the tumor was visualized. There were vessels both superior and inferior to the tumor.

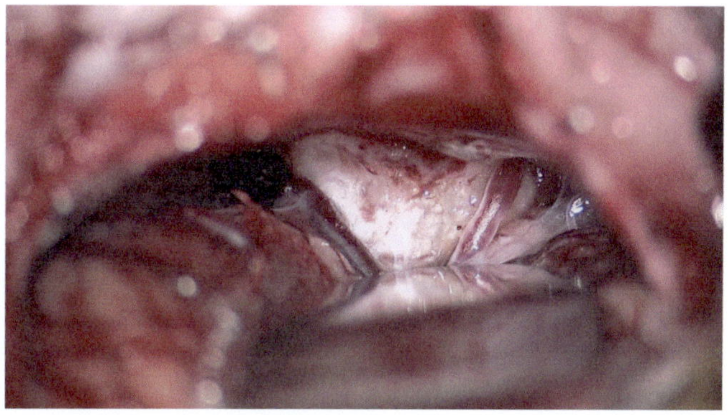

120. An 11 blade scalpel was used to incise the capsule.

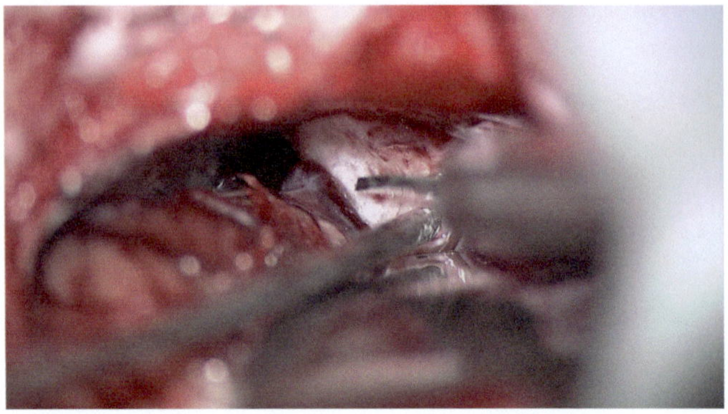

121. Curved microscissors were used to remove a section of the posterior tumor capsule. Care must be taken so as to not lose the interface between the tumor and the cerebellum. An edge of the tumor capsule should always be maintained. This is helpful in maintaining the proper plane of dissection.

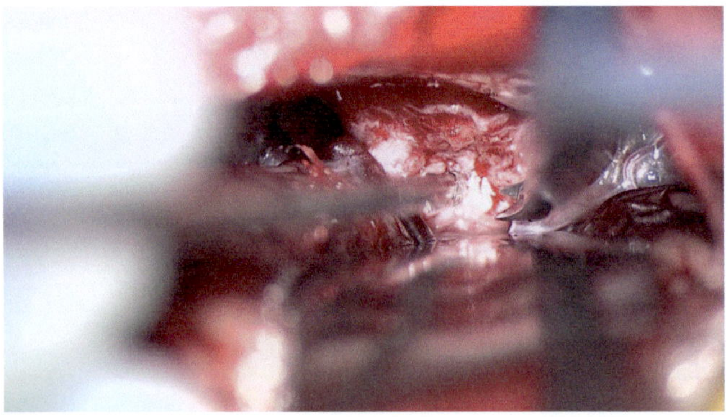

122. After partial debulking, the superior face of the tumor could be mobilized to expose the deeper structures. Here, the nerve stimulator was on the motor branch of CN V. The larger sensory branch can be seen directly to the right of the stimulator probe.

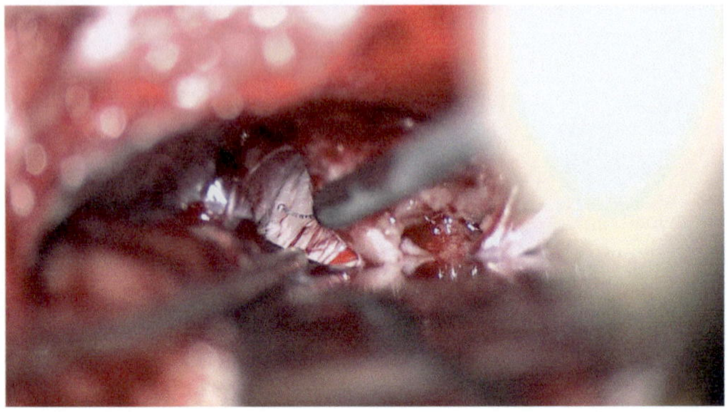

123. With further debulking, the medial face of the tumor could be collapsed inward, separating much of the tumor from the brainstem.

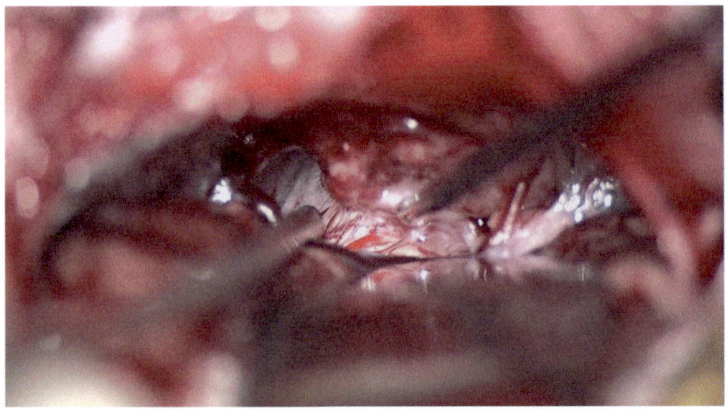

124. The inferior capsule of the tumor was then dissected off the vessels and arachnoid around the cerebellar peduncle.

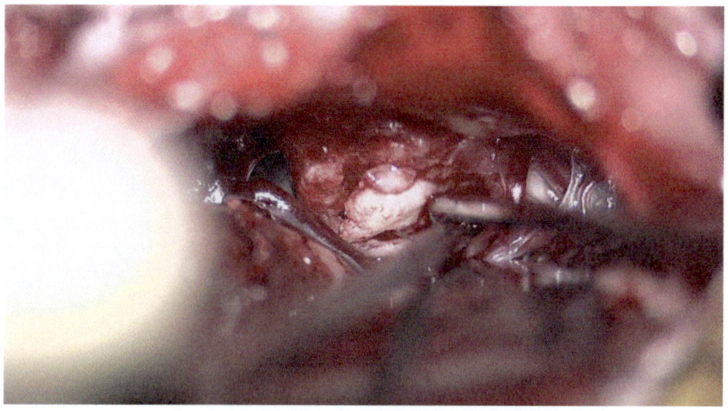

125. Attention was then turned to the lateral aspect of the tumor. Gelfoam was placed on the brainstem to protect it and a right angle probe used to identify the porus acusticus (*PA*).

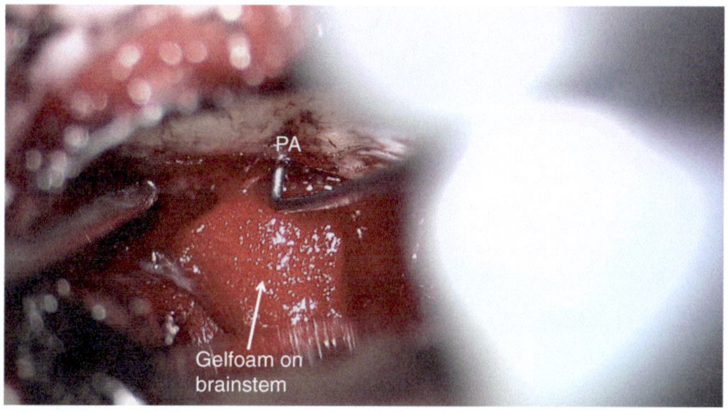

126. A cutting burr was used to begin drilling away the posterior face of the temporal bone. Diamond burrs were used when the drilling proceeded deeper.

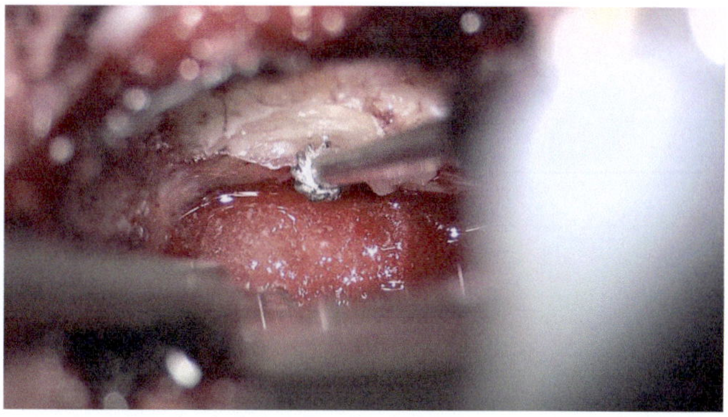

127. A superior trough (*ST*) and inferior trough (*IT*) were drilled, and about half the distance of the internal auditory canal was opened. This was all that was needed for this patient because the lateral aspect of the tumor could be seen (*arrow*).

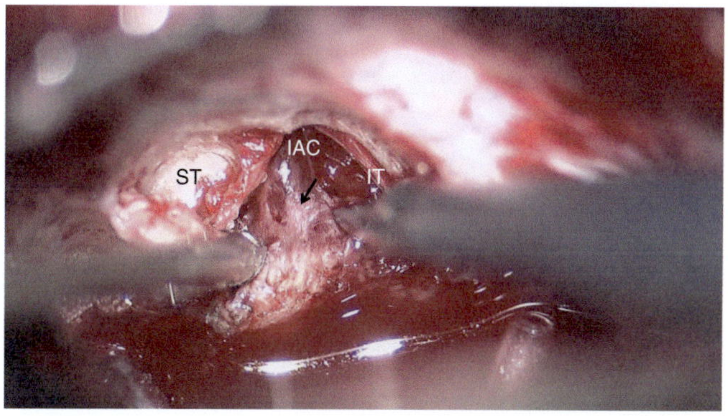

128. The lateral aspect of the tumor was elevated off the underlying nerves. In this example, the individual nerves were not visible because they are contained within their own arachnoid. This made hearing preservation possible. If the auditory nerve is infiltrated with tumor, there is no way to preserve hearing.

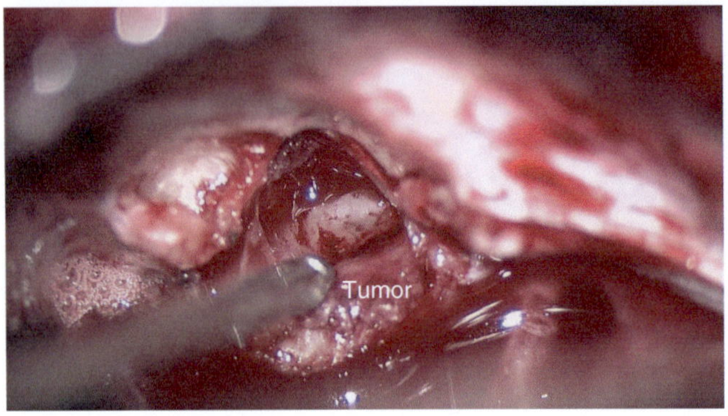

129. The tumor was then rotated superiorly to separate it from the auditory and facial nerves.

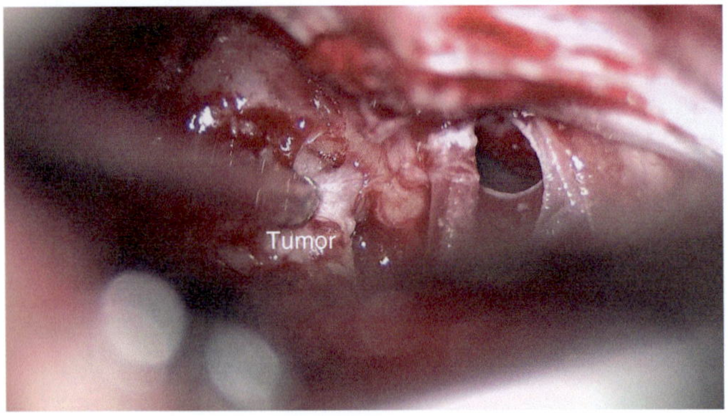

130. After total tumor removal. The remaining tissue was the auditory and facial nerves contained within their arachnoid (*tissue between arrows*).

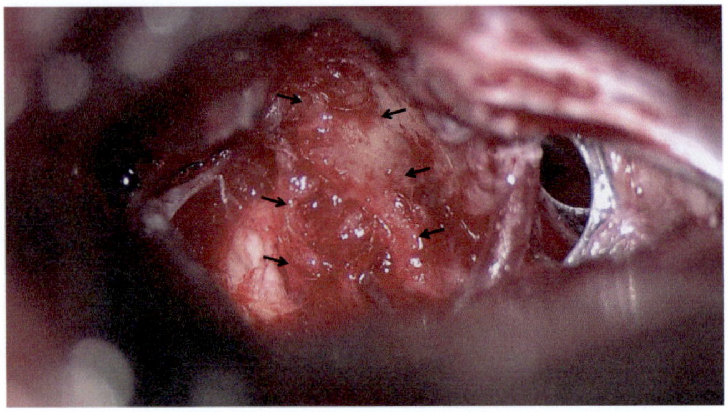

131. Bone wax was applied to the drilled-out areas of the temporal bone to help prevent cerebrospinal fluid leak.

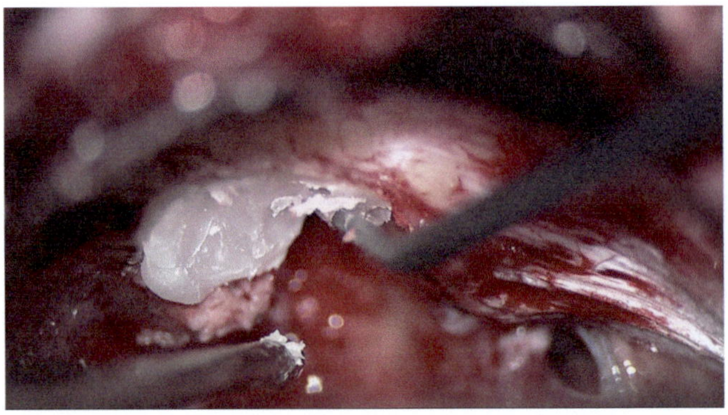

132. After removing the retractor, the cerebellum relaxed. The extent of the drilled-out area around the internal auditory canal can be appreciated.

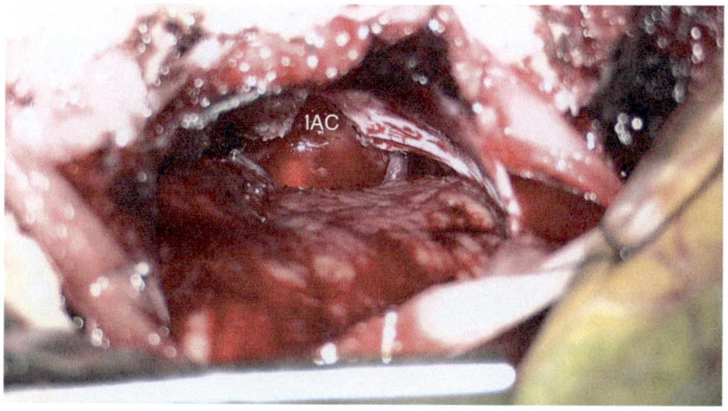

133. In this example, a layer of Surgicel (*arrow*) was placed directly on the cerebellum to aid hemostasis. Interrupted sutures were used to close as much of the dura primarily as possible.

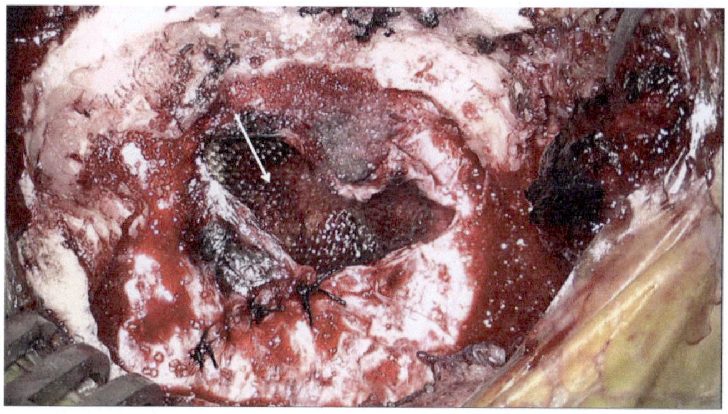

134. A dural patch was then used to close the rest of the opening.

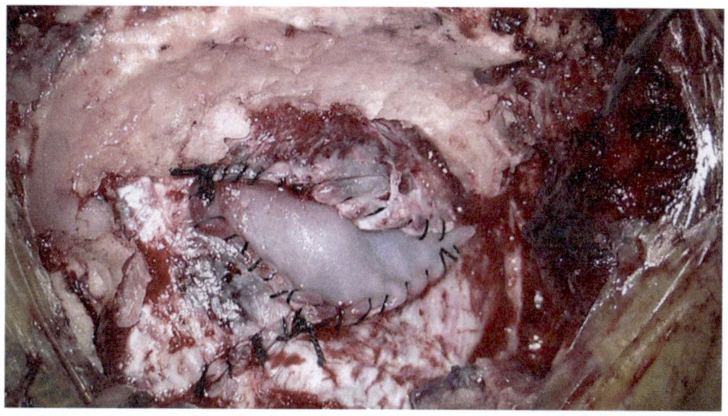

135. Tisseal was applied to help form a watertight closure.

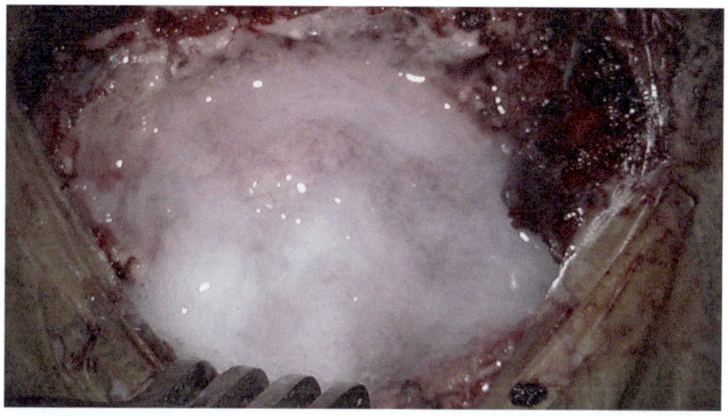

136. The bone flap was plated back in place, with burr-hole covers used to bridge the gap at the transverse-sigmoid junction.

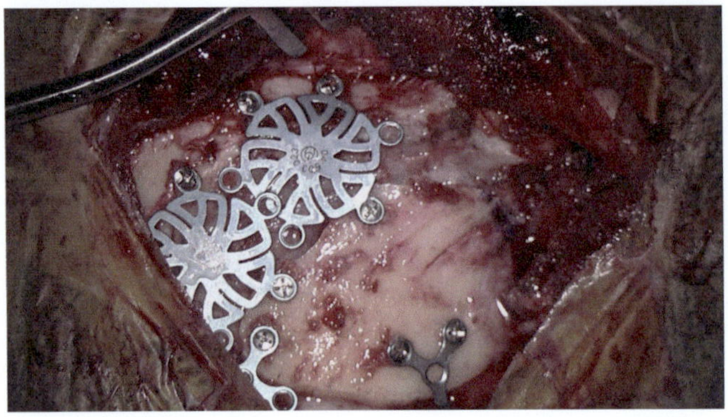

137. Immediate post-op MRI demonstrated complete tumor removal. There was no change in hearing, and facial nerve function was normal.

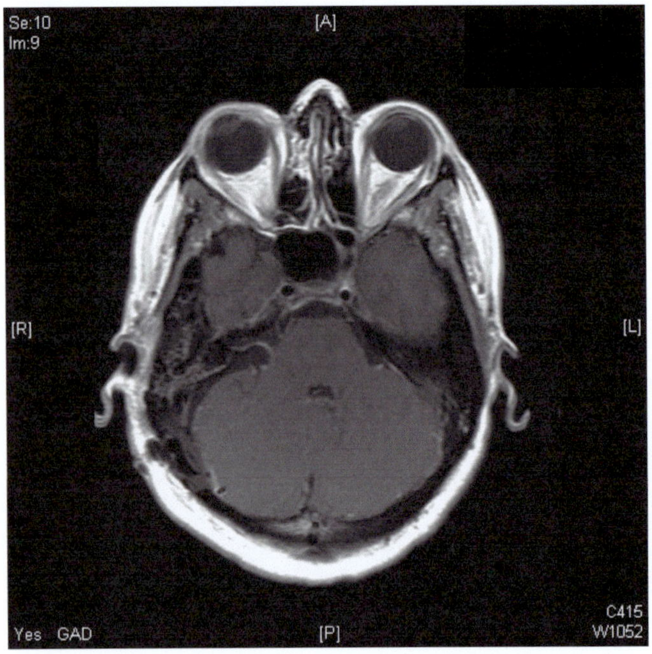

138. T2 MRI highlights the amount of bone removed around the internal auditory canal (*arrow*). Notice how much additional bone could be removed before entering the posterior semicircular canal.

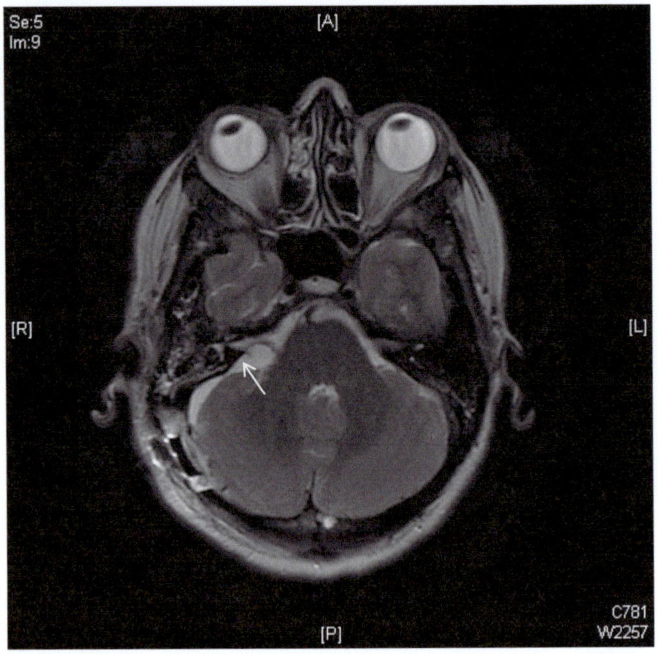

139. Case 2. A 1.8 cm right vestibular schwannoma that was removed via the retrosigmoid approach. After opening the dura and releasing CSF, the tumor was exposed. A piece of Gelfoam was placed on top of a small bleeding vessel on the posterior surface of the tumor.

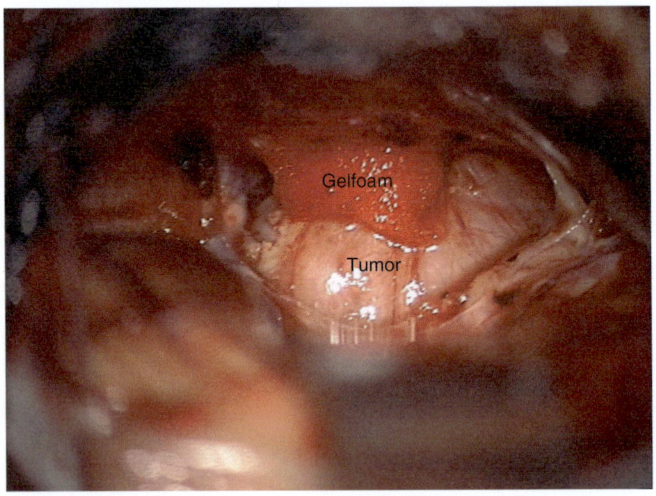

140. After partial debulking, the inferior pole of the tumor was mobilized. The jugular foramen nerves (CN IX, X, and XI) can be seen.

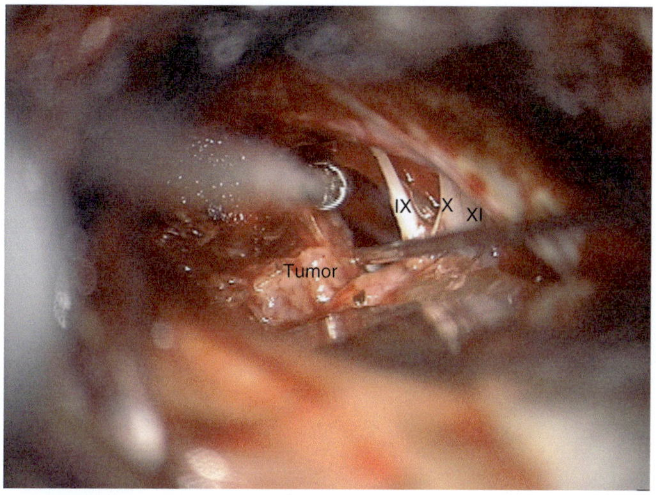

141. Deep to the superior pole of the tumor, CN V was visible.

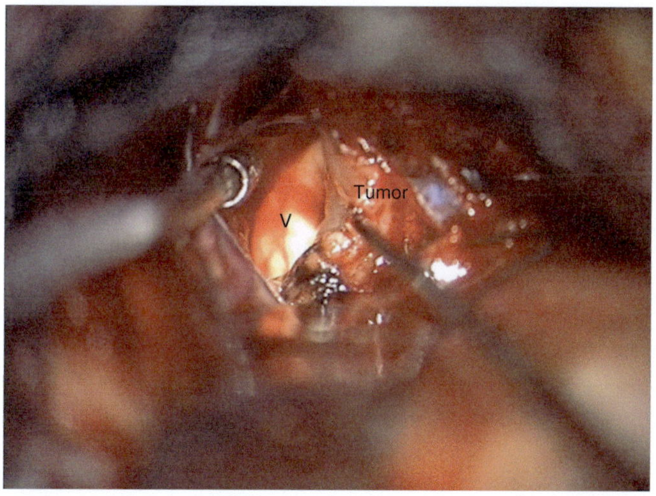

142. After drilling the temporal bone to expose the internal auditory canal (*IAC*). The tumor extended quite laterally.

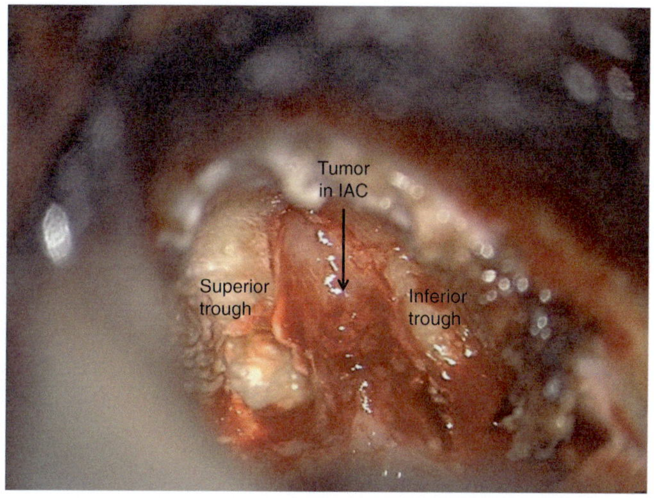

143. The lateral aspect of the tumor was microdissected out of the internal auditory canal and the cochlear nerve (*C*) and facial nerve (*F*) left down.

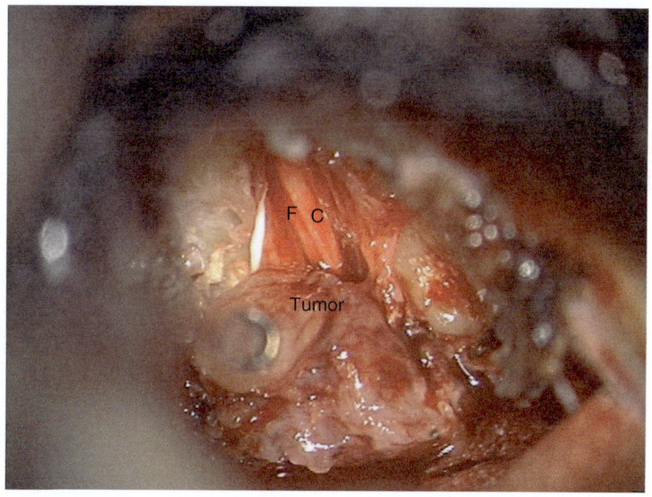

144. During tumor removal, the cochlear nerve was found to be infiltrated by tumor near the porus acusticus and was sacrificed (*arrow*). The facial nerve (*F*) was intact and covered in arachnoid within the cerebellopontine angle.

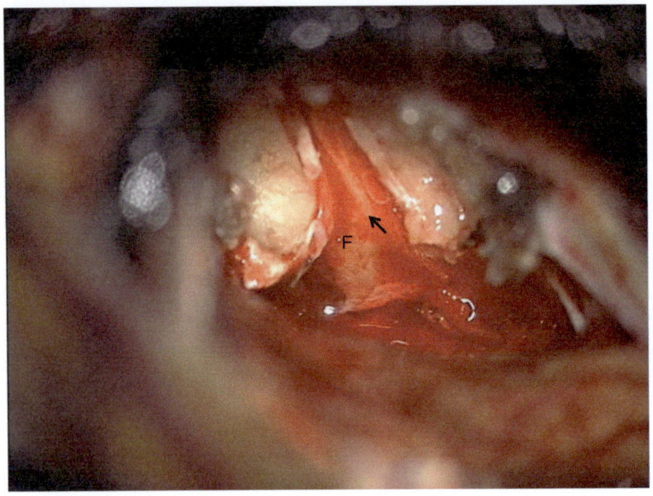

145. Case 3. Axial MRI of a left vestibular schwannoma.

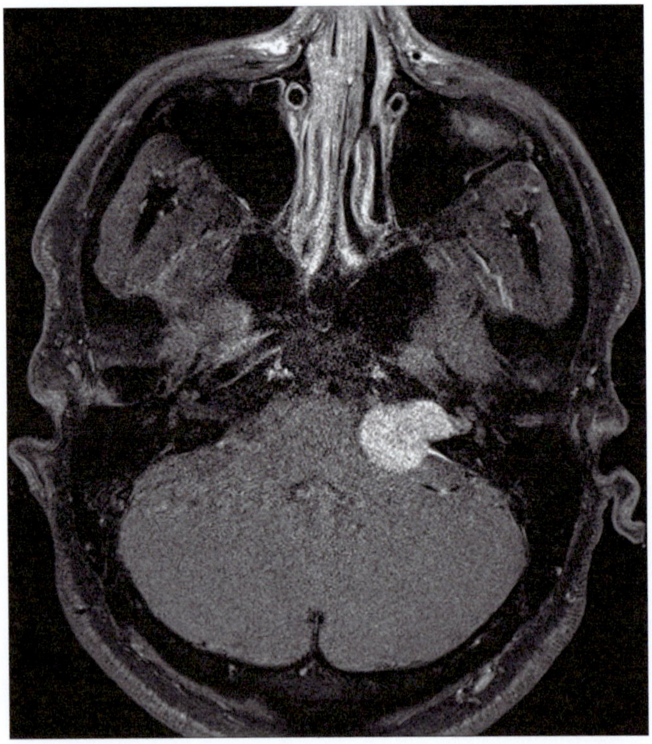

146. T2 MRI demonstrates cerebrospinal fluid at the fundus of the internal auditory canal (*arrow*). This makes direct visualization of the distal end of the tumor and hearing preservation more likely. Tumors that extend to the fundus require more drilling for exposure and are associated with a higher risk of hearing loss and leaving residual tumor.

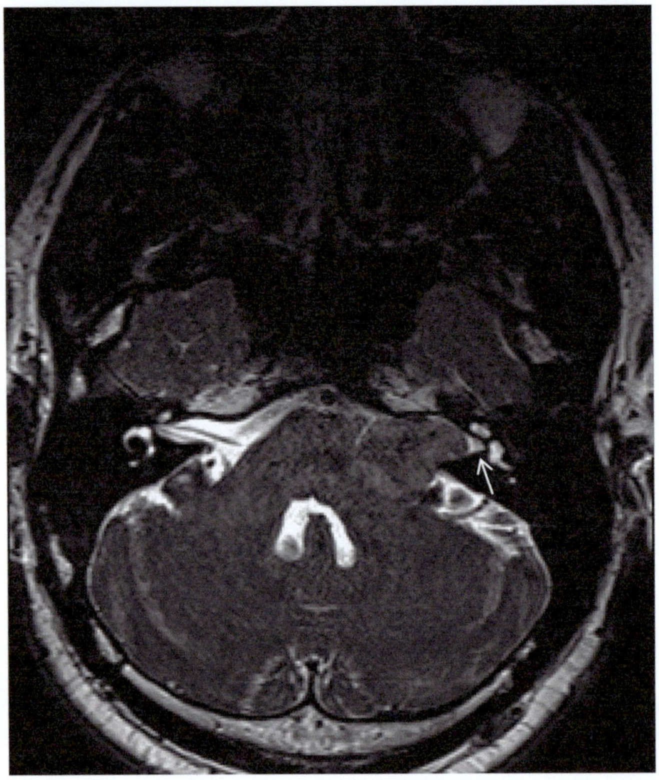

147. Post-op MRI demonstrating complete tumor resection after retrosigmoid craniotomy.

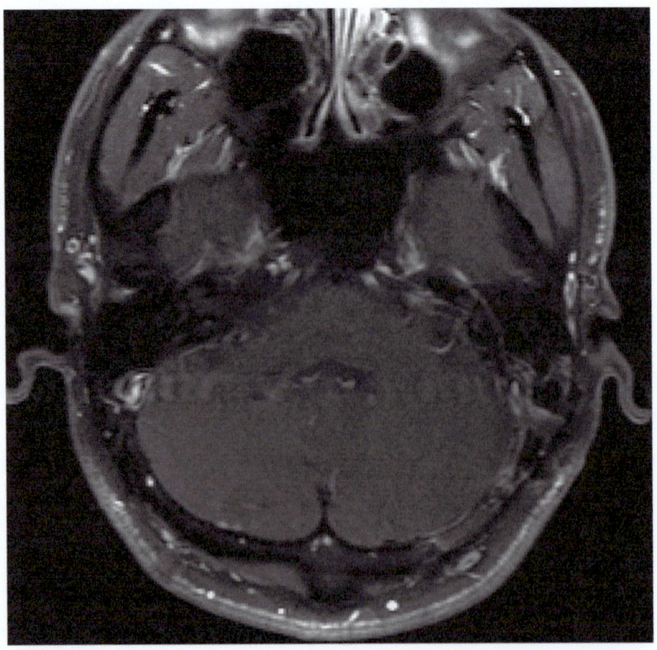

148. Post-op T2 MRI demonstrates the amount of bone removed to expose the length of the internal auditory canal (*arrow*). Almost the entire length was exposed. This is a good example of how anatomy varies between patients. It is commonly stated that the fundus of the internal auditory canal cannot be directly visualized through the retrosigmoid approach and that tumor resection requires some blind dissection. This case illustrates that not only can it be exposed but that it can even be done in some cases without entering the labyrinth, allowing the possibility of hearing preservation. The fundus can be fully exposed in all cases, but most often, this will require opening into the labyrinth. When hearing preservation is not a goal, the dissection should be carried far enough laterally to assure complete tumor removal even if this results in entering the vestibule or posterior semicircular canal.

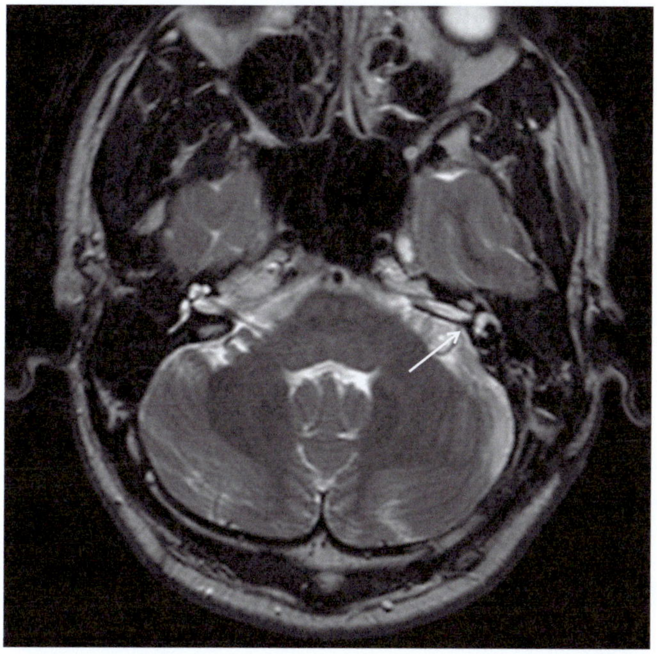

149. Case 4. Axial MRI with gadolinium of a patient with a large posterior fossa meningioma.

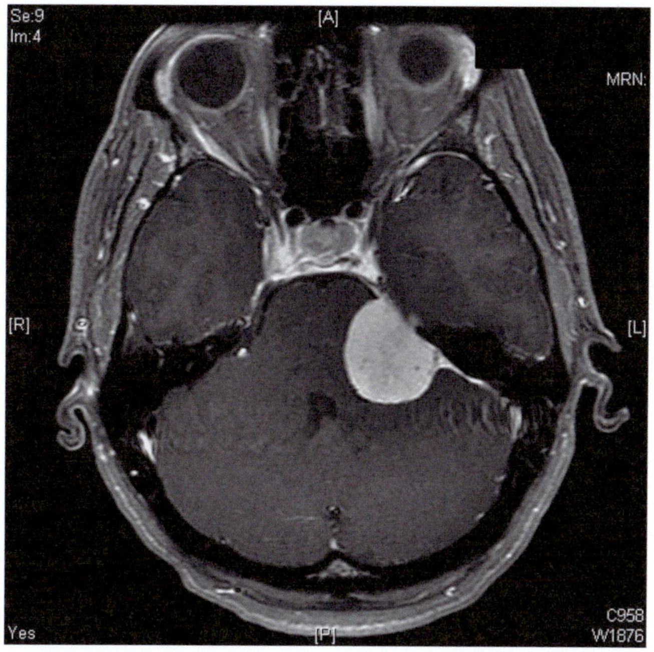

150. Coronal imaging demonstrated that this tumor was based from the tentorium. This tumor could thus be expected to be pushing CN VII and VIII inferiorly.

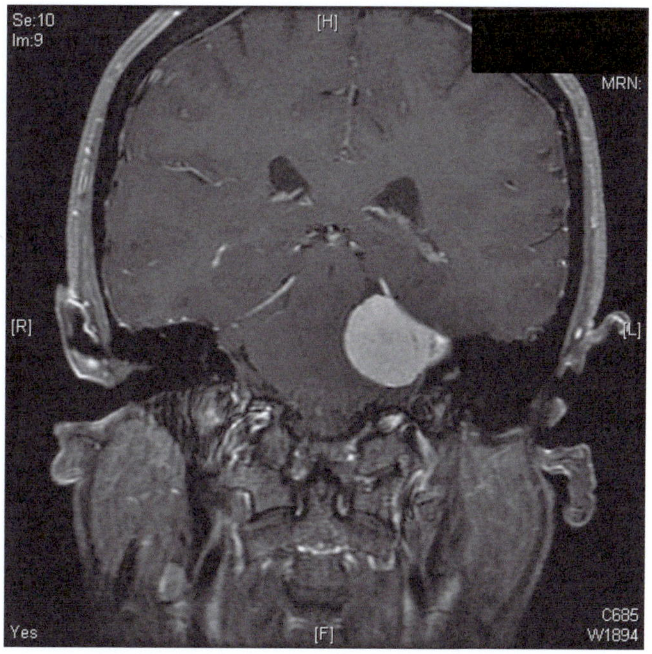

151. T2 MRI demonstrated minimal extension into the internal auditory canal. The retrosigmoid approach was chosen to resect this tumor. The retrosigmoid approach provides the most expeditious exposure and ability to preserve hearing and balance function. Regardless of tumor size, the facial and cochlear nerves can typically be easily separated from meningiomas.

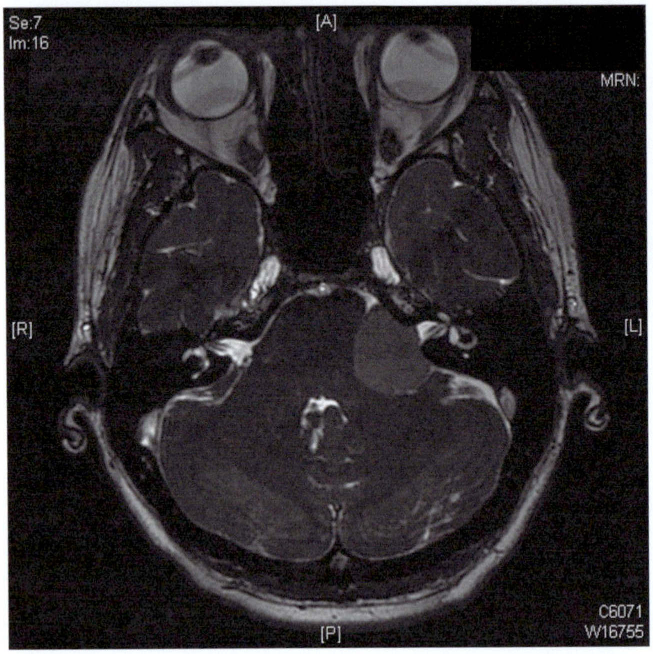

152. Post-op MRI demonstrated near-complete tumor removal. The enhancement of the dura along the left clivus may represent residual tumor infiltration (*arrow*). It is difficult to remove all tumor from a patient with a large meningioma because of this type of dural infiltration. However, not all dural enhancement represents residual tumor nor do all small remnants result in recurrence.

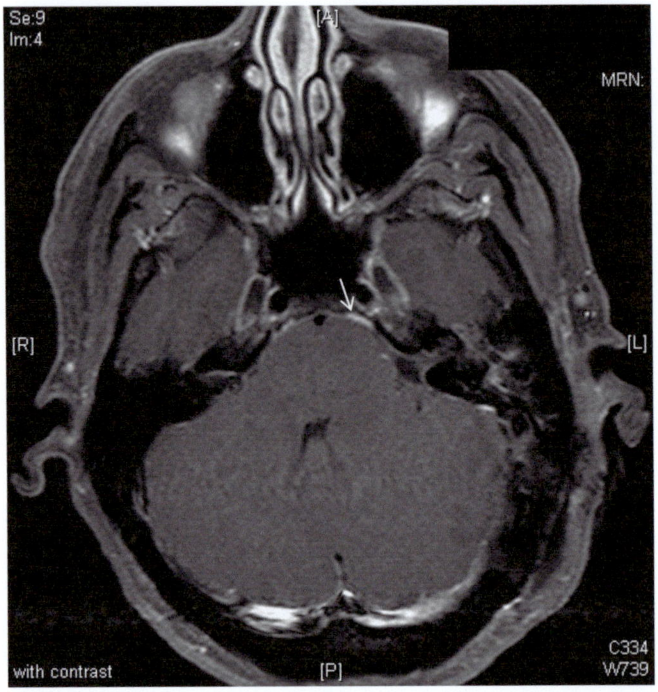

153. Case 5. An epidermoid of the left posterior fossa that was compressing the brainstem (*arrow*). It had CSF density on T1 MRI.

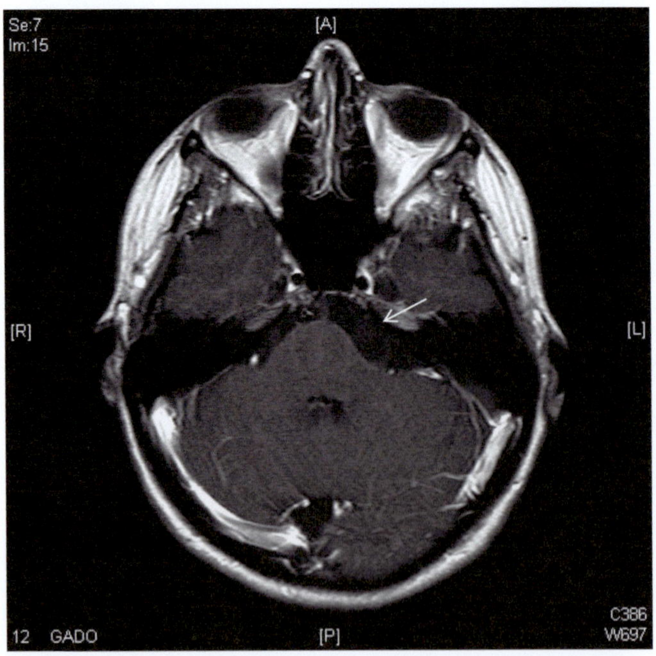

154. T2 MRI demonstrated similar findings (*arrow*).

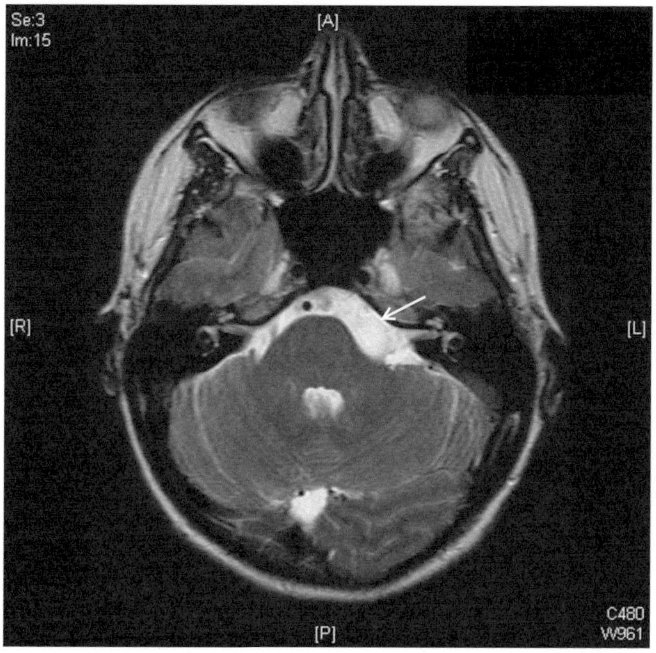

155. Flair imaging demonstrated that the lesion had brain density (*arrow*). Unfortunately, no diffusion-weighting images were performed. However, this lesion would be bright on diffusion weighting. For an example of this, please see Chap. 5.

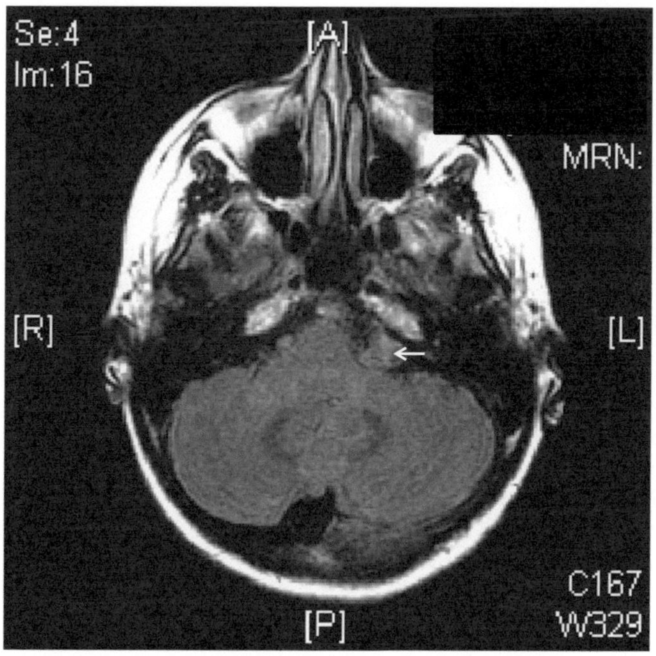

156. Post-op T2 MRI. After resection via the retrosigmoid approach, the brainstem compression was relieved.

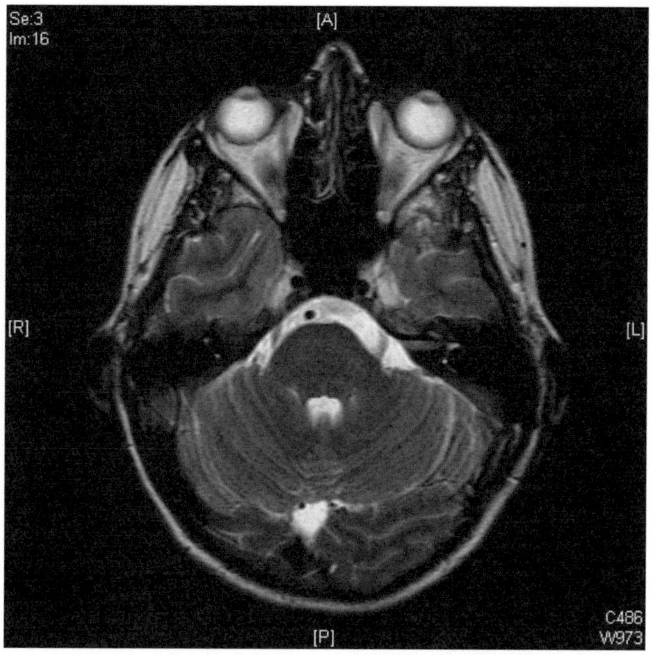

157. Post-op flair imaging demonstrated reduction in the size of the epidermoid. It may be impossible to remove all the lining of epidermoids like this because it is adherent to the vessels and cranial nerves. However, substantial debulking of the mass to relieve brain compression is relatively easy to achieve.

Conventional wisdom states that we cannot cure epidermoid tumors, but this is not true, particularly in the case of smaller lesions and those in more favorable locations. During cholesteatoma surgery, otologists routinely remove squamous epithelium from delicate structures in the ear such as the facial nerve, the stapes footplate, or the endosteum of a lateral canal fistula. The same meticulous dissection techniques can be applied intracranially. Patience, irrigation, small suctions, and microhooks can result in cure. The first operation is the best opportunity to achieve complete removal. If entire lesions are not curable, it may be possible to at least "clear" some areas of disease and thus decrease long-term risk to structures in those areas.

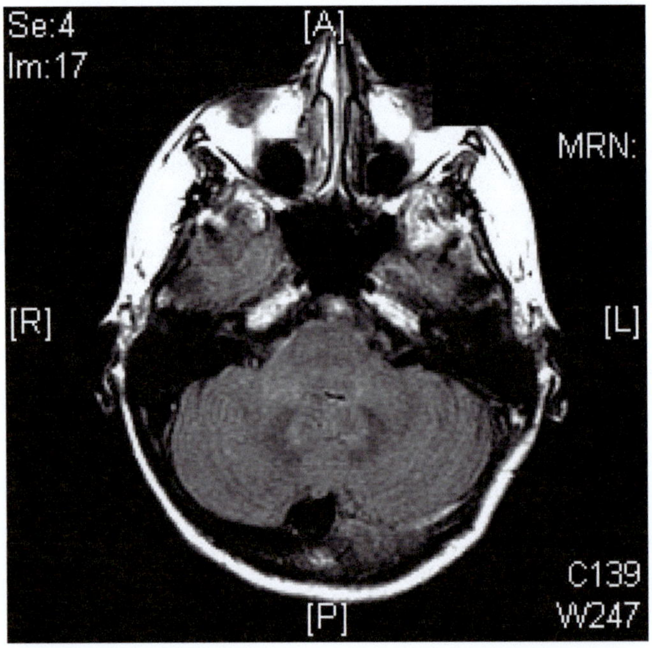

Far Lateral Approach

- *Concept*
  - The far lateral approach begins as the retrosigmoid approach, but the craniotomy is extended inferiorly to open foramen magnum and expose the cervical spinal cord.
- *Conditions treated*
  - Tumors involving foramen magnum or upper cervical spinal cord such as meningiomas
  - Hypoglossal nerve schwannomas with intracranial disease
- *Risks*
  - Brainstem or cervical spinal cord injury producing dysmetria or paralysis
  - Dysphagia, possibly with aspiration
  - Vocal cord paralysis
  - Hearing loss
  - Facial nerve injury
  - Shoulder weakness
  - CSF leak
- *Benefits*
  - Allows decompression of the medulla and spinal cord at foramen magnum
  - Clear visualization of the intracranial hypoglossal foramen

158. Overview of the bone to be removed (*gray*).

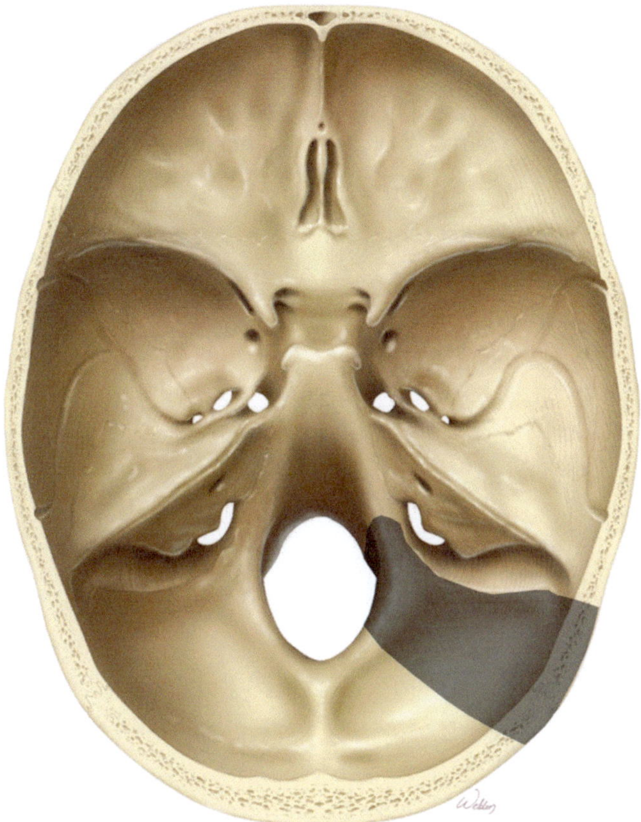

159. The incision for the far lateral approach has an inverted U-shape.

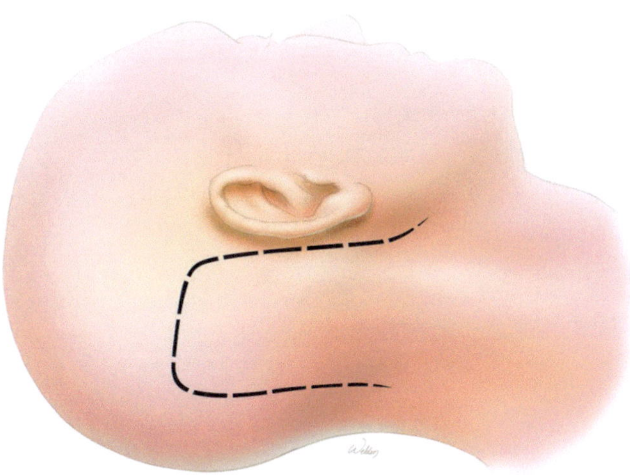

160. The soft tissues and periosteum are dissected off the skull. Foramen magnum is identified as are the lamina of C1 and C2. The vertebral artery (*arrow*) should be carefully identified. It runs through the bony transverse foramen, and there is no need to mobilize it. In our opinion, mobilizing the vertebral artery offers no advantage in exposure and puts the artery at risk of damage. The first and second cervical nerve (*1* and *2*) are shown.

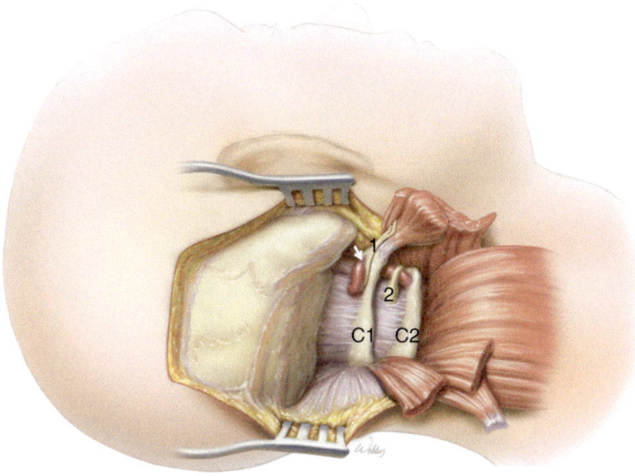

161. A retrosigmoid craniotomy is then performed. It is important to clearly find the transverse sinus and sigmoid sinus during this process to obtain adequate exposure.

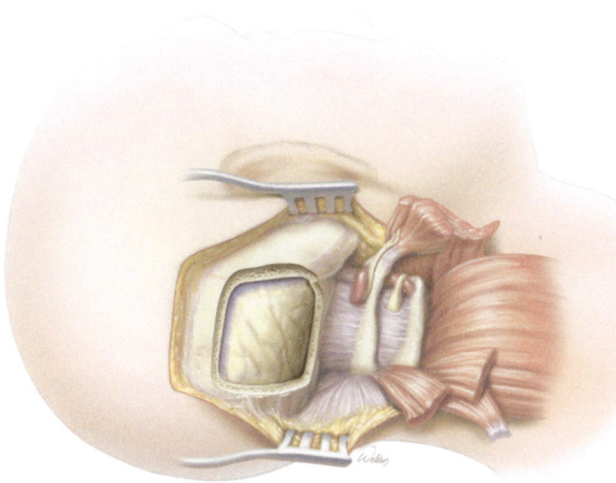

162. A mastoidectomy can be performed to identify the vertical segment of the facial nerve that can then be traced to the stylomastoid foramen (*arrow*). This early identification of the facial nerve decreases the risk of injury when widening the craniotomy anteriorly and inferiorly along the sigmoid sinus. The sigmoid sinus is followed inferiorly to the point where it courses medial to the facial nerve. This is important to obtain adequate exposure of the hypoglossal foramen.

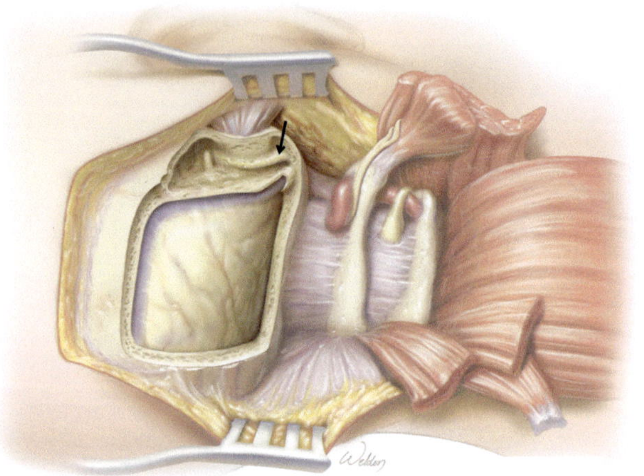

163. A rongeur is used to remove the rest of the skull to open foramen magnum. The marginal sinus (*MS*) runs within the dura of foramen magnum. It should be dissected free from the bony rim of the skull before removing the bone to prevent injury.

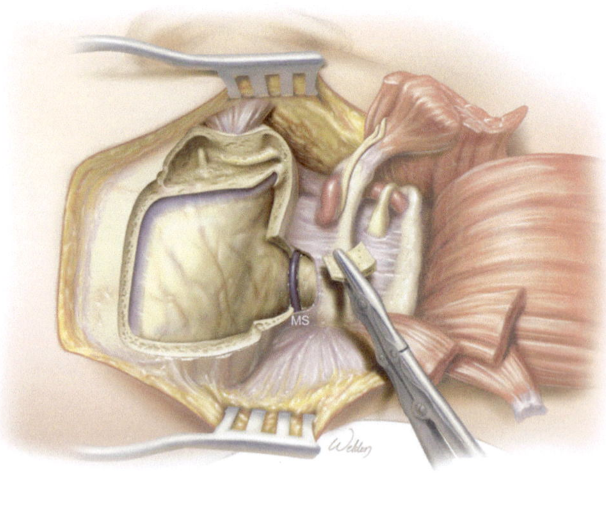

164. A malleable retractor is used to protect the posterior fossa dura and the occipital condyle drilled away with a diamond burr. The posterior half of the condyle can be safely removed without need for head stabilization hardware. Care should be taken not to damage the vertebral artery as it makes the transition from being extradural to intradural at this location.

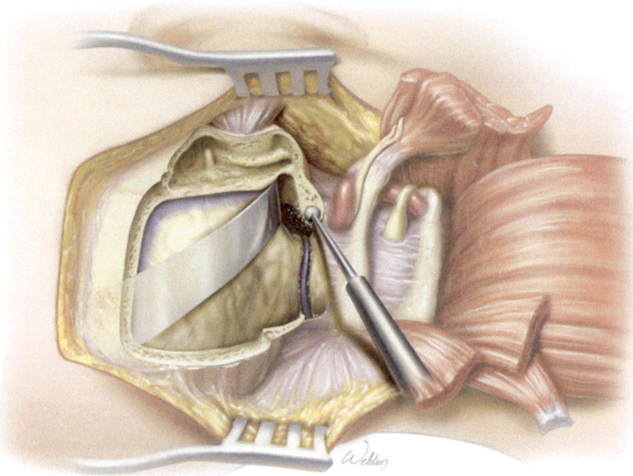

165. The cervical spinal cord dura is dissected off the underside of the lamina of C1 and C2. A malleable retractor is used to protect the dura while the bone is removed with a drill or a ronguer. The first and second cervical nerves (*1* and *2*) are preserved and the vertebral artery carefully left untouched.

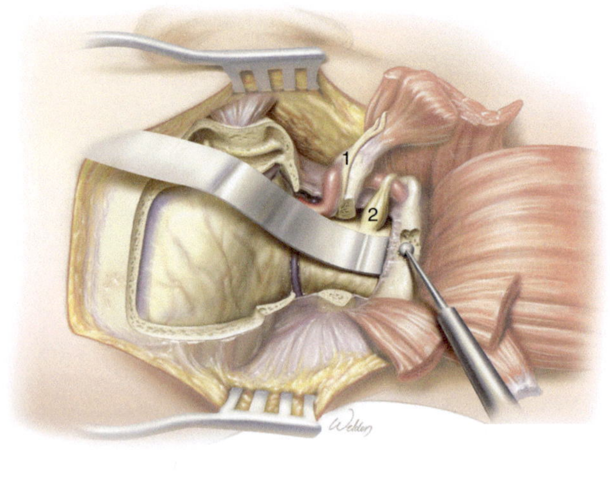

166. The dural opening is shown. The marginal sinus should be well cauterized with a bipolar before opening across it.

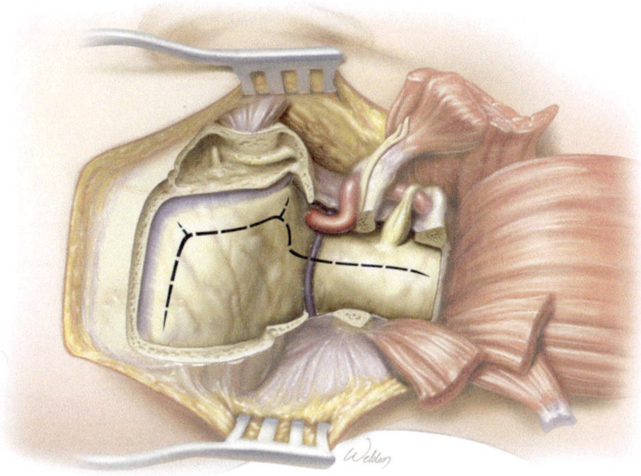

167. The dura is opened and the edges tacked up with sutures. The rootlets of the first (*1*) and second (*2*) cervical nerves, CN XI, and the intradural vertebral artery (*arrow*) are visible.

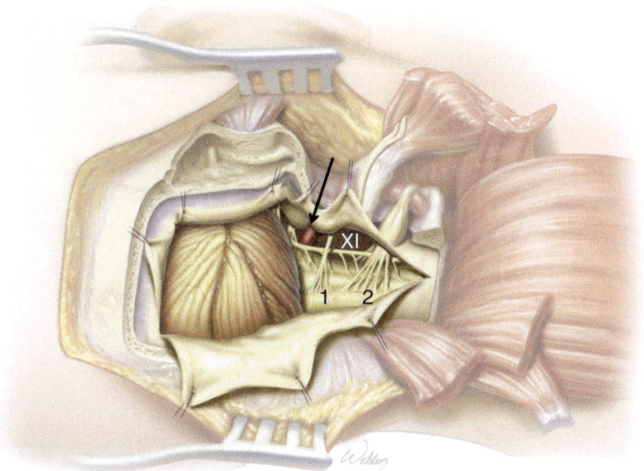

168. A malleable is used to retract the cerebellum to see the lateral brainstem. A Telfa strip is always used between the retractor and the brain to reduce trauma, but it is left out of this illustration for simplicity. CN VII and VIII complex, the jugular foramen CN IX, X, and XI, and the cervical rootlets for C1 are visible. The rootlets of CN XII are visible anterior to them.

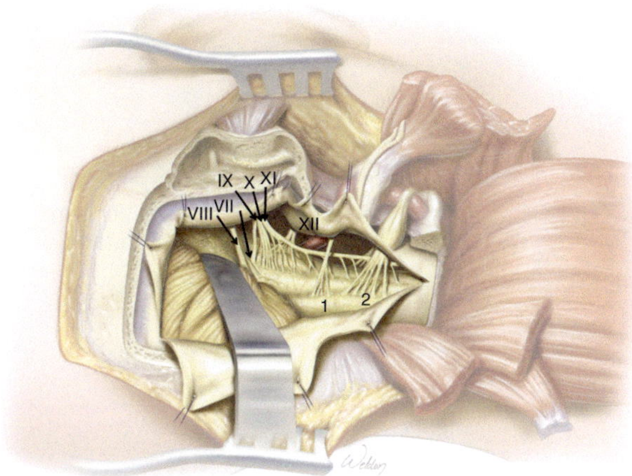

169. An illustration of what a hypoglossal nerve schwannoma or meningioma in this area looks like. Usually, cranial nerves IX, X, and XI are displaced posteriorly, and the brainstem and cervical spinal cord are compressed. Tumor removal is performed by dissecting between these fine rootlets. If too many rootlets are disturbed, dysphagia, vocal cord paralysis, aspiration, and shoulder weakness develop.

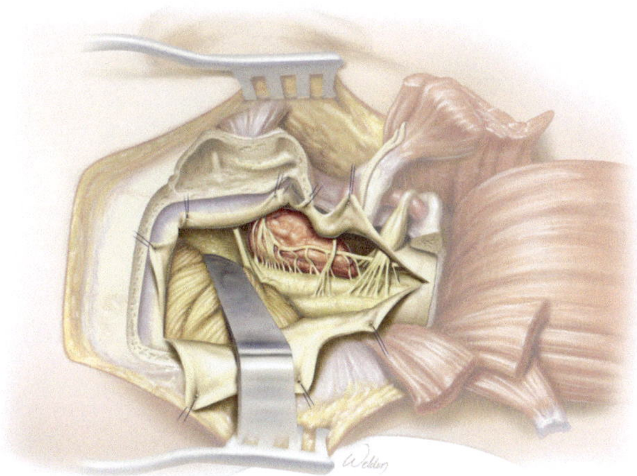

170. In order to access the hypoglossal foramen, the jugular tubercle is drilled away from the intracranial side of the skull.

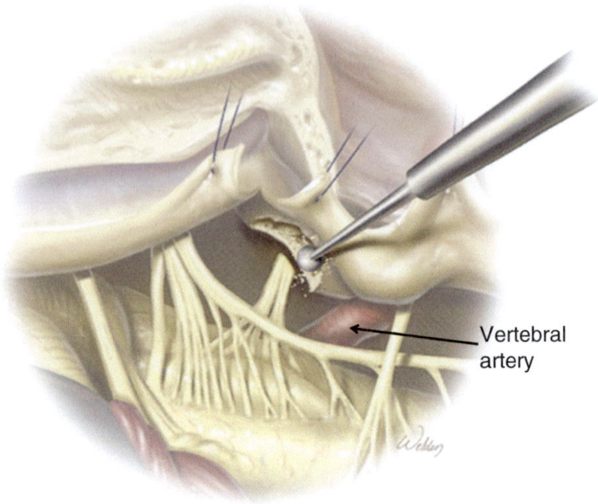

171. Case 1. A left bilobed hypoglossal schwannoma with both intracranial and extracranial components. There is significant compression of the medulla and a cyst within the intracranial component of the tumor.

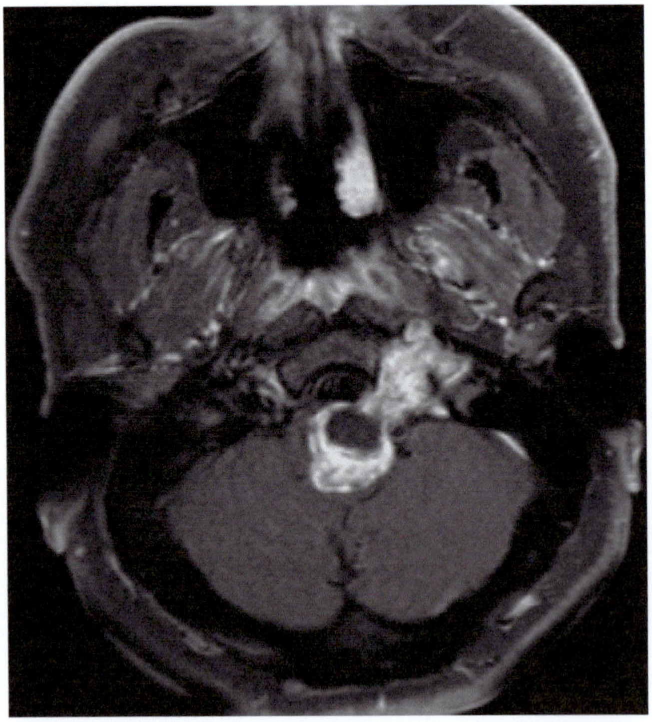

172. Coronal view demonstrates the compression of the brainstem at the craniocervical junction.

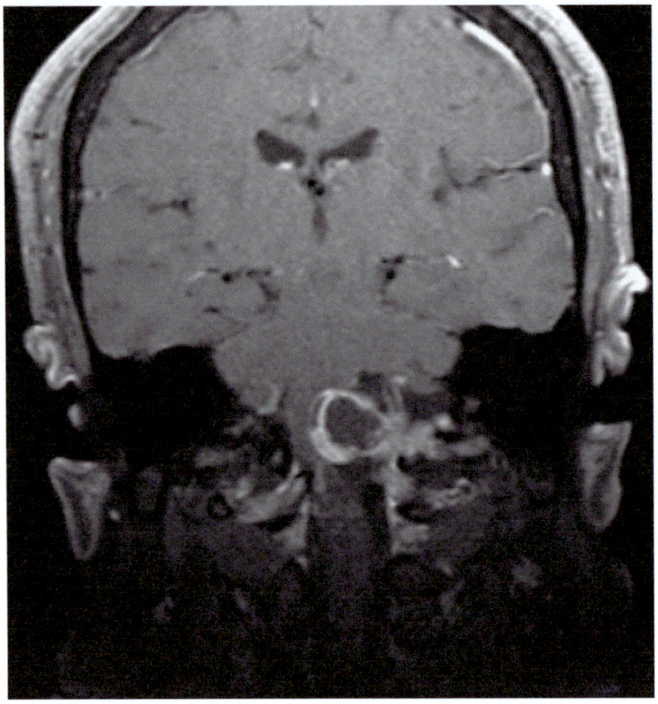

173. CT demonstrates that the hypoglossal canal is expanded (*arrow*).

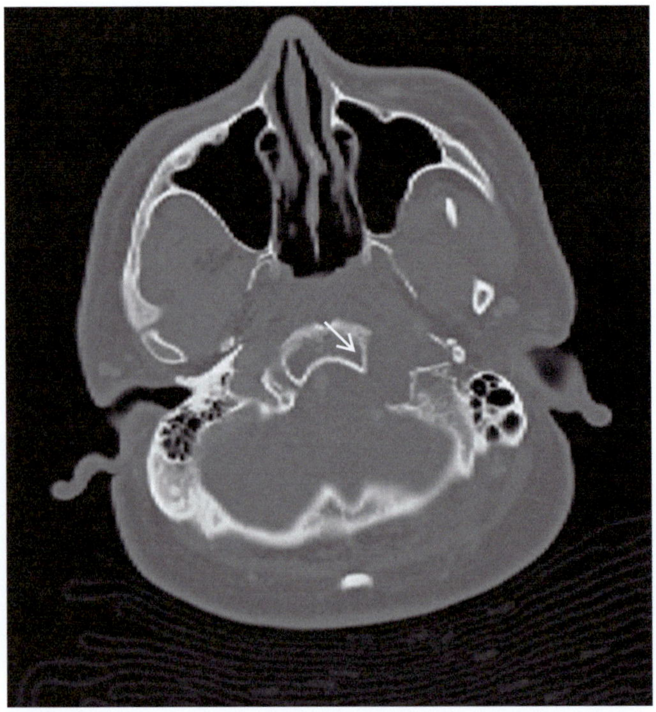

174. We approached the tumor via a far lateral approach to remove the intracranial portion of the tumor. The patient was placed in the lateral decubitus position. The head was held in a Mayfield head holder. The Stealth computer-guided navigation system was being set up.

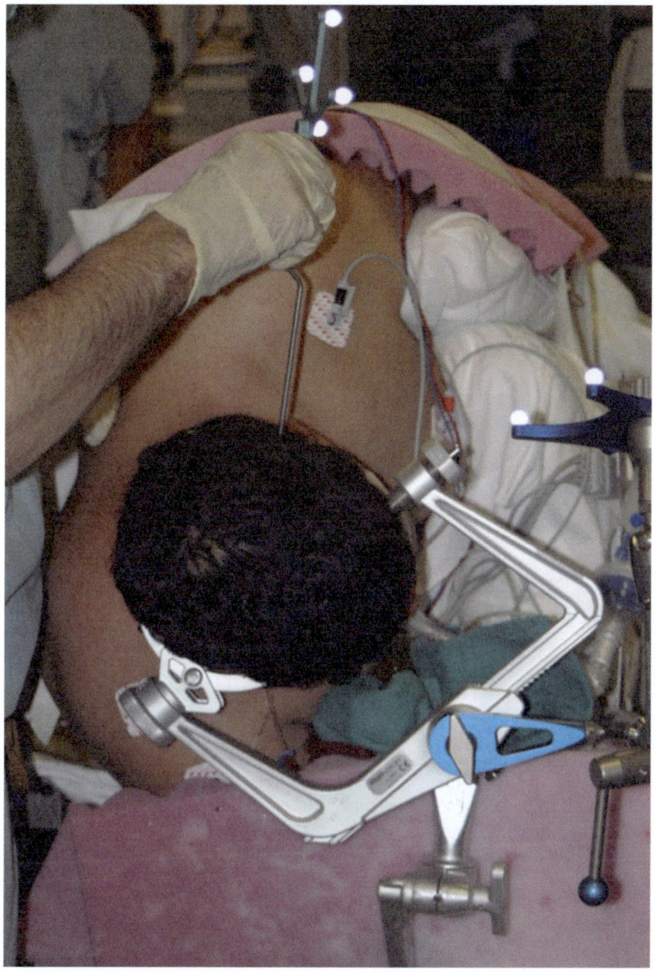

175. After shaving and prepping the field. The inferiorly based U-shaped flap was outlined.

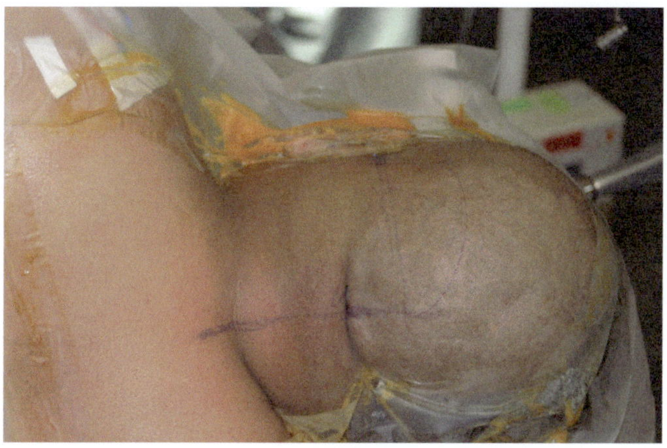

176. The skin was opened, the muscles were reflected, and the retrosigmoid dura was exposed.

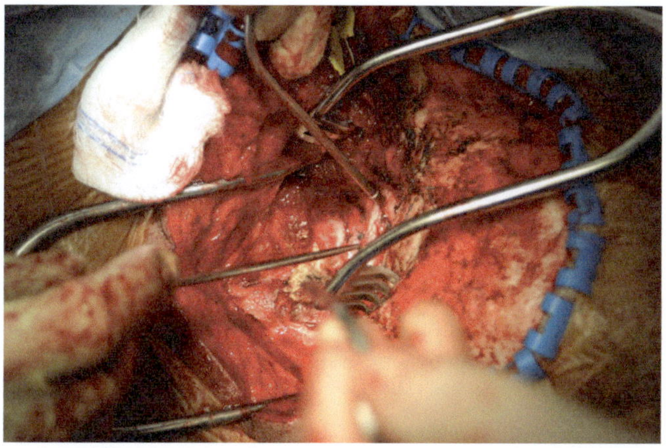

177. Dissection continued inferior to foramen magnum. The lamina of C1 and C2 were removed.

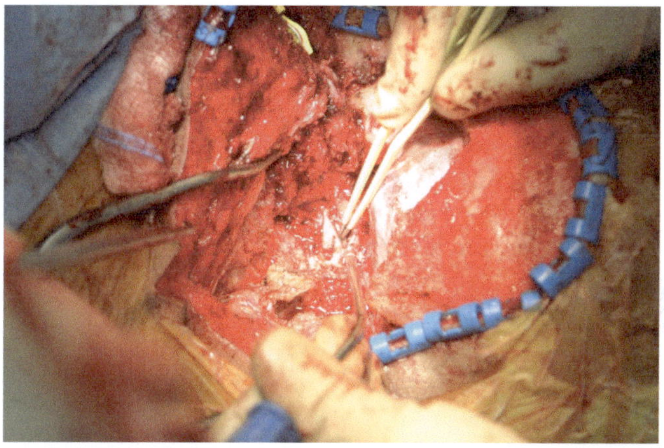

178. After exposure of the dura of the posterior fossa and cervical spinal cord. Only the lamina of C1 was removed for this case. The vertebral artery (*V*) was in the soft tissue between the transverse processes of C1 and C2 (*1* and *2*, respectively). The first cervical nerve was visible (*arrow*).

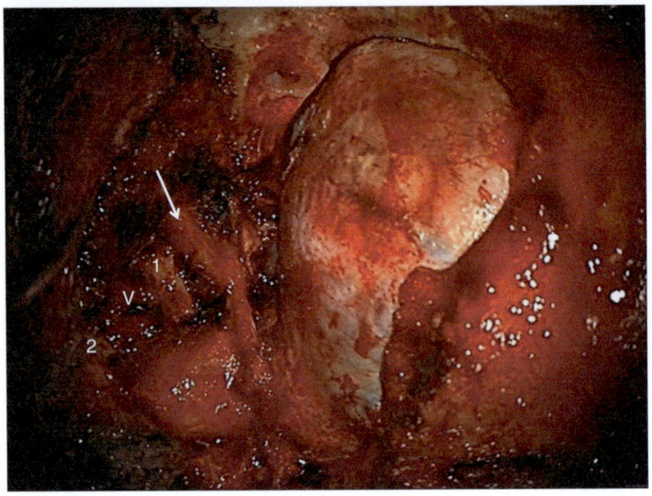

179. More anterior exposure was achieved by drilling away the posterior portion of the occipital condyle. This was done by first using a malleable to protect the posterior fossa dura and then drilling away the mastoid tip to follow the posterior edge of the sigmoid sinus.

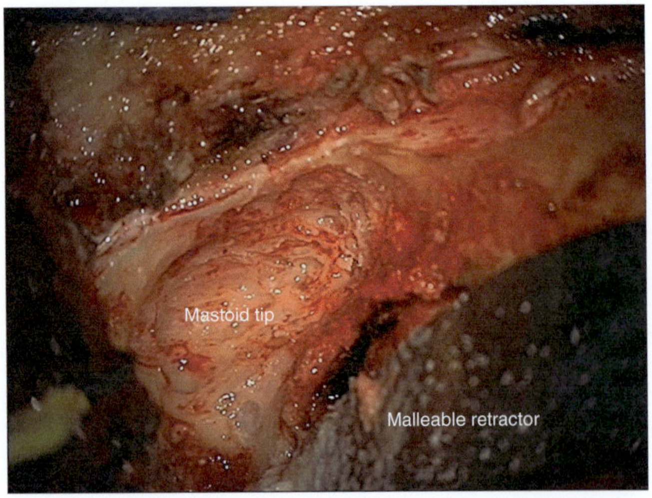

180. The occipital condyle was drilled then away. Again, the malleable retractor was used to protect the dura.

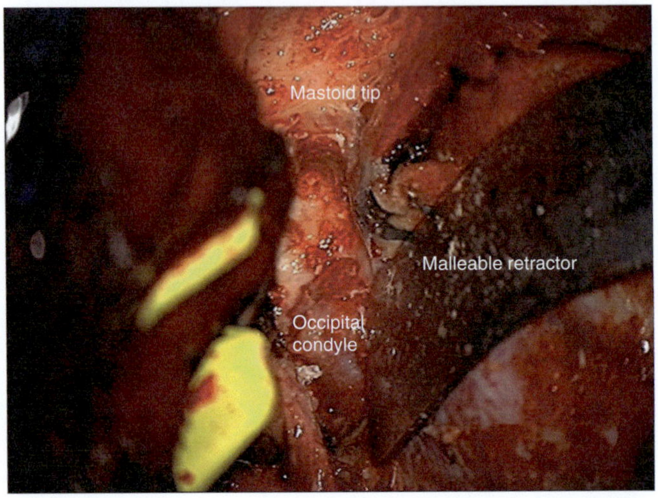

181. Completed exposure. The dura was then opened and tumor dissection performed.

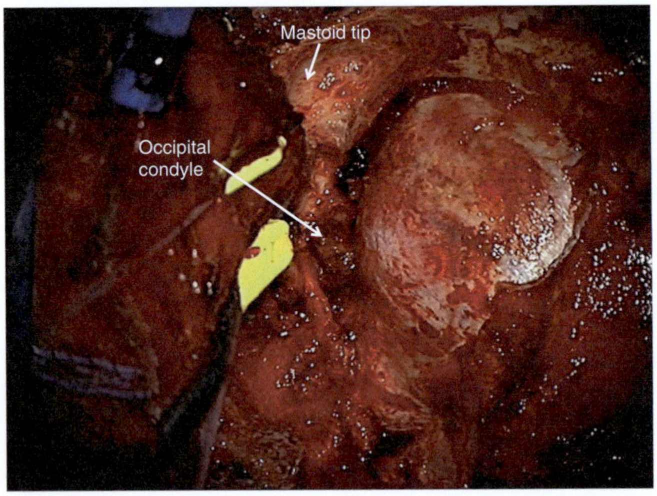

182. Post-op MRI. We used a two-stage approach to remove the tumor. The far lateral approach was used first to remove the intracranial disease and an infratemporal fossa approach used to resect the extracranial disease 6 months later. While there was still a small amount of disease within the hypoglossal canal itself, the vast majority of the tumor was removed. The brainstem compression was relieved.

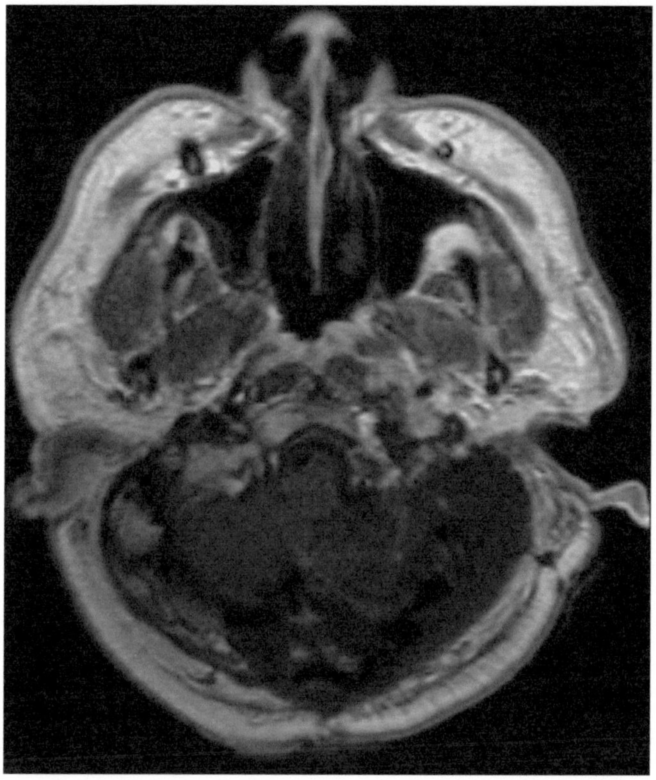

183. Case 2. A left posterior fossa meningioma at the craniocervical junction.

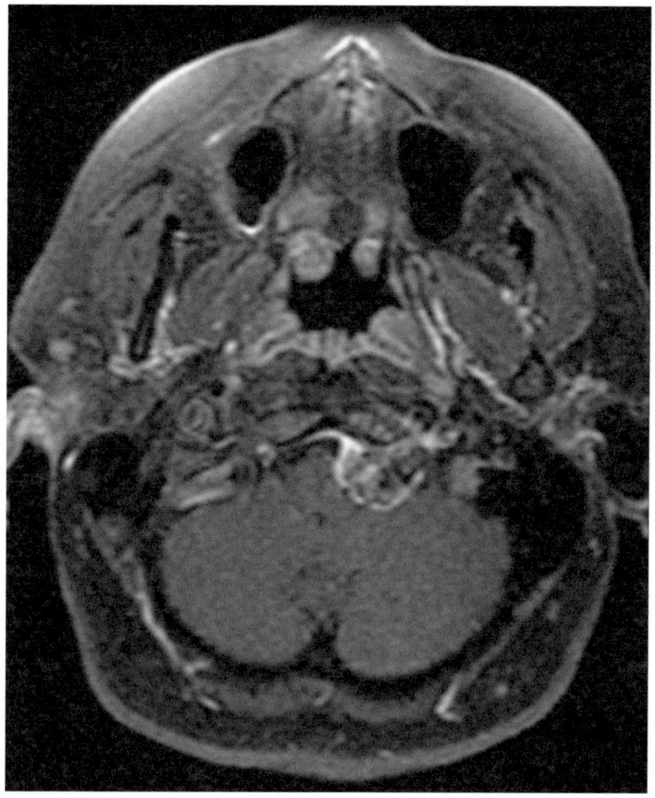

184. Coronal MRI demonstrated compression of the medulla and upper spinal cord (*arrow*).

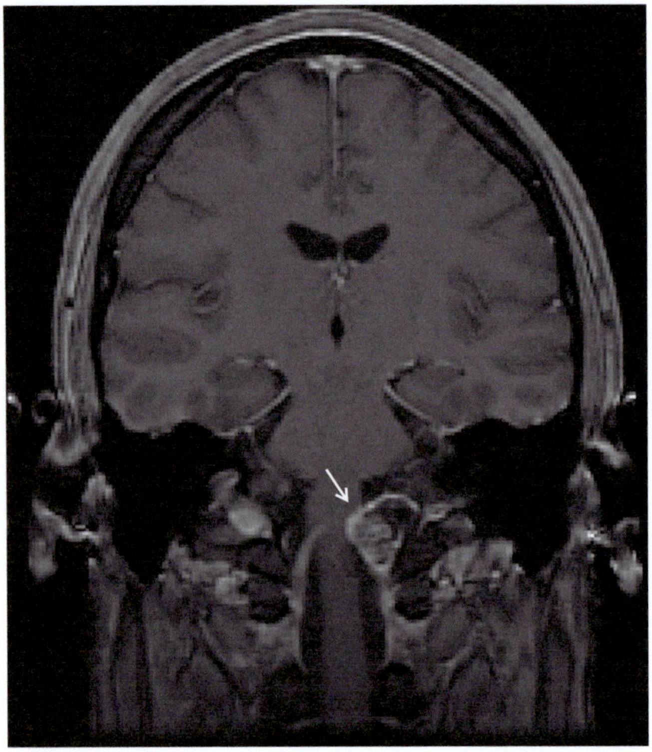

185. T2 MRI demonstrated that the mengioma was calcified, as noted by the dark regions within the tumor (*arrow*).

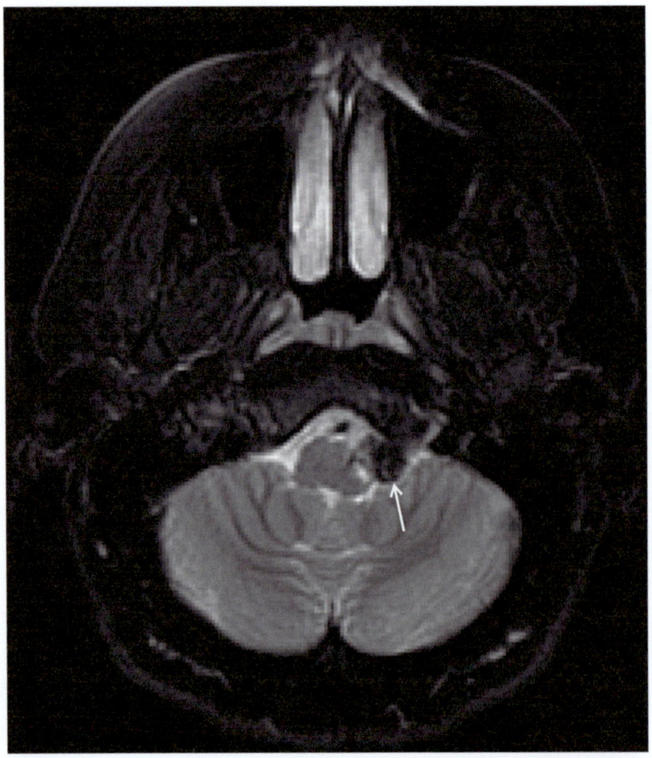

186. After the initial part of the opening was performed, the sigmoid sinus and the retrosigmoid dura were exposed. The mastoid antrum was opened, although that is not typically necessary. However, it can be helpful in the identification of landmarks. While not formally identified, the region of the vertical portion of the facial nerve is shown.

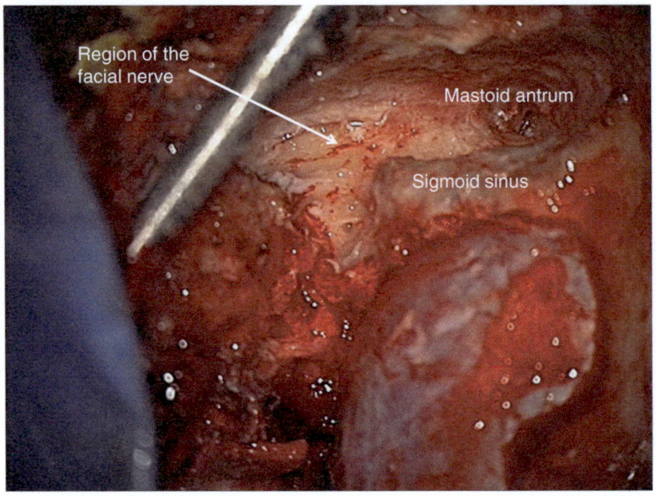

187. Further drilling deep to the mastoid tip was performed to remove the posterior portion of the occipital condyle.

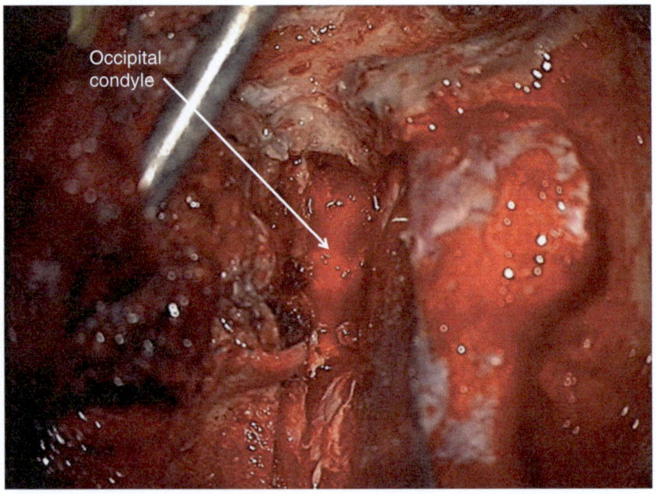

188. Complete dural exposure of the posterior fossa and upper cervical spinal cord.

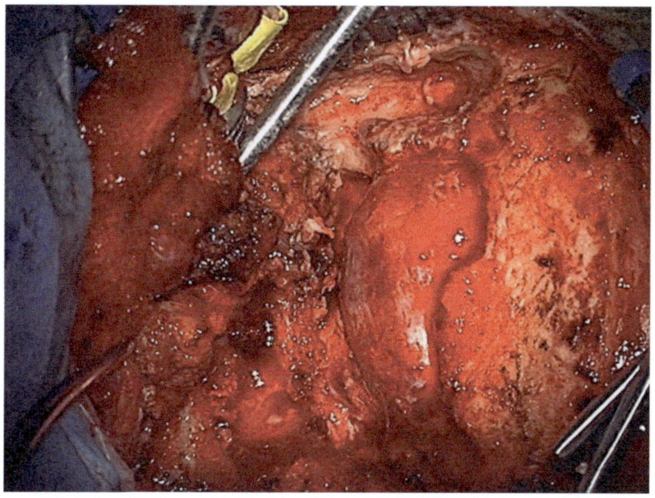

189. The dura was opened posterior to the sigmoid sinus, beginning superiorly and coursing inferiorly through foramen magnum down to the cervical spine.

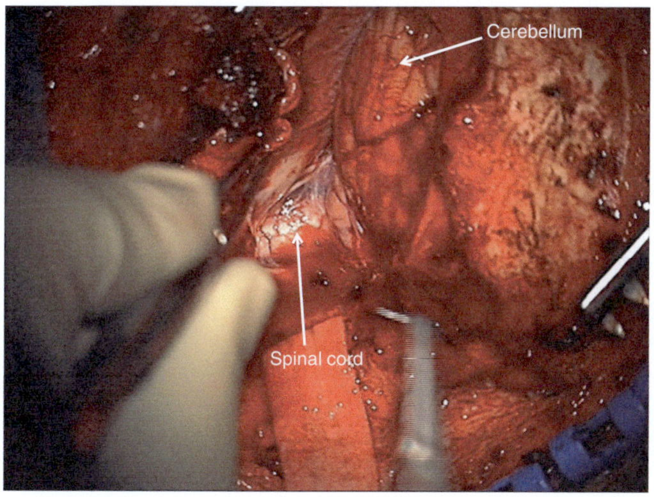

190. The meningioma was seen anterior to the nerve rootlets of the spinal accessory nerve and the hypoglossal nerve. Tumor dissection was performed between these rootlets with the goal of minimizing trauma to them.

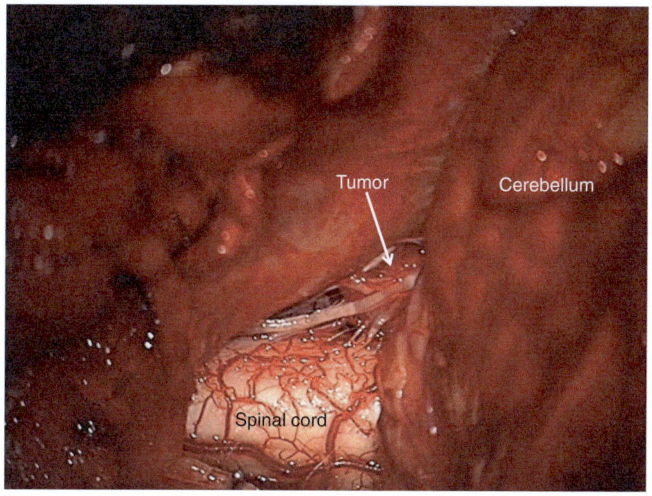

191. Elevation of the cerebellum with a malleable retractor permitted better visualization of the tumor.

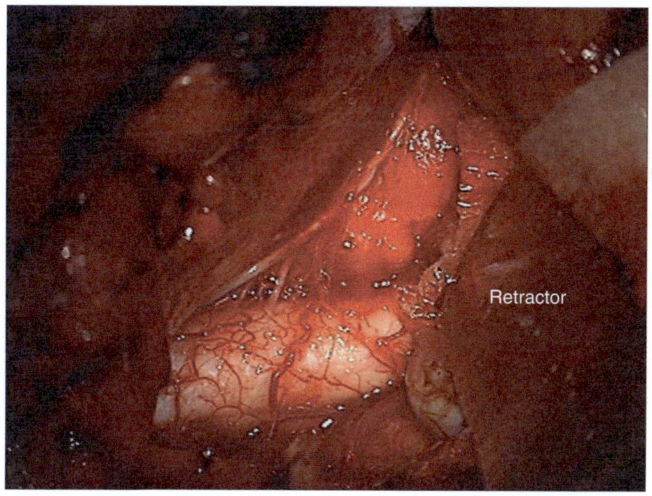

192. Tumor debulking was performed through a window in the posterior face of the tumor (*arrow*).

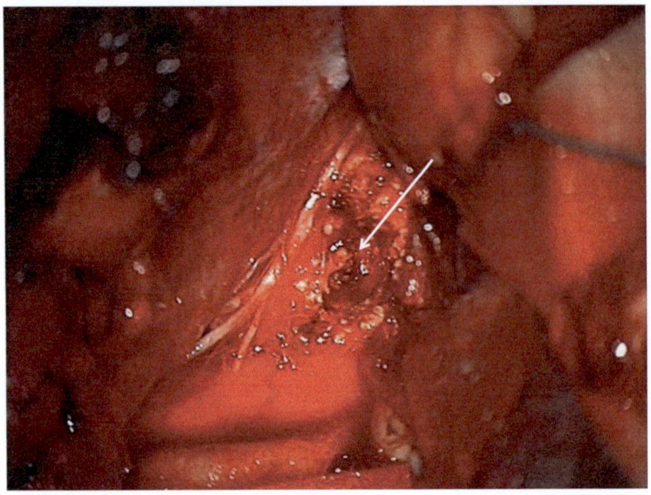

193. The jugular foramen nerves (CN IX, X, and XI) could be seen to enter pars nervosa just medial to the jugular bulb.

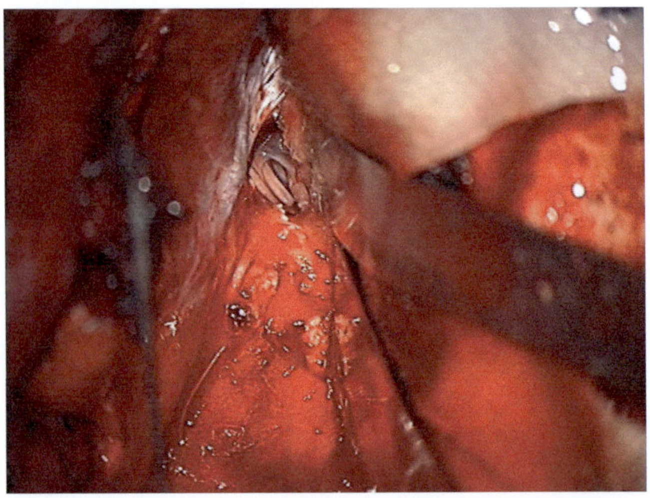

194. The meningioma was dissected off the bone by gently elevating the nerve rootlets.

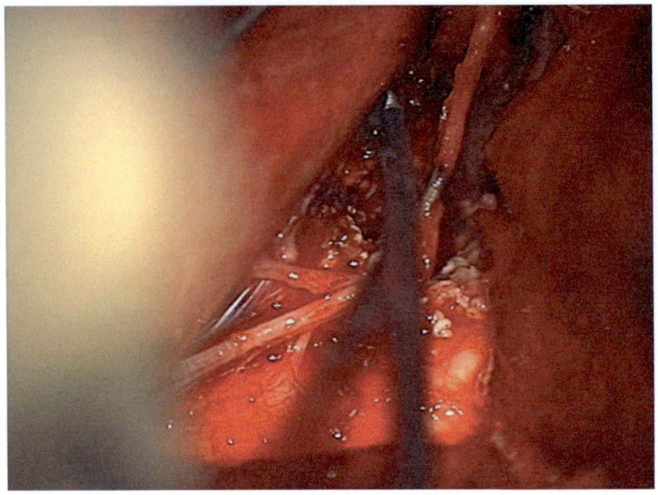

5 Combined Approach to the Middle and Posterior Fossa

- *Concept*
  - The approach combines a presigmoid, retrolabyrinthine craniotomy with a middle fossa craniotomy.
  - The two craniotomies are connected by splitting the superior petrosal sinus and dividing the tentorium.
- *Conditions treated*
  - Petroclival meningiomas
  - Trigeminal schwannomas
  - Epidermoids of the cerebellopontine angle and ventral pons
  - Other lesions that extend into both the middle and posterior fossa
- *Risks*
  - Labyrinthine injury with hearing loss and dizziness
  - Facial nerve injury
  - Palsy of CN III, IV, VI
  - Damage to the vein of Labbé, which could produce temporal lobe infarction
  - Seizure
  - CSF leak
- *Benefits*
  - Excellent exposure of the posterior fossa and middle fossa is provided. The view extends from the posterior communicating artery within the Circle of Willis and CN III superiorly to the jugular foramen and CN XI inferiorly.
  - Hearing, balance, and facial nerve function can be preserved.

J.S. Oghalai, C.L.W. Driscoll, *Atlas of Neurotologic and Lateral Skull Base Surgery*,
DOI 10.1007/978-3-662-46694-0_5, © Springer-Verlag Berlin Heidelberg 2016

1. Overview of the bone to be removed (*gray*). Additional bone can be removed posterior to the sigmoid sinus to allow for greater retraction and exposure in the posterior fossa. This additional exposure also improves the trajectory to the internal auditory canal, jugular bulb, and petrous apex as viewed posteriorly. It helps with seeing "around" the intact semicircular canals to address tumor in the temporal bone.

2. The incision is marked so as to course around the temporalis muscle boundaries yet still end up in the preauricular crease to reduce visible scarring and prevent injury to the frontal branch of the facial nerve. For tumors that do not extend far anteriorly in the middle fossa, it can be adequate to omit the descending part of the anterior limb of the incision.

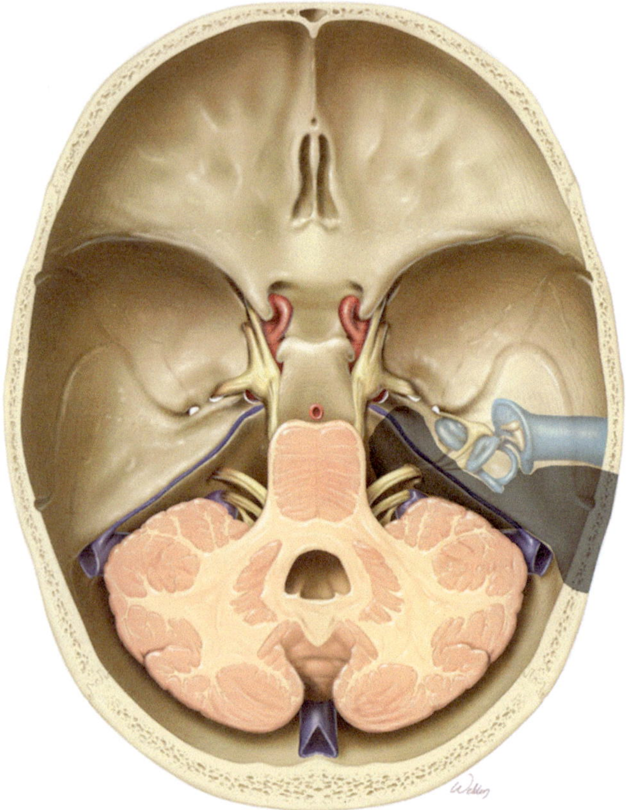

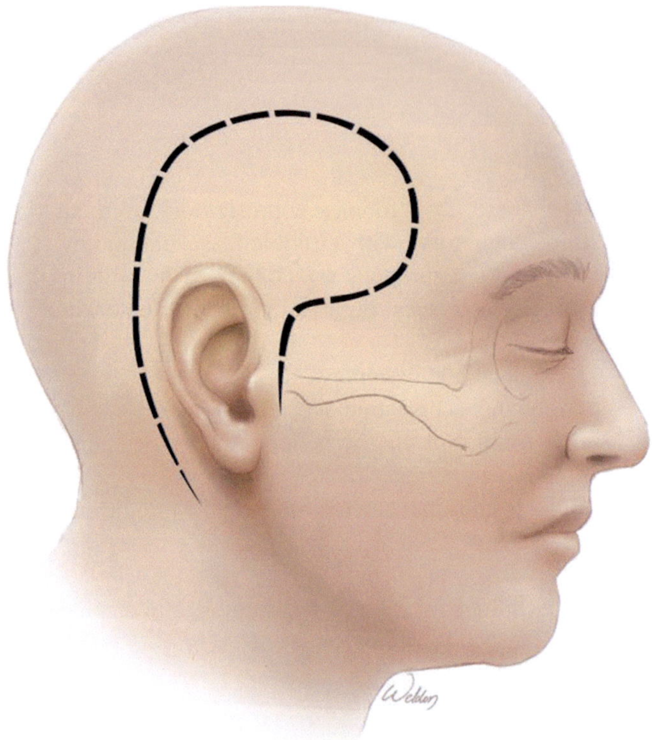

3. The superficial tissues are elevated off the mastoid and temporalis muscle and retracted anteriorly and inferiorly. The ear canal tethers this tissue, and it is important not to tear into it and contaminate the sterile field.

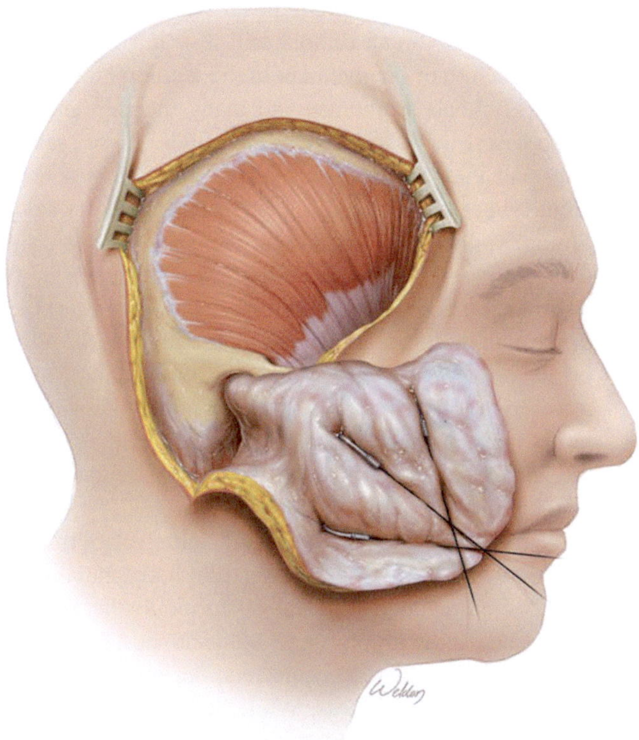

4. The temporalis muscle is then elevated and retracted anteriorly. If desired, it could be left attached to the skin flap and the entire mass of tissue elevated off the skull at once.

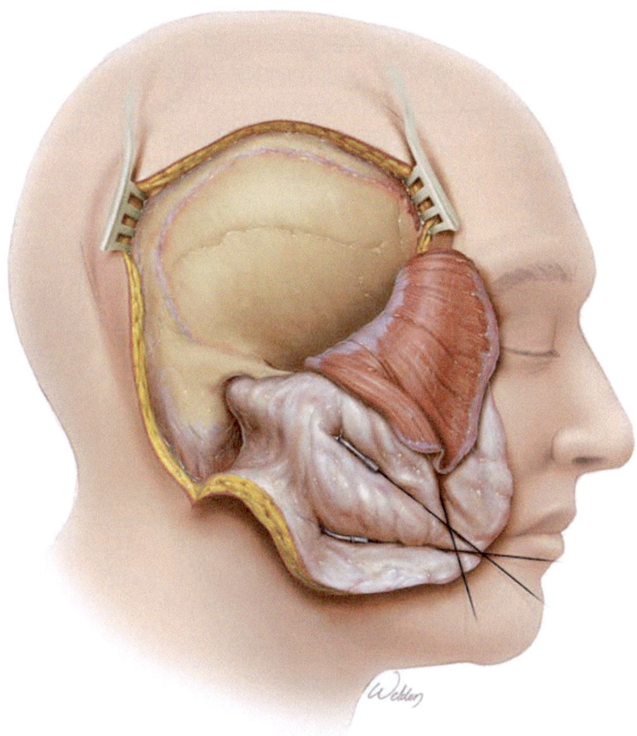

5. A mastoidectomy with sigmoid sinus decompression is performed. The middle fossa and posterior fossa dura is exposed. The additus ad antrum is seen but not widely opened as it will have to be sealed off at the end of the procedure to prevent CSF leak. These steps are exactly the same as the initial steps in the translabyrinthine approach. One difference is that all three semicircular canals must be clearly delineated and the bone around them thinned. The canals do not need to be "blue lined," but every millimeter of bone removal is critical for achieving excellent exposure.

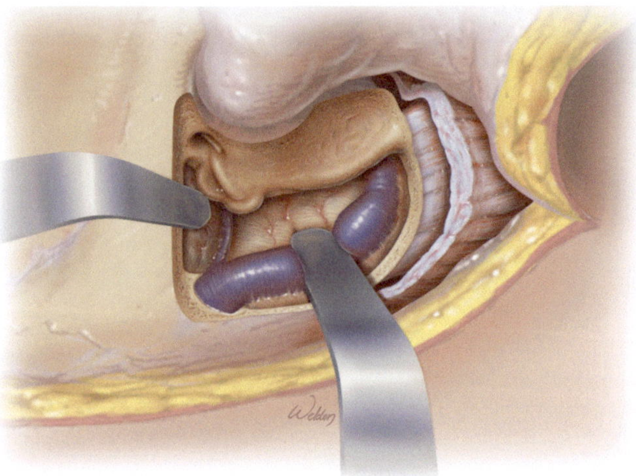

6. The temporal lobe dura is dissected away from the inner surface of the skull with a Penfield elevator and a craniotome then used to turn a bone flap in one piece.

   For tumors that do not involve the temporal bone such as a bilobed trigeminal nerve schwannoma, this amount of temporal bone removal will provide acceptable exposure. Some tumors will also have significant extension into or involvement of the temporal bone, particularly chondrosarcomas and many meningiomas. In these cases, one can perform the middle fossa craniotomy and then remove bone in the petrous apex, even identifying and skeletonizing the internal auditory canal. Similarly, one can work around the endolymphatic sac/duct, removing bone deep into the petrous apex in the retrofacial and retrolabyrinthine areas when needed. Some meningiomas and epidermoids may have tumor extension in the internal auditory canal that can be exposed in this manner. In both situations, removing the tumor in the temporal bone prior to opening the dura has the added advantage of decreasing the vascular supply of the remaining tumor.

   Achieving adequate retrofacial/retrolabyrinthine exposure to visualize the internal auditory canal often requires more bone removal posterior to the sigmoid sinus to have the proper view. Some advocate removing the posterior semicircular canal and occluding with bone wax to gain added access. While hearing might be preserved, it is certainly put at increased risk, and we have not found it to be necessary.

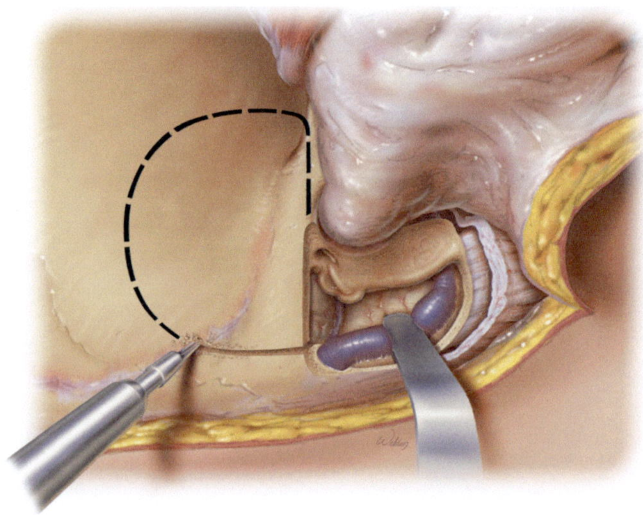

7. The dural incisions are shown. For optimal exposure, the inferior limb of the incision needs to go all the way down to the sigmoid "crotch" (*arrow*). This is the region where the sigmoid sinus curves around to rise up to the jugular bulb. Also, the dural opening should cross the superior petrosal sinus midway between the transverse-sigmoid junction and the petrous apex bone (*arrowhead*). Dividing this too far posteriorly may impact temporal lobe venous drainage, particularly if the vein of Labbé joins with the superior petrosal sinus, a frequent anatomic variant.

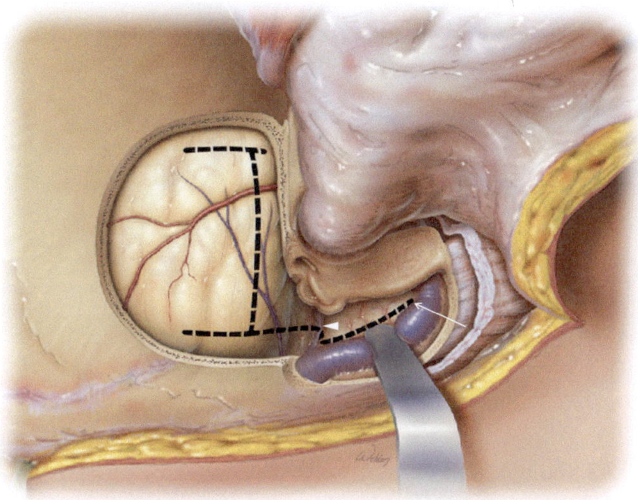

8. Typically, the posterior fossa opening is performed first to release CSF. The middle fossa opening is then performed. Retractors are used on top of moistened Telfa strips to protect the brain. Importantly, the vein of Labbé should be identified prior to connecting the two dural openings (See Chap. 8, images 98 & 99 for an example of how to identify the vein of Labbé). It is critical to not inadvertently transect it while opening the dura around the superior petrosal sinus. Once the vein of Labbé has been protected, the superior petrosal sinus can be either cauterized with a bipolar or clipped prior to transaction. The remaining dural incision can then be safely performed.

   Following this, the tentorium is divided. There are veins within the tentorium, particularly medially and anteriorly, that anastomose with the cavernous sinus. Thus, the tentorium should be incised in a stepwise fashion by first cauterizing a section with a bipolar and then cutting that section with a scissors.

   When nearing the tentorial notch, CN IV (*arrow*) should be identified within the surrounding arachnoid and dissected free of the tentorium so it is not damaged when cutting the tentorium. It is usually superior to the notch slightly but may also be found inferior to it occasionally.

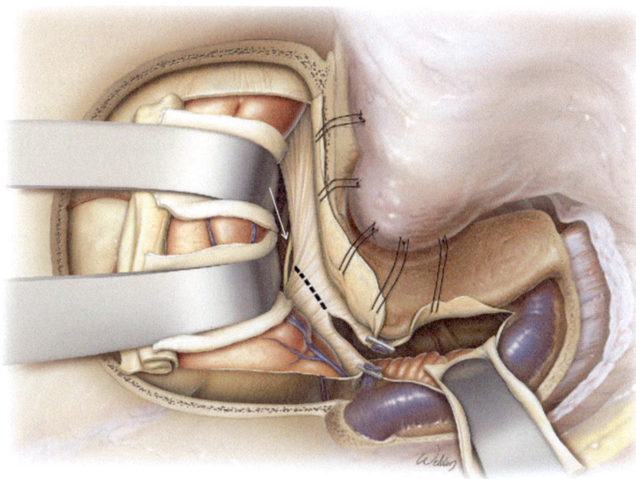

9. After dividing the tentorium, the retractors work much more effectively, and visualization of the petroclival junction is substantially enhanced. This illustration indicates all the structures that can be seen after the opening has been completed. However, in reality, these structures cannot all be seen simultaneously as shown. The microscope will need to be positioned at different viewing angles to see them all.

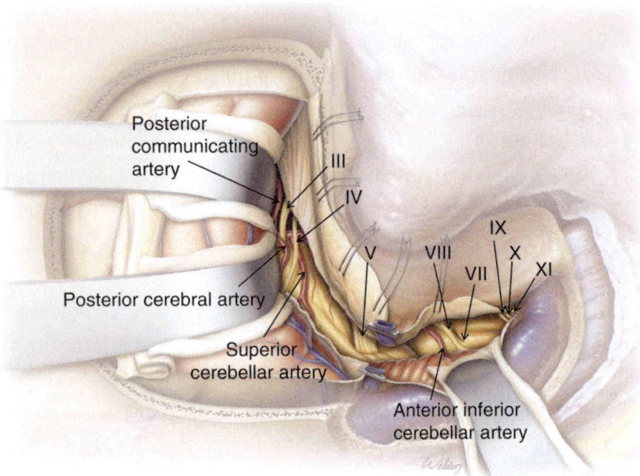

10. Case 1. Epidermoid of the cerebellopontine angle. Axial T1 MRI with gadolinium revealed a hypointense lesion exerting mass effect upon the pons. It originated from the left side.

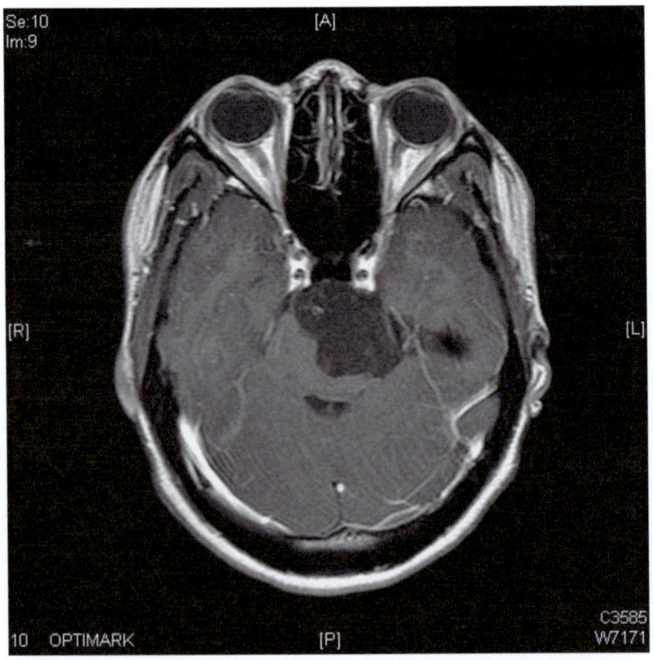

11. Coronal T1 MRI with gadolinium demonstrated that it extended superiorly to impact the midbrain as well.

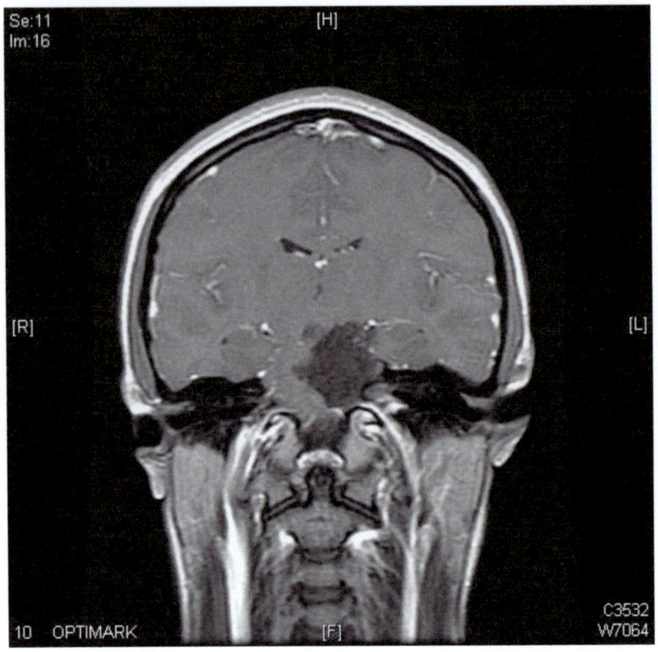

12. Axial T2 MRI demonstrated that the lesion was bright, similar to CSF. The basilar artery (*arrow*) was deviated to the right side.

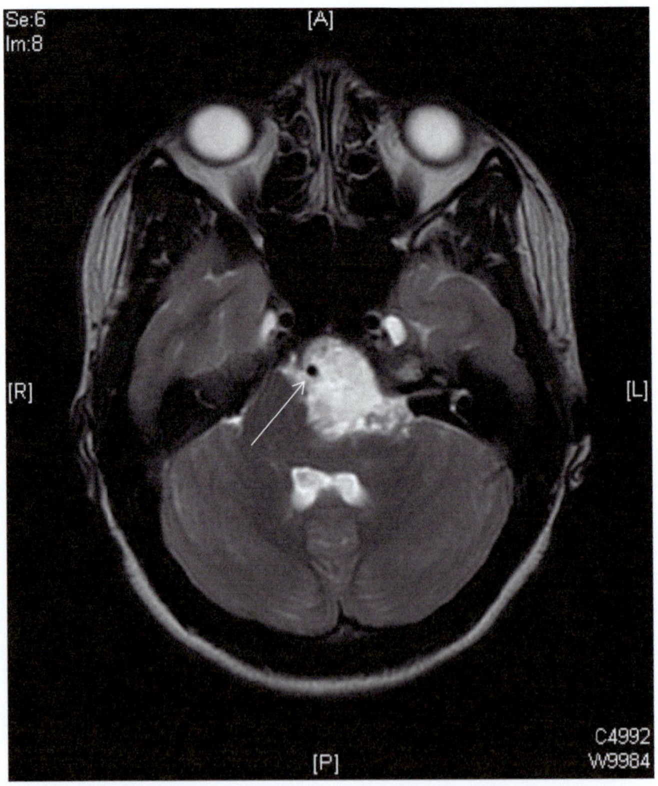

13. Another axial T2 MRI at a higher level showed that the epidermoid involved the posterior circulation within the Circle of Willis.

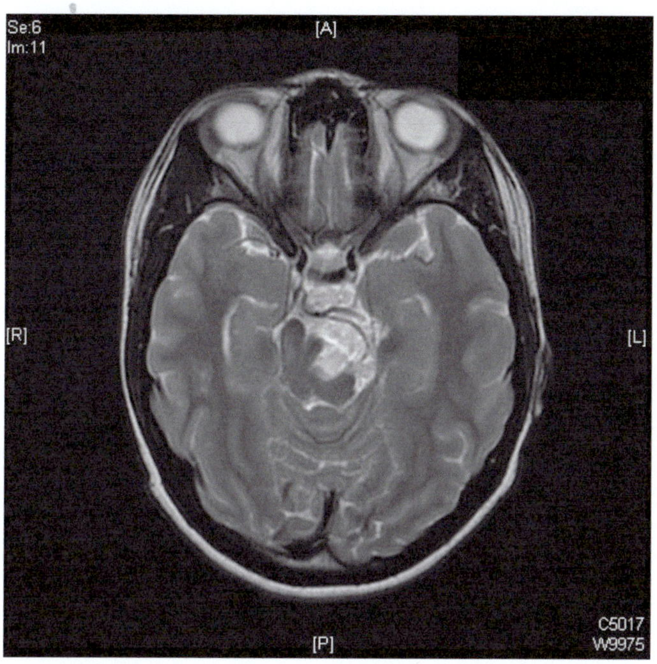

14. Diffusion-weighted MRI demonstrates that the mass was bright (i.e., it had restricted diffusion) and was thus consistent with an epidermoid.

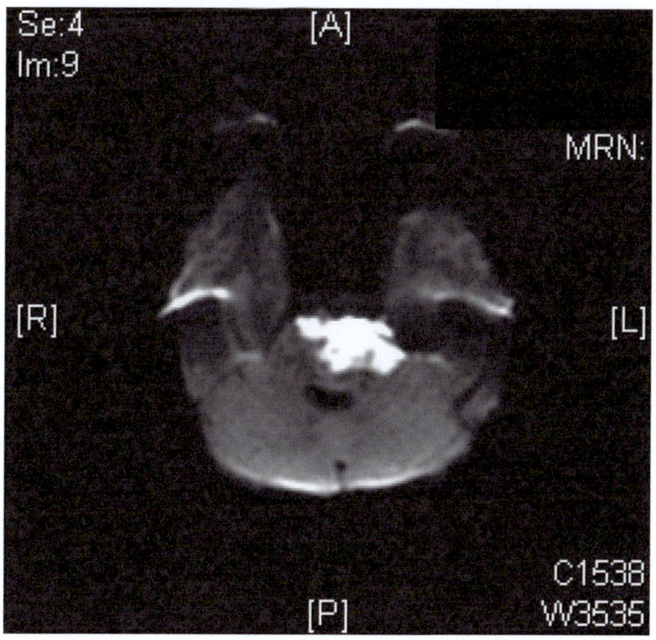

15. Because of the degree of brainstem compression, surgery was planned. The incision was marked on the patient. Note that an earphone (*arrow pointing to the blue tube*) was placed in the ear in order to measure intraoperative auditory evoked potentials. Tegaderms were used to seal off the ear so that blood and/or fluid would not seep in and affect these measurements.

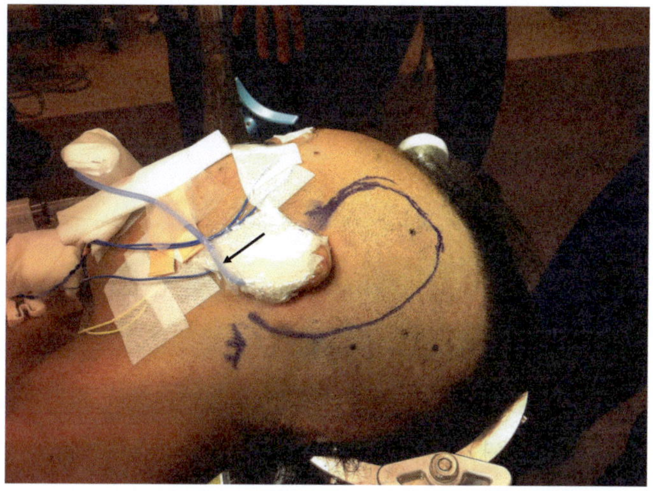

16. We elevated the skin and temporalis muscle up as one flap, covered it with a moist sponge, and retracted the flap using yellow fishhook retractors (also known as Lone Stars).

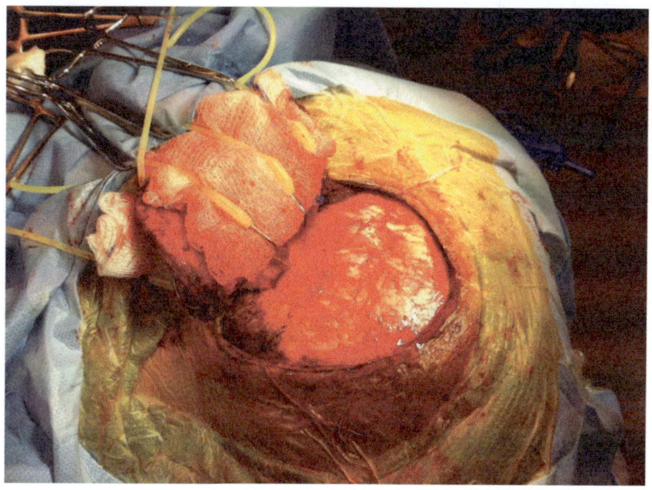

17. A standard mastoidectomy was performed to expose the antrum. At this point, the sigmoid sinus and tegmen were still covered in bone.

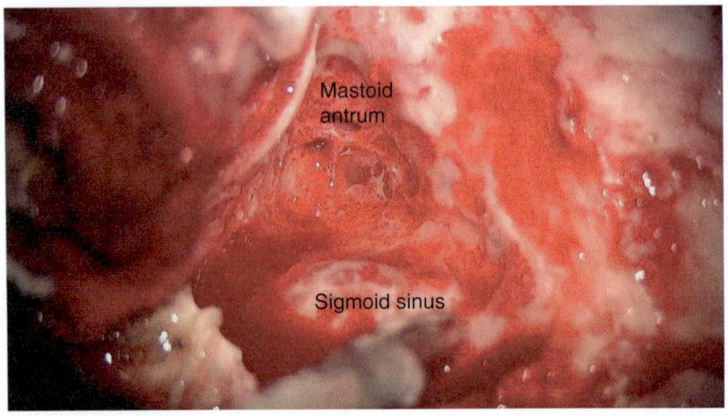

18. The sigmoid sinus, posterior fossa dura, and middle fossa dura were exposed. Malleable retractors were placed on each. The superior petrosal sinus was visible between them (*arrow*). The lateral semicircular canal (*LSCC*) and the posterior semicircular canal (*PSCC*) were identified.

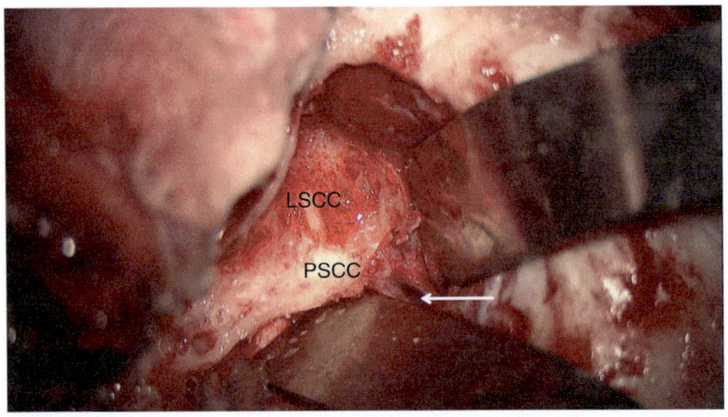

19. A trough was drilled to expose the dura to the root of the zygomatic arch (*arrows*).

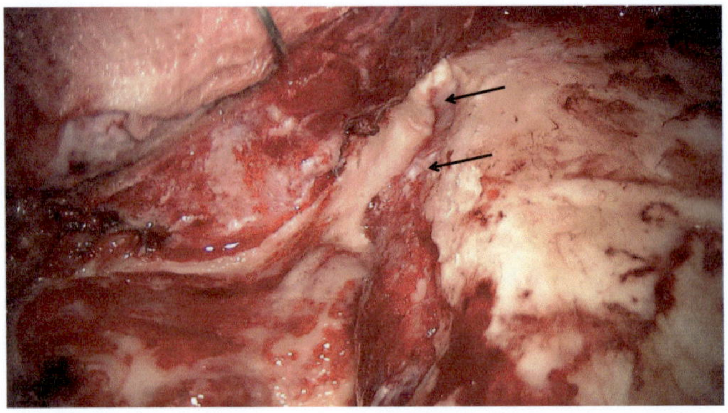

20. A Penfield 1 elevator was used to dissect the dura away from the inner table of the skull. This reduces the risk of tearing the dura with the craniotome.

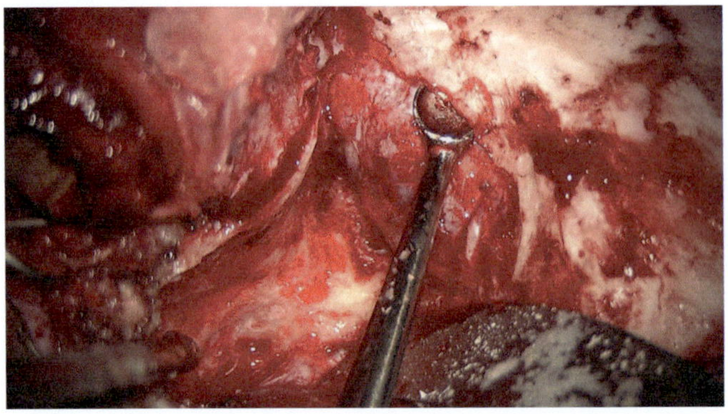

21. A view after using the craniotome to remove the lateral skull. Note that we chose not to remove as much bone as was originally marked. It is not necessary to remove that much bone because it does not improve the deep exposure. The angle of the retractors which will eventually be used is actually much more critical.

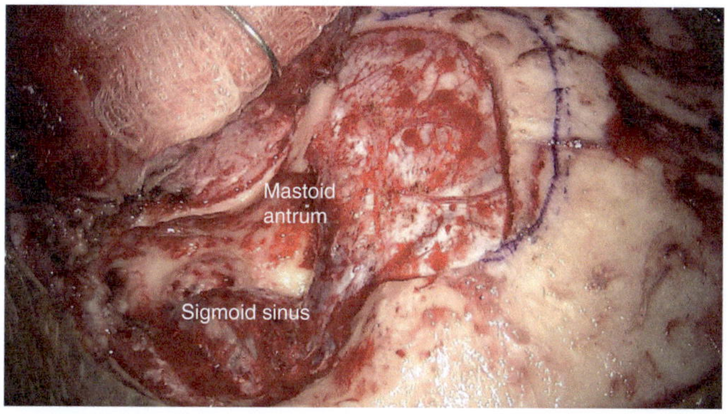

22. The superior petrosal sinus was cauterized with a bipolar. Another option is to open the dura first, identify the vein of Labbé, and then clip and divide the superior petrosal sinus.

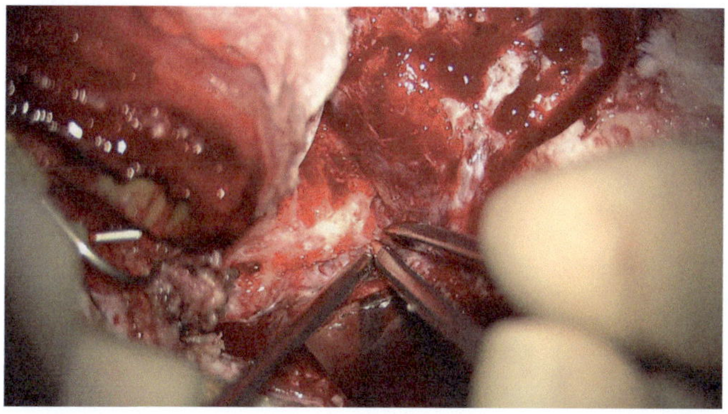

23. The presigmoid posterior fossa dura was opened from just inferior the superior petrosal sinus to the sigmoid crotch (*arrow*). The dural incision follows the course of the sigmoid sinus to avoid injury to the endolymphatic sac. Leave a cuff of dura along the sinus for suture closure at the end of the case. A Telfa strip was placed through the opening to protect the cerebellum.

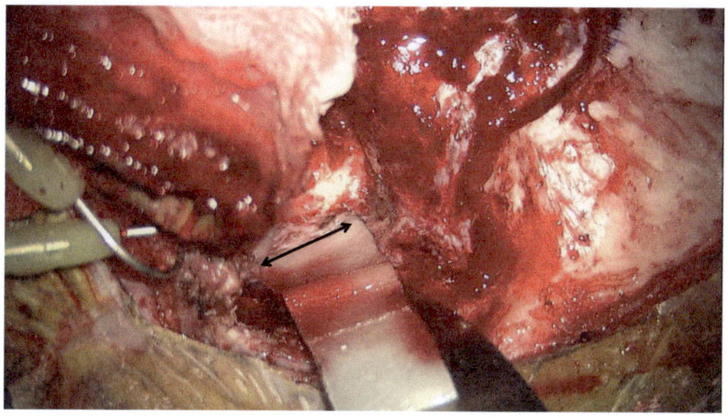

24. The middle fossa dura was opened at the lateral aspect to expose the temporal lobe. Again, a Telfa strip was placed on the brain.

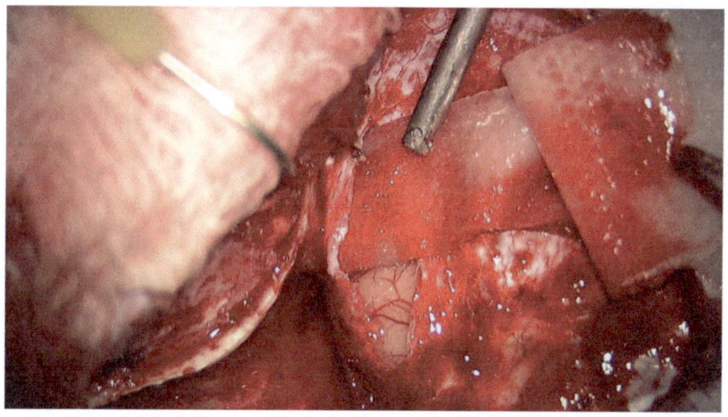

25. The middle fossa dura incision was then extended medially down to the superior petrosal sinus (*SPS*). While not shown in this picture, care must be taken to trace out and protect the vein of Labbé during this process. In this case, the vein of Labbé was safely covered by the Telfa strip.

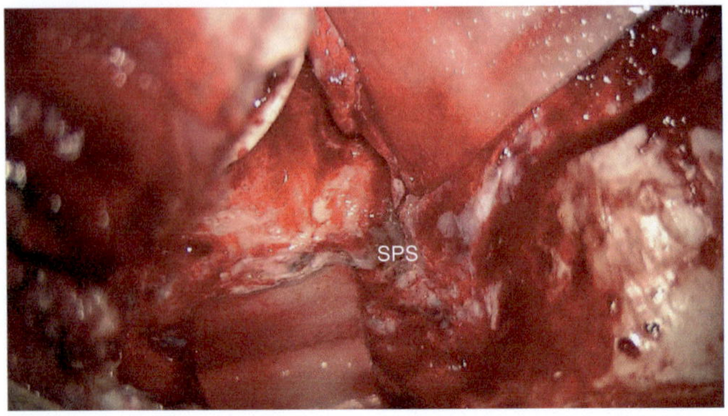

26. The superior petrosal sinus was then divided. The beginning of the tentorium is the deep dural layer that formed the trifurcation with the posterior fossa and middle fossa dura.

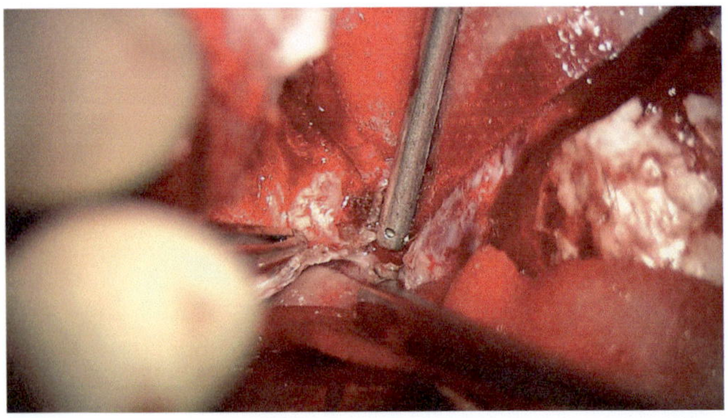

27. The cerebellum and temporal lobe were gently retracted away from the tentorium. The tentorium was cauterized with the bipolar and then cut in a stepwise fashion. We often find that the turbinate scissors are helpful for this portion of the procedure as they are stronger than microscissors and can cut through the tough dura of the tentorium more easily.

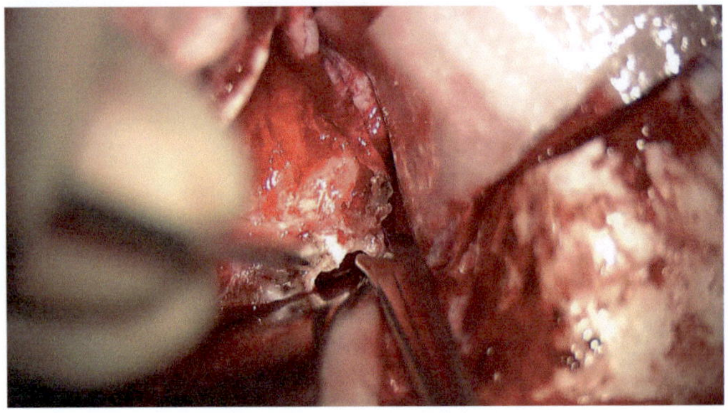

28. When proceeding medially, veins from the temporal lobe are often found entering the superior aspect of the tentorium. These should be preserved to reduce the risk of venous infarct. In this example, we angled our incision anterior to the vein (*arrow*) to allow it to continue to drain into the transverse sinus.

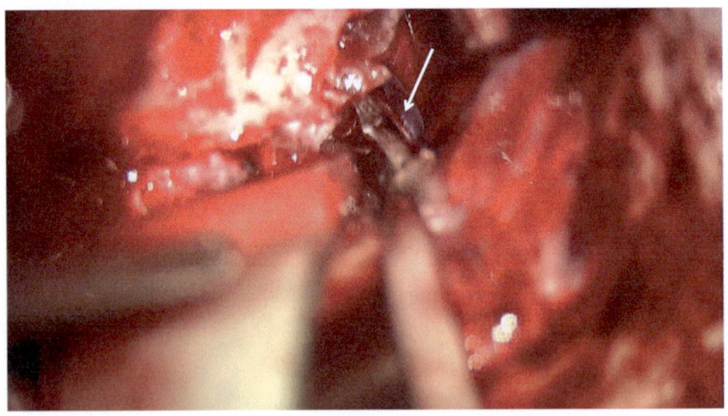

29. After cutting the notch of the tentorium, the white epidermoid was visible. Typically, CN IV should be identified and separated from the tentorium prior to cutting the notch as it often is adherent to it in a fold of arachnoid. However, in this case, CN IV was displaced by the epidermoid and not visible.

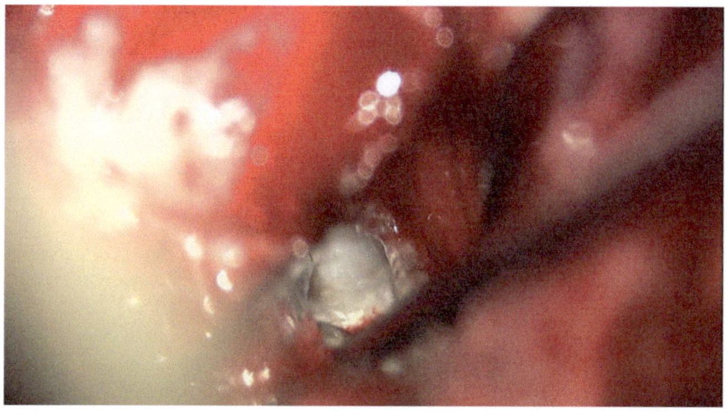

30. Dissecting out the epidermoid (*asterisk*) using a suction and a curette. CN V was inferior to the tip of the suction.

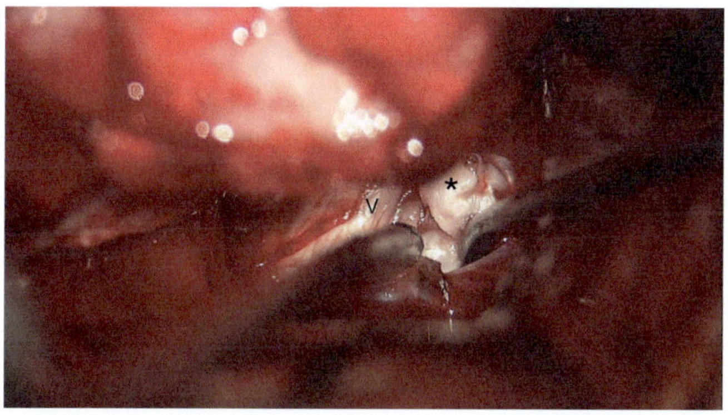

31. A cavity was developed in the center of the lesion.

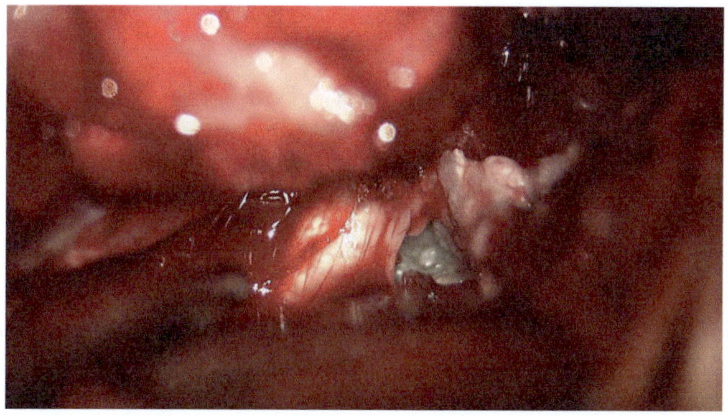

32. A portion of the wall is microdissected out.

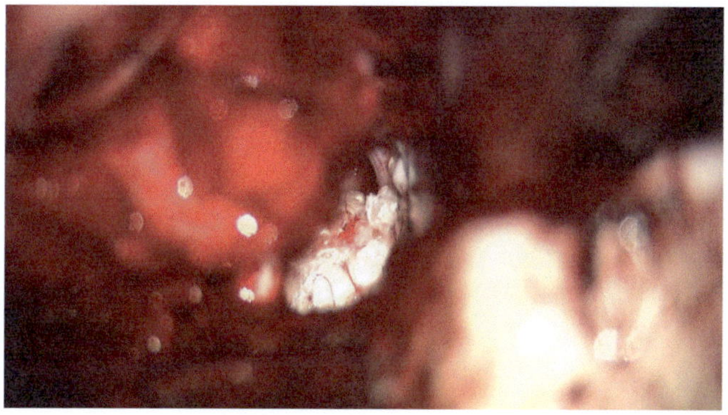

33. Residual epidermoid that was adherent to the brain and thus was not removed.

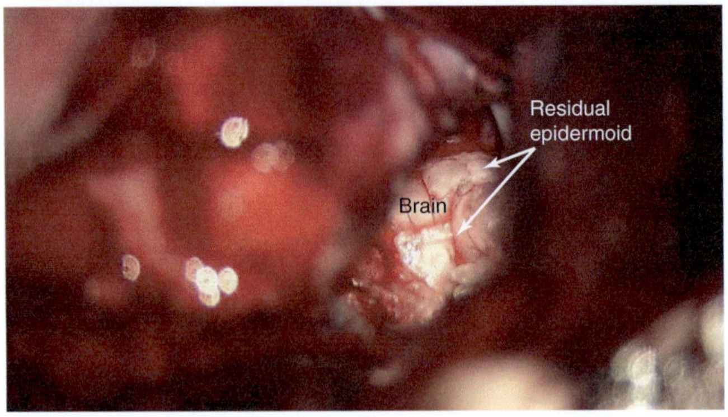

34. A view of the posterior fossa, looking between CN V and the CN VII/VIII complex. Much of the epidermoid has been debulked.

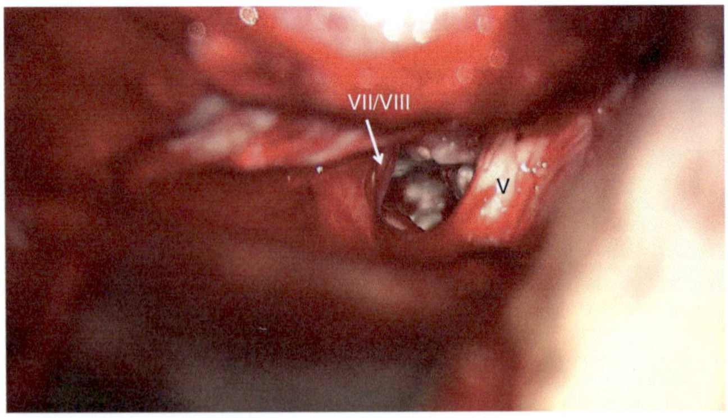

35. After further resection, this section was free of residual disease.

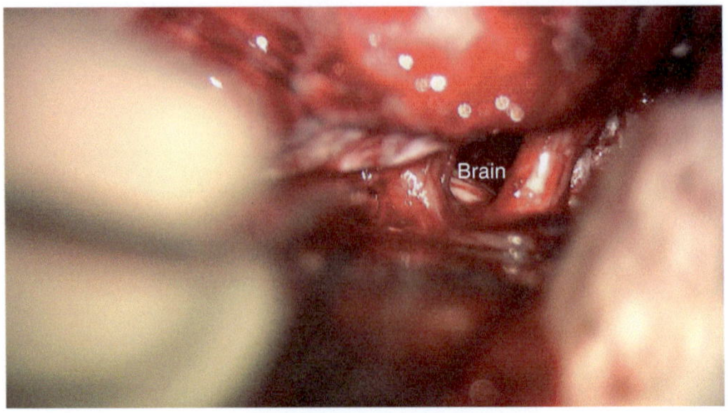

36. After removing as much epidermoid as possible, this was the overall view of the wound. While it is never possible to remove all of a large epidermoid such as this one, the vast majority of the core can be removed, and often much of the lining can safely be removed as well. Disease that is adherent to the brain is left behind in order to reduce morbidity. Note how the dural flaps were tacked up with sutures to keep them from obstructing the view of the intracranial cavity during the dissection process. They are moistened with saline periodically during the procedure to keep them healthy.

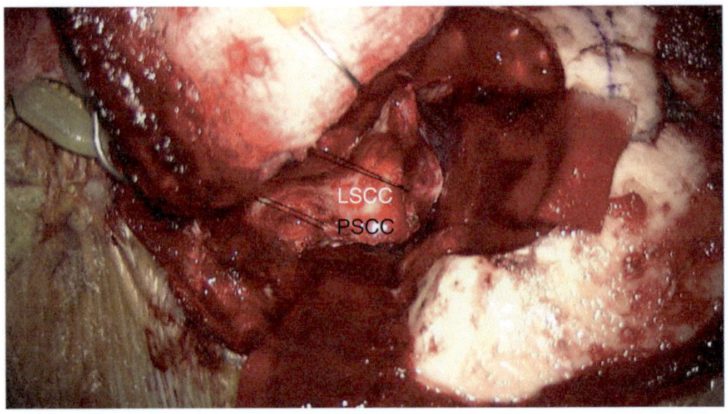

37. The Telfa strips were removed, the wound was irrigated, and all bleeding was stopped. Then, interrupted sutures were used to close as much of the dural opening as possible. Keeping the dural flaps moist throughout the procedure helped to keep them pliable enough to close most of the incision. The region at the trifurcation could not be closed (*arrow*). A piece of Duragen was inserted into this opening and sealed with Tisseal.

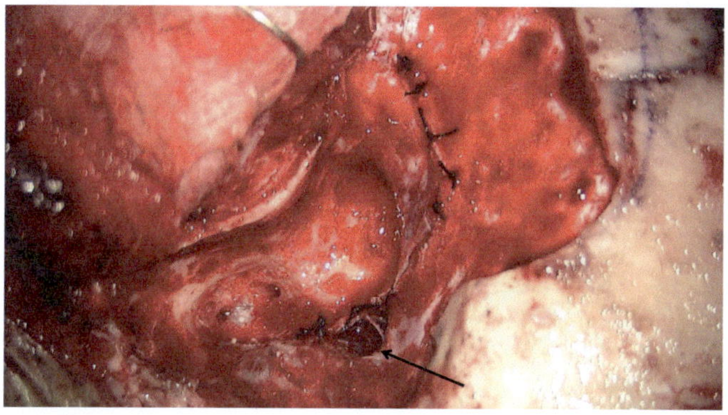

38. A piece of temporalis fascia was laid over the aditus ad antrum and sealed with Tisseal to separate the middle ear from the mastoid cavity. Then, an abdominal fat graft was harvested and placed in the mastoid cavity as shown here.

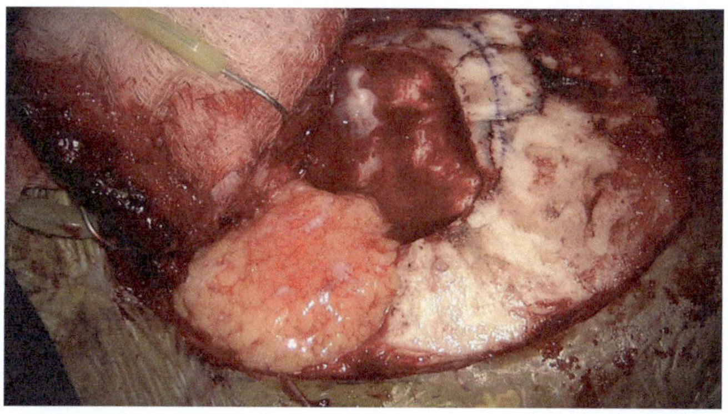

39. The bone flap was then plated back in place.

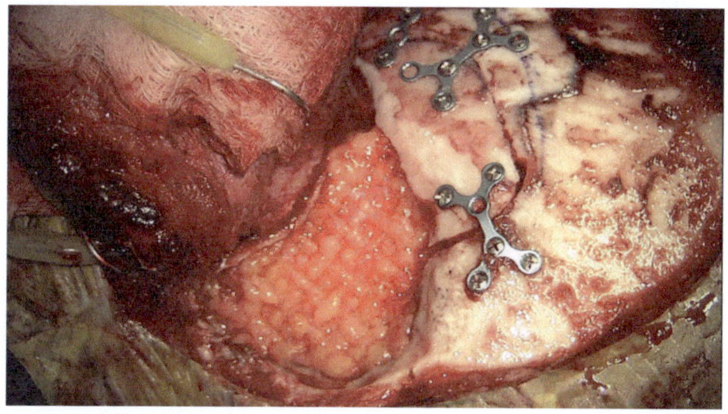

40. Postoperative T1 MRI with gadolinium showed significantly less mass effect on the brainstem.

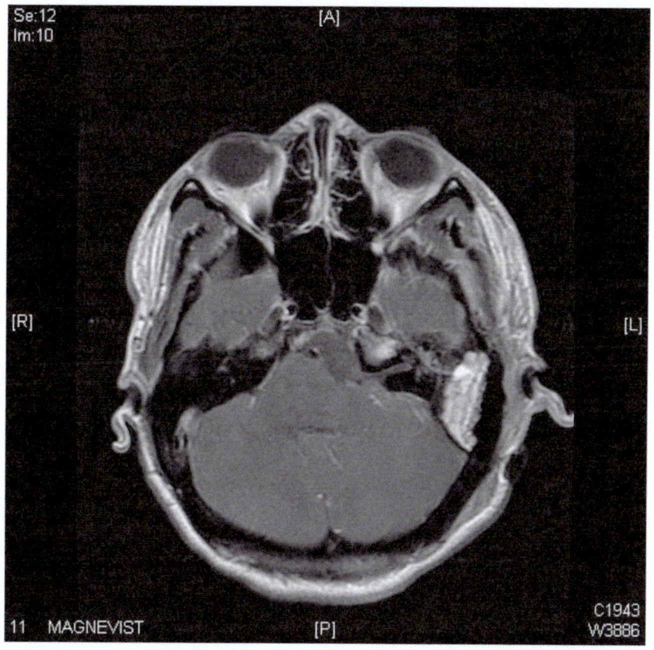

41. Postoperative T2 MRI.

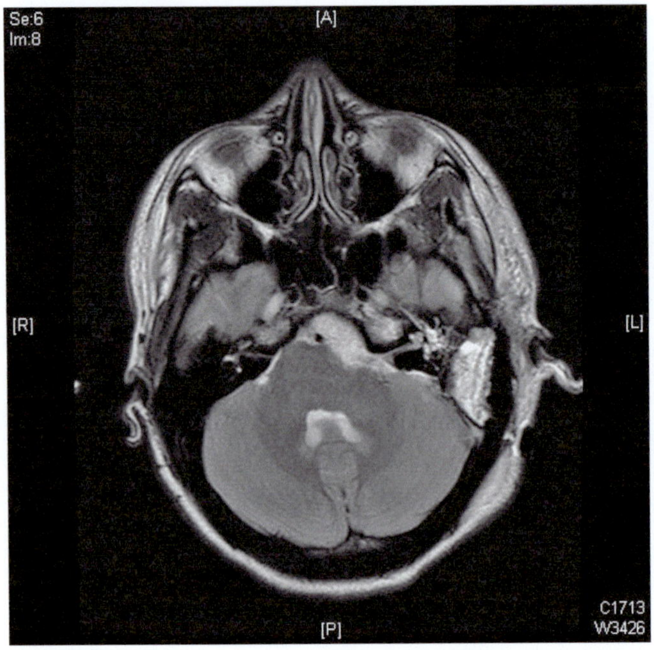

42. Postoperative diffusion-weighted MRI showed no evidence of a residual mass. This patient had no complications and had normal extraocular movements, hearing, and facial nerve function following surgery.

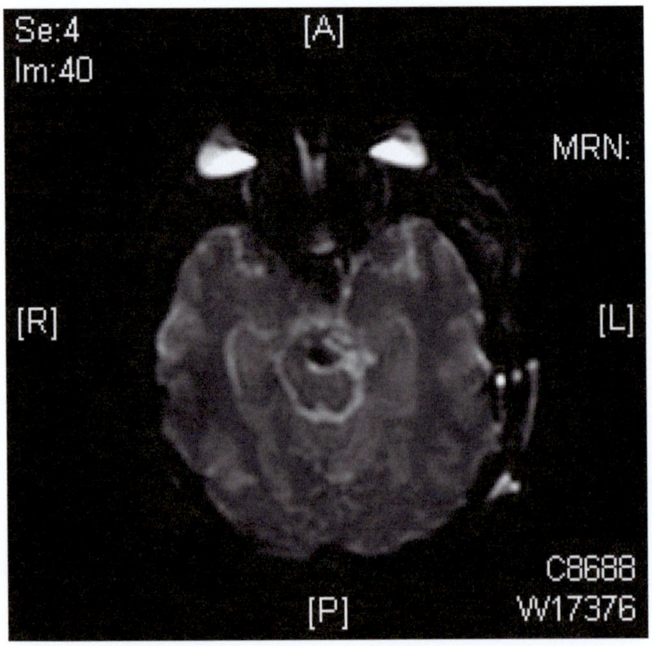

43. Case 2. T1 MRI with gadolinium of a patient with a petroclival meningioma that is appropriate for resection using the combined approach. It is based anterior to the internal auditory canal and exerts significant brainstem compression.

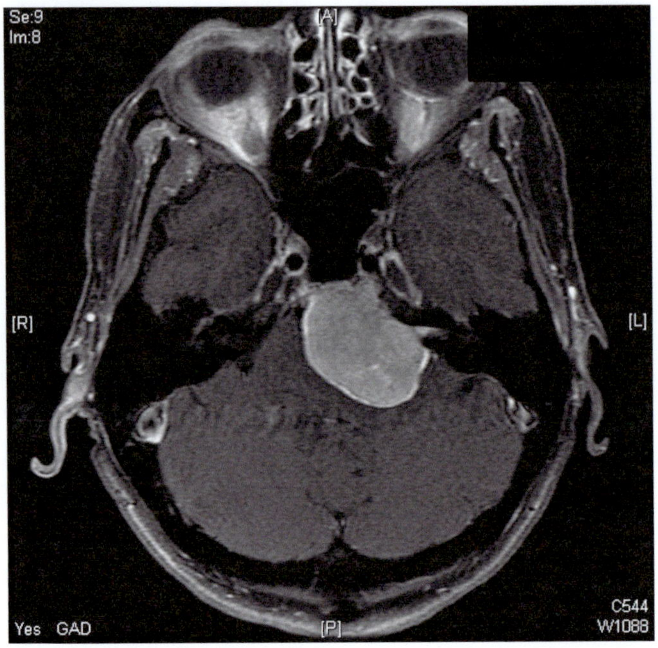

44. T2 MRI of the same patient. The internal auditory canal has only a small region of disease along its anterior aspect. Most of the tumor is within the posterior fossa, within the cerebellopontine angle, and ventral to the brainstem.

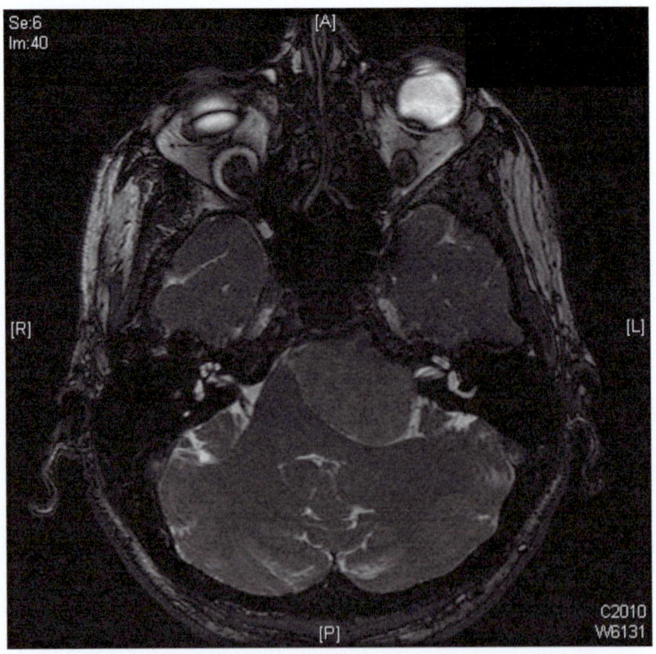

45. Coronal T1 MRI with gadolinium demonstrates that the tumor is inferior to the tentorium and does extend a little bit into the internal auditory canal. It extends inferior to the jugular bulb.

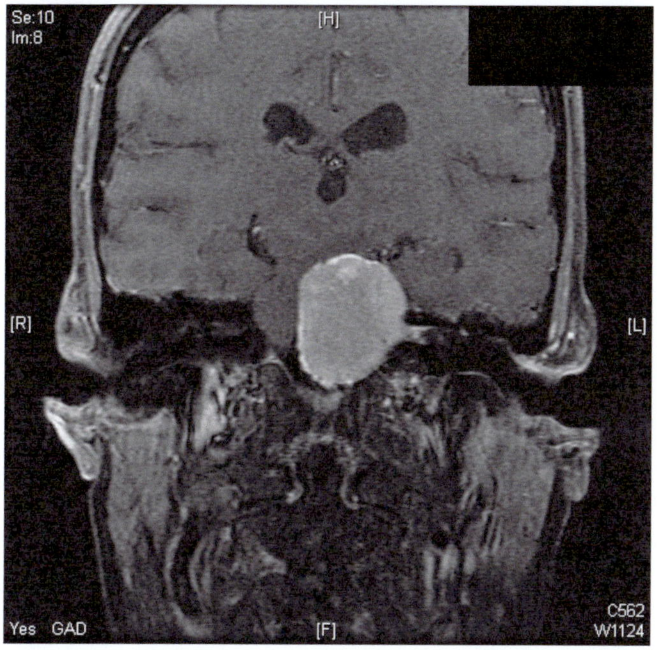

46. Postoperative axial T1 MRI with gadolinium. A combined approach was performed and a gross-total resection achieved intraoperatively. However, a small bit of disease may still present within the dura of the anterior internal auditory canal.

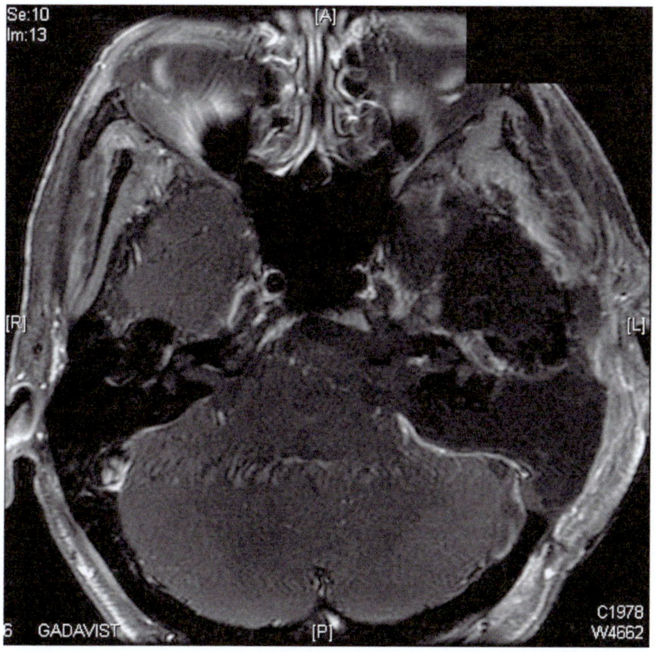

47. Postoperative coronal T1 MRI with gadolinium.

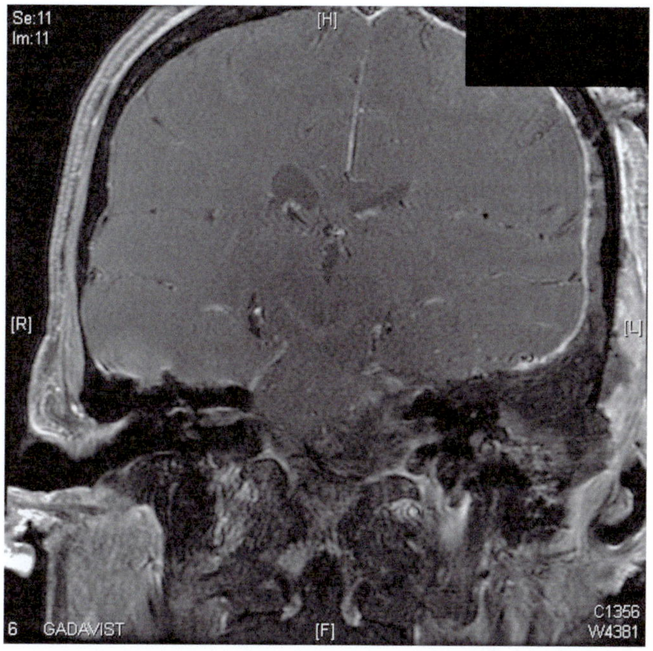

48. Postoperative axial T2 MRI demonstrates placement of fat graft within both the drilled-out mastoid and along the temporal floor.

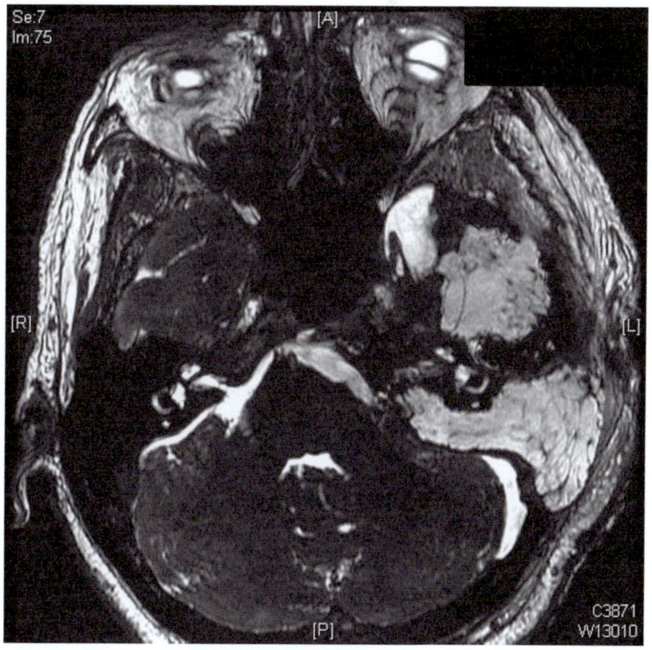

49. Postoperative CT demonstrates the amount of bone removal within the mastoid and petrous apex.

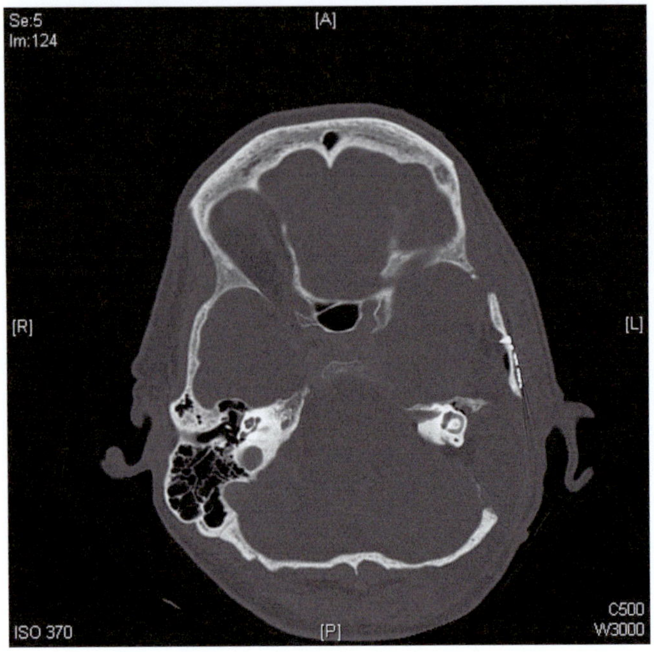

50. Case 3. Another patient with a petroclival meningioma that is appropriate for resection using the combined approach.

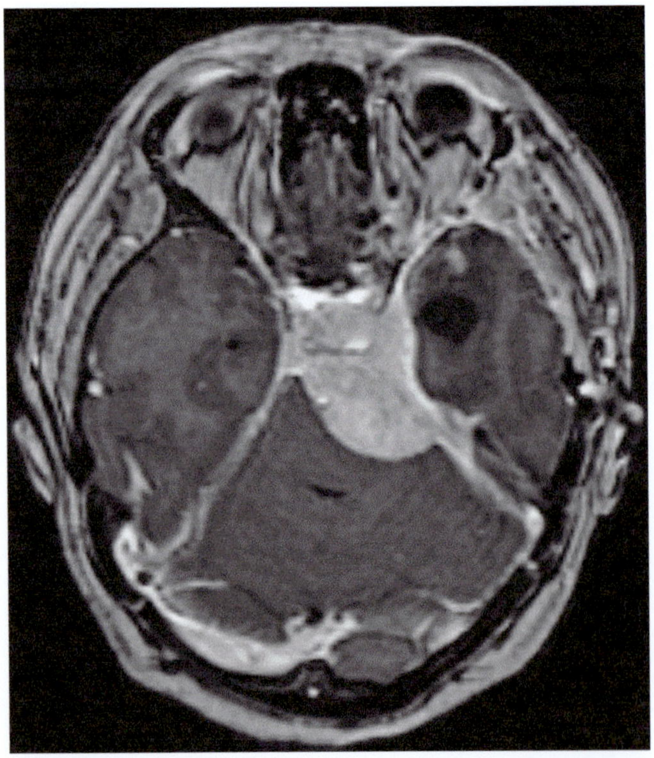

51. A lower cut from the same patient showing that the tumor had both middle and posterior fossa components.

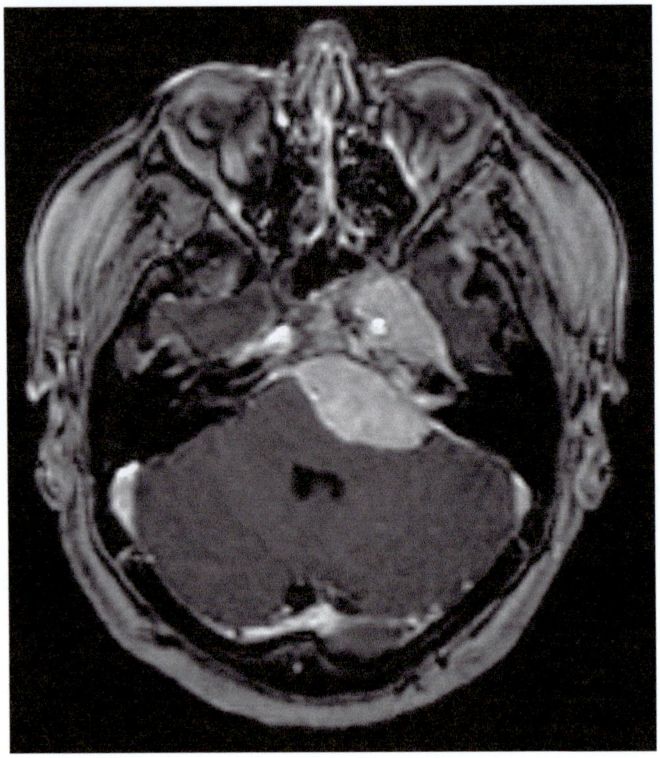

6 Infratemporal Fossa Approaches

Postauricular Approach to the Infratemporal Fossa

- *Concept*
  - Classically, this approach traverses the mastoid to reach the jugular foramen (termed a Fisch type A). It can be extended to reach the internal carotid artery, clivus, upper parapharyngeal space, and nasopharynx (Fisch types B, C, and D).
  - There are several different options for handling the facial nerve. These include
    - Leaving the nerve in place covered in a thin sleeve of bone (the fallopian bridge technique)
    - Rerouting the nerve in the lower half of the vertical segment just over the bulb (micro rerouting)
    - Rerouting the entire vertical segment from the second genu (short rerouting)
    - Rerouting the horizontal and vertical segments (long rerouting)
  - While the fallopian bridge technique causes no change in facial function, rerouting can create facial paralysis. The degree of facial paresis increases as more of the nerve is rerouted. With a long rerouting, complete facial paralysis in the immediate postoperative period should be expected. This will usually partially recover to reach a House–Brackmann grade III-IV functional level.
  - The postauricular infratemporal fossa approach can be tailored to provide as much exposure as needed to remove the tumor. These additional steps include
    - Removal of the ear canal with closure of the meatus
    - Translabyrinthine/transcochlear removal of the otic capsule
    - Decompression of carotid artery
    - Division of the GSPN followed by complete facial nerve rerouting (from the internal auditory canal to the stylomastoid foramen)
  - If the tumor extends through the dura of the jugular foramen, the procedure can be extended into a transjugular craniotomy. In this case, the sigmoid sinus is resected and the posterior fossa dura opened.
- *Conditions treated*
  - Glomus jugulare
  - Jugular foramen schwannoma
  - Jugular foramen meningioma
  - Other tumors involving the jugular foramen and lateral skull base
- *Risks*
  - Hearing loss
  - Facial nerve injury
  - Palsy of CN IX, X, XI, or XII
  - Injury to the internal carotid artery
  - Cerebral venous infarction or intracranial hypertension
- *Benefits*
  - There is excellent exposure of the entire course of the sigmoid sinus, jugular bulb, and internal jugular vein.
  - Exposure of the internal carotid artery at skull base and into the petrous temporal bone.
  - CN VII, IX, X, XI, and XII can be traced all the way from the skull out into the face and neck.

J.S. Oghalai, C.L.W. Driscoll, *Atlas of Neurotologic and Lateral Skull Base Surgery*,
DOI 10.1007/978-3-662-46694-0_6, © Springer-Verlag Berlin Heidelberg 2016

1. Diagram of the venous outflow of the brain. Note the multiple intra- and extracranial anastomostic pathways between the cavernous sinus and the jugular vein.

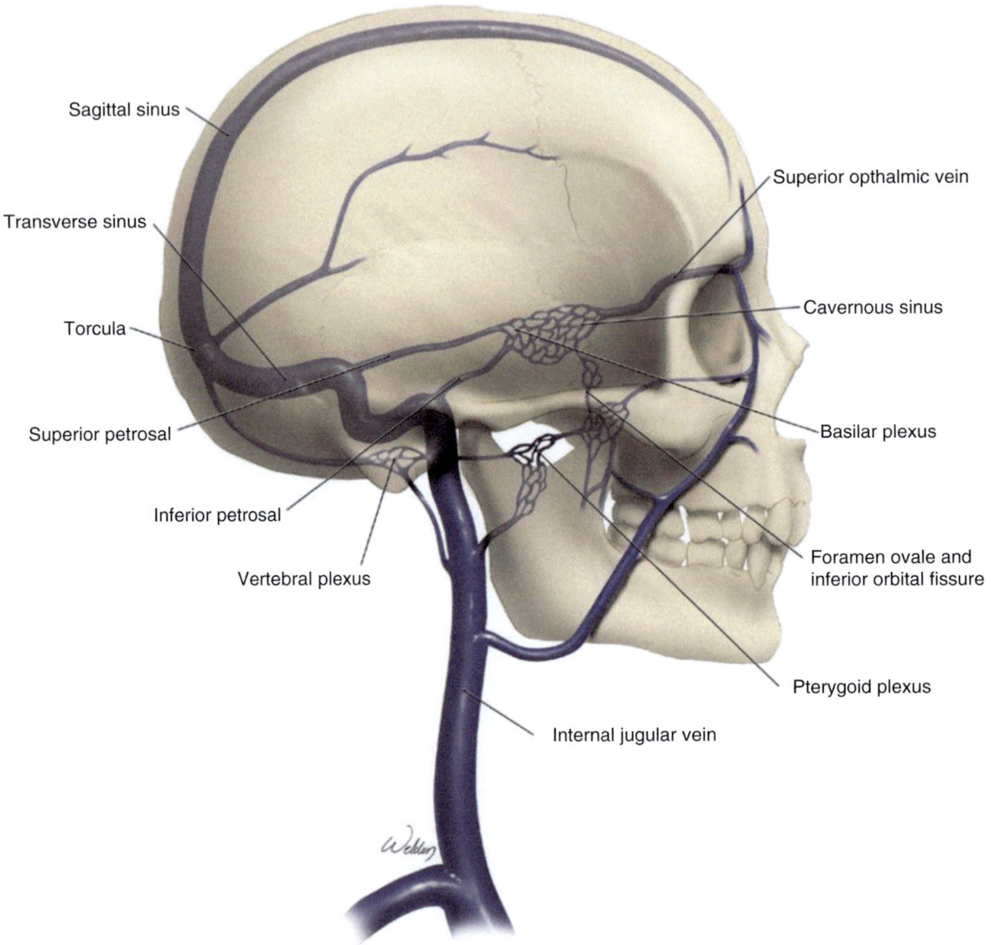

2. There are also many congenital variants in the anatomy of the sigmoid sinus. (A) Most common is that one side is dominant. (B) Rarely, one side may be absent (C, D). Other anatomic variations are also occasionally found. Surgical planning should take this into consideration. For example, one would not want to resect a sigmoid sinus unless the sigmoid sinus on the other side is present and large enough to be able to handle the additional blood flow.

   In otolaryngology residency training and in the clinical practice of general otolaryngology, little attention is paid to preservation of venous structures because of the robust collateral flow throughout the head and neck. It is even possible to remove both jugular veins with a relatively low risk of complications due to inadequate venous drainage. This is clearly a different environment than what we face within the skull base and intracranially. Cerebral venous infarction can be devastating, and even transient increased intracranial pressure can result in a CSF leak, pseudomeningocele, or need for a shunting procedure. It is critical to carefully assess venous flow prior to intervention. We often obtain an angiogram during the evaluation (assess tumor vascularity, status of carotid) and treatment (embolization) of these tumors, and this provides an opportunity to assess venous drainage. This is complementary to the MR venogram or CT angiogram. We may alter our surgical approach or aggressiveness of tumor removal based on venous drainage patterns. In vestibular schwannoma surgery, we will avoid a translabyrinthine approach when compromise of the sigmoid sinus could be catastrophic. Even without injury, the sinus can occlude after a translabyrinthine approach. Some tumors involving the jugular foramen that have partially or completely compressed the sigmoid sinus or jugular bulb/vein can be removed with preservation of the vein so even in cases with no flow through the vein, we may attempt to preserve the vein.

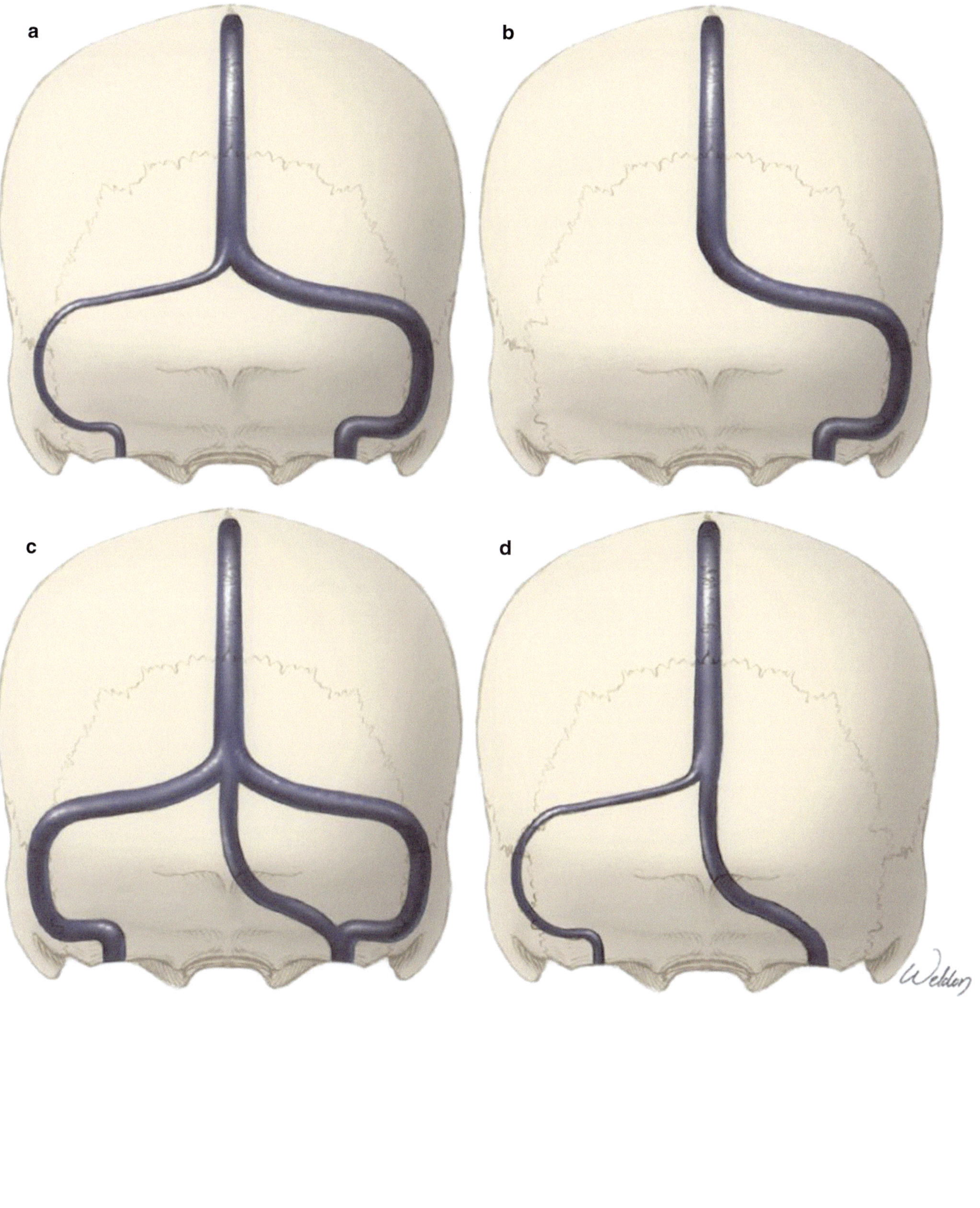

3. The postauricular approach involves resecting much of the bone within the dotted lines in order to expose the jugular bulb.

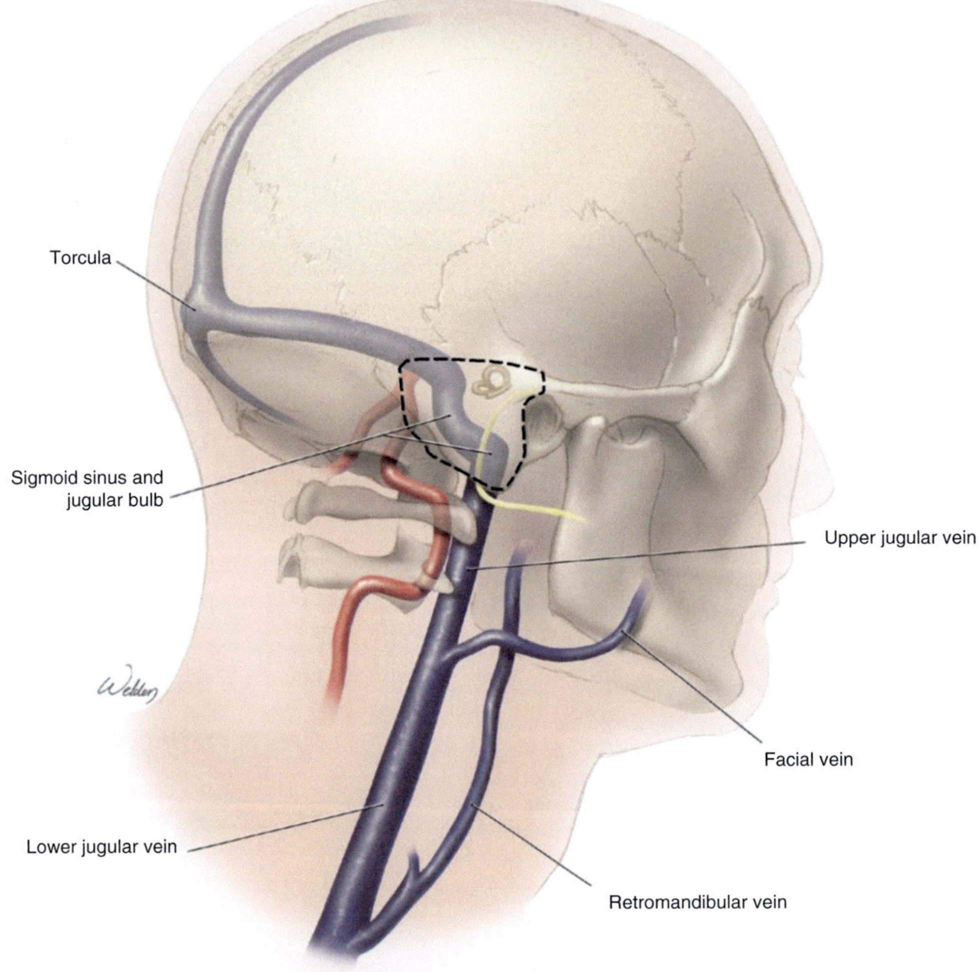

4. The incision should be carried down onto the neck to allow for exposure and control of the jugular vein and carotid artery. When planning to open dura, it is possible that CSF may leak down into the neck postoperatively and form a pseudomeningocele. Therefore, it is best to limit the dissection in the neck to minimize the potential space for fluid to collect.

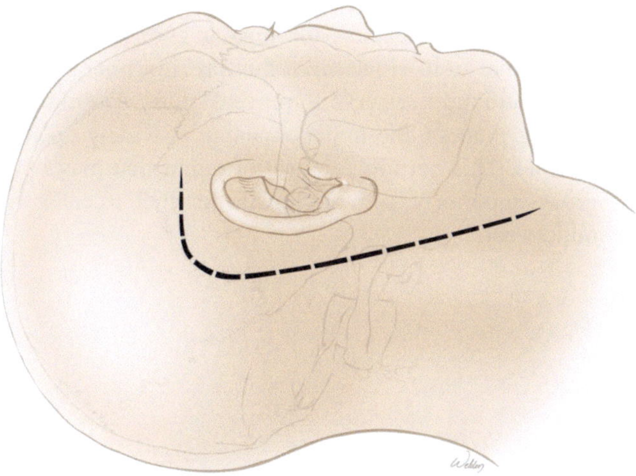

5. The soft tissues are reflected off the mastoid and the parotid gland identified. Dissection is carried along the anterior border of the sternocleidomastoid muscle and the digastric muscle identified. Deep and inferior to the digastric, the internal carotid artery and internal jugular vein are identified. Rubber slings are wrapped circumferentially around the vessels with the ends held together with a hemostat. The slings should be kept loose so as not to compress the vessels. However in an emergency (i.e., rupture of the vessel), the slings can be pulled tight to control the bleeding. The vessel loops can also be placed around the artery and vein without circumferential looping. This still permits the surgeon a way to quickly pull up and clamp the vessel if needed. While perhaps not as secure as circumferential looping, there is less risk of traction on the loop causing inadvertent tightening around the vessel during the procedure.

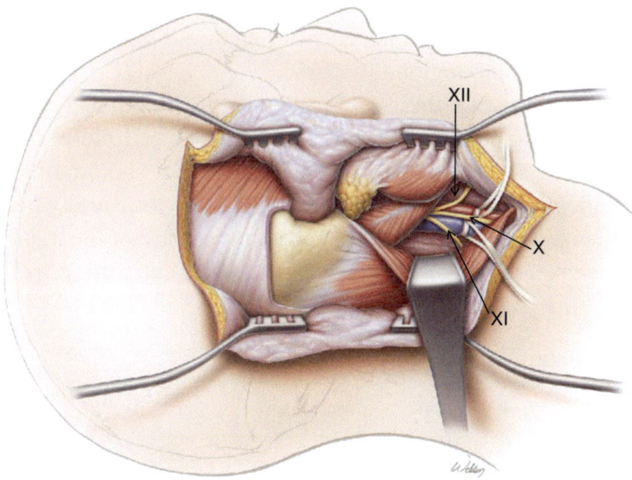

6. A standard mastoidectomy has been performed and the ear canal wall preserved. The bone covering the inferior half of the sigmoid sinus has been removed (see the translabyrinthine approach for details on this technique). The facial nerve is identified at the second genu and followed down to the stylomastoid foramen. The main trunk of the extracranial facial nerve is identified but does not need to be dissected out to the pes anserinus.

   The key point of this entire operation is to expose the tissues inferior to the sigmoid sinus. This is performed by first releasing the sternocleidomastoid muscle (*SCM*) from its attachment to the mastoid process, retracting it posteriorly and then drilling away the entire mastoid tip. Next, the digastric muscle is divided near its attachment to the skull base and retracted anteriorly. The bone inferior to the sigmoid sinus (the area of the digastric muscle attachment) is drilled away. Sometimes, a condylar emissary vein is found draining into the sigmoid sinus. This should be divided and occluded at this stage as it will decrease bleeding later during tumor removal in the jugular bulb region.

   Removing these muscles and the bone that they attach to permits the great vessels to then be followed up to the skull base. CN IX, X, XI, and XII should all be identified during this dissection. The vertebral artery lies within the fascia along the posterior surface of the transverse process of C1; there is no need to enter this area.

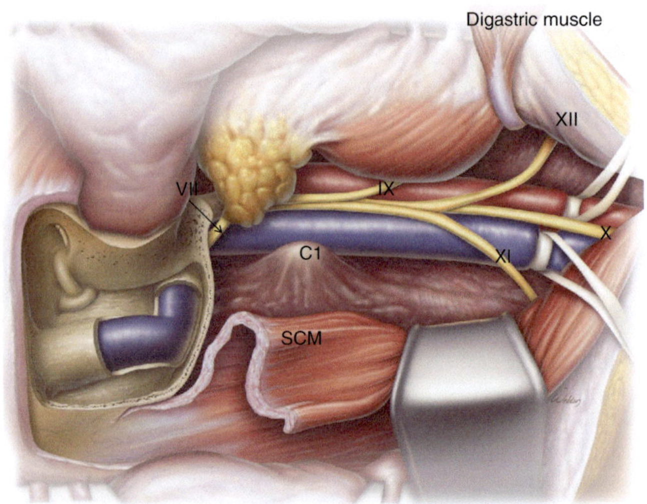

7. In this example, a canal wall up procedure with the fallopian bridge technique is shown. A facial recess approach is performed and then extended inferiorly. Dividing the chorda tympani nerve should be done sharply rather than with the drill to prevent traction injury to the facial nerve. Note that the ossicular chain should be left intact to maintain hearing with this approach.

   The facial nerve is skeletonized circumferentially (*arrowheads*) to expose the jugular bulb (*JB*), which lies medial to it. However, a thin layer of bone should be left around the nerve to prevent injury. During this drilling process, the hypotympanum is widely opened (*arrow*). This permits removal of tumor that may have grown superiorly from the jugular foramen to enter the middle ear.

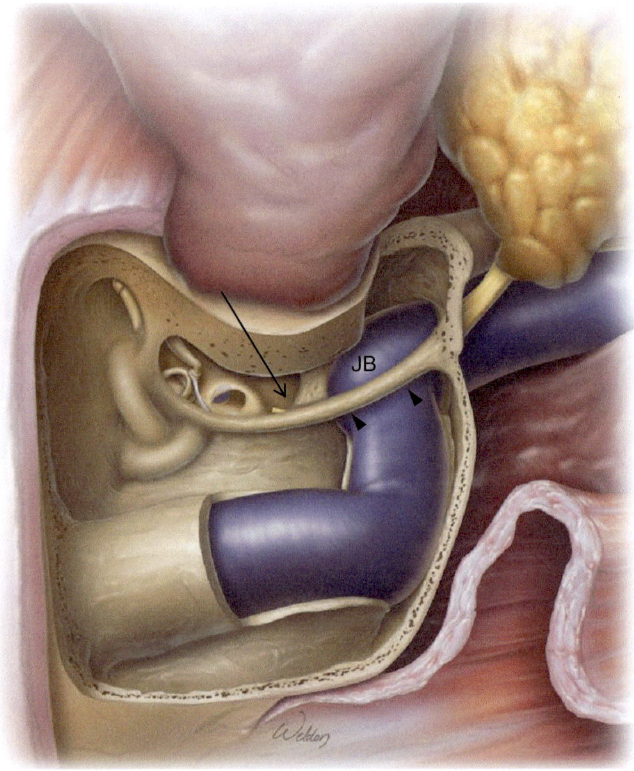

8. Alternatively, a canal wall down procedure can be performed as shown in this example. The ear canal is transected at the bony cartilaginous junction and most of the ear canal drilled away. Only the anterior canal wall is left intact. In order to remove the tympanic membrane, the incudostapedial joint is separated and the incus removed. Cutting the tensor tympani tendon then permits removal of the entire tympanic membrane and malleus. All ear canal skin is carefully removed using a round knife. Finally, the anterior ear canal bone is drilled smooth to verify that all epithelial remnants within it have been removed. Closure of this wound involves plugging the Eustachian tube, closing off the ear canal, and filling the defect with a fat graft (see the section on temporal bone resection in Chap. 8 for details). In this example, the fallopian bridge technique is still used. Alternatively, rerouting of the facial nerve may be performed to more completely expose the jugular bulb. To do this, the bone overlying the nerve should be carefully removed and the nerve elevated out of the fallopian canal (see Chap. 9 for details).

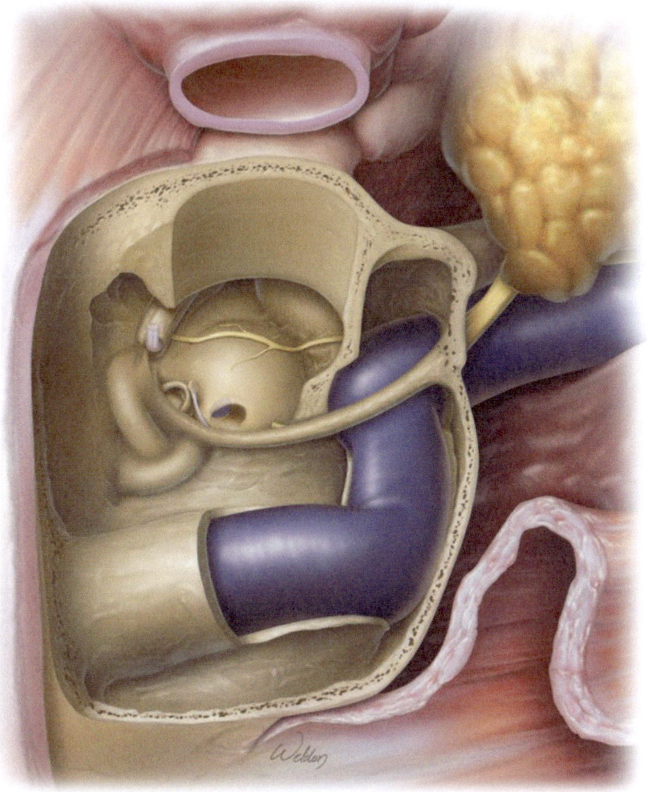

9. Venous flow through the sigmoid sinus is blocked by extraluminal packing of Surgicel between the bone and the lateral sinus wall. Next, the internal jugular vein is divided and ligated in the neck.

   The sinus can then be opened with a scissors to expose the jugular bulb. If there is a large tumor within the jugular bulb, bleeding is usually minimal at this stage. If there is only a small tumor or it is not fully occluding the bulb, bleeding from the condylar emissary vein and the inferior petrosal sinus can be significant. This bleeding can be partially controlled with Surgicel, cottonoid pledgets, and pressure. However, there is no way to completely stop this bleeding without full exposure of the bulb, removal of all tumor within it, and then packing of the bulb with Surgicel to occlude the inferior petrosal sinus collaterals and the condylar emissary vein. Care should be taken to not pack too tightly and risk injury to the underlying lower cranial nerves.

   An alternative to extraluminal compression of the vein is to use a 6-0 nylon suture to sew across the vein tacking the anterior wall of the sinus to the posterior wall. While theoretically this can be done without opening the dura, it is significantly easier to do with opening of the dura. However, we would only do this if we were already planning to open the dura for tumor removal. The benefit of this method is that when opening the dura across the sigmoid sinus, it can be tough to get adequate pressure from extraluminal surgical packing. Also, it allows us to block the vein more distally, which may decrease the risk of occluding the superior petrosal sinus or vein of Labbé.

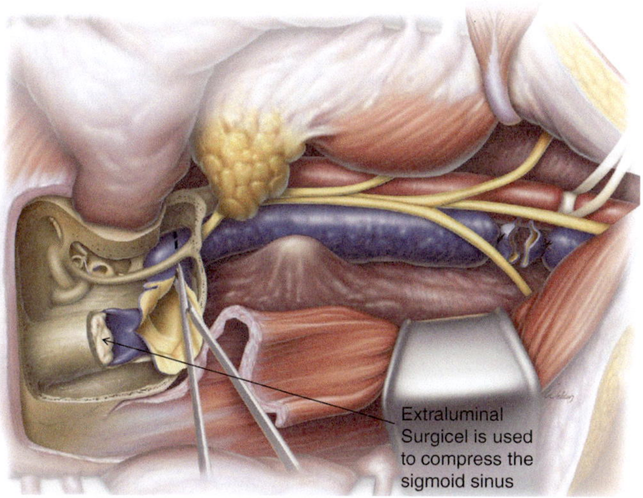

10. In this example, a canal wall down technique has been used together with long rerouting of the facial nerve. The internal carotid artery has been exposed to the petrous temporal bone, and tumor within the opened jugular bulb is visible. The tumor is adjacent to the genu of the internal carotid artery. This tumor can now be carefully microdissected off the carotid artery and removed from the jugular bulb. There are often small branches emanating from the carotid artery at the genu, and this portion of the artery seems particularly vulnerable to injury. It is sometimes wise to leave a small amount of adherent tumor in this area.

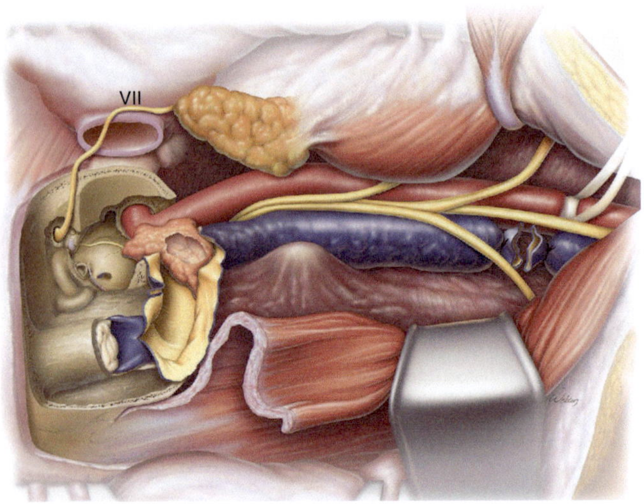

11. If the tumor extends into the intradural space, a transjugular craniotomy can be performed. Rather than simply compressing the sigmoid sinus, it can be suture ligated and the dura across the sigmoid opened. This allows resection of intra- and extradural tumor. Watertight closure of the dura is needed if the canal wall up approach is used as shown here in order to prevent cerebrospinal fluid leak into the middle ear and down the Eustachian tube. Typically, we use an artificial dural patch, a dura sealant, and then pack off the mastoid with a fat graft. A lumbar subarachnoid drain is often beneficial as well for larger dural defects.

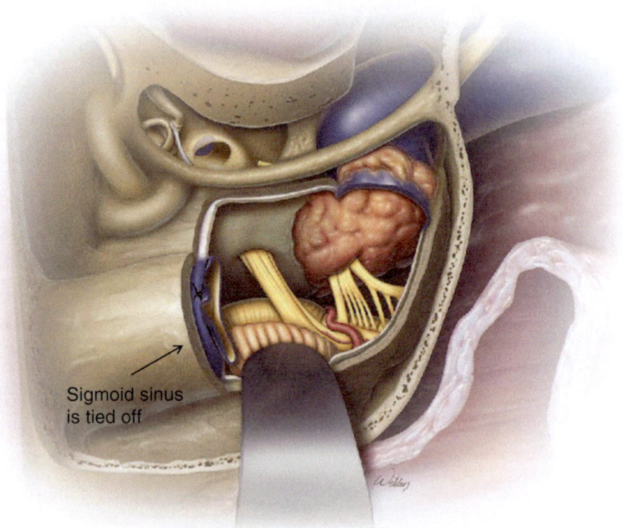

12. Case 1. Axial CT of a cholesteatoma involving the jugular bulb. On exam, the squamous epithelium was visible within the hypotympanic region (*arrow*).

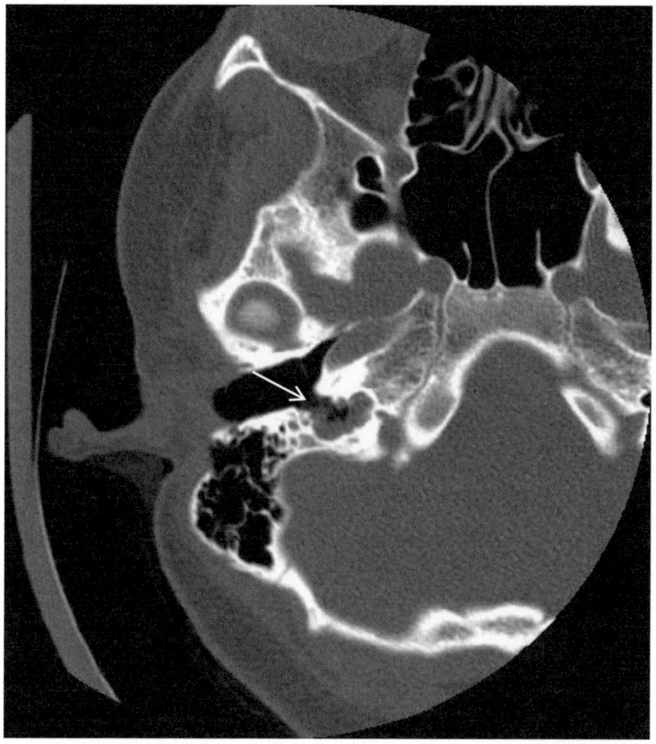

13. A fallopian bridge technique was used to access the cholesteatoma and dissect it off the jugular bulb. The vertical segment of the facial nerve with a thin layer of bone seems to be floating in midair (*arrowhead*).

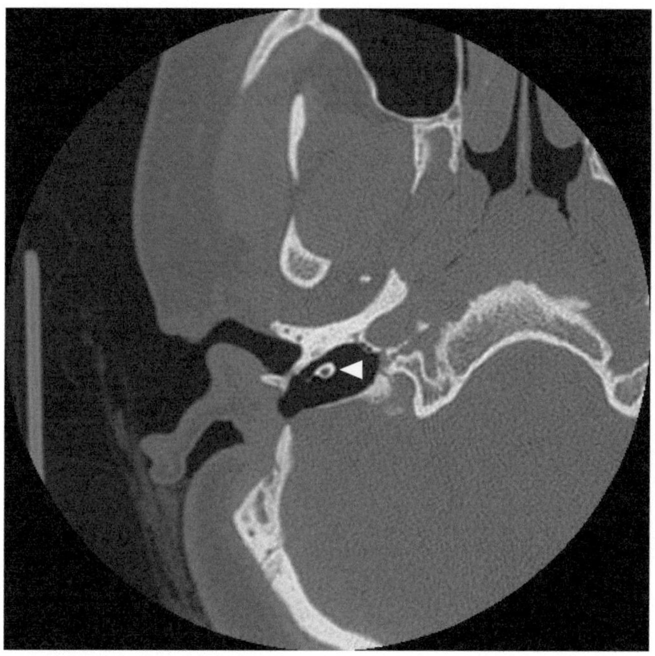

14. More superiorly, a standard canal wall up with facial recess approach was performed. Ossicular chain reconstruction with a PORP was performed.

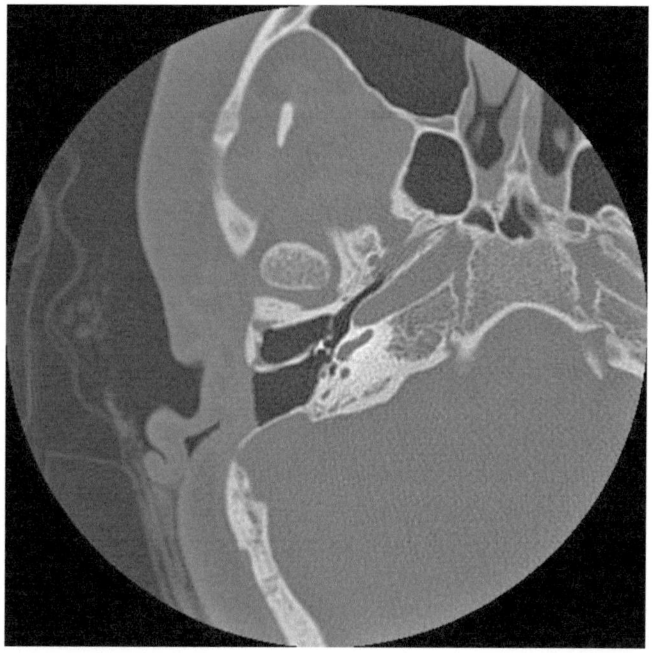

15. Case 2. Axial T1 MRI with gadolinium demonstrated a left posterior fossa schwannoma.

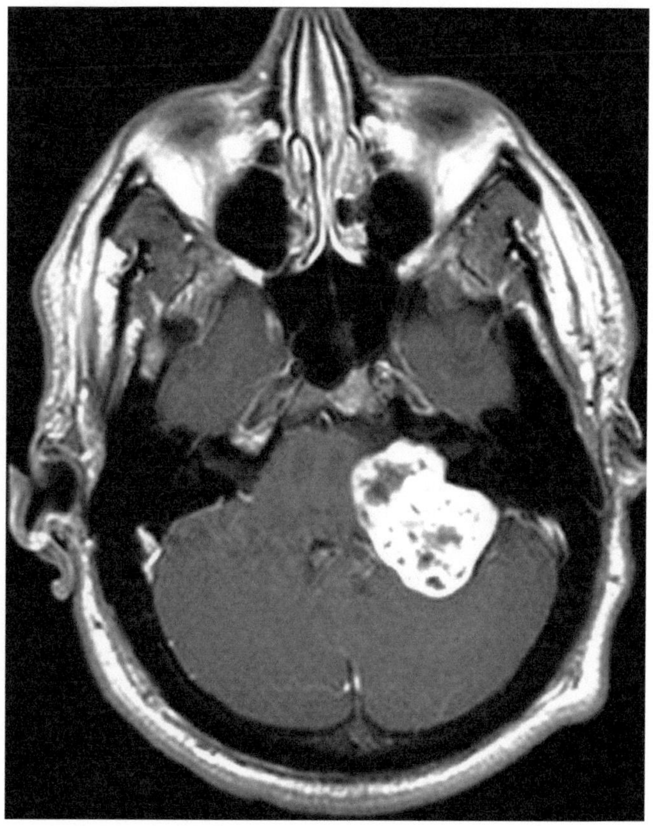

16. A more inferior cut revealed that the tumor entered the jugular foramen. Thus, the tumor originated from CN IX, X, or XI. Exam demonstrated weakness of the left vocal cord consistent with a schwannoma of CN X.

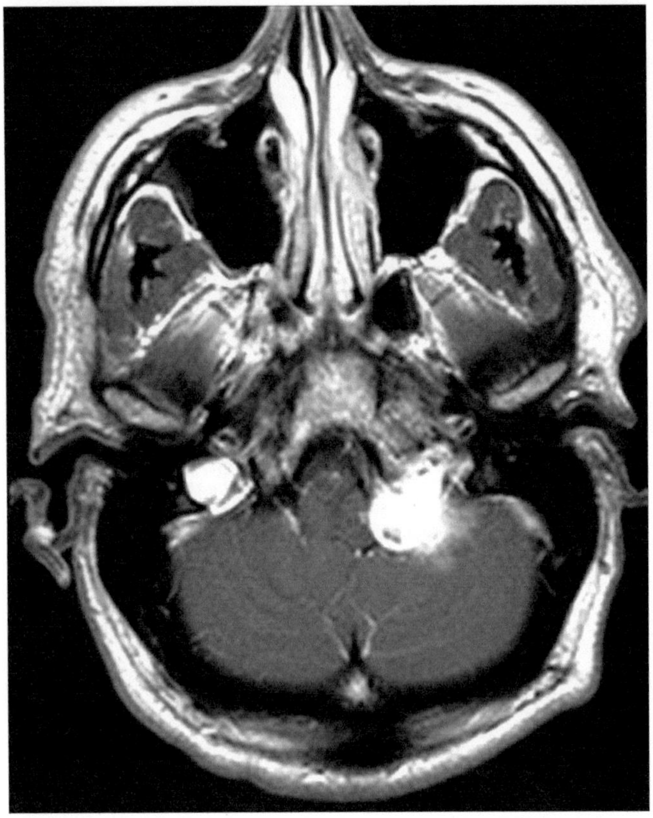

17. The coronal MRI clearly demonstrated how the schwanomma entered the jugular foramen. Because the tumor was primarily intradural with only minimal skull base bone involvement, a retrosigmoid approach was used as opposed to a formal postauricular infratemporal fossa approach.

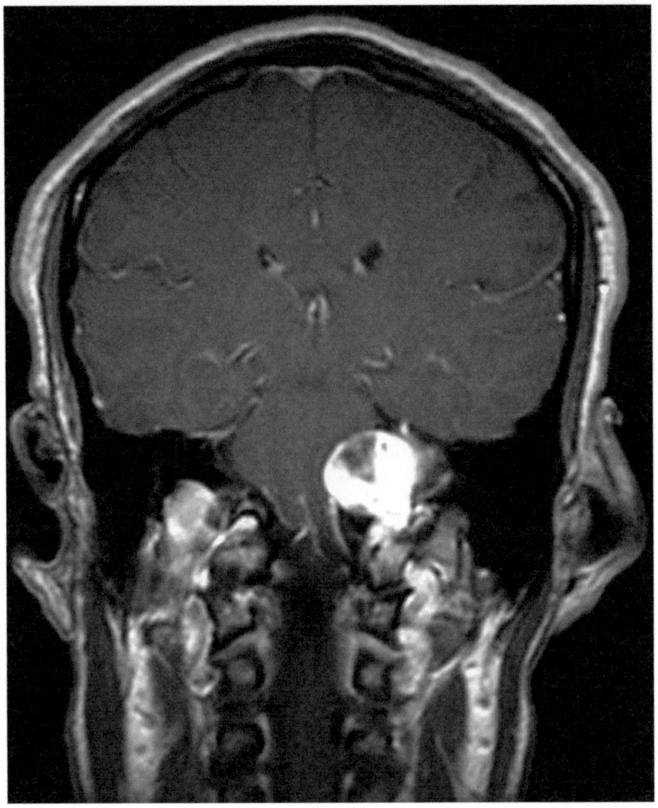

18. Postoperative T1 MRI with fat saturation demonstrates a near-total resection of the tumor. A small stub of tumor (*arrow*) was left in the jugular foramen to preserve the function of CN IX and XI. If we had wanted to remove this remnant, we could have drilled away the posterior lip of bone covering the jugular foramen. However, this would undoubtedly have affected function of these lower cranial nerves.

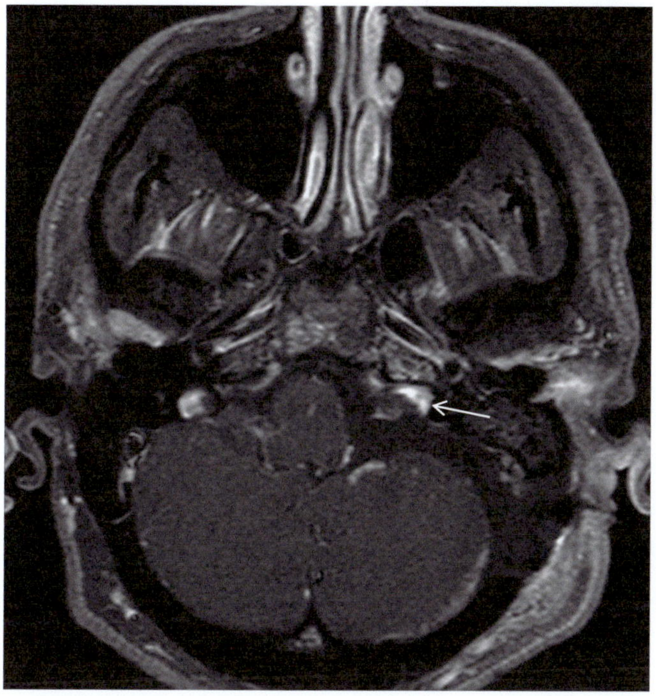

19. Case 3. A skull base meningioma that involved the temporal bone, otic capsule, and jugular foramen. There were hyperostotic changes to the posterior face of the temporal bone (*arrows*), and the internal auditory canal was narrowed. The dura enhanced from the sigmoid sinus all the way across the clivus. The enhancement lateral to the internal auditory canal was meningioma that infiltrated into the middle ear (*arrowhead*) and was visible on otoscopy in clinic as a white mass behind the tympanic membrane.

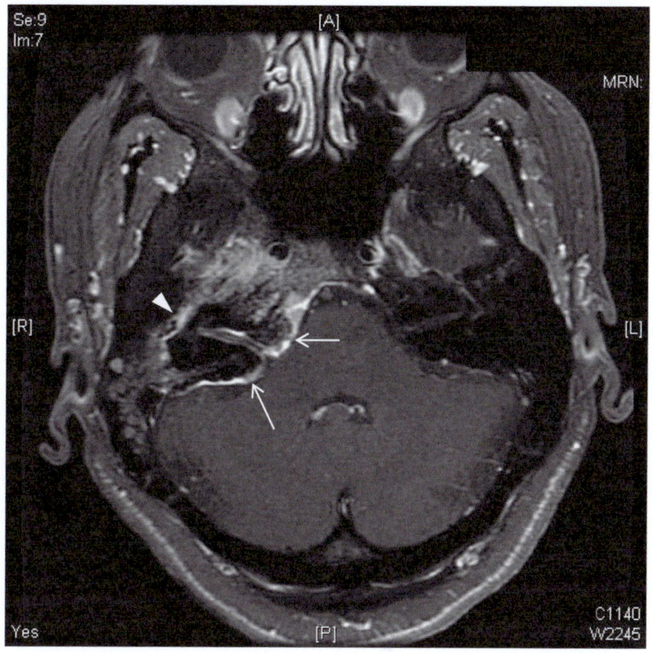

20. Coronal T1 MRI of the same patient. The middle fossa dura was also involved.

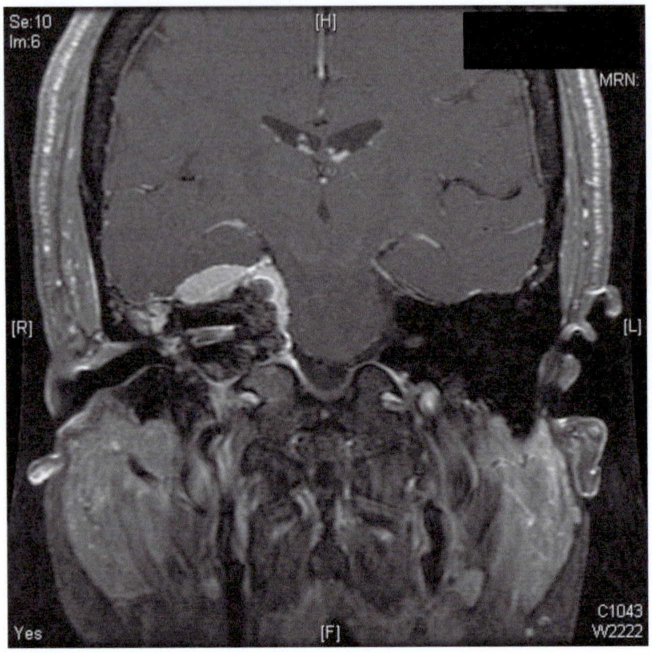

21. A pink mass was visible behind the right tympanic membrane in the posterior portion of the middle ear cavity. There was no serviceable hearing in the ear, thus a combined transjugular/transcochlear procedure was performed for access to the primary areas of tumor involvement: the middle fossa dura, the posterior fossa dura, the middle ear, the internal auditory canal, and the petrous apex. CN VII, IX, X, XI, and XII all had normal function. Therefore, we planned a subtotal resection with the goal of sparing their function while debulking the majority of the tumor.

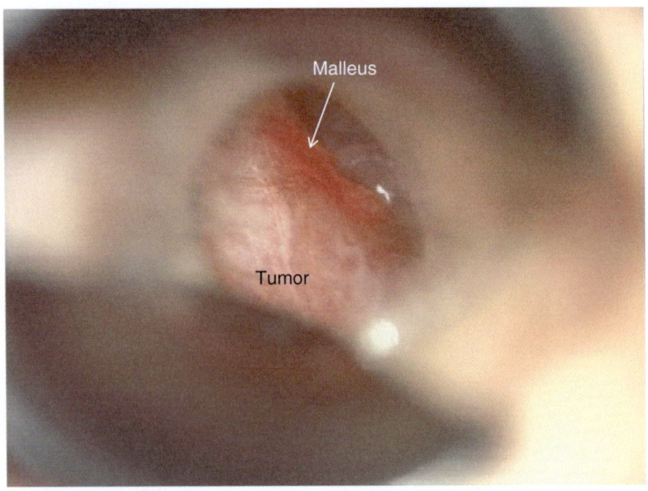

22. The ear canal was transected and a standard mastoidectomy performed. The retrosigmoid dura was exposed and the malleable retractor placed on the sigmoid sinus.

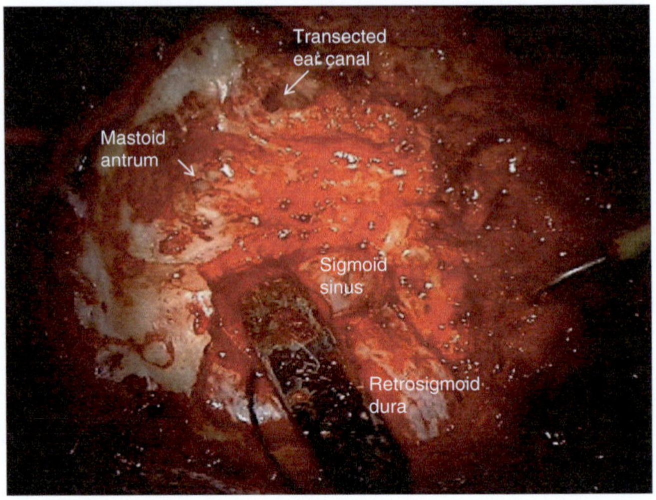

23. Another retractor was placed on the middle fossa dura. The otic capsule bone of the semicircular canals (*arrow*) can be seen to be irregular and invaded with tumor.

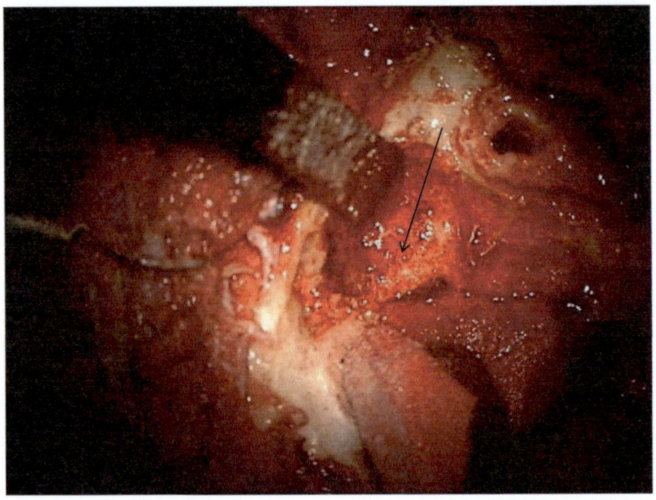

24. Looking through the ear canal with the tympanic membrane removed, the tumor within the middle ear can be seen.

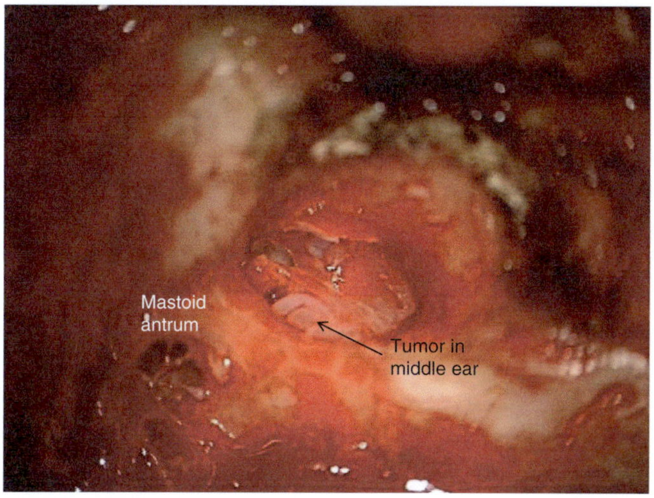

25. The canal wall was removed and all the ossicles resected. A labyrinthectomy was performed and the facial nerve skeletonized around the second genu, leaving a thin bony fallopian canal intact. Note that all the skin of the ear canal has been removed. The Eustachian tube is visible (*arrow*).

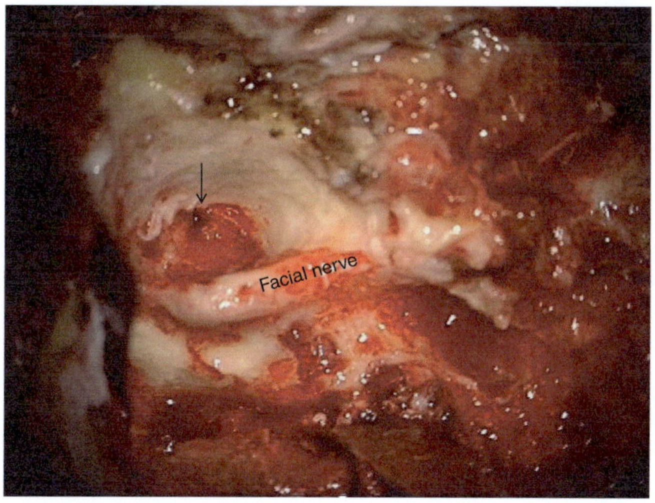

26. The promontory was then drilled, and tumor can be seen within the cochlea (*arrow*).

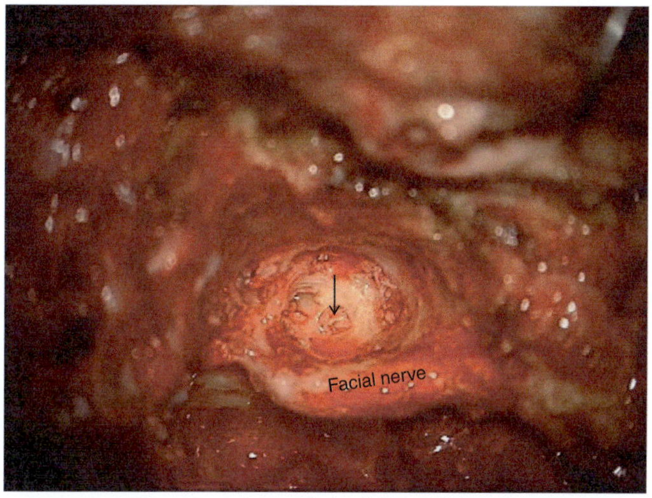

27. After removal of the cochlea, the facial nerve fallopian bridge can be appreciated.

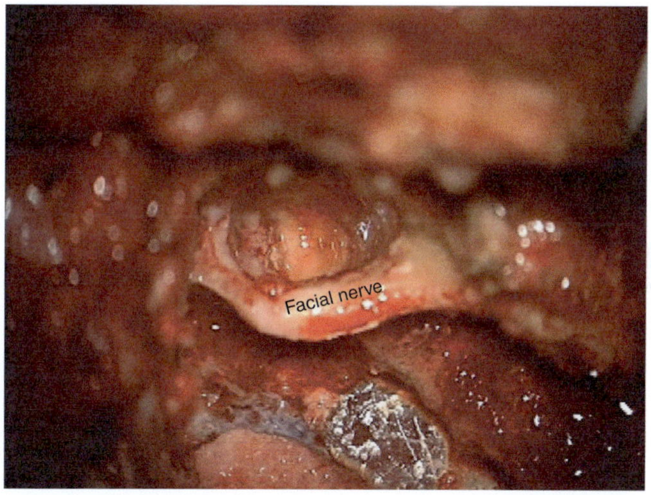

28. The suction is visible around the facial nerve, demonstrating 360° skeletonization of the fallopian canal.

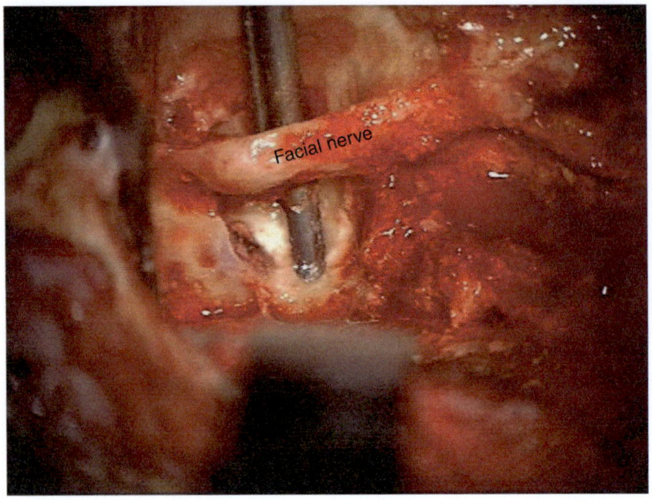

29. The internal jugular vein (*IJV*) was identified in the neck and retracted with a rubber sling.

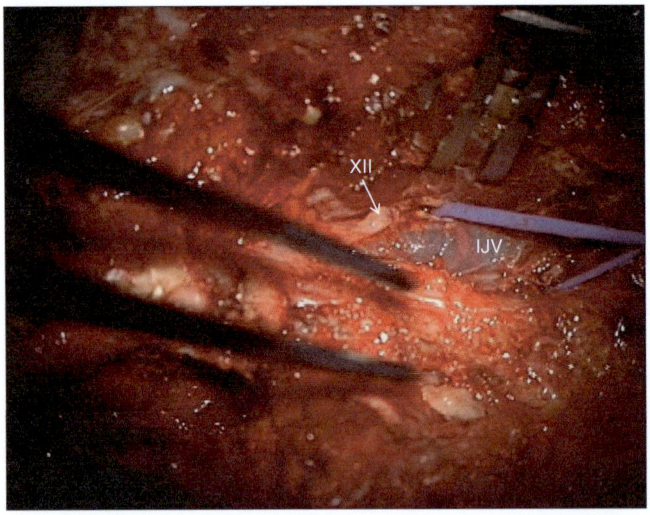

30. A small stitch was placed through the outer leaflet of the retrosigmoid dura to use for retraction.

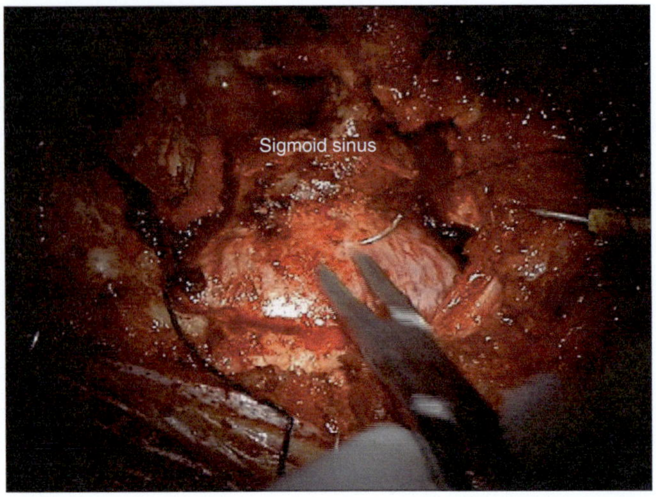

31. The dura was lifted up with the suture to prevent injury to the cerebellum when opening the dura with an 11 blade scalpel. Once an initial opening was made, scissors were used to enlarge the opening.

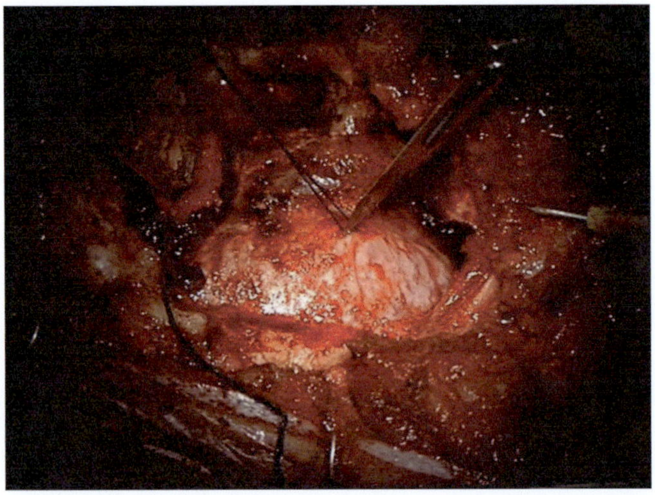

32. The cerebellum was exposed, and a moist Telfa strip is placed on it for protection.

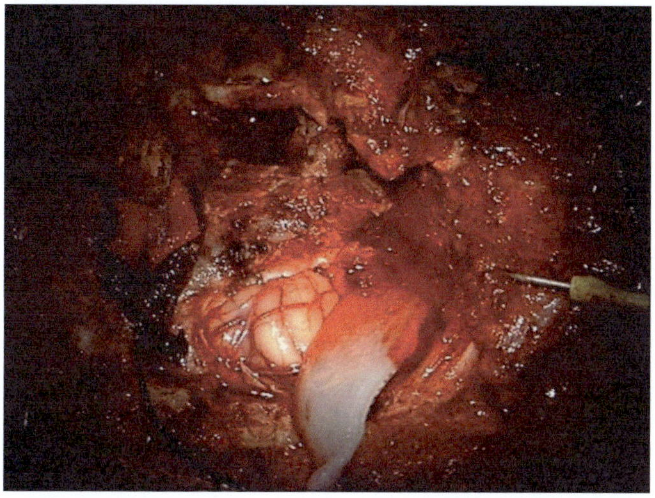

33. More Telfa strips were placed on the cerebellum to help with retraction. The meningioma involved the sigmoid sinus and presigmoid dura. We did not need to tie the proximal sigmoid sinus because it was involved with tumor all the way to the junction of the transverse sinus and sigmoid sinus.

    Since we did not plan a complete tumor resection, we elected to leave a little tumor in the sigmoid-transverse sinus junction. The benefit of this was that we did not need to work in this region and risk damaging the vein of Labbé. Complete tumor removal is not always achievable, and strategic decisions must be made regarding where tumor is left behind by assessing the potential morbidity of additional tumor removal versus the long-term risk of leaving residual tumor in this area. Should a small tumor remnant grow, it should be easily treated with stereotactic radiosurgery or possibly even external beam radiation.

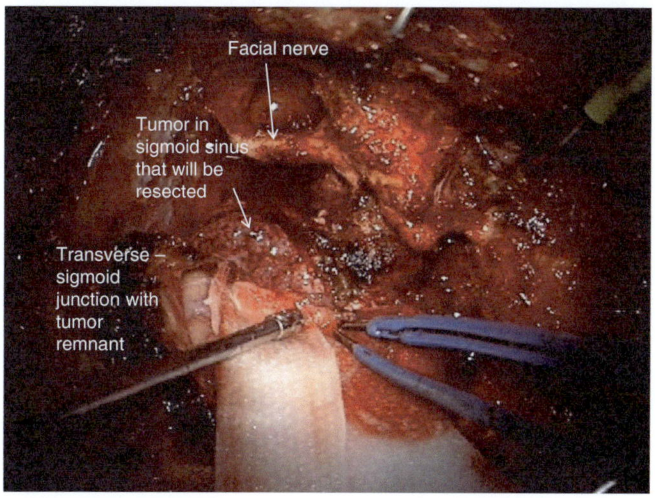

34. In this view, the superior portion tumor was removed, while the tumor around the jugular foramen remained. CN V can be seen.

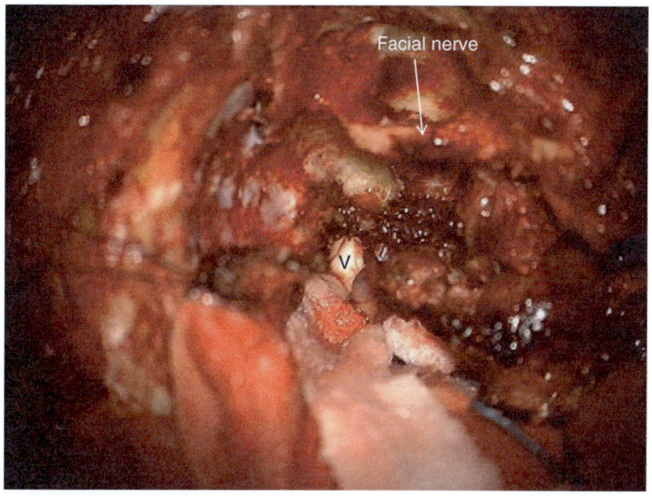

35. Nerve rootlets of CN IX, X, and XI entered the jugular foramen, and the tumor remnant was reduced in size so as to not cause brain compression. We elected to leave this pad of tumor to spare cranial nerve function.

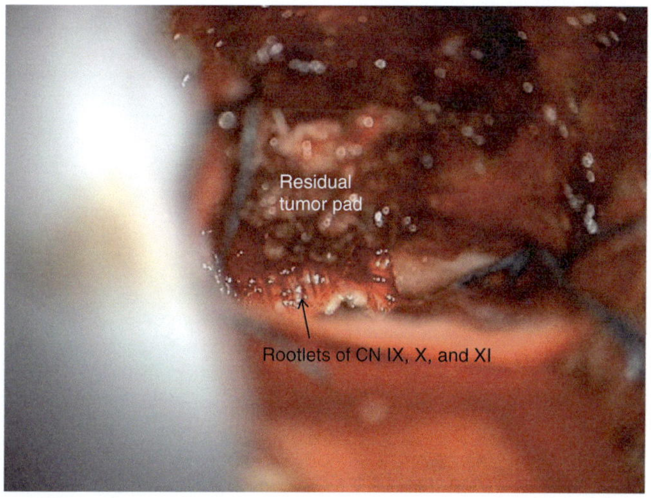

36. The view at the conclusion of tumor resection. The pad of well-cauterized tumor remnant was visible at the jugular foramen. The ear canal was closed, the Eustachian tube was plugged (*arrow*), and a fat graft was placed into the cavity.

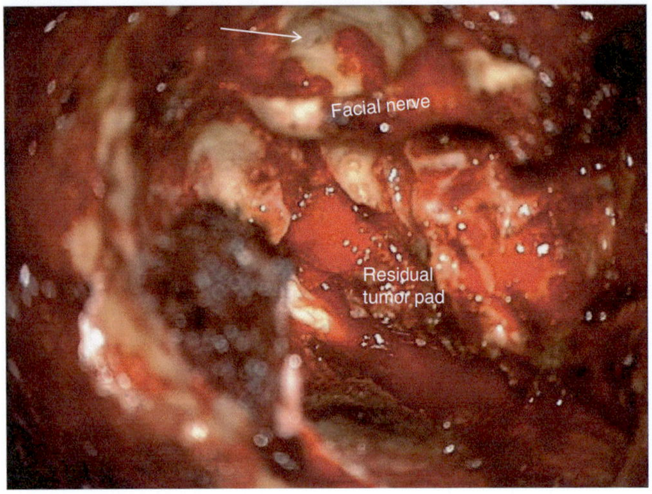

37. Immediate postoperative axial MRI demonstrated that a complete temporal bone resection with resection of the jugular bulb was performed. The pad of residual tumor was visible (*arrow*).

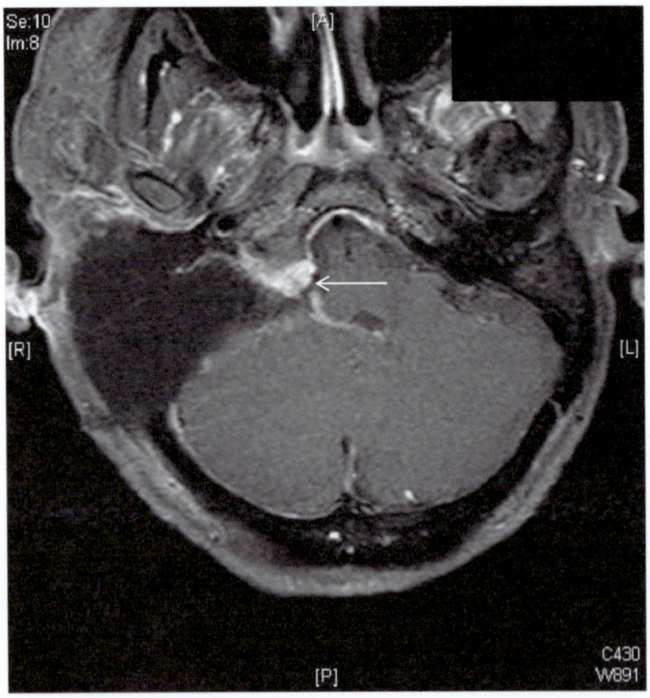

38. A more superior cut.

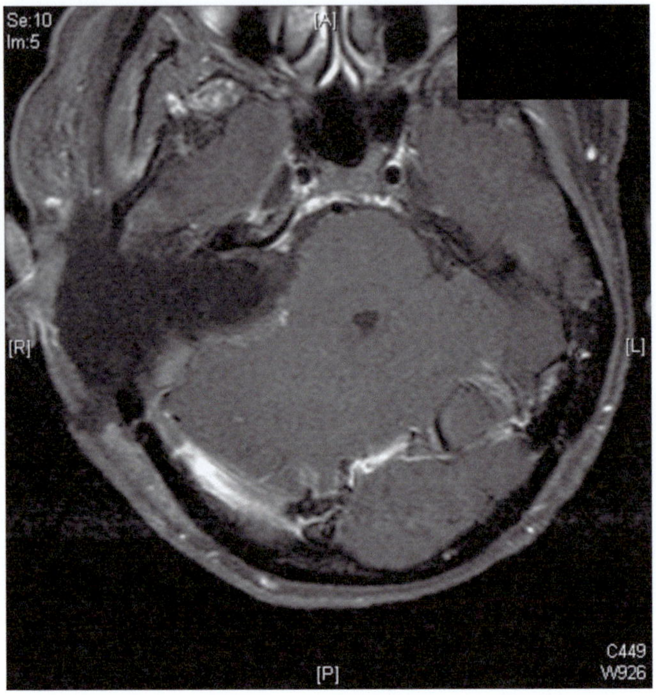

39. Coronal view demonstrated the tumor remnant (*arrow*) in the jugular foramen.

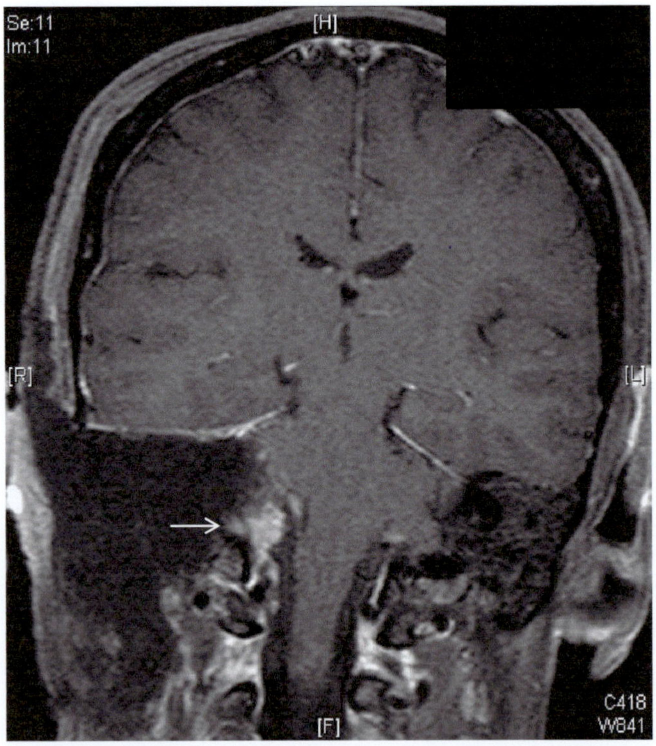

40. Axial CT demonstrated the extent of bone removal and the fallopian bridge encompassing the vertical portion of the facial nerve (*arrow*).

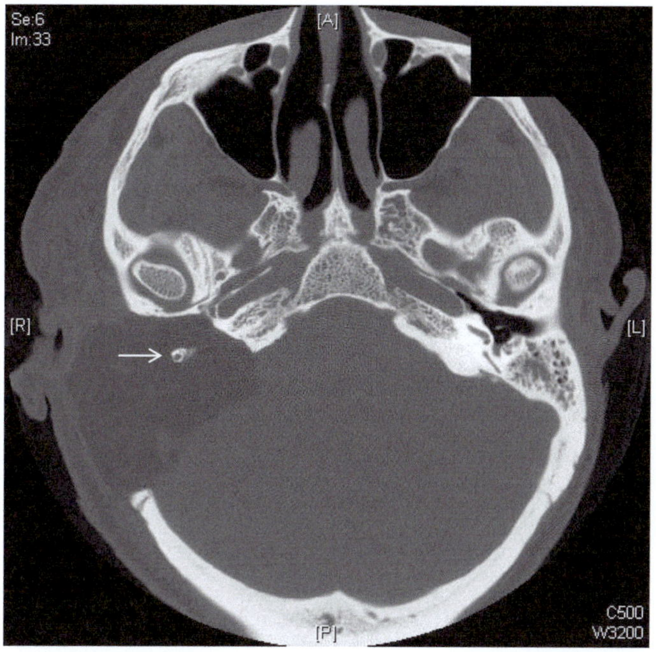

41. A lower cut demonstrated resection of the jugular bulb.

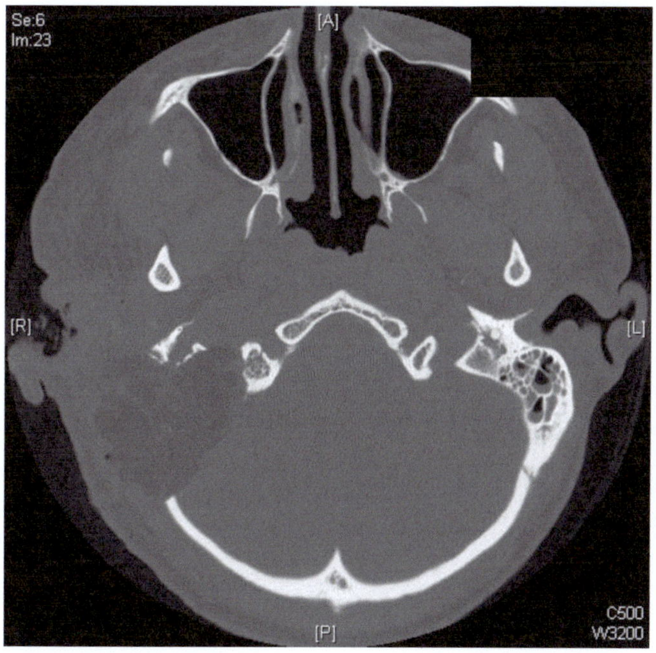

42. Three months postoperatively, the fat graft was scarred in, and the tumor remnant remained unchanged.

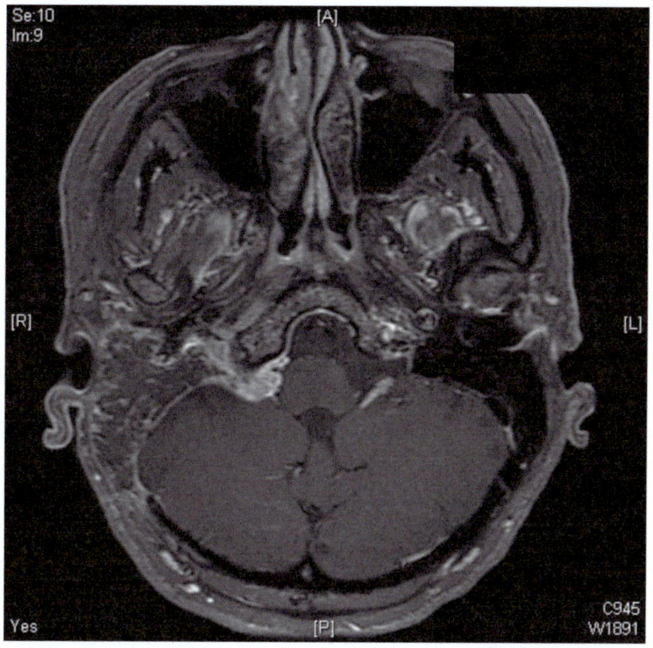

43. Axial T2 view demonstrated the fat graft and new dura that formed between it and the cerebellum (*arrowheads*).

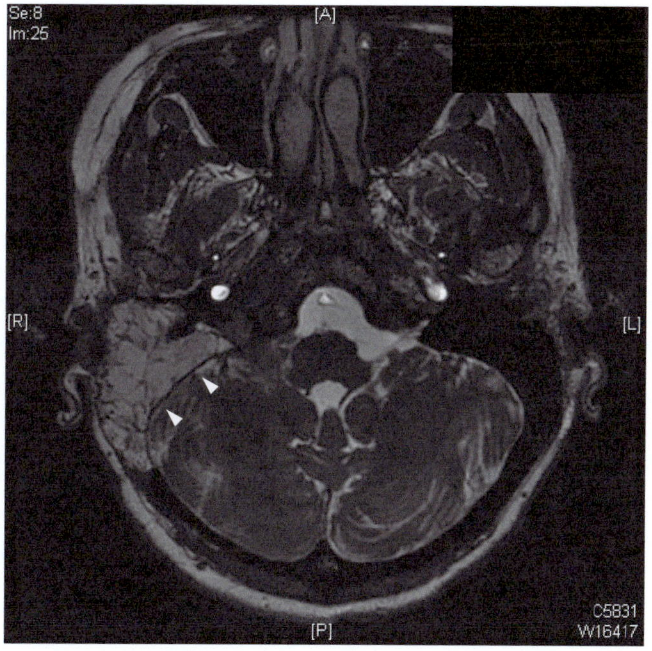

44. Case 4. Axial MRI with gadolinium of a child with recurrent neuroblastoma of the skull base and infratemporal fossa. She had failed chemotherapy and radiotherapy. Note that the tumor involved the left jugular foramen (*arrow*) and the internal carotid artery (*arrowhead*).

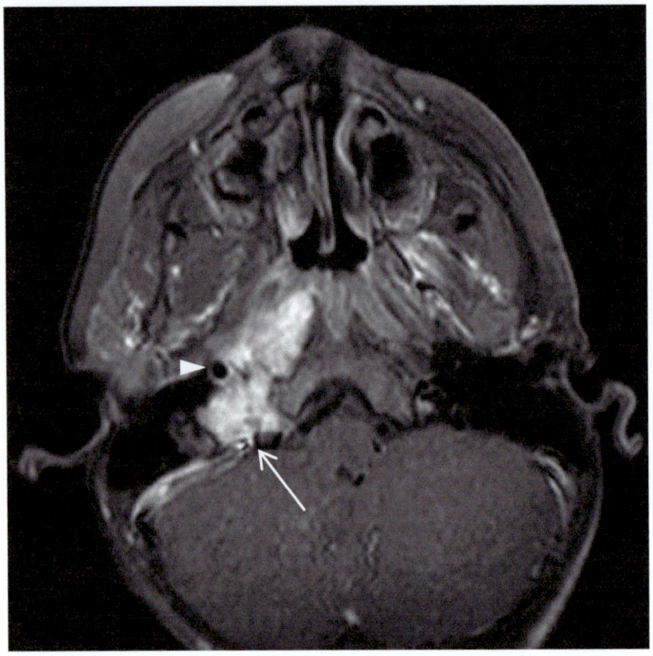

45. A more inferior image demonstrates that the tumor encompassed the internal carotid artery and partially enveloped the prevertebral musculature (*arrow*).

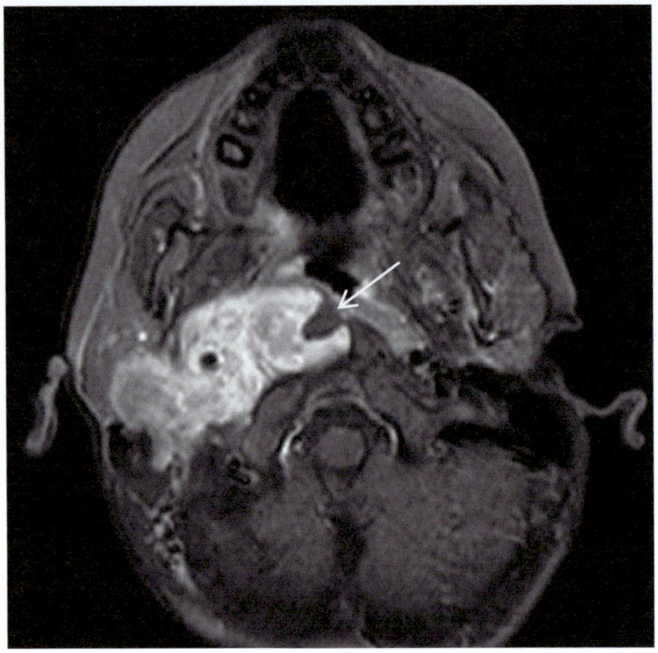

46. Coronal view demonstrates the tumor surrounding the internal carotid artery (*arrow*).

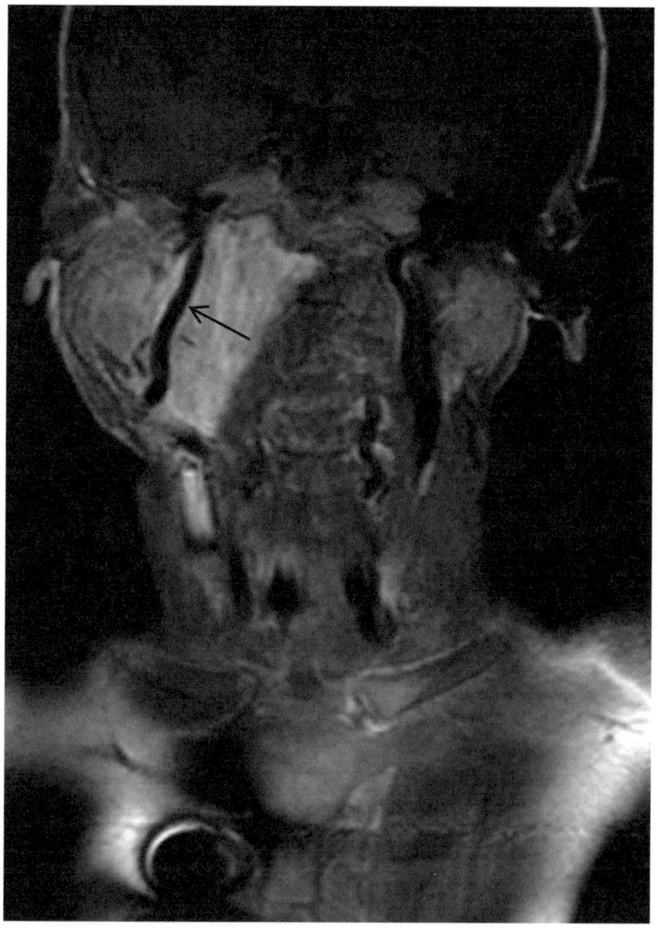

47. Axial CT with contrast identifies that tumor was occluding the jugular bulb (*asterix*).

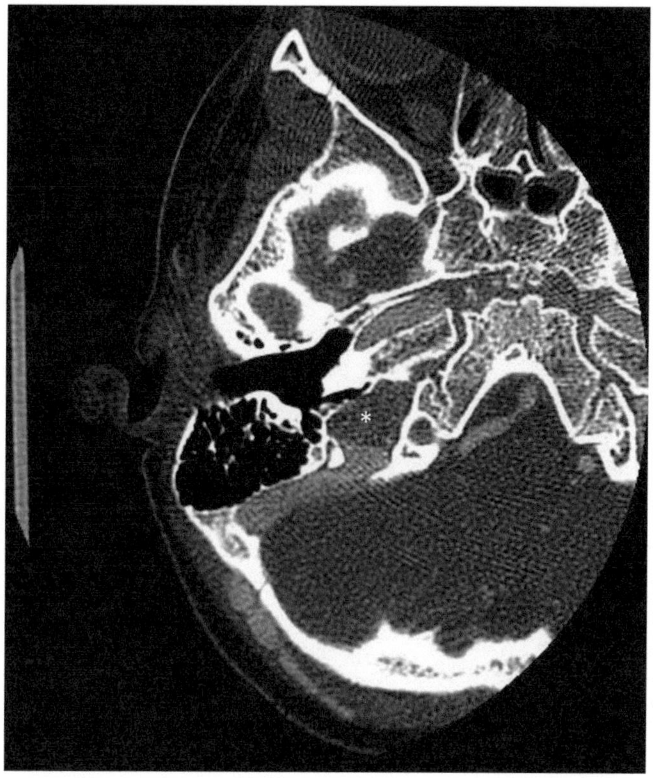

48. A postauricular approach to the infratemporal fossa was performed to resect this tumor. A canal wall up mastoidectomy was first performed.

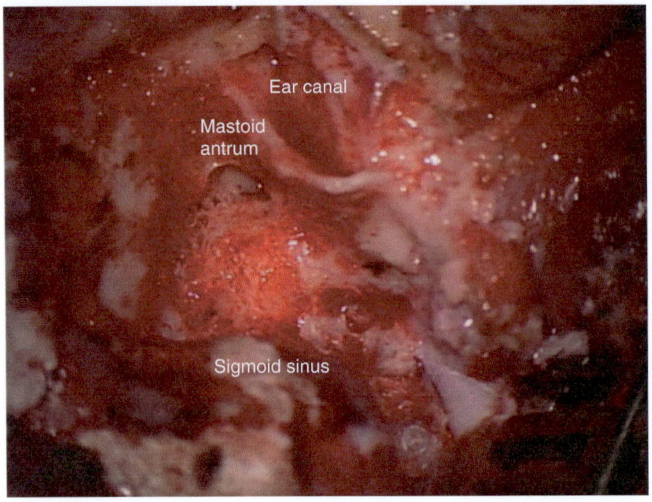

49. The bone overlying the sigmoid sinus was removed along its inferior half. Bone was left superiorly (*dotted line separates the two regions*).

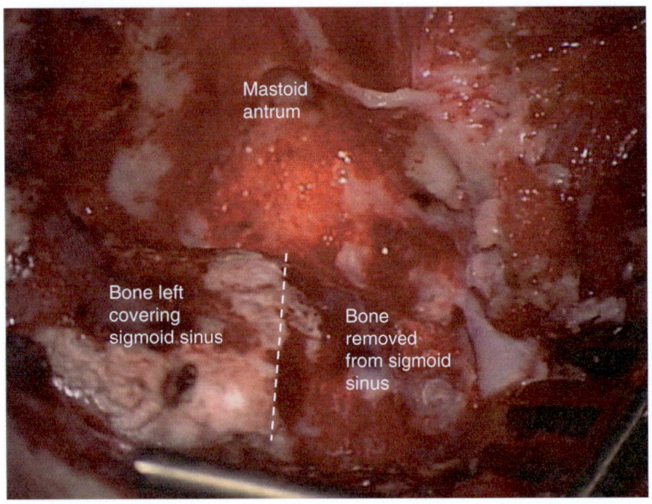

50. The facial nerve was identified at the second genu and followed inferiorly. The sigmoid sinus was traced inferiorly to the jugular bulb (*JB*). A fallopian bridge was developed around the vertical facial nerve.

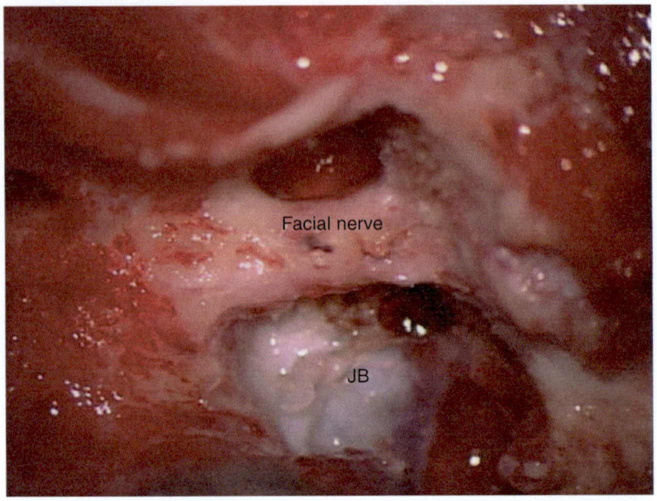

51. The internal jugular vein (*IJV*) was ligated in the neck and traced up to the skull base. The sigmoid sinus was occluded under the ledge of bone (*arrow*) and the sigmoid sinus opened to the bulb. A wad of Surgicel is sitting on top of the jugular bulb (*arrowhead*).

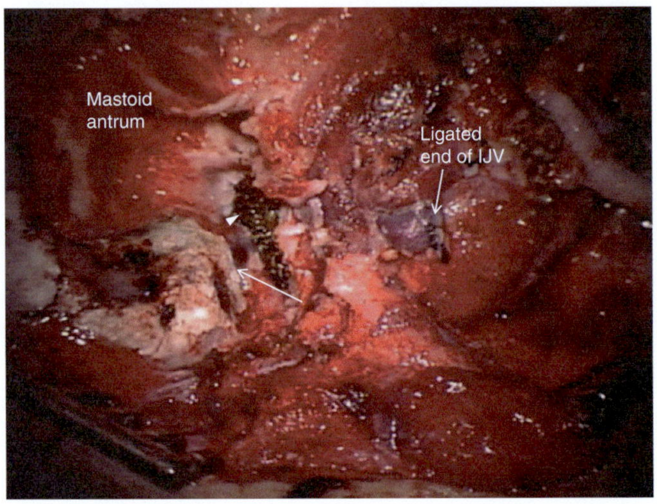

52. After removing the bulb together with the internal jugular vein (*course highlighted by the dotted line*), the tumor in the infratemporal fossa is visible. The internal carotid artery (*ICA*) has been partially dissected free and has a tortuous course over the residual tumor.

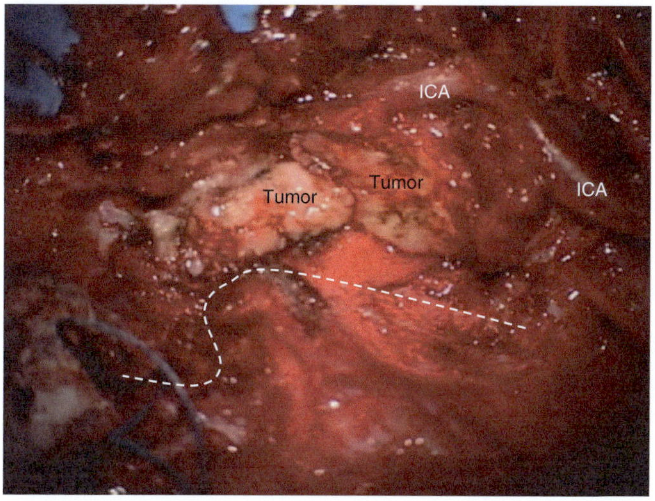

53. Tumor was dissected off the posterior fossa dura.

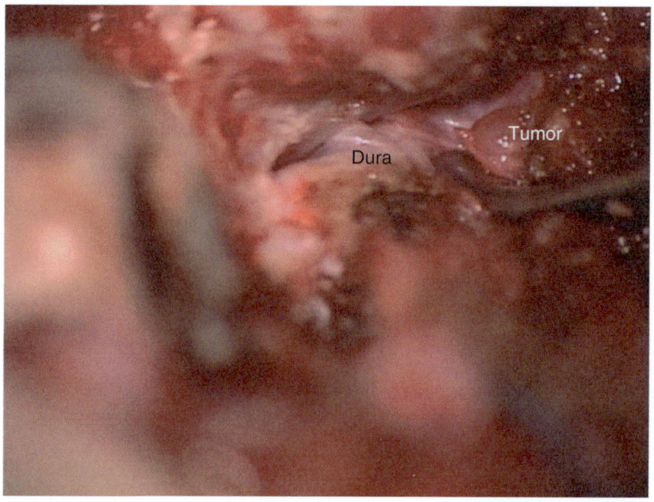

54. After removing all the rest of the visible tumor, the internal carotid artery (*ICA*) and external carotid artery (*ECA*) were clearly visible. The blue fishhook retractor was elevating up the mandible. To close, a fat graft was placed into the defect to help protect the vessels and provide some bulk for reconstruction.

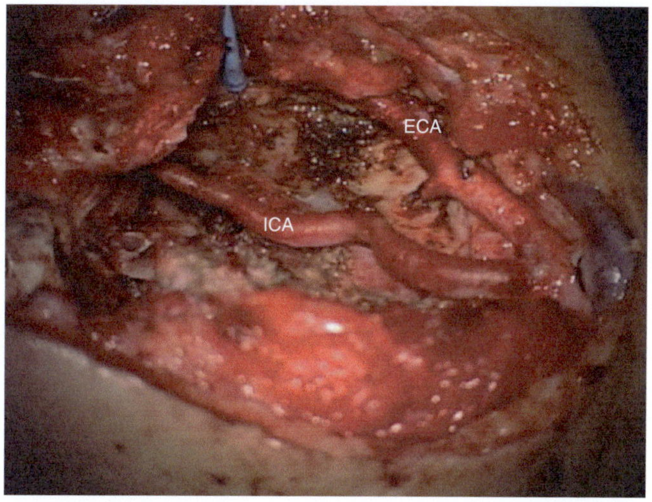

55. Immediate postoperative MRI demonstrated tumor resection.

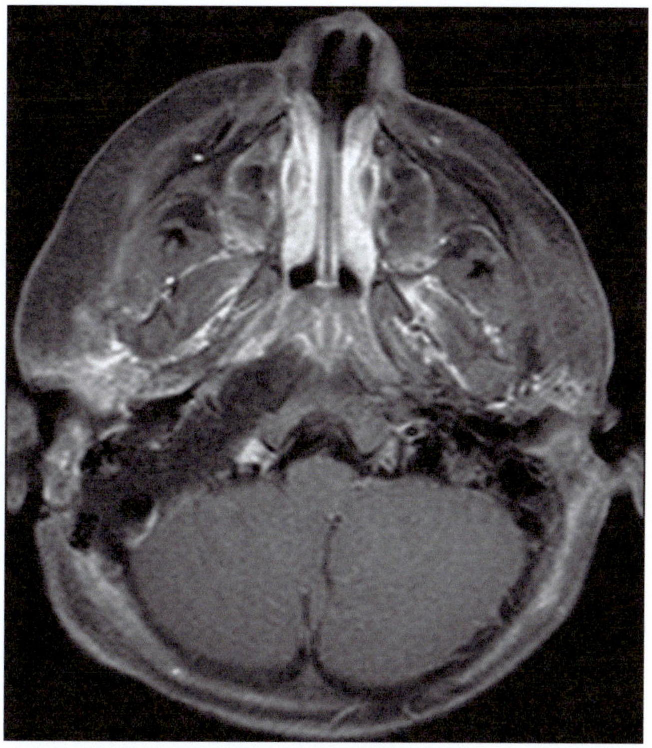

56. A lower cut demonstrating the fat graft (asterisk) protecting the internal carotid artery.

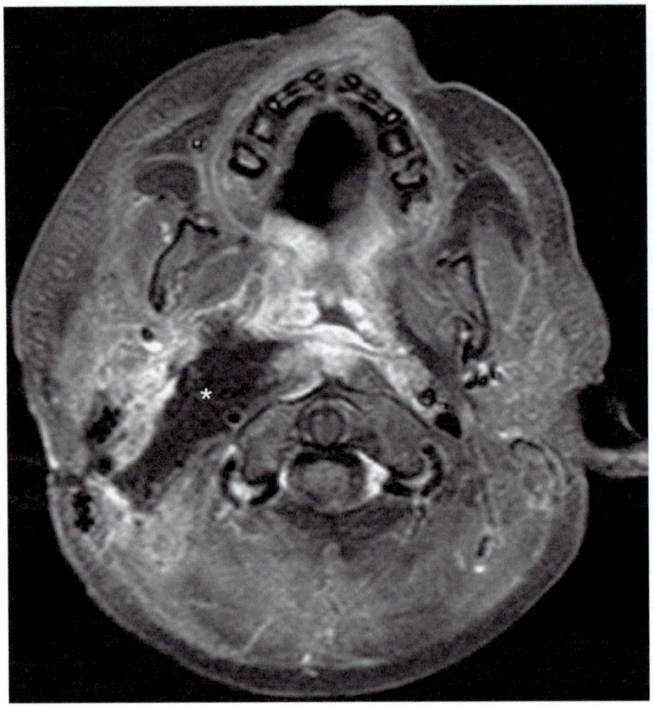

57. Axial CT demonstrated the mastoidectomy defect. The inner ear and ossicular chain were preserved. A drain (*arrow*) was visible within the mastoid space.

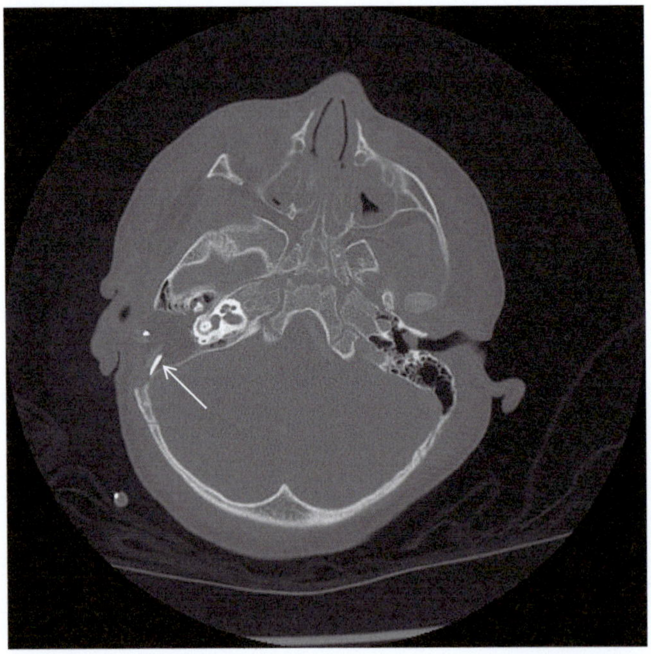

58. A lower cut demonstrating preservation of the ear canal.

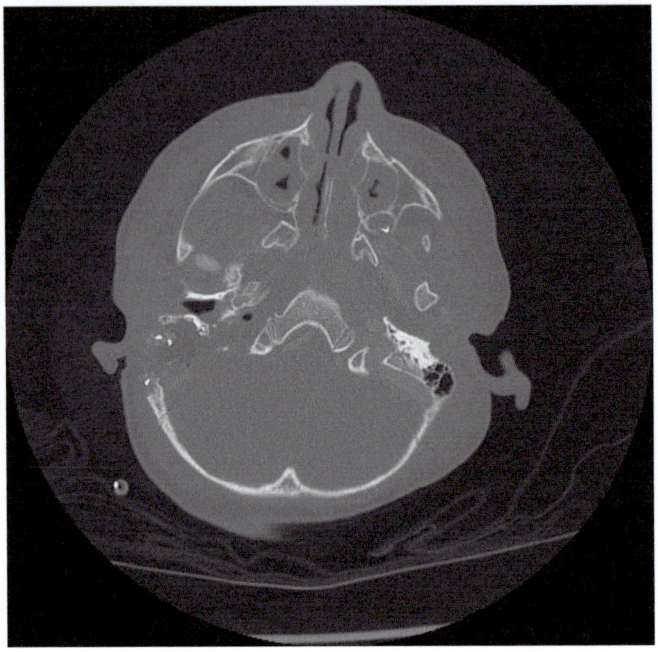

59. An even lower cut demonstrating preservation of the fallopian bridge (*arrow*) and resection of the jugular bulb.

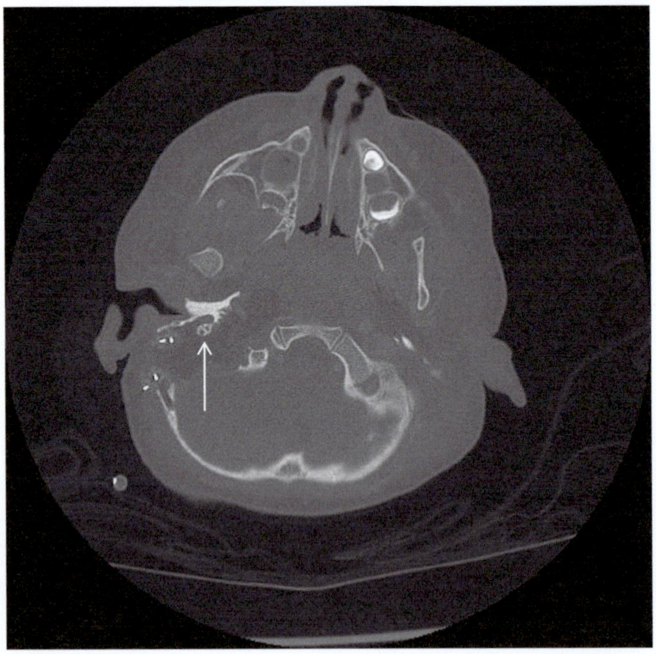

60. Seven months later, a follow-up MRI demonstrated no tumor regrowth. There was scar formation (*arrow*) within the resected region.

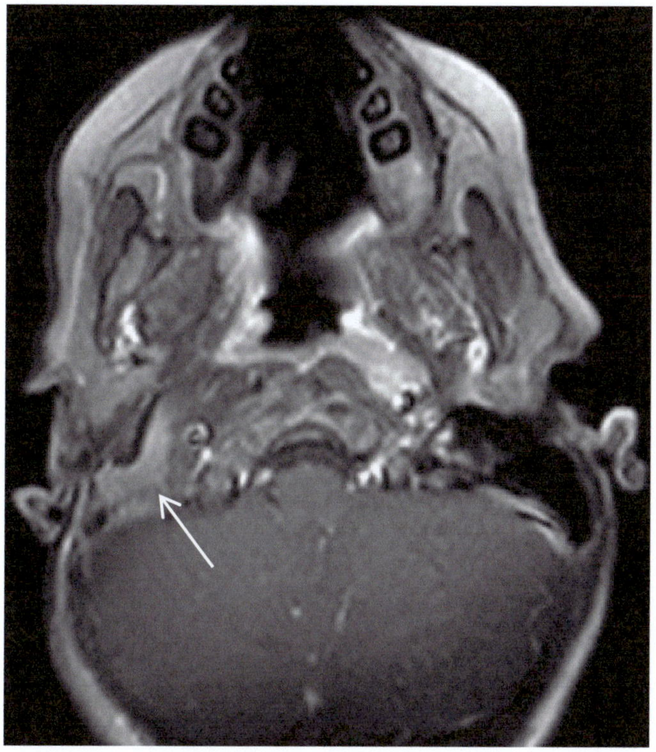

61. Without fat suppression or contrast administration, the fat graft around the internal carotid artery was obviously visible.

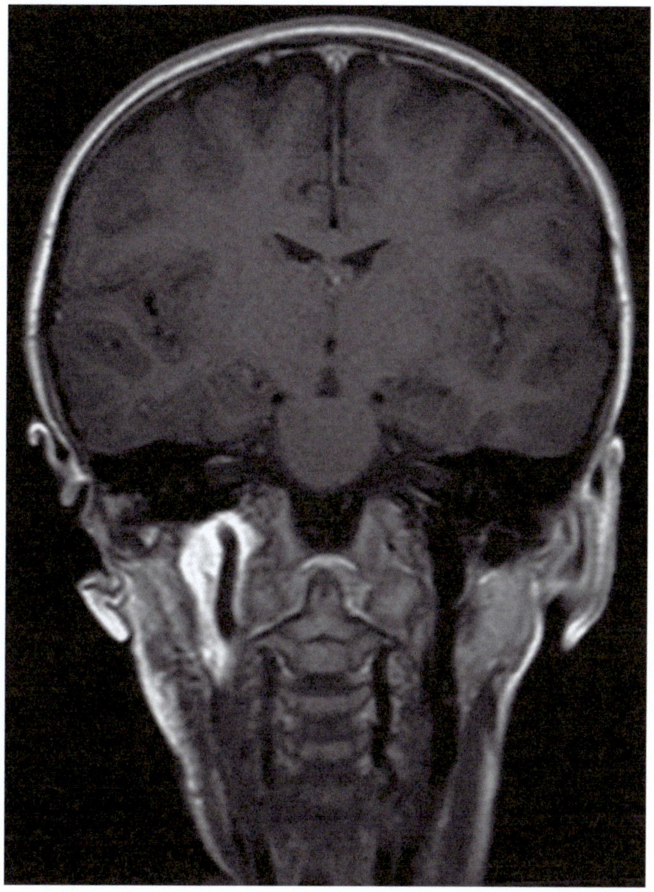

62. Case 5. Axial MRI with gadolinium of a teenage boy with a clival chordoma (*arrows*). It involved not only the clivus but also the right petrous apex. He had sixth and seventh cranial nerve palsies, complete hearing loss in the right ear, and severe headaches.

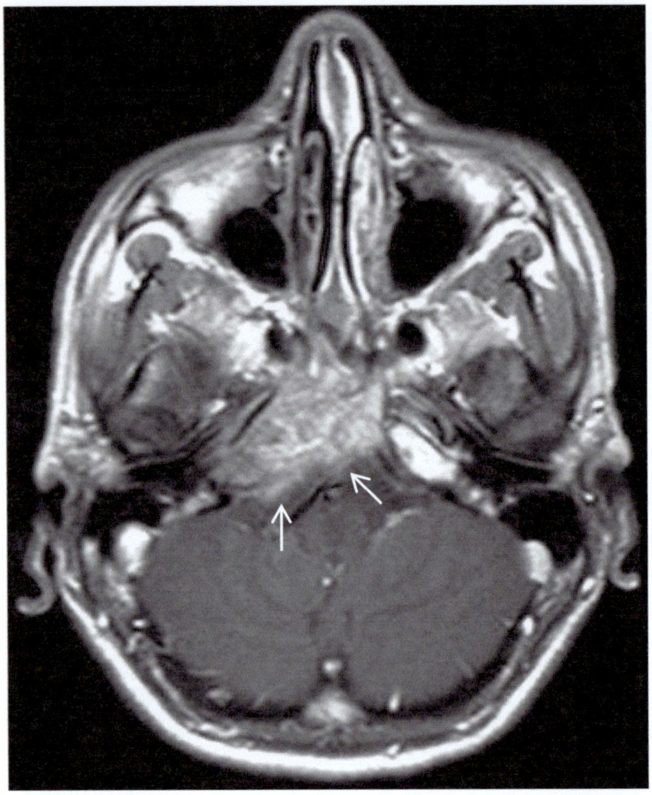

63. More superiorly, it was noted to compress the internal carotid artery within the cavernous sinus (compare the two sides; *arrowheads*).

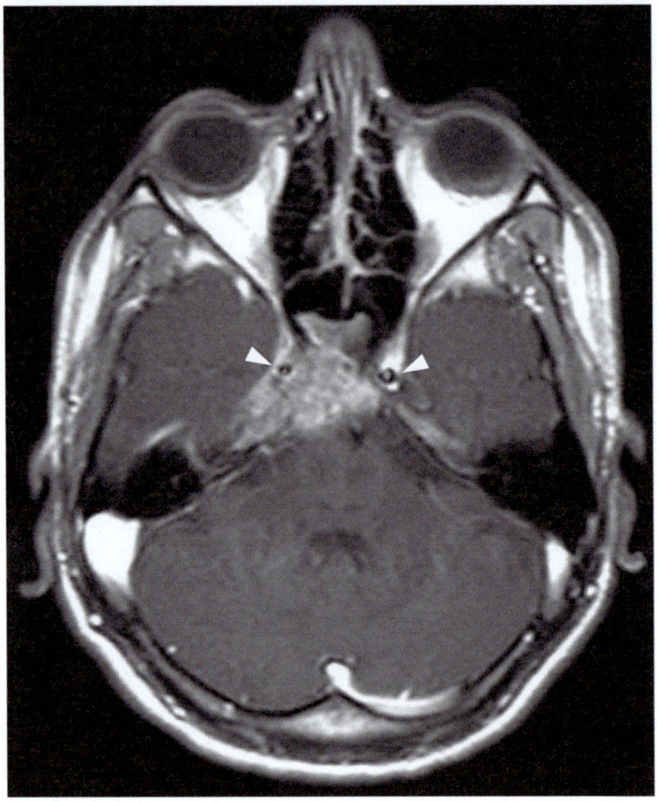

64. The sagittal view suggested it was an extradural tumor because there was a thin rim of CSF between the clivus and the pons (*arrowhead*).

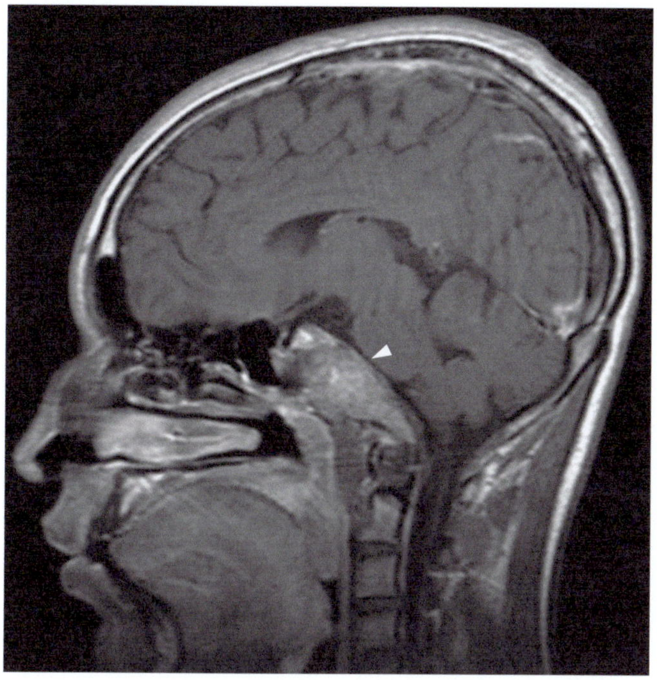

65. The coronal view demonstrated mild compression of the temporal lobe (*arrow*).

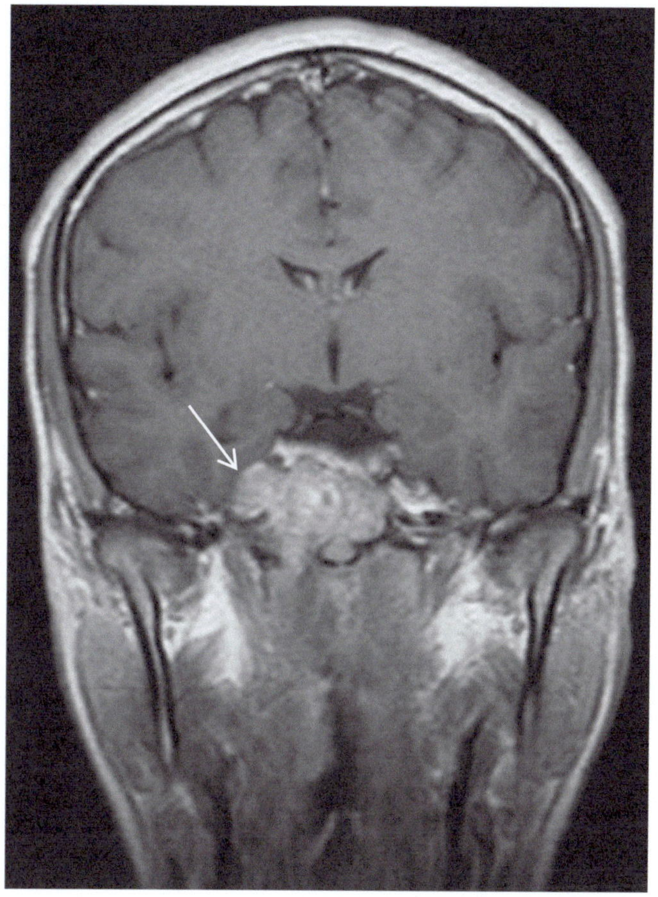

66. Axial CT demonstrates an erosive lesion of the lower clivus. Note that an endoscopic biopsy through the sphenoid sinus had already been performed (*arrow*).

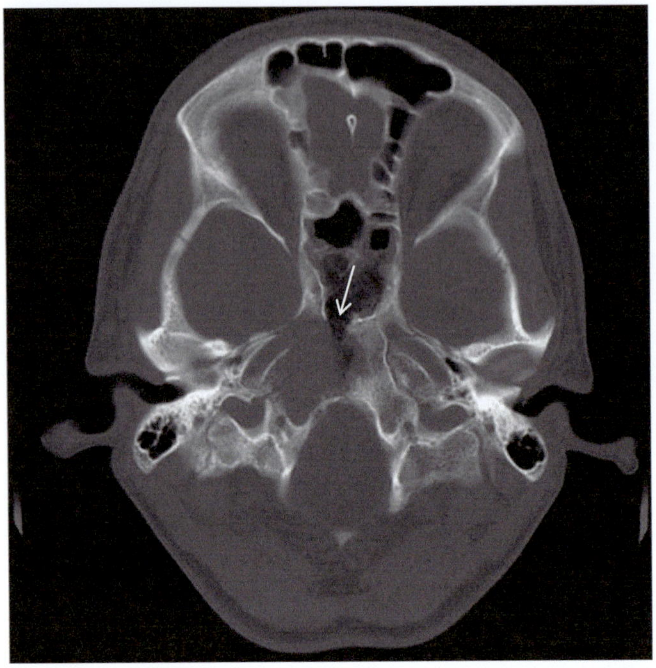

67. A postauricular transcochlear approach to the infratemporal fossa was selected to remove as much of this tumor as possible to be followed by proton beam radiotherapy. A large C-shaped incision was used.

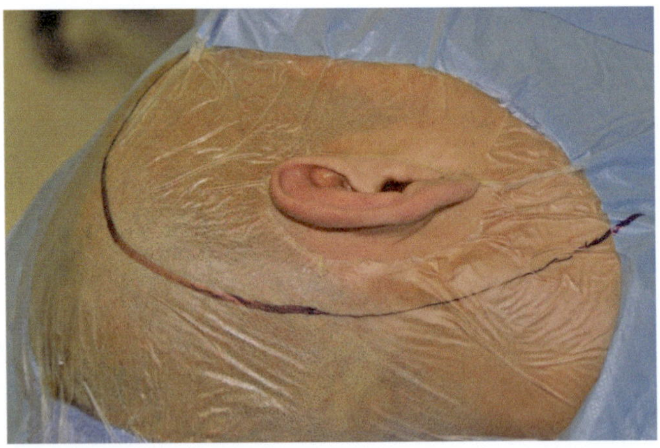

68. The ear canal was transected, the soft tissues were reflected anteriorly, and the internal jugular vein (*IJV*) and internal carotid artery (*ICA*) were identified in the neck. The zygomatic arch was dissected in a subperiosteal fashion.

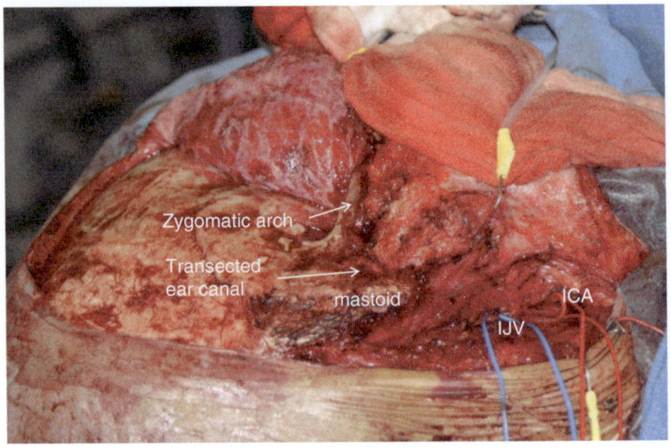

69. The zygomatic arch was resected. A complete mastoidectomy was performed to expose the temporomandibular joint (*TMJ*). The sigmoid sinus was skeletonized and a bone flap removed from the middle fossa.

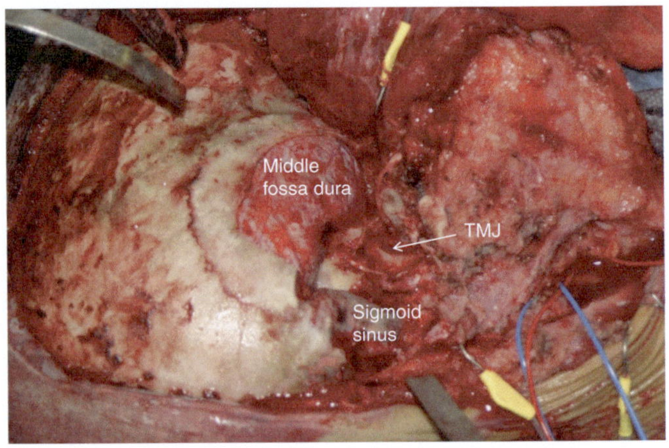

70. The internal carotid artery (*ICA*) was identified inferiorly and then traced up as it curved anteriorly. Note the tumor adjacent to the artery at the suction tip.

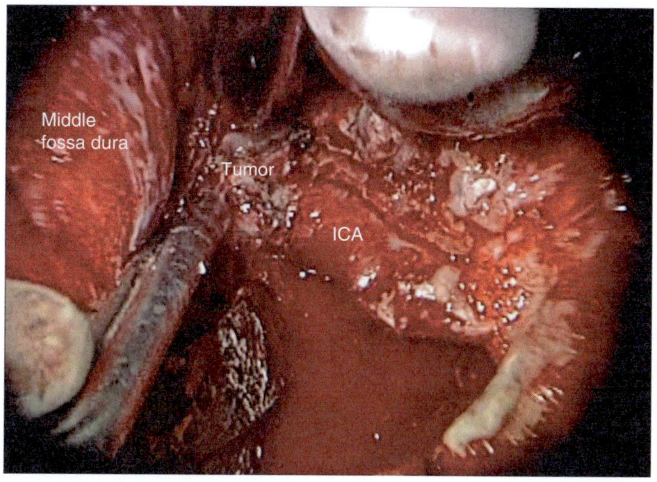

71. After removing as much gross tumor as possible, residual tumor that was adherent to the adventitia of the internal carotid artery was carefully cauterized with a bipolar in an effort to devitalize it. While carotid resection with or without reconstruction can be performed technically, the risks often outweigh the benefits. Tumors that are aggressive enough to infiltrate the wall of the carotid are usually infiltrative everywhere and thus can never be completely resected.

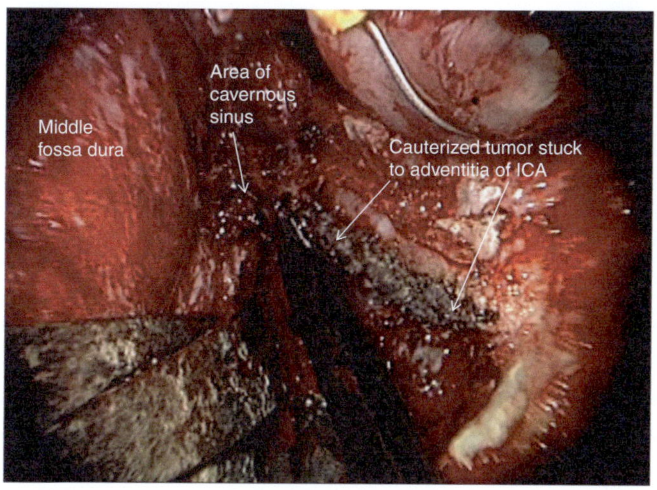

72. In order to remove as much disease within the clivus as possible, a rhinologist skilled in endoscopic skull base surgery can be quite helpful. While many small chordomas can be completely removed endoscopically, in this case we felt that a team approach would be beneficial. In this case, the rhinologist removed a portion of the tumor within the sphenoid sinus and clivus that was difficult to remove from the lateral approach because the position of the internal carotid arteries blocked visualization.

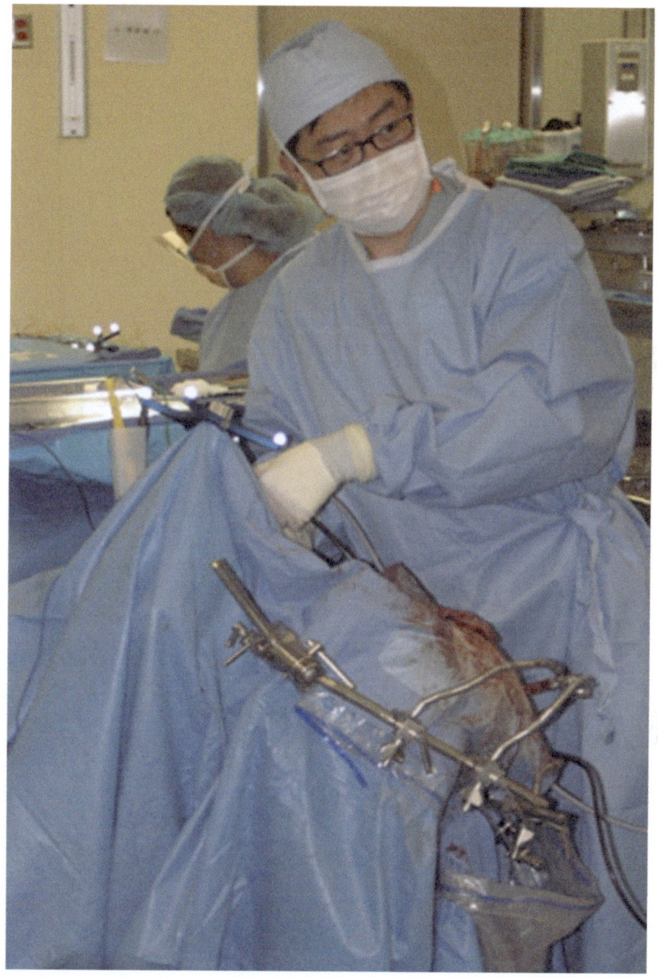

73. Endoscopically, the tumor within the sphenoid sinus was visible.

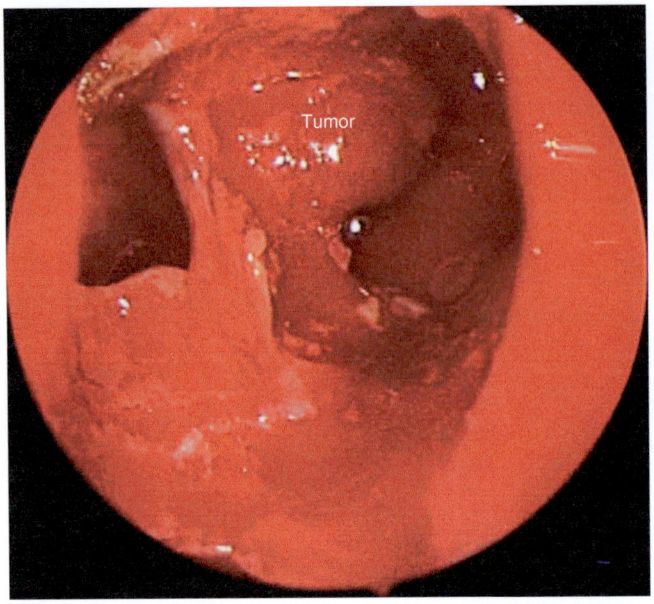

74. This tumor was removed.

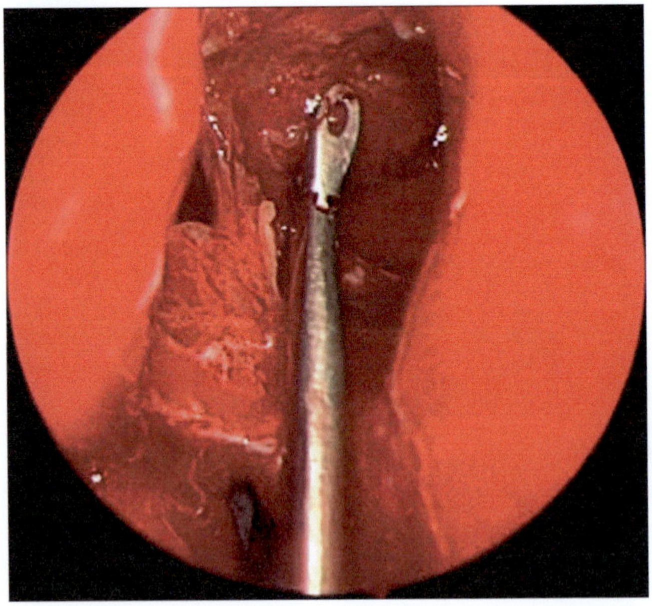

75. Drilling to remove tumor within the clivus was then performed.

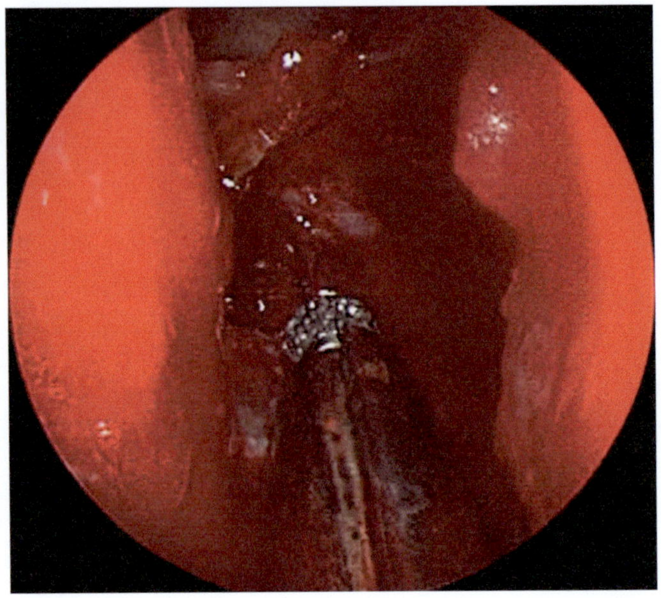

76. Once as much tumor as possible was removed, a temporalis muscle flap was used for reconstruction. We pulled it into the sphenoid siunus through the lateral defect, plugging the connection between the ear and the nose and covering the internal carotid artery.

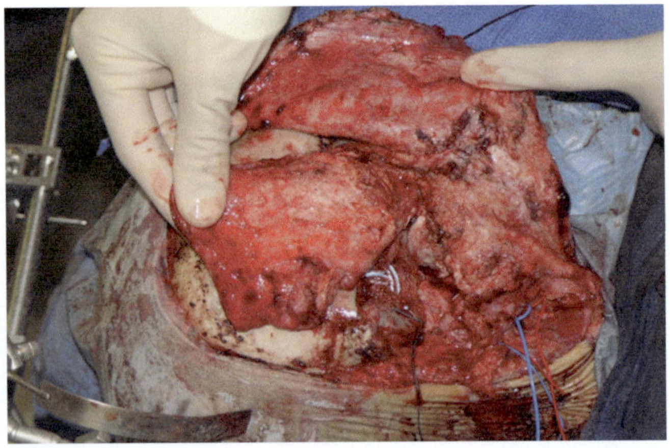

77. An endoscopic view of the forceps from the ear passing a suture tied to the tip of the temporalis muscle flap to a cup forceps.

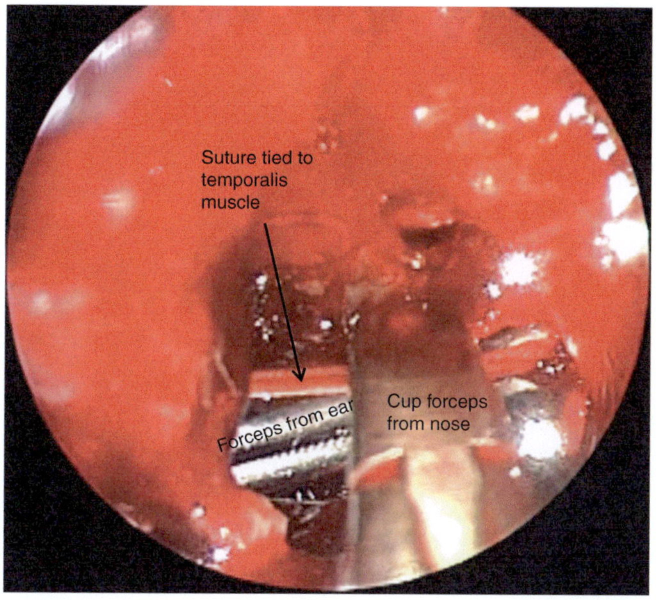

78. The suture was then pulled back out the nose so that the temporalis muscle filled the sphenoid sinus and covered the internal carotid artery. The bone flap and zygomatic arch were plated back in place during wound closure.

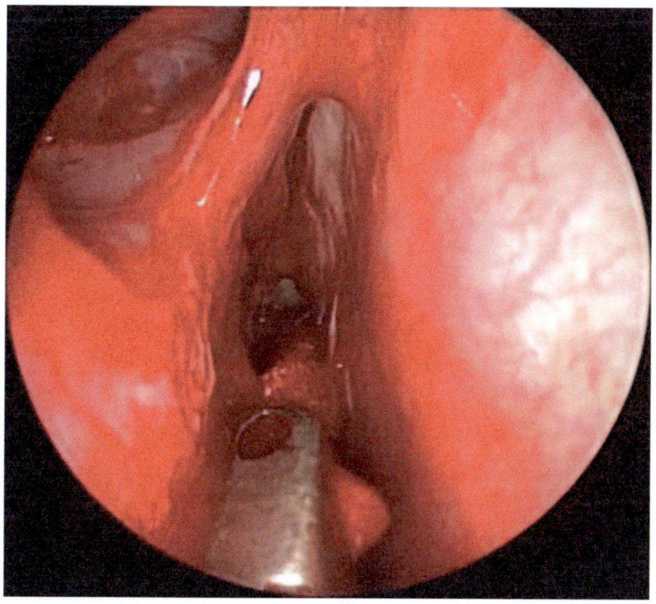

79. Postoperative MRI demonstrated the temporalis muscle flap filling the defect.

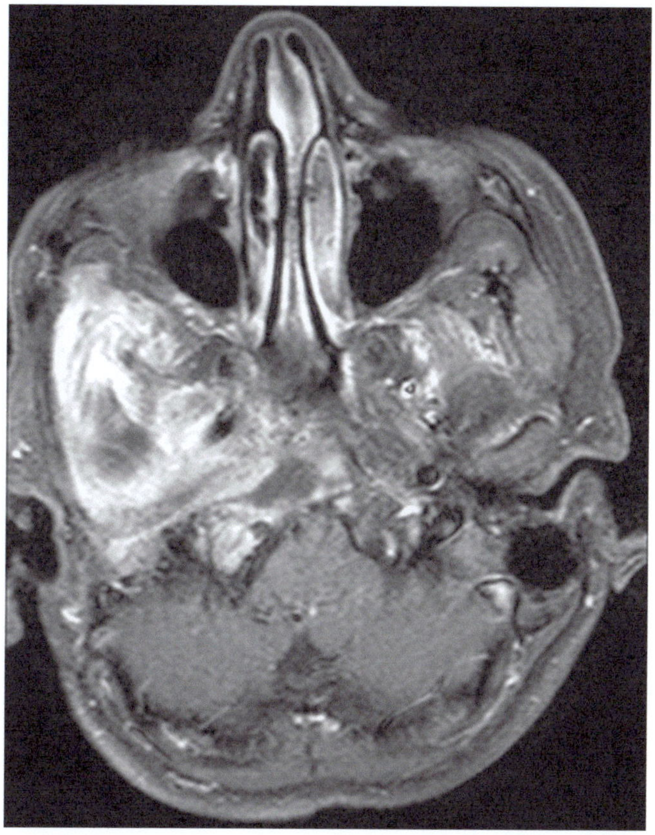

80. The muscle within the sphenoid sinus was visible (*arrow*). Also, note that the carotid artery was no longer compressed (*arrowhead*).

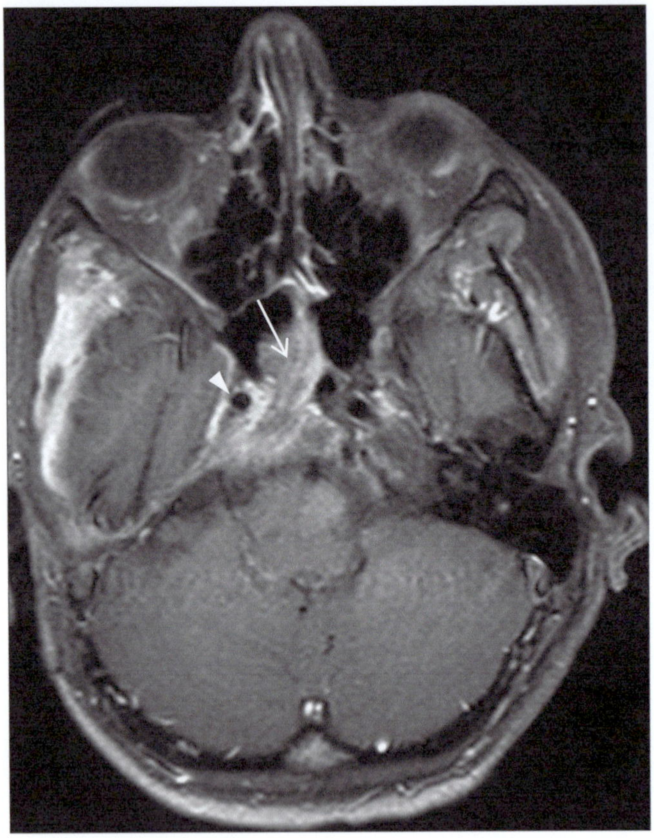

81. Postoperative CT confirmed that the temporal bone and clivus were resected. Radiotherapy was used postoperatively.

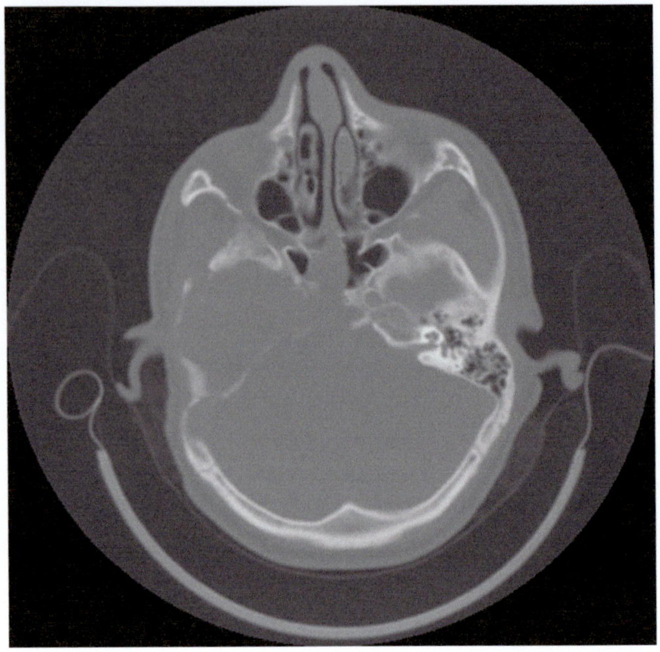

82. Case 6. Axial CT of a glomus jugulare tumor that presented as an aural polyp. There was extensive bone destruction within the ear canal and mastoid.

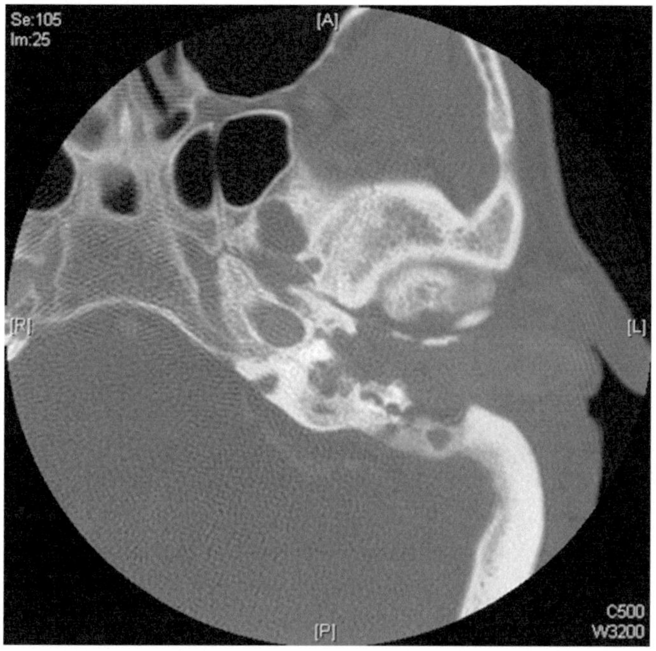

83. Coronal CT demonstrated a connection between the dome of the jugular bulb and the erosive mass in the middle ear (*arrow*). The tumor also grew superiorly into the middle cranial fossa (*arrowheads*).

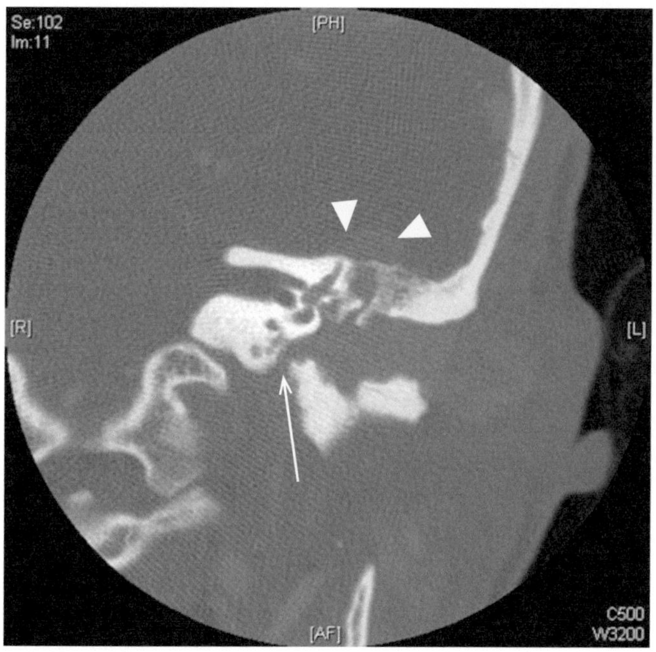

84. Axial MRI with gadolinium demonstrated enhancing tumor within the jugular bulb, middle ear, and ear canal. The aural polyp can be noted (*arrow*).

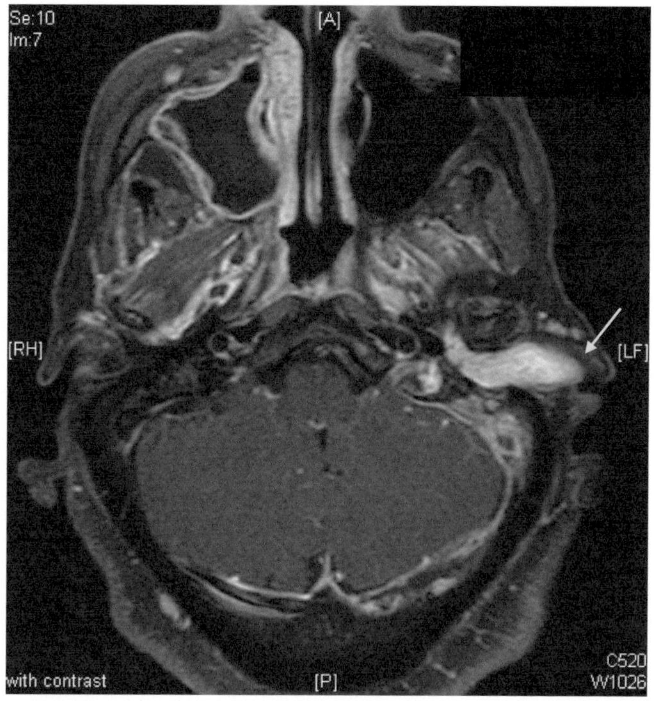

85. The tumor also grew down the Eustachian tube and was visible within the nasopharynx during flexible examination (*arrow*). A postauricular approach would work well for resecting this tumor.

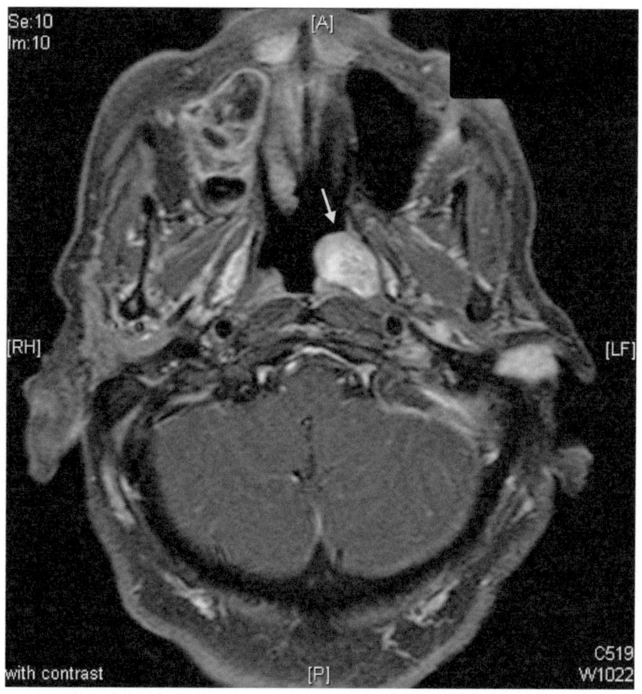

Preauricular Approach to the Infratemporal Fossa

- *Concept*
  - This approach provides exposure to the upper parapharyngeal space, foramen ovale, and the nasopharynx (Fisch B, C, D) without exposure of the middle ear or jugular bulb.
  - It can be performed with or without a middle fossa craniotomy.
- *Conditions treated*
  - Extensive, infiltrative tumors of the infratemporal fossa and parapharyngeal space
  - Cavernous sinus tumors such as meningioma
  - Life-threatening skull base infections
  - Recurrent nasopharyngeal carcinoma
  - Juvenile nasopharyngeal angiofibroma with intracranial extension
- *Risks*
  - Conductive hearing loss due to Eustachian tube obstruction
  - Facial nerve injury
  - Palsy of CN III, IV, V, or VI
  - Internal carotid artery injury
- *Benefits*
  - As opposed to the transcervical approach or mandible-splitting approach, this approach provides excellent exposure of tumors that have both middle fossa and infratemporal fossa components. The view is from both above and below the tumor, increasing the safety profile of the procedure.

86. The incision is marked. The lower limb is essentially a standard parotid incision. The upper limb can be tailored to the desired exposure. For example, it can course around the posterior and superior borders of the temporalis muscle like the incision used for the orbitocraniozygomatic approach. Alternatively, the incision may be shortened in situations where the tumor does not require such a large exposure.

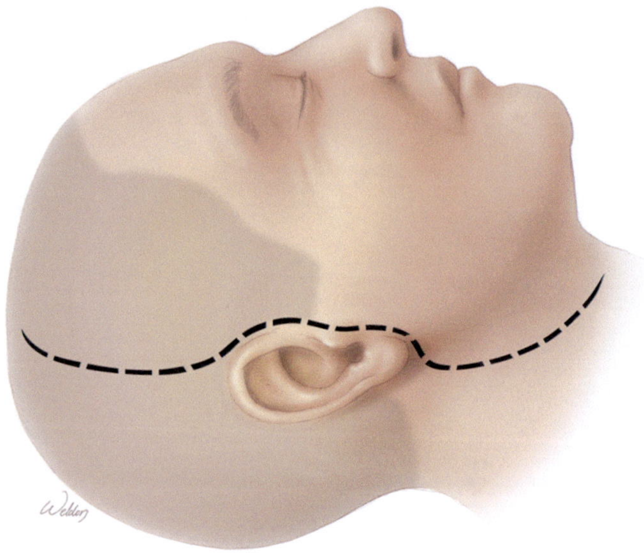

87. The superior limb of the incision is taken down to the skull, and the skin flap and temporalis muscle are elevated anteriorly as a unit. The medial/superior side of the zygoma is identified first, and then the periosteum is elevated over its lateral surface from posterior to anterior. This preserves the zygomatic branch of the facial nerve. The temporalis muscle tendon is mobilized but left connected to the coronoid process of the mandible.

After opening the inferior limb of the incision, a standard parotid approach is performed. However, there is no need to extensively develop a skin flap over the lateral surface of the parotid unless the gland will be removed. If the goal is just to get deep to the parotid, the skin can be left attached to the lateral surface of the parotid. The sternocleidomastoid muscle (*SCM*) and digastric muscle (*DM*) are identified. Then, the main trunk of the facial nerve (*VII*) is identified and traced out to the pes anserinus.

The styloid process should be palpable. The masseter muscle, temporomandibular joint capsule, and deep skull base musculature (i.e., the stylohyoid muscle, stylomandibular ligament, etc.) are all found medial to the main trunk of the facial nerve. Care should be taken during the retraction process as stretch injury can occur to the facial nerve.

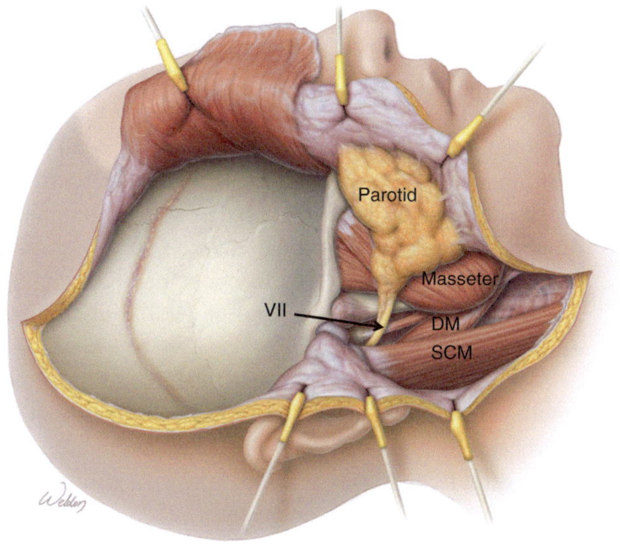

88. The zygoma is cut anteriorly and posteriorly (as described in Chap. 3, orbitocraniozygomatic approach). The temporomandibular joint capsule is incised, allowing the mandibular condyle to be retracted anteriorly with a large retractor such as a Weitlaner. To increase the anterior displacement of the mandible, the stylomandibular and sphenomandibular ligaments should be divided. This greatly enhances the exposure of the upper parapharyngeal space, infratemporal fossa, and underside of the lateral skull base.

Note that there may be a lot of bleeding from small veins within the infratemporal fossa fat. It is nearly impossible to identify these and cauterize them effectively. The use of Surgicel and gentle pressure from a cottonoid patty is the best way to control this bleeding when this area is being dissected. Also, the internal maxillary artery and its branches may be visible.

The skull base should be followed from lateral to medial to identify foramen spinosum. The middle meningeal artery entering it should be divided. Just anterior and medial to foramen spinosum is foramen ovale. The mandibular branch of CN V can be divided in order to permit further medial exposure. There is a plexus of veins that carry blood through foramen ovale. These can be cauterized with the bipolar prior to sectioning the nerve but still often bleed. To stop this bleeding, a piece of Surgicel can be stuffed into foramen ovale and sealed with bone wax.

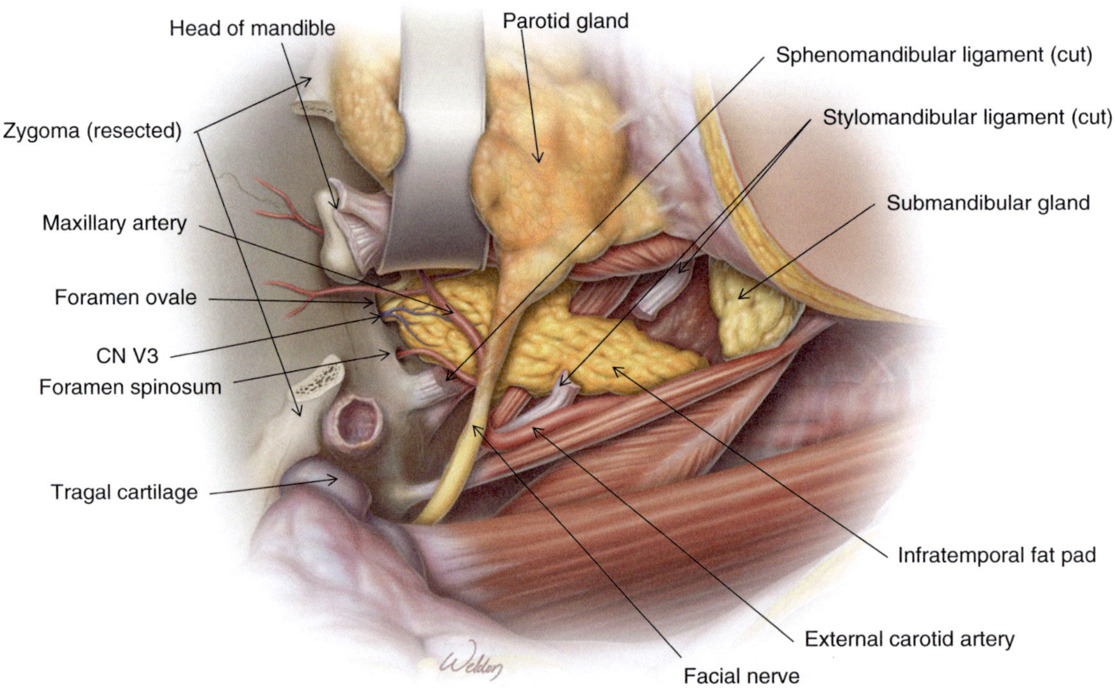

89. After removing more soft tissue and the medial pterygoid muscle, the nasopharynx will be entered. The contralateral Eustachian tube will be visible.

While not illustrated in this series, a middle fossa craniotomy can also be performed with extradural dissection to reach the cavernous sinus (see Chap. 3, orbitocraniozygomatic approach). When combined with the preauricular infratemporal fossa approach, extensive disease of the skull base that involves both the intracranial cavity and the infratemporal fossa can be safely resected.

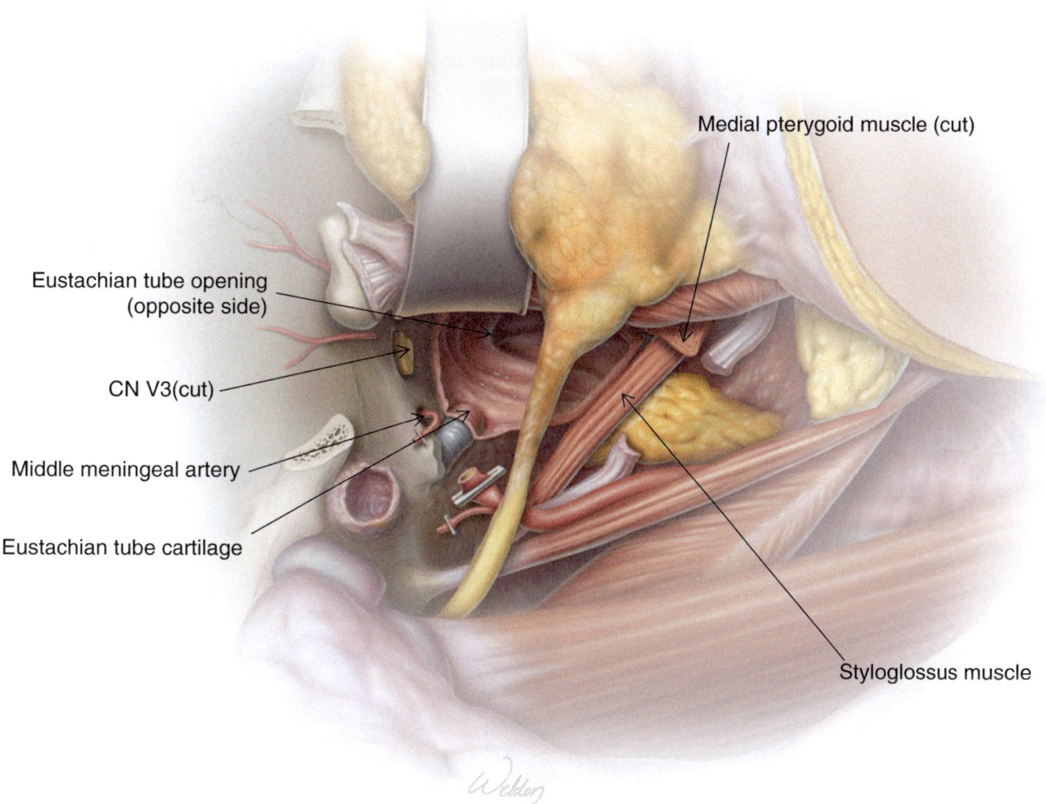

90. Case 1. A diabetic patient who presented with invasive fungal sinusitis that spread to the muscles of mastication and left skull base. Culture demonstrated the organism was aspergillus. Axial MRI with gadolinium demonstrates extensive enhancement of the soft tissues within the infratemporal fossa.

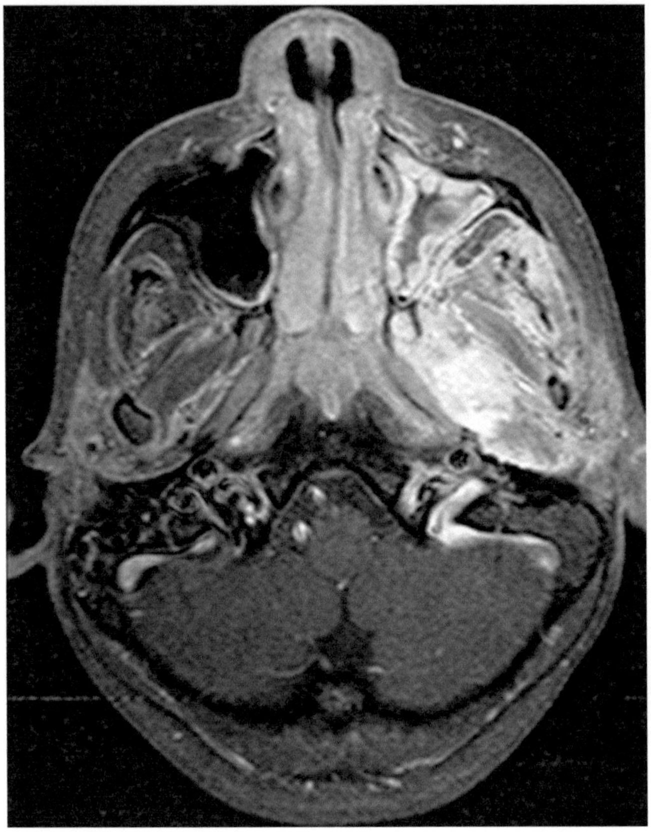

91. Coronal MRI demonstrates that the disease extended through foramen ovale (*arrow*) to the cavernous sinus. This patient had left ophthalmoplegia due to dysfunction of CN III, IV, and V.

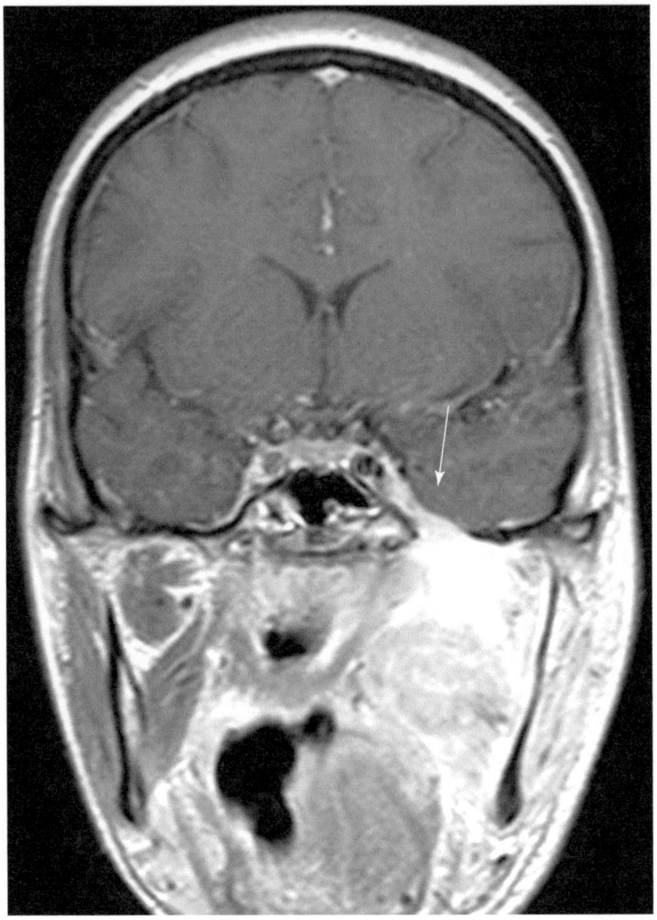

92. Axial CT scan demonstrates that there was also erosion of the left mandibular ramus (*arrow*). Inpatient medical management of the infection and careful blood sugar control did not stem the progression of the disease. Because of the life-threatening nature of the disease, we elected to surgically debride as much devitalized tissue as possible with the hope that this would allow the antifungal therapy to treat the residual disease more effectively.

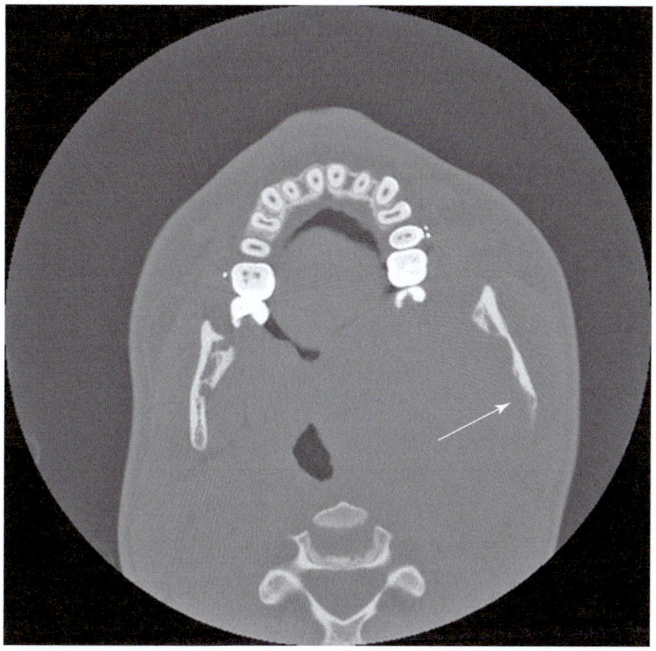

93. The preauricular incision extended from the neck to the top of the head.

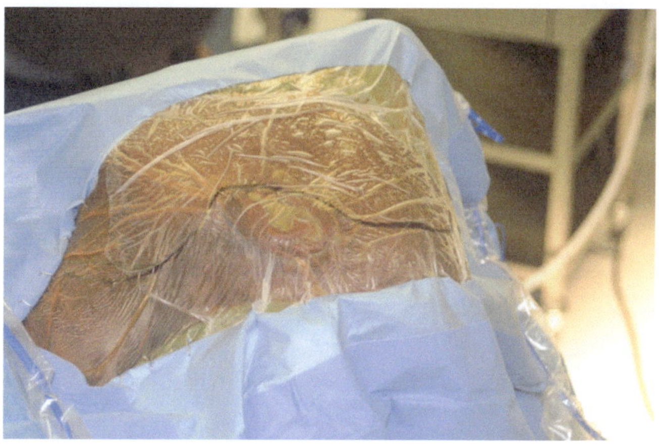

94. The incision was opened down to the skull.

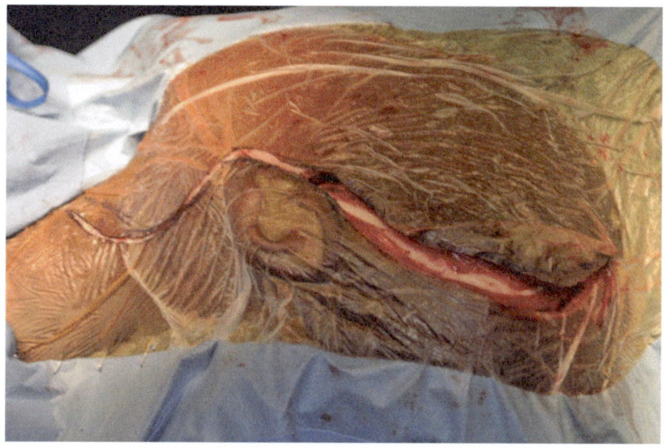

95. The superior aspect of the flap was elevated directly off the skull and the zygoma (*arrowhead*) delineated. Most of the temporalis muscle was necrotic and had to be resected. Inferiorly, a standard subplatysmal flap was elevated and the angle of the mandible identified (*arrow*).

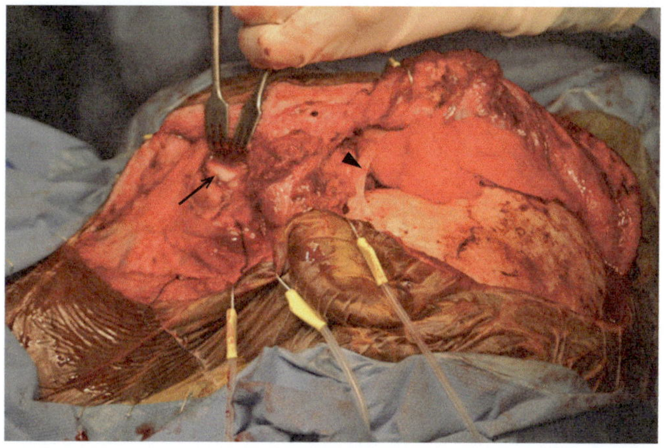

96. The facial nerve was traced out from the stylomastoid foramen to the pes anserinus (*arrow*).

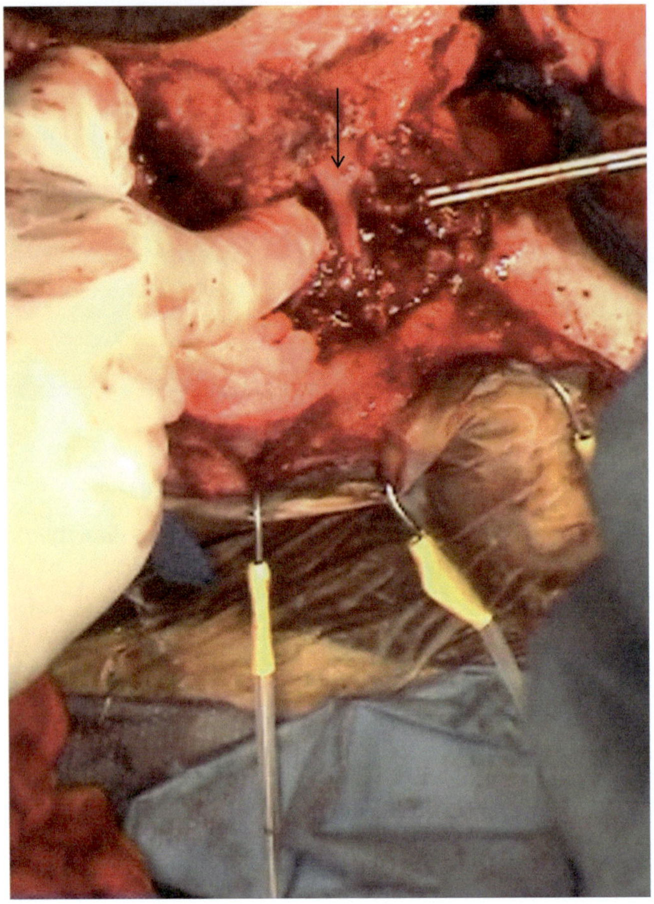

97. The deep lobe of the parotid was then removed, leaving the facial nerve (*VII*) in place. This opened up access to the infratemporal fossa medial to the facial nerve.

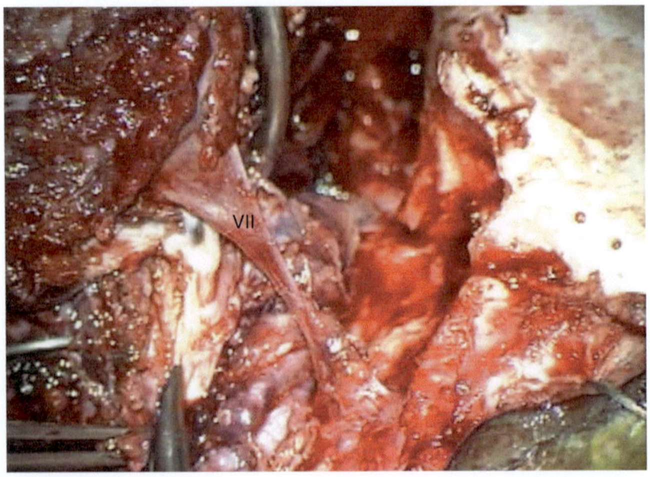

98. Next, a middle fossa craniectomy was performed using a craniotome.

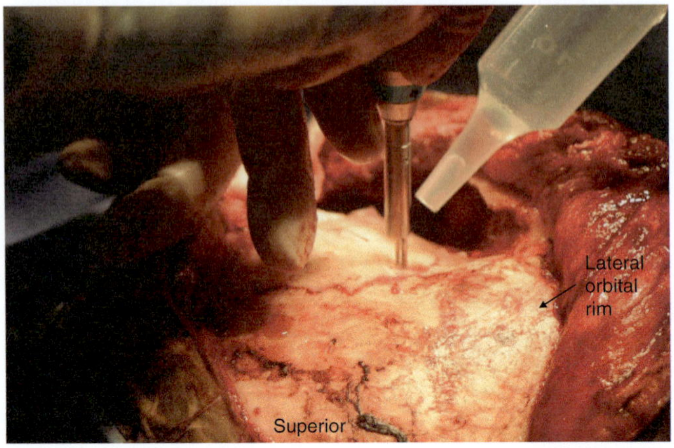

99. The middle fossa dura was elevated off the skull base bone.

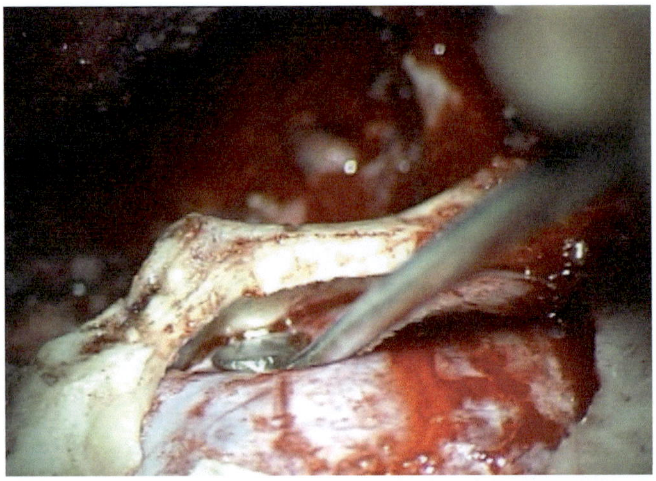

100. Necrotic tissue was found at foramen ovale (*arrow*).

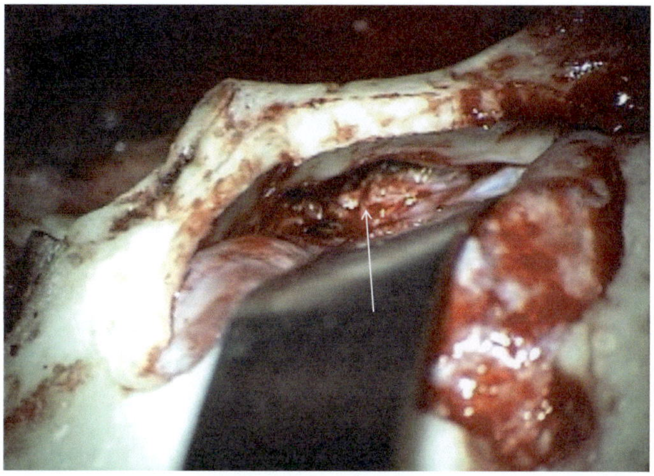

101. Microscissors were used to divide V3.

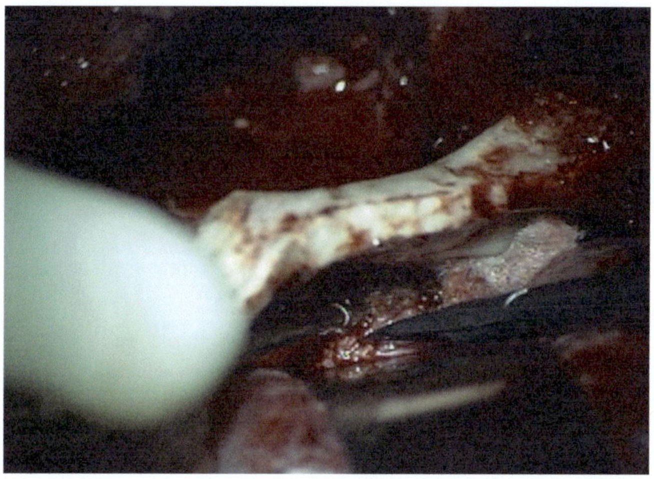

102. This permitted dissection to continue medially to reach the cavernous sinus. In this image, the forceps were reaching through a large defect in the bone in the area of foramen ovale. The tips were in Meckel's cave.

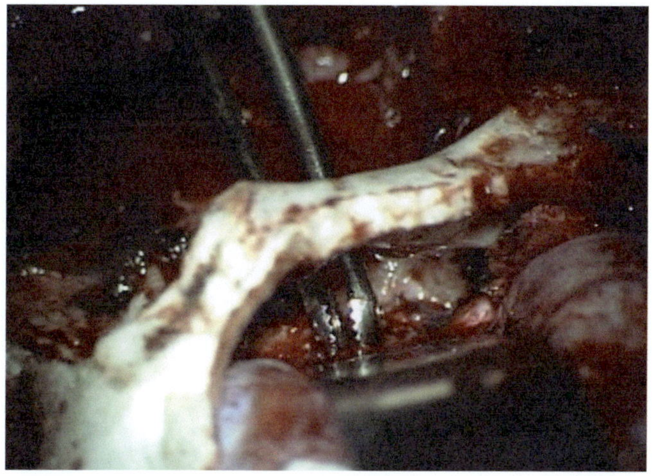

103. After resection of the disease, the facial nerve remained anatomically intact, but all the infratemporal fossa, the muscles of mastication, and the mandibular ramus were resected. The necrotic skull base bone around foramen ovale was drilled away (*arrow*). One black suture is on the stump of the facial artery and the other on the stump of the external jugular vein. These were used for free flap reconstruction of the defect.

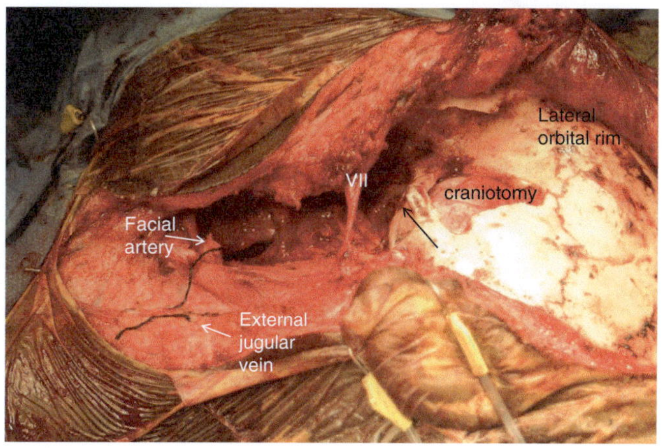

104. A muscular free flap was used to fill and bring healthy, vascularized tissue to the defect. The goal was for this tissue to bring antifungal drugs in close approximation to residual disease in the cavernous sinus and skull base bone. The flap was inset under the main trunk of the facial nerve.

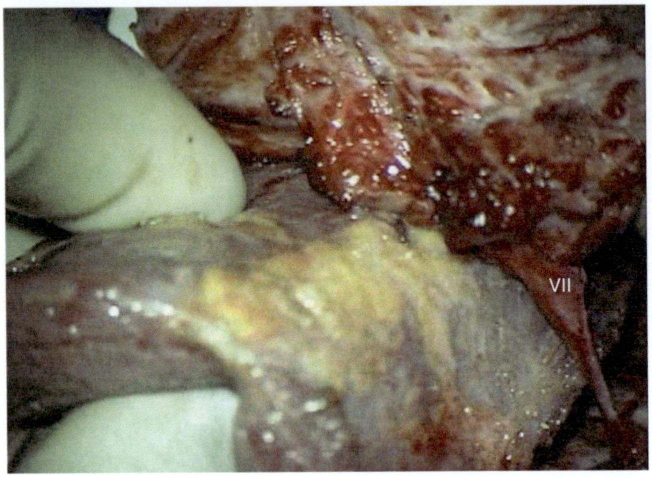

105. The arterial anastamosis is shown.

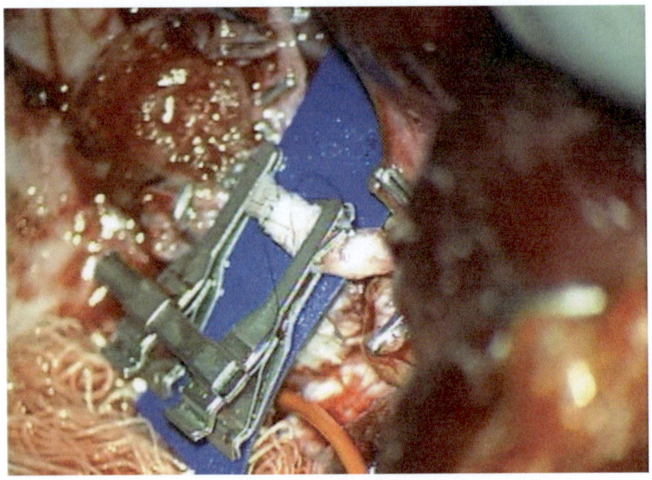

106. Post-op axial MRI demonstrating the free flap filling the defect.

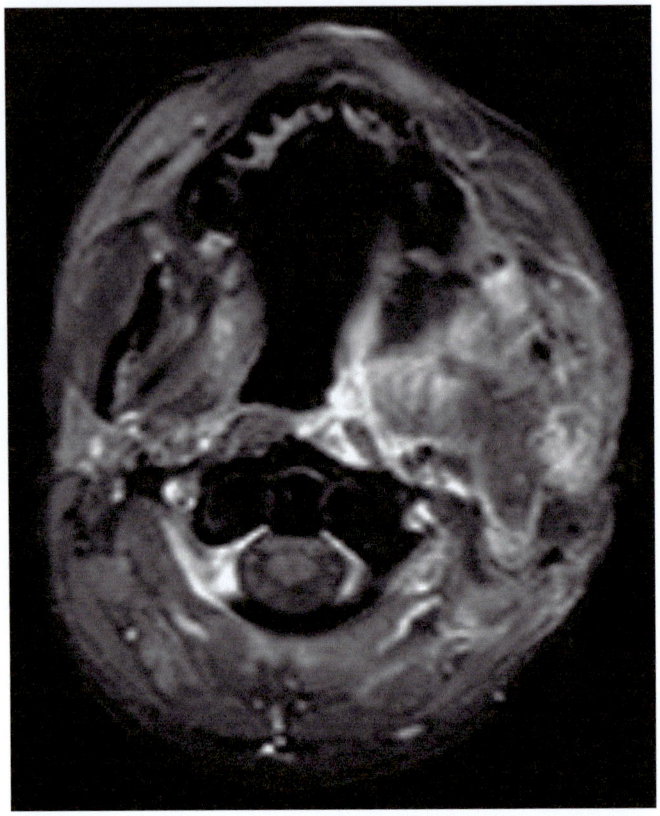

107. Post-op coronal MRI

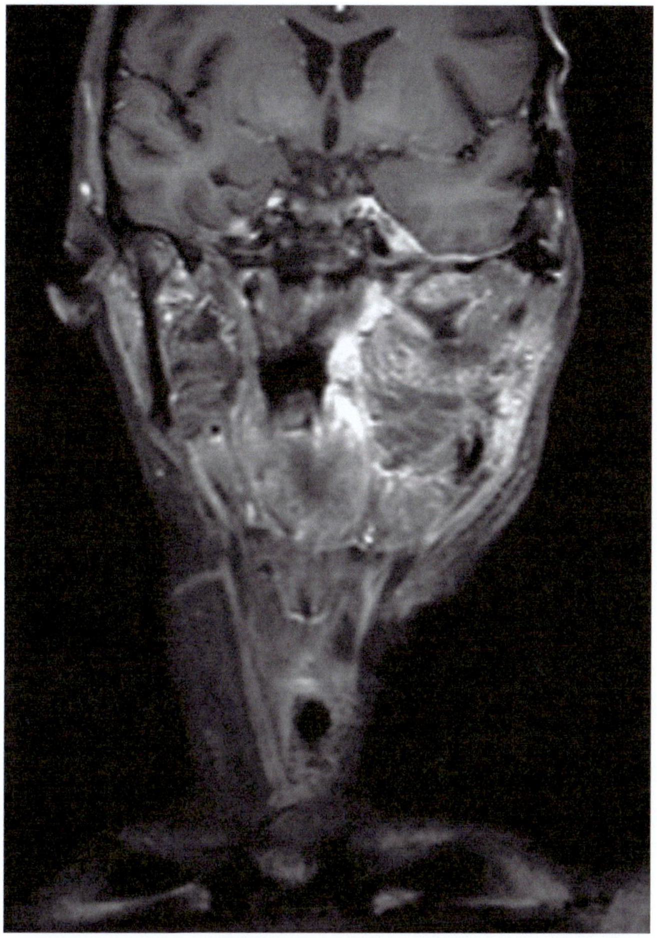

108. Post-op axial CT demonstrating that the mandibular ramus and the pterygoid plates were removed.

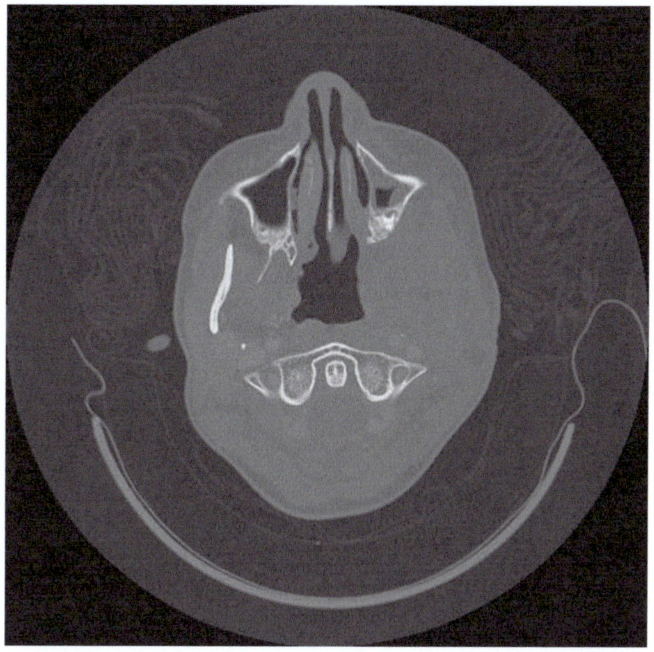

109. Post-op coronal CT demonstrating the resection of the skull base bone around foramen ovale (*arrow*).

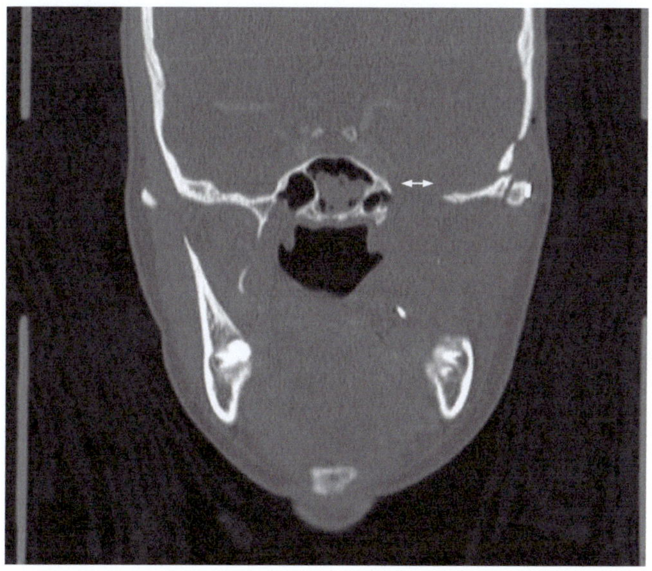

110. Case 2. This child had a teratoma of the upper jugular region resected as an infant. She then presented with recurrent disease at the skull base that extended inferiorly and into the ear canal as an aural polyp. The axial T1 MRI with gadolinium demonstrated that this lesion was cystic (*arrow*).

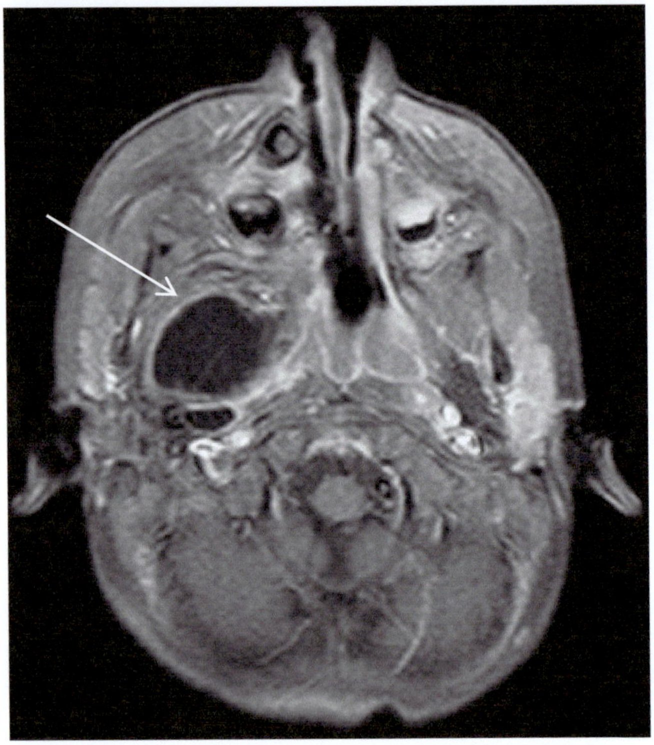

111. Coronal T1 MRI demonstrated that there was erosion of the skull base bone around foramen ovale (*arrow*).

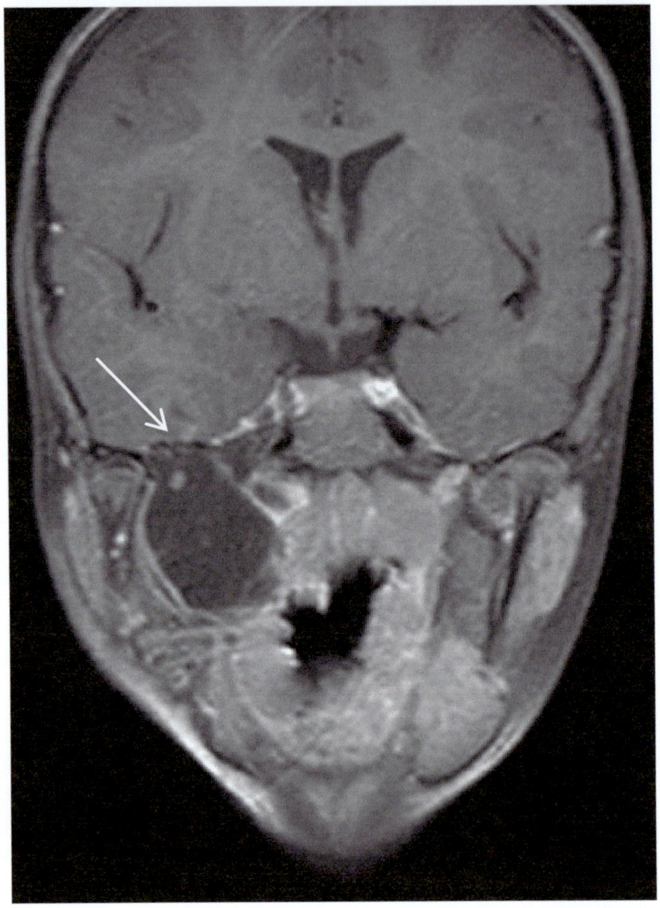

112. Sagittal T1 MRI also demonstrated the extension into the skull base.

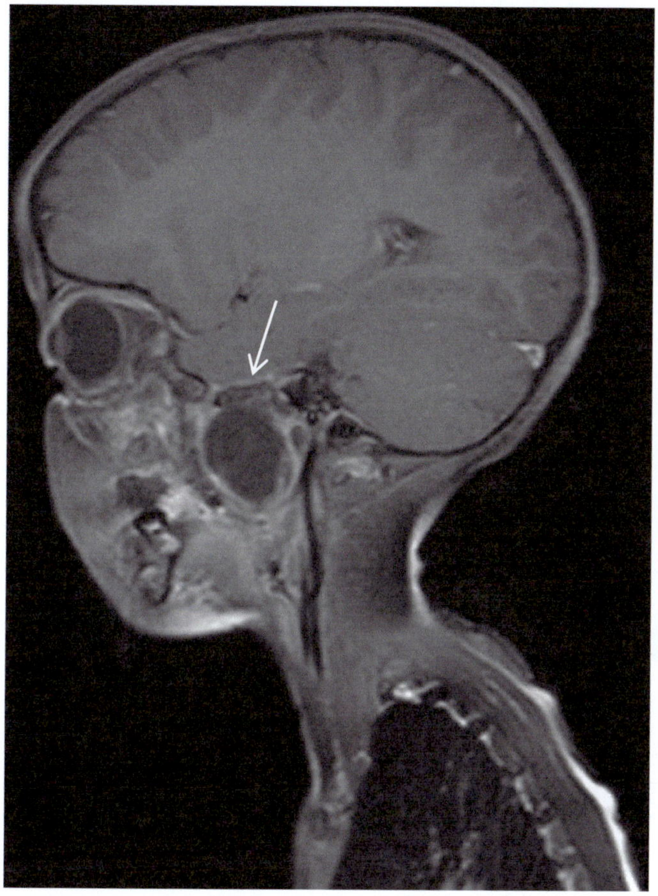

113. Coronal T2 MRI demonstrated the cystic nature of the tumor and suggested that the tumor didn't penetrate the dura.

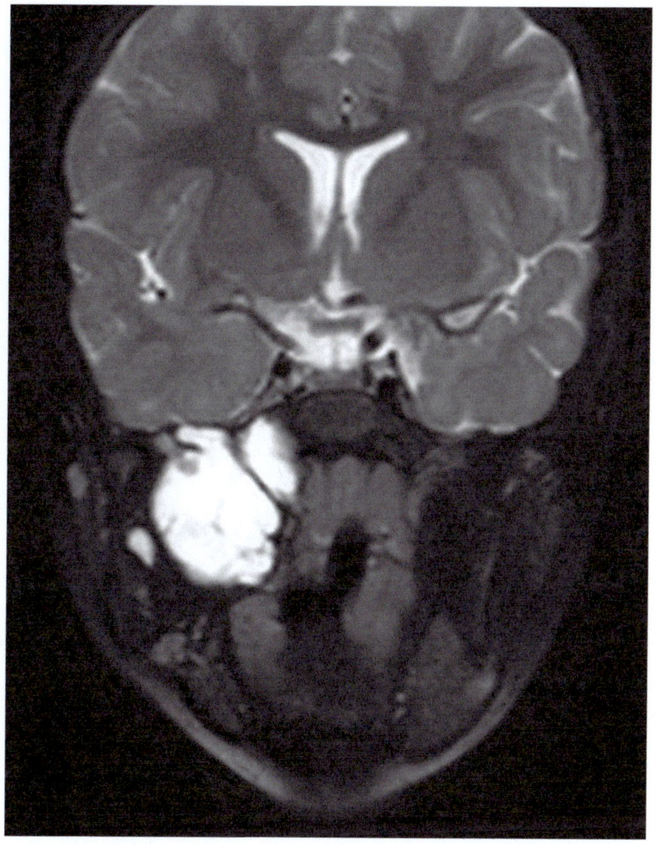

114. Axial CT scan demonstrated that the tumor eroded the anterior medial ear canal bone (*arrow*) and entered the middle ear space.

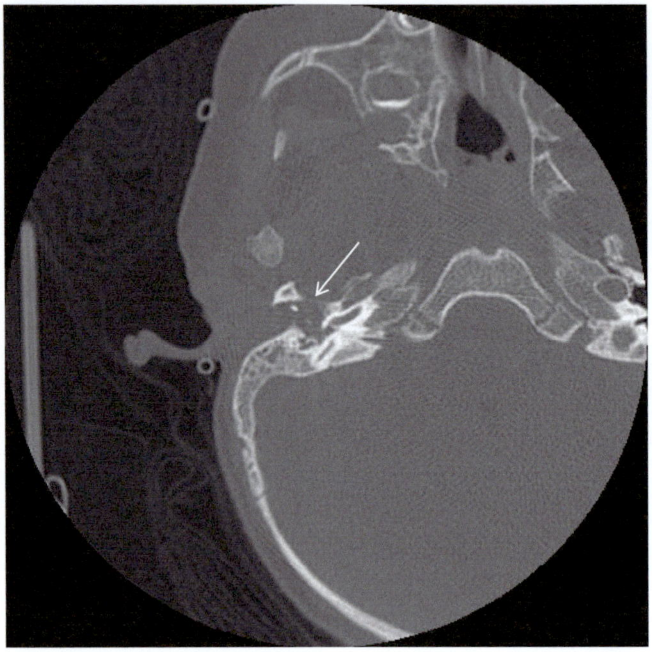

115. A preauricular incision was designed. Scars from the previous resection were visible, as was the polyp in the ear canal.

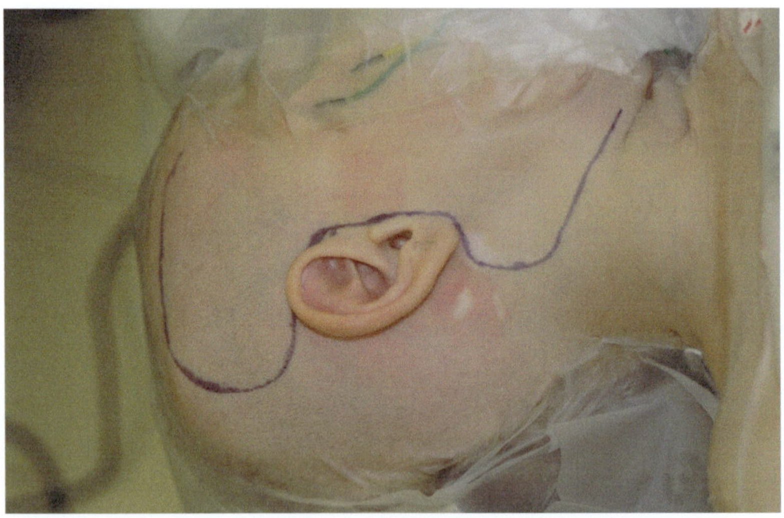

116. The great vessels in the neck were identified. The cystic tumor was just anterior to them (*asterisk*). The blue vessel loop is around the internal jugular vein, and the yellow vessel loop is around the internal carotid artery.

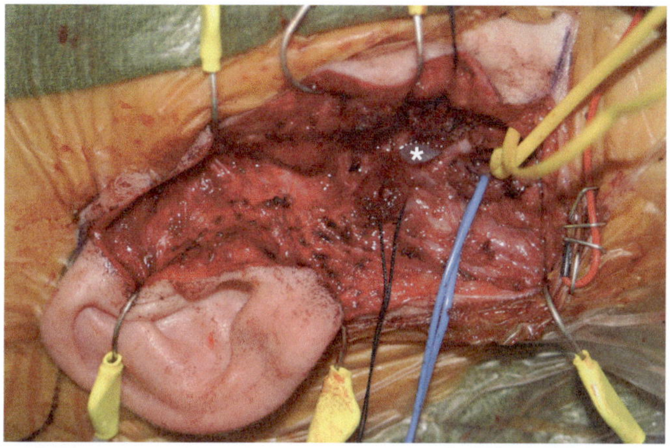

117. The temporalis muscle was elevated and the ear canal transected at the bony cartilaginous junction with the plan to obliterate the middle ear space after removing the tumor. The tympanic membrane, with tumor growing out of its superior aspect (*arrow*), was visible. The main trunk of the facial nerve was dissected out to the pes anserinus (*VII*).

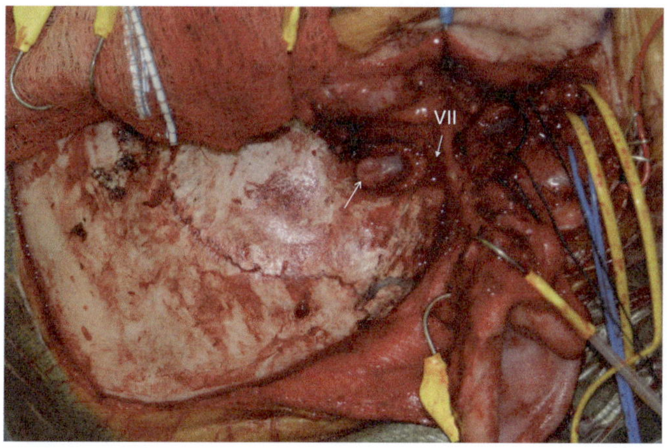

118. A mastoidectomy with delineation of the vertical segment of the facial nerve (*VII*) was performed. All squamous epithelium was carefully removed from the ear canal and tympanic annulus. The bony ear canal was resected. A middle fossa craniectomy was performed and the defect in the skull base bone superior to the ear canal (*arrow*) opened. This allowed access to separate the upper pole of the tumor from the middle fossa dura.

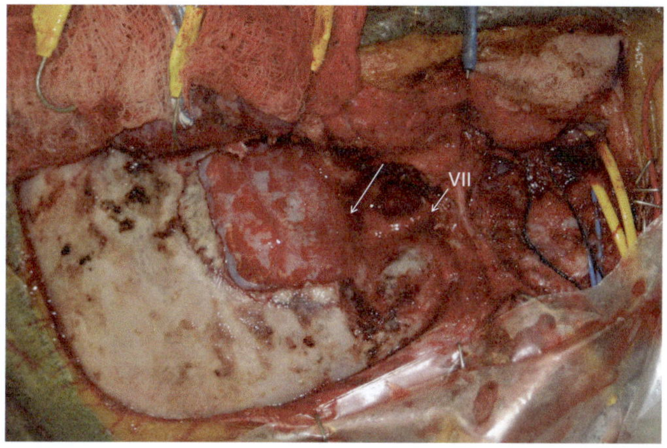

119. The tumor was resected out from the infratemporal fossa, sparing the facial nerve (*VII*).

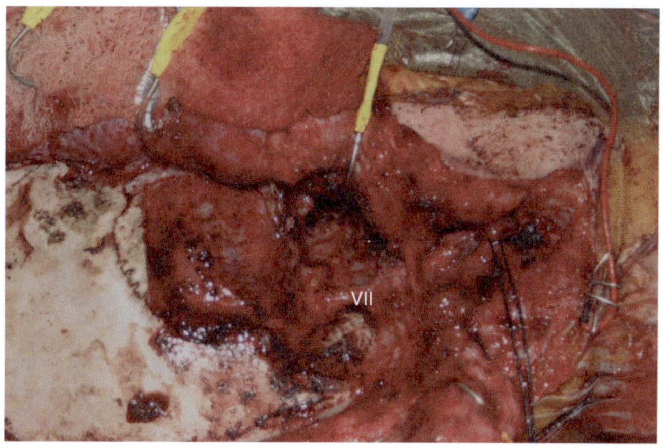

120. After resection, the defect was filled with a fat graft. The bone flap was cut in half and the posterior portion of the bone flap plated back. We used a hydroxyapatite bone cement to fill in the anterior gap. The anterior portion of the bone flap was used to reconstruct the tegmen defect.

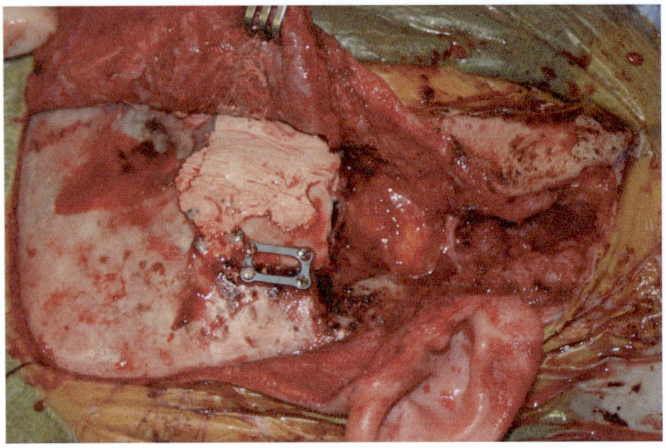

121. The ear canal was everted and oversewn (*arrow*). The wound was closed.

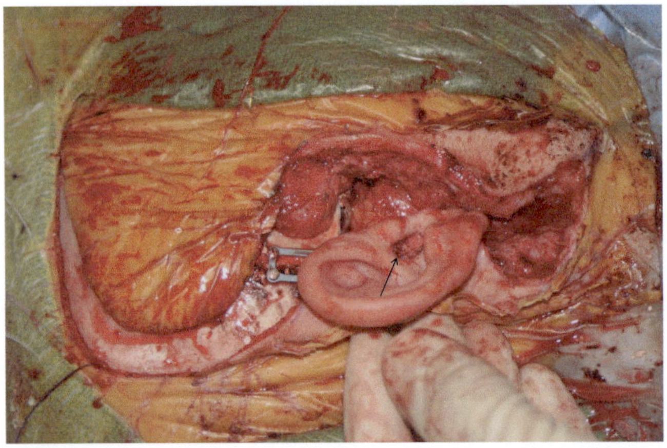

122. Post-op coronal MRI. The black tissue in the infratemporal fossa is the fat graft and the bone flap (*arrow*) reconstruction of the tegmen defect can be seen.

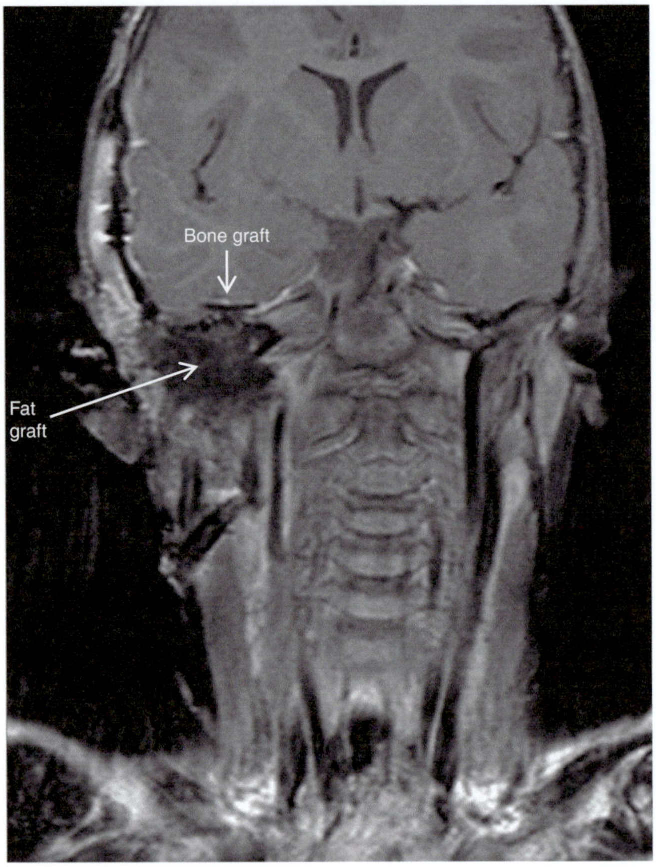

123. Post-op T2 MRI demonstrating the fat graft filling the space in the infratemporal fossa.

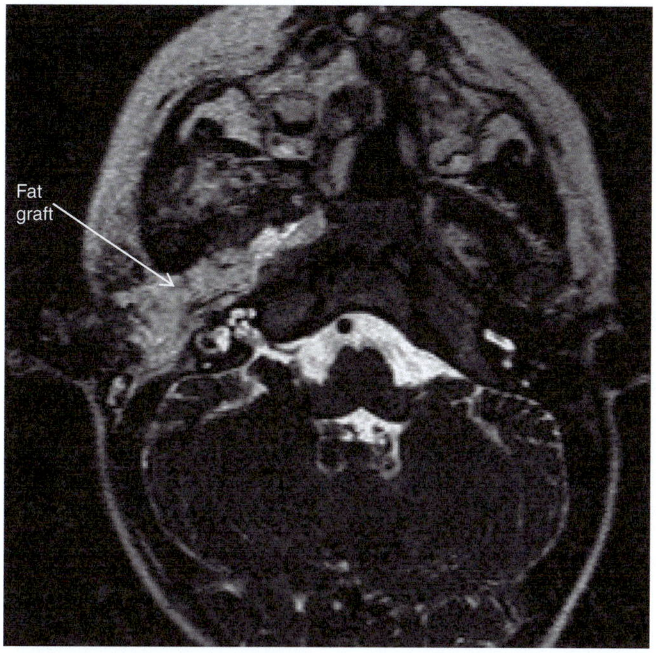

124. Post-op coronal CT demonstrating the reconstruction of the tegmen defect.

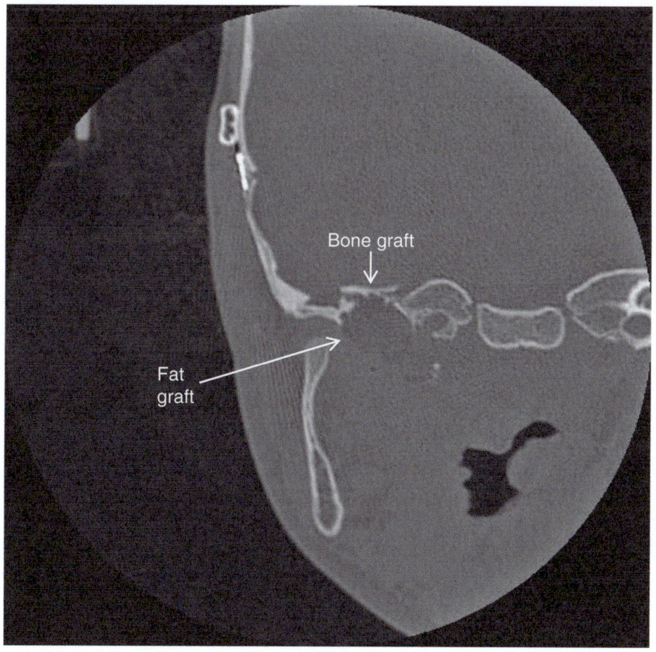

125. Case 3. A patient presented with a CN VI palsy. T2 MRI demonstrated a bright lesion within the right petrous apex (*arrow*) that extended slightly into the posterior fossa.

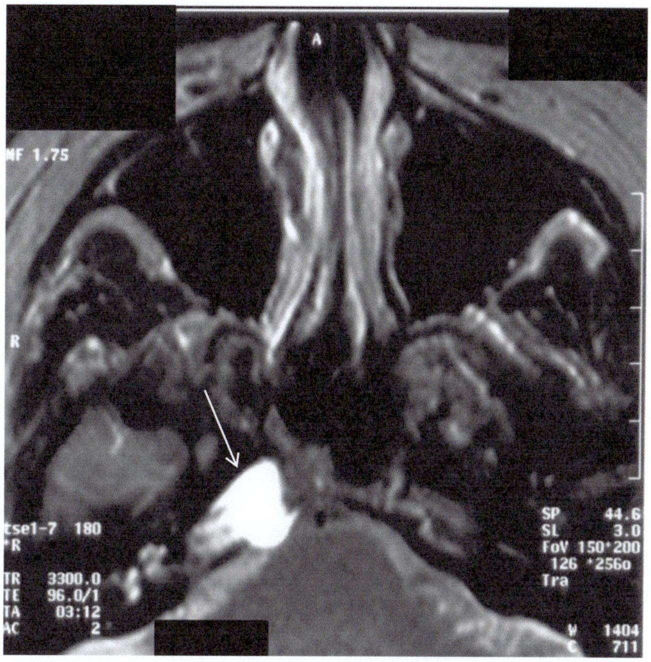

126. T1 MRI without gadolinium demonstrated that the lesion had similar intensity to brain and muscle. This was inconsistent with a cholesterol granuloma (which would be bright on T1 without gadolinium).

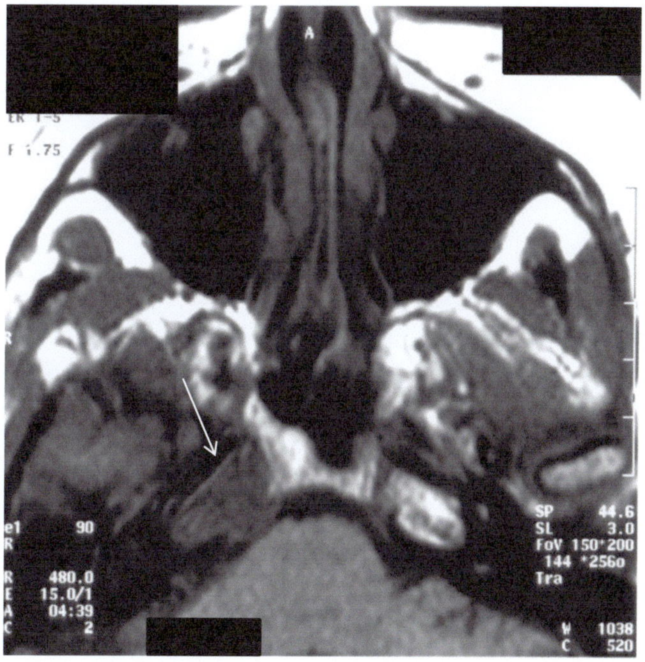

127. T1 MRI with gadolinium demonstrated moderate enhancement of the lesion. Taken together, these imaging characteristics suggested that the lesion was neoplastic.

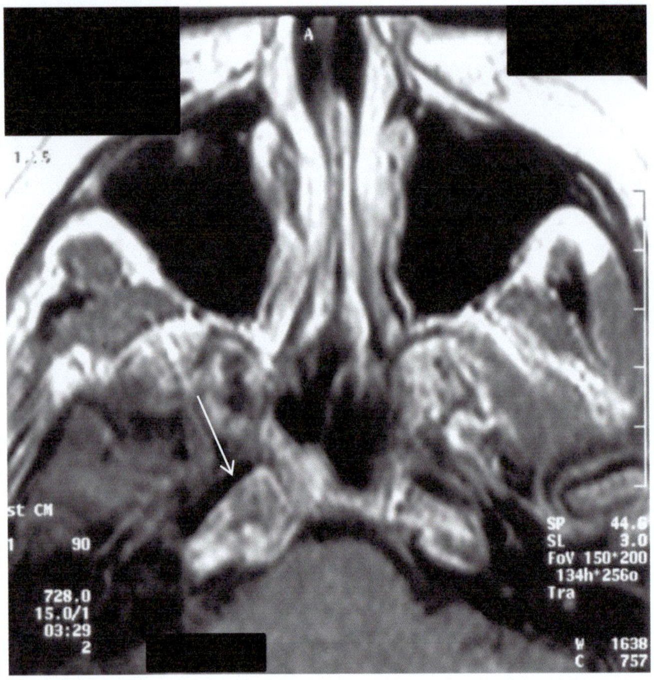

128. CT demonstrated that the lesion eroded the petrous apex and abutted the medial aspect of the internal carotid artery. The borders were not smooth as would be expected with a cholesterol granuloma. This further suggested the lesion was neoplastic. In this area, the most common tumor with these characteristics is a chondrosarcoma. We performed a gross total tumor resection of the lesion using a preauricular infratemporal fossa approach and pathology confirmed the diagnosis of chondrosarcoma.

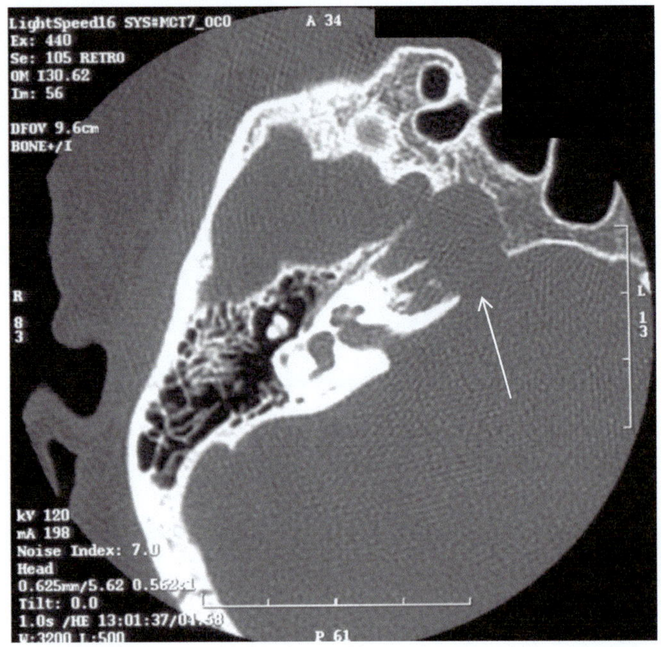

129. Case 4. MRI of a child with a large plexiform neurofibroma of the parotid gland, infratemporal fossa, and parapharyngeal space. She had multiple cutaneous neurofibromata and had NF1.

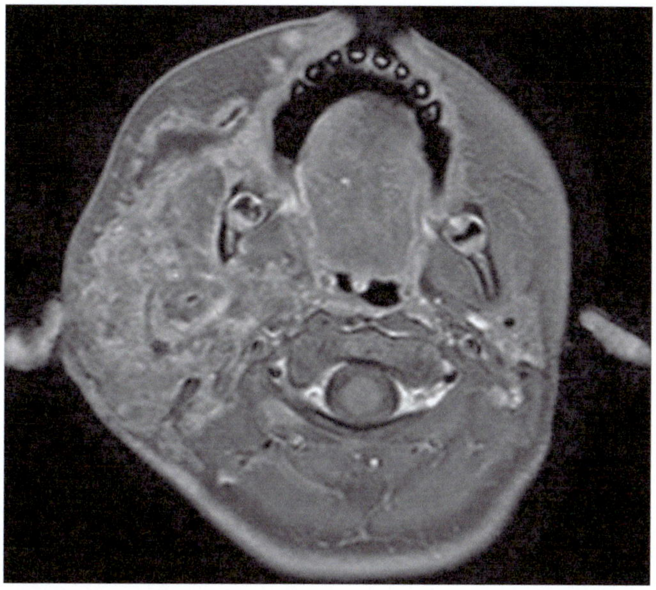

130. Coronal MRI of the patient. Note the compression of the upper aerodigestive tract (*arrow*). The best management option for neurofibromas is usually conservative observation as it is impossible to resect the entire tumor. Furthermore, the patient has a genetic disease affecting every cell in his/her body, and the disease will recur, with neurofibroma continuing to form regardless of the extent of surgical resection. In this patient's case, however, the child began having difficulty swallowing and had obstructive sleep apnea from the airway compression. Thus, we elected to debulk the tumor.

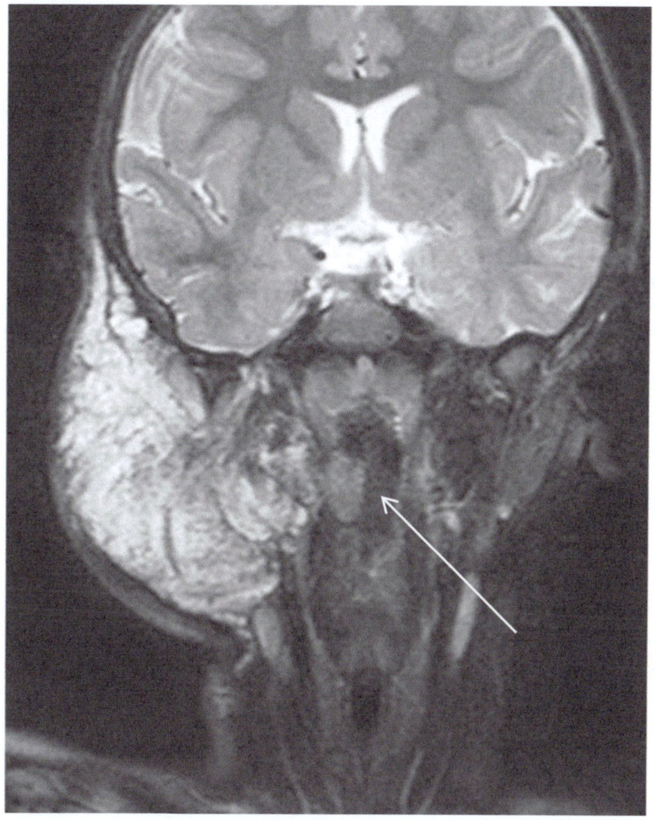

131. The incision. We did not need to extend it superiorly because the lesion only involved the infratemporal fossa and did not involve the dura.

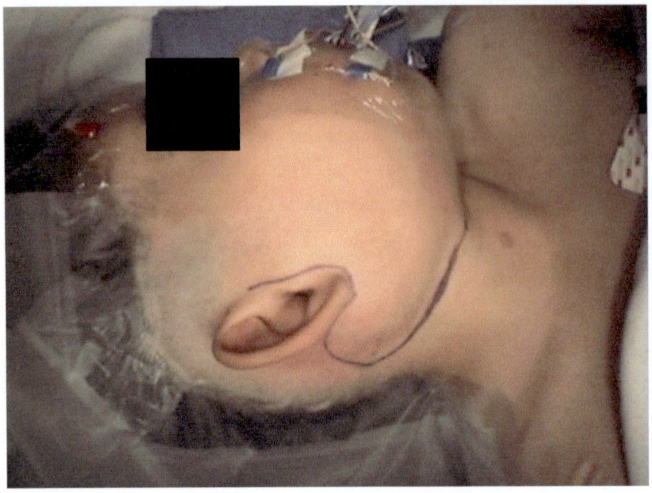

132. A standard parotid skin flap was developed in this case because the entire parotid was involved with tumor.

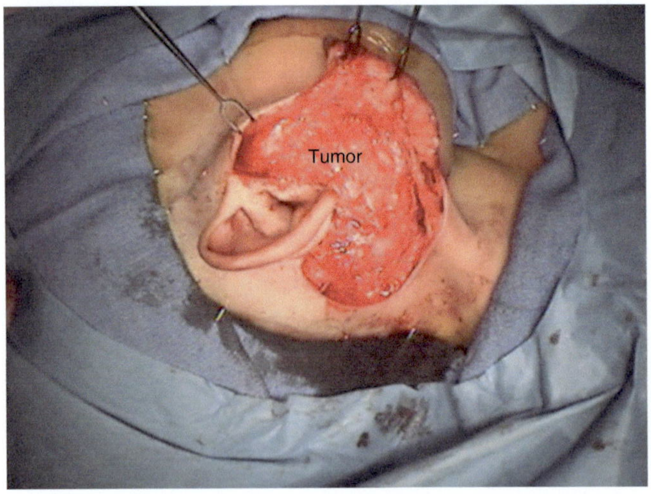

133. The hypoglossal nerve (*arrow*) was identified and preserved. It appeared normal and not part of the neurofibroma.

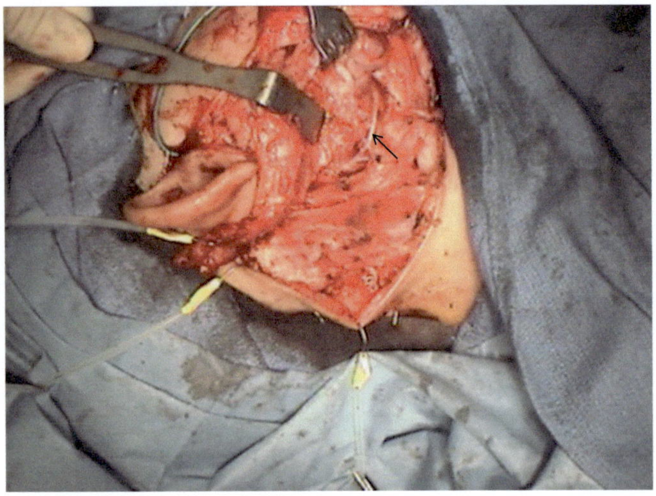

134. The main trunk of the facial nerve was identified and traced out to the pes anserinus (*arrow*). It was greatly thickened and involved with neurofibroma. Thus, this neurofibroma originated from the facial nerve. The upper branches could not be traced out because of the extensive tumor involvement.

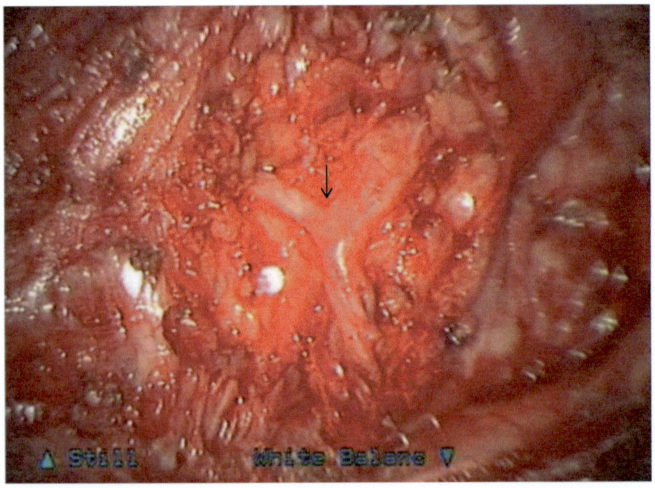

135. The wound after the resection. All of the parotid gland together with much of the subcutaneous and deeper tumor from the infratemporal fossa was resected. The lower division of the facial nerve was preserved (*arrow*). Tumor was left in the anterior cheek near the mouth and nose.

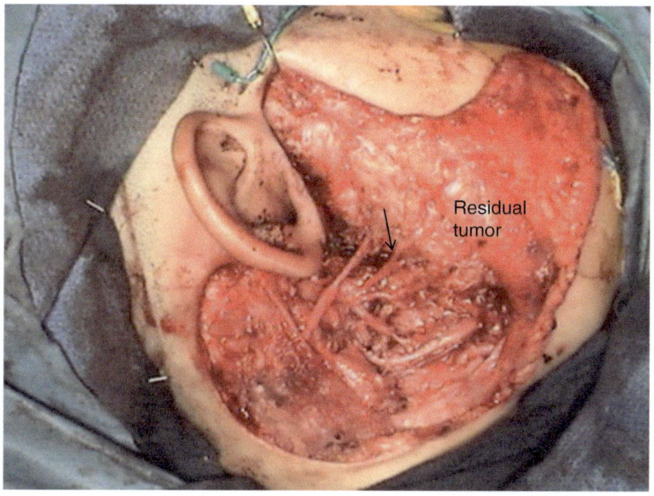

136. After closure of the wound. Two drains were used because the raw surface of residual neurofibroma tends to weep profusely. After resecting a neurofibroma, we recommend drainage for longer-than-normal period of time to reduce the risk of seroma formation.

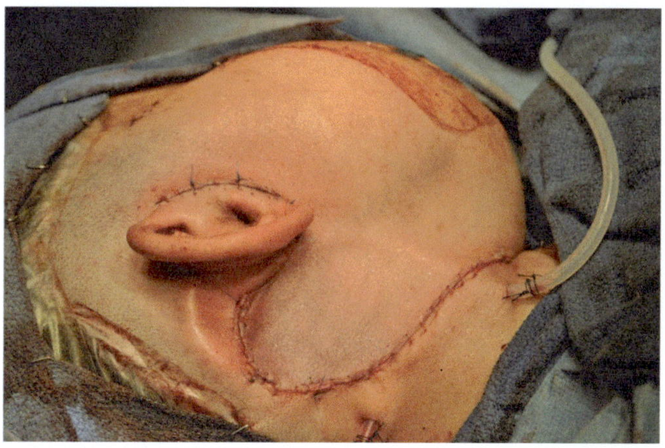

Pre- and Postauricular Approach to the Infratemporal Fossa

- *Concept*
  - Like the preauricular approach, this approach provides exposure to the upper parapharyngeal space, foramen ovale, and the nasopharynx. However, it also permits exposure of the hypoglossal foramen and jugular foramen.
- *Conditions treated*
  - Extracranial hypoglossal nerve schwannoma
  - Extensive, infiltrative tumors of the infratemporal fossa and parapharyngeal space
- *Risks*
  - Conductive hearing loss due to Eustachian tube obstruction
  - Palsy of CN V, VII, IX, X, XI, or XII
  - Internal carotid artery injury
- *Benefits*
  - Exposure of the infratemporal fossa without entering the middle ear

137. Diagram of the vascular supply to the head. This approach involves accessing the region where the internal carotid artery and internal jugular vein enter the skull base.

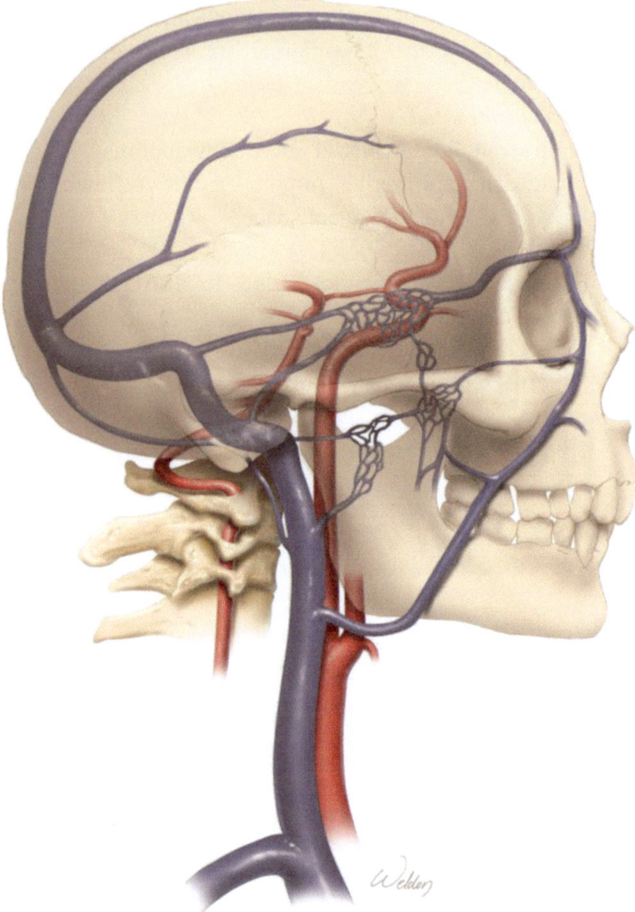

138. The nerves of the jugular foramen (*IX*, *X*, *XI*) and the hypoglossal nerve (*XII*) are overlaid on the vascular supply.

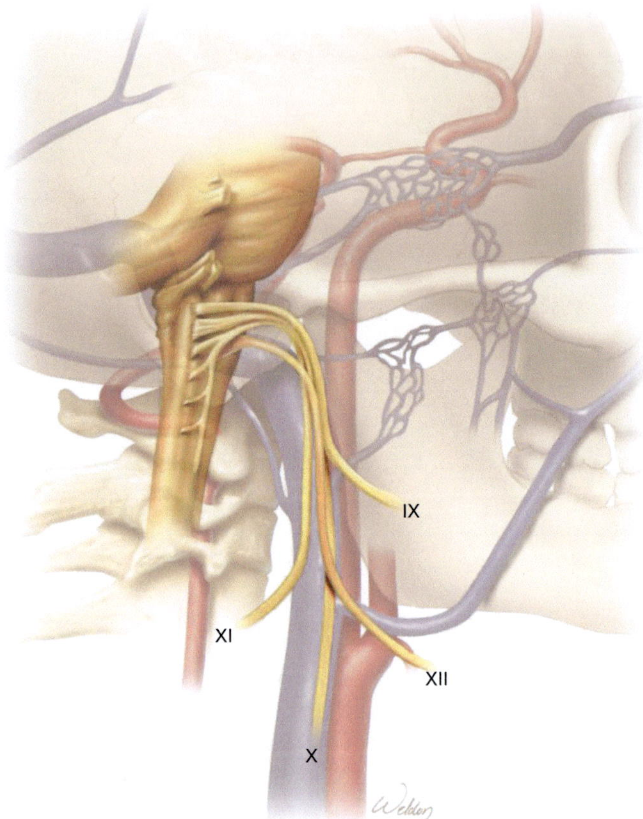

139. The same diagram viewed anteriorly. The jugular foramen (*arrow*) and hypoglossal foramen (*arrowhead*) are shown in gray. Hypoglossal nerve tumors can be extracranial (*top inset*), intracranial (*middle inset*), or dumbbell shaped (*bottom inset*). The pre- and postauricular approach permits resection of extracranial disease. A far lateral approach is needed to resect intracranial disease.

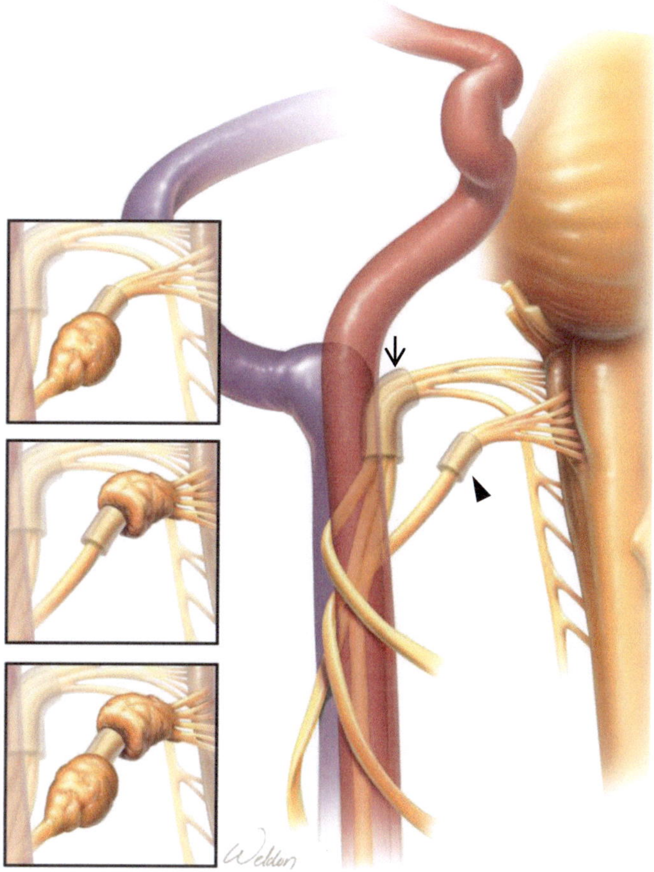

140. The incision for a pre- and postauricular approach is outlined.

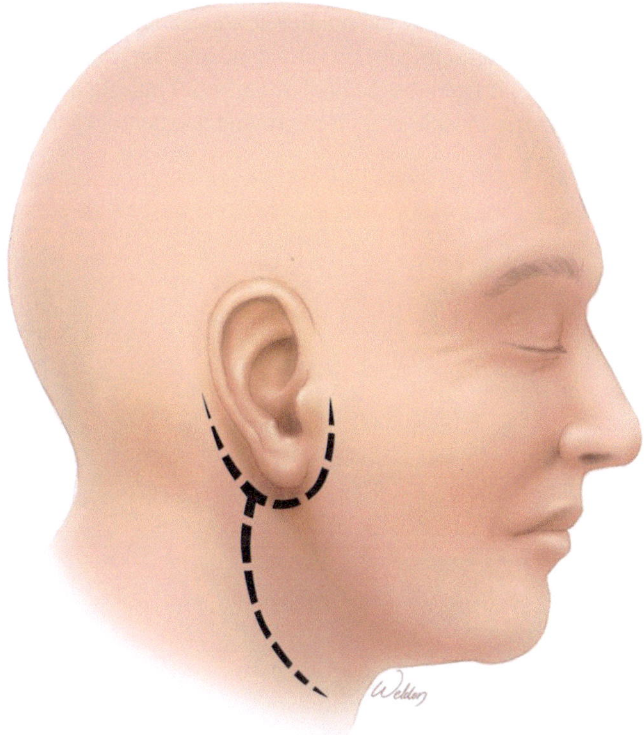

141. The main trunk of the facial nerve is identified and the parotid gland retracted anteriorly to expose the infratemporal fossa, which lies deep into it. Dissecting the facial nerve out to the pes anserinis aids exposure but is often not needed for smaller and more lateral tumors. Simply retracting the parotid gland anteriorly after separating it from the sternocleidomastoid muscle and the digastric muscle will often provide adequate exposure.

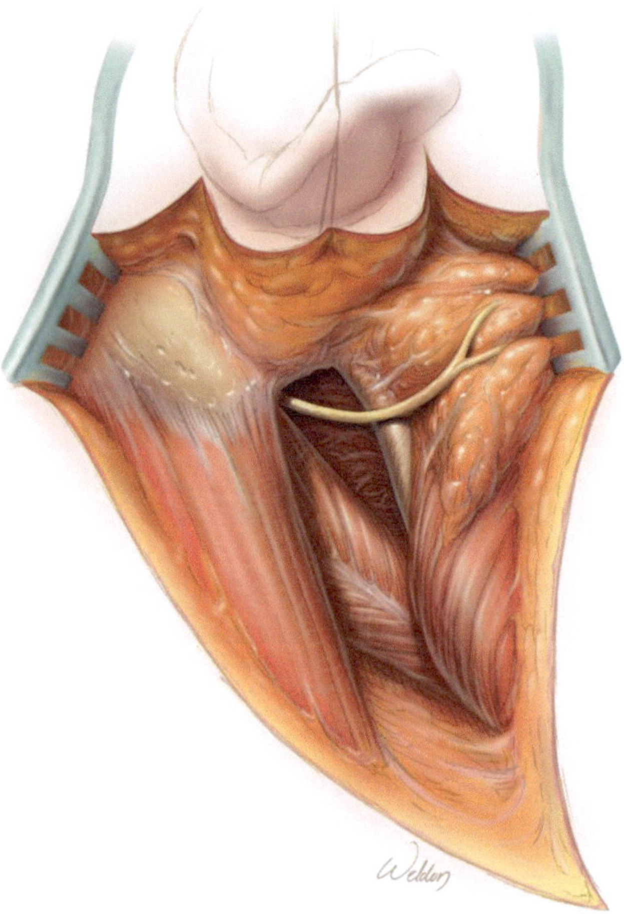

142. The sternocleidomastoid muscle is separated from the mastoid tip, the digastric muscle is divided, and the transverse process of C1 is identified. The fibrous tissue surrounding C1 is left in place to protect the vertebral artery. The internal jugular vein lies just anterior to the transverse process, as do cranial nerves X, XI, and XII. The stylohyoid muscle (*arrow*) covers the superior course of these nerves.

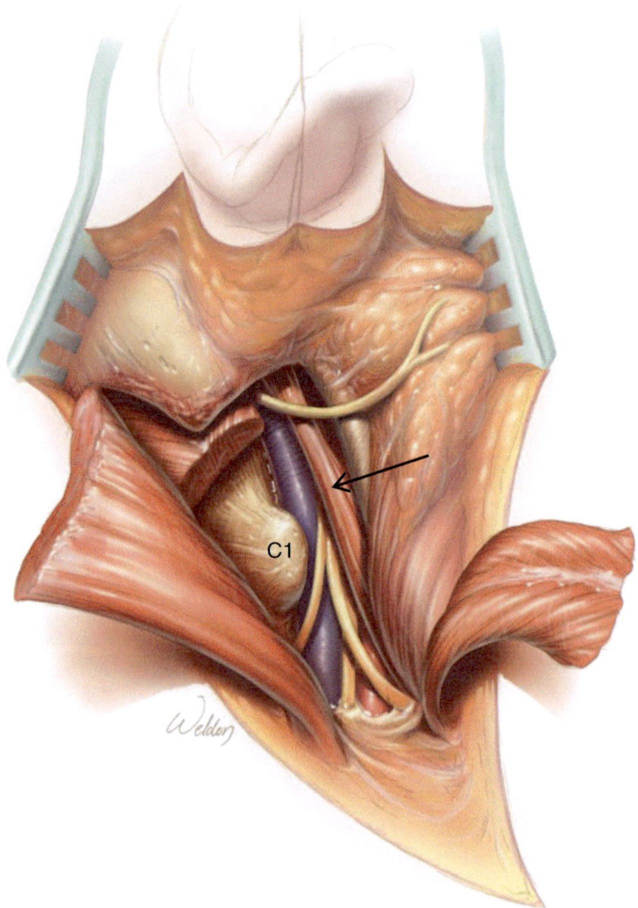

143. The stylohyoid muscle is divided permitting anterior displacement of the mandible with a retractor. While handheld retractors can be used, a self-retaining retractor (such as a Weitlaner) works well. Retraction opens up the infratemporal fossa, and CN IX can then be found. In this illustration, CN IX is covered by the retractor. After developing adequate retraction, the hypoglossal nerve is traced up the hypoglossal foramen (*arrow*).

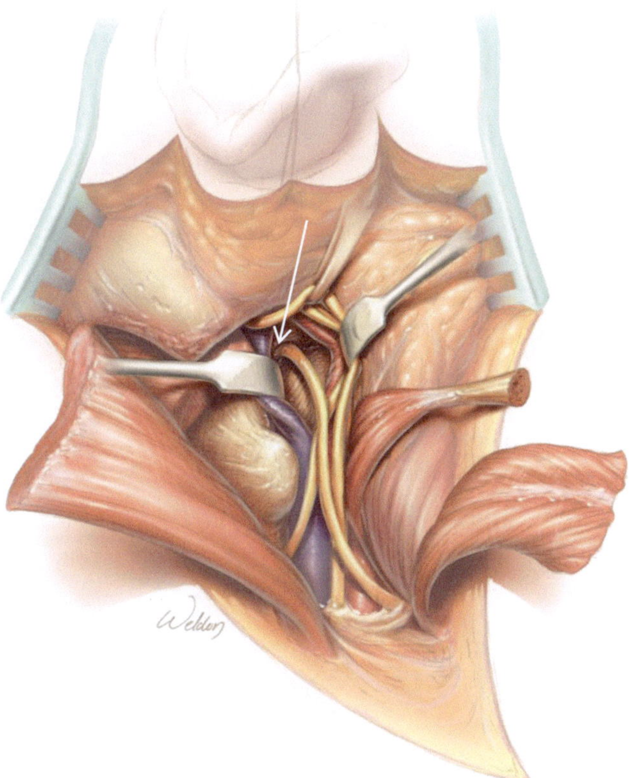

144. An extracranial hypoglossal nerve schwannoma is illustrated.

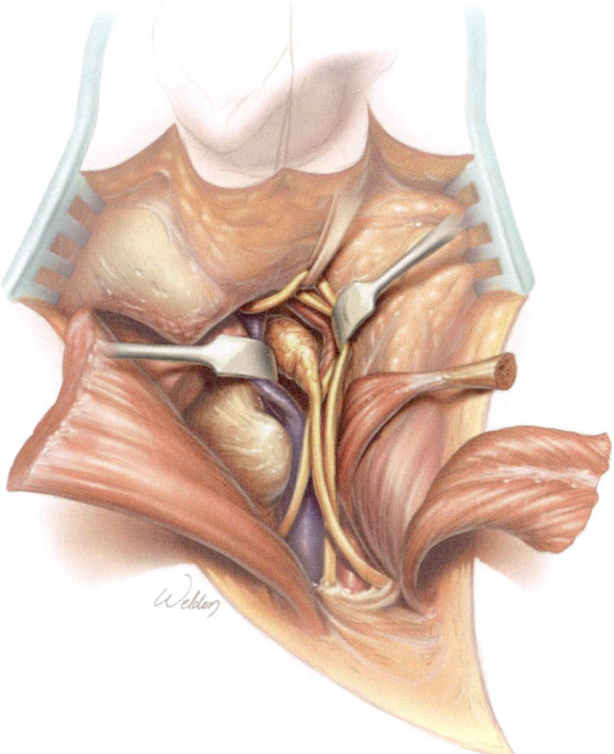

145. Case 1. Axial T1 MRI with gadolinium of a patient with a left bilobed hypoglossal schwannoma who had already had a far lateral approach for resection of the intracranial tumor. In this image, the extracranial tumor was visible (*arrow*).

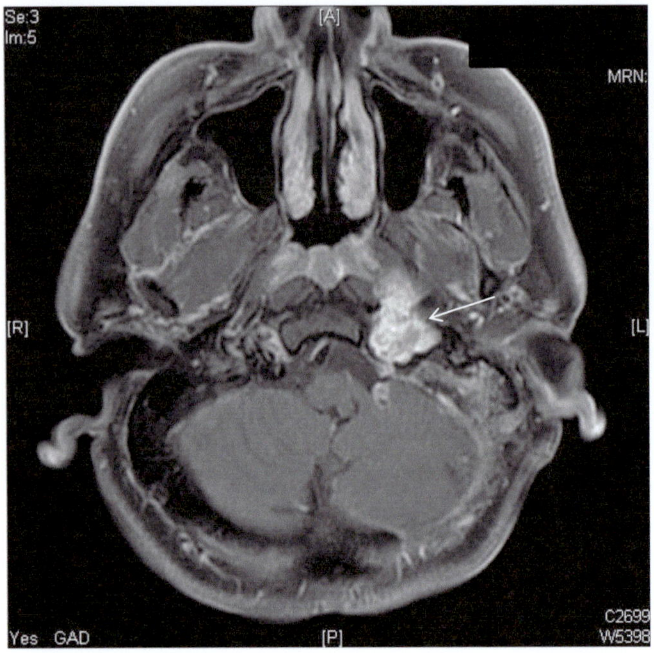

146. Coronal MRI demonstrated the residual extracranial hypoglossal schwannoma.

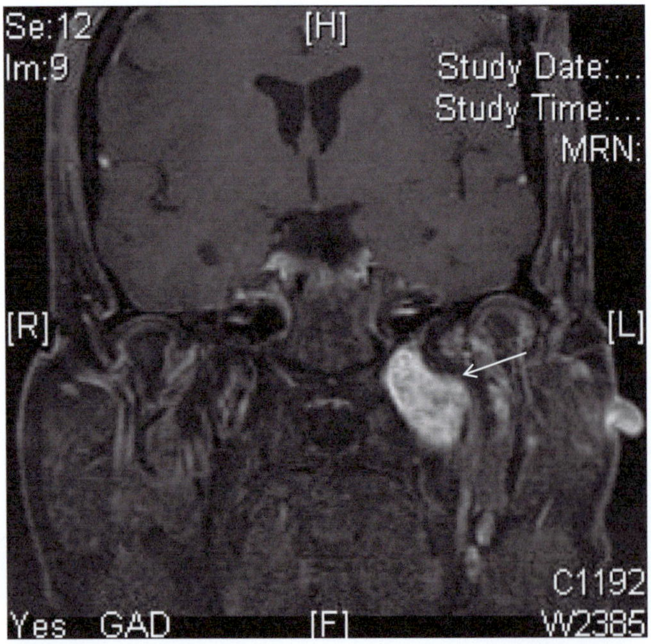

147. A pre- and postauricular approach was performed to resect the residual tumor. After opening the wound, the main trunk of the facial nerve (*arrow*) was traced out to the pes anserinus (*arrowhead*).

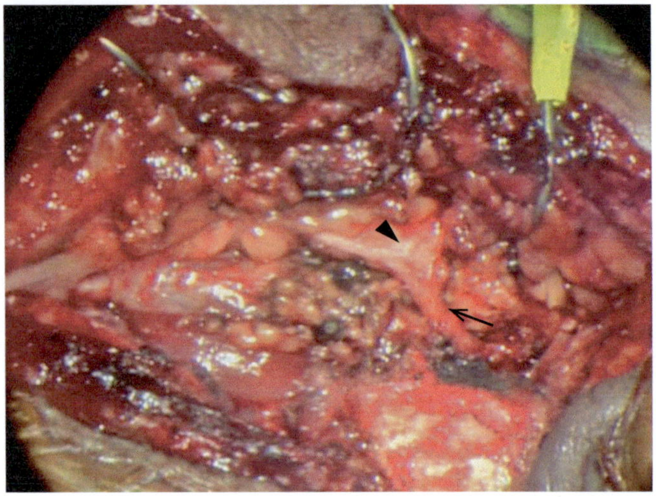

148. The internal jugular vein was identified and controlled with vessel loops.

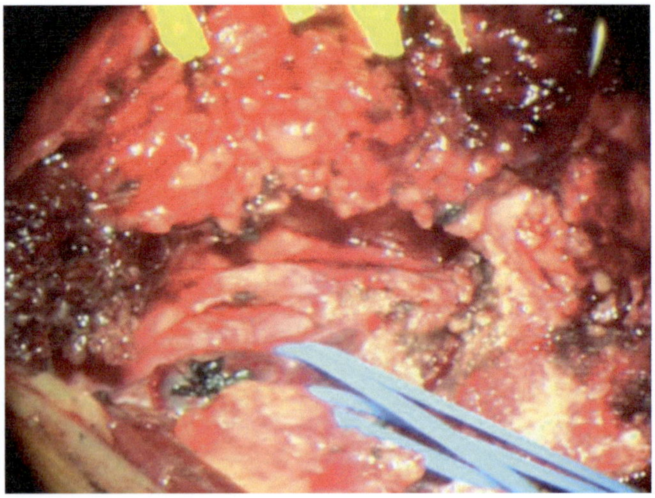

149. The internal carotid artery was also identified and controlled with a vessel loop. The hypoglossal nerve was identified anteriorly (*arrow*).

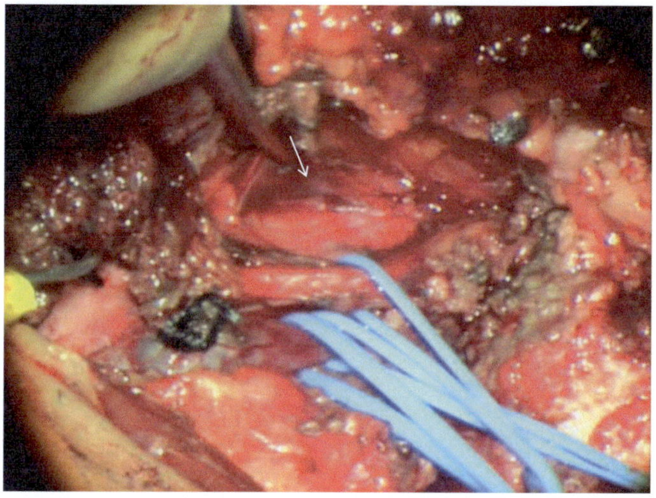

150. The hypoglossal nerve was then traced superiorly and the inferior aspect of the tumor found.

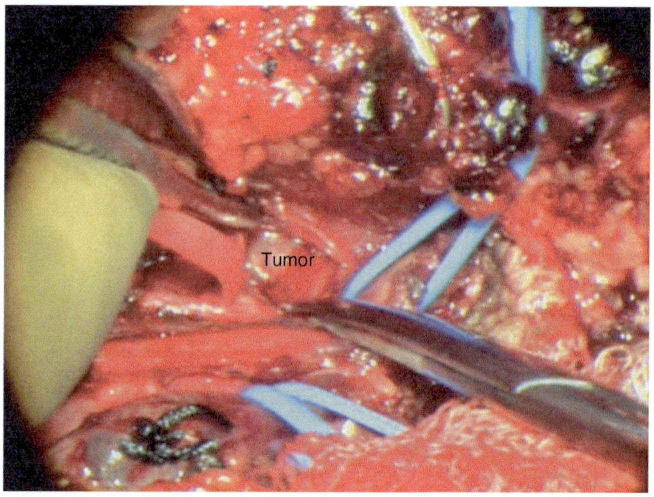

151. After resecting the tumor, there was a large space in the infratemporal fossa (medial to the deep lobe of the parotid gland).

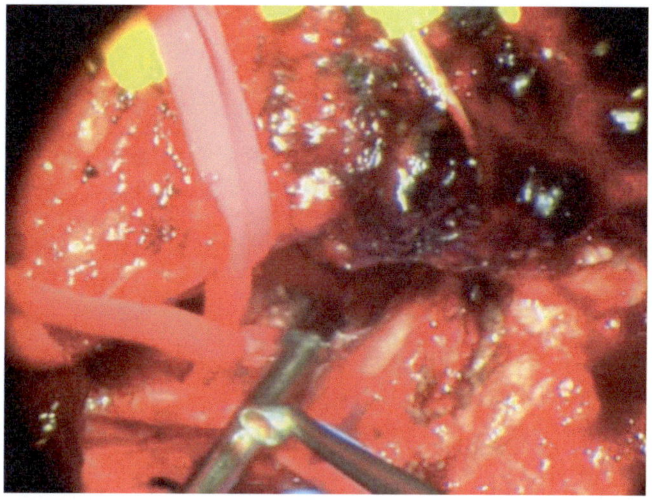

152. Post-op axial MRI with gadolinium demonstrated resection of the extracranial tumor. A small remnant (*arrow*) remained within the hypoglossal foramen, which we planned to observe conservatively.

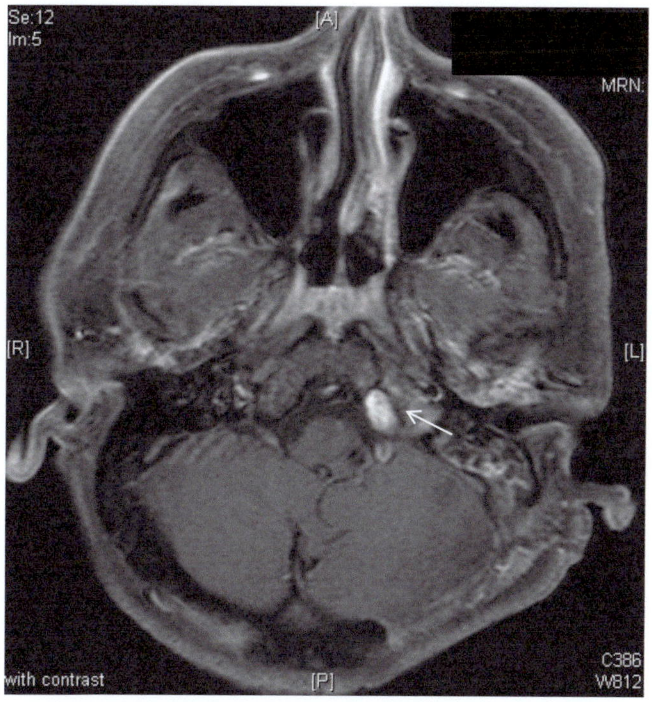

153. Post-op coronal MRI demonstrated the small focus of residual tumor (*arrow*).

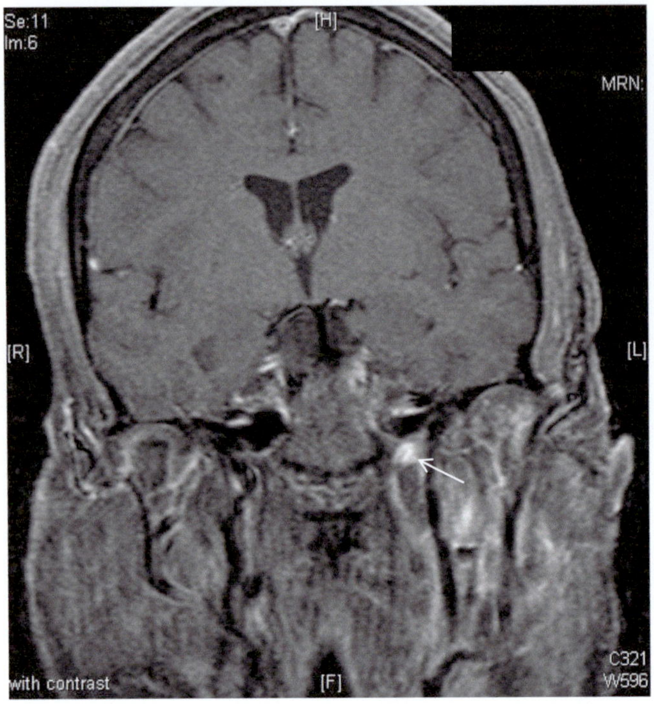

154. Case 2. Coronal MRI with gadolinium of a patient with a small extracranial hypoglossal schwannoma (*arrows*). This patient presented with deep upper neck pain, and right-sided tongue atrophy was noted on exam. While stereotactic radiation was considered, the patient chose surgical resection with the hope of pain relief.

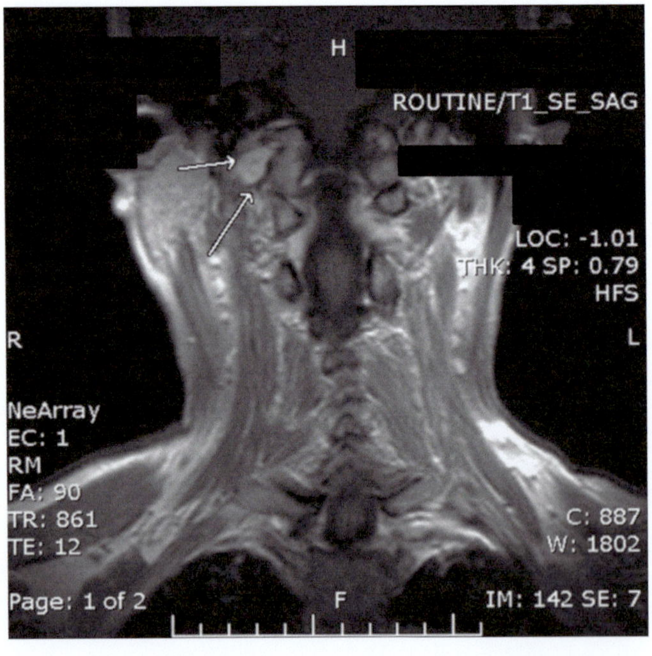

155. Axial MRI demonstrated the lesion within the infratemporal fossa/parapharyngeal space (*arrow*).

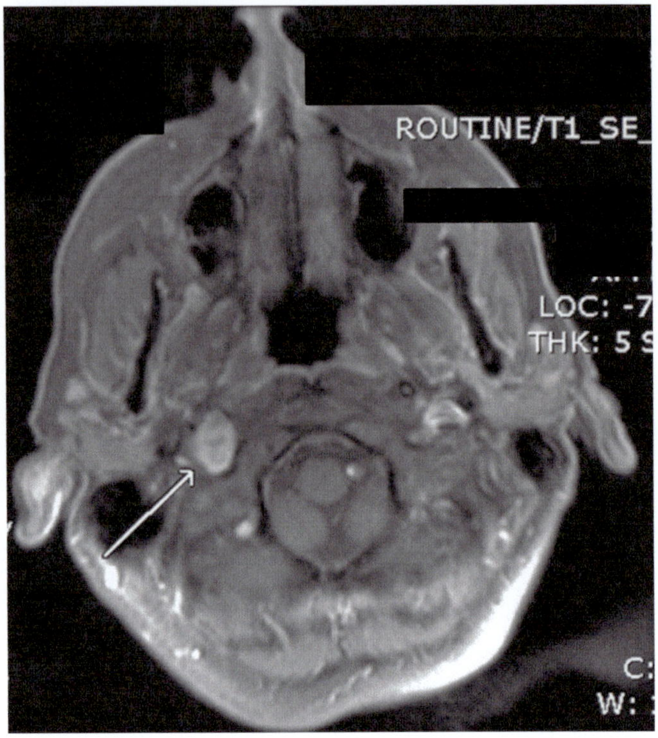

156. Axial CT demonstrated the tumor extending into the hypoglossal canal (*arrow*).

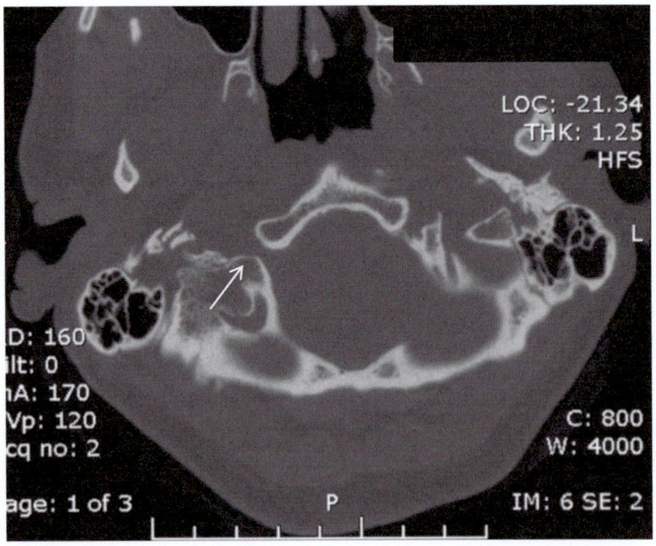

157. The surgical incision was marked.

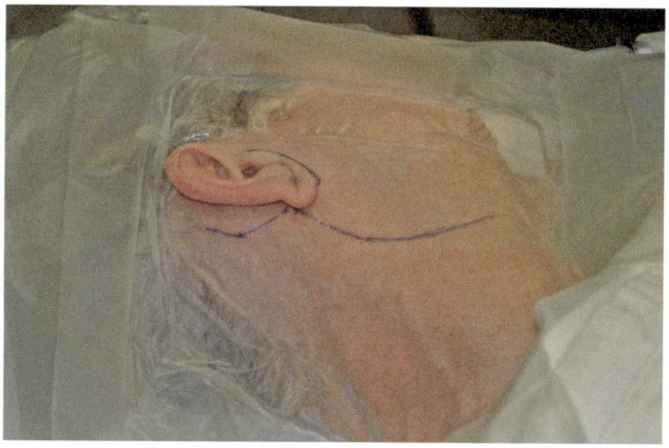

158. The muscular attachments to the mastoid tip were removed and the digastric muscle (*arrow*) skeletonized.

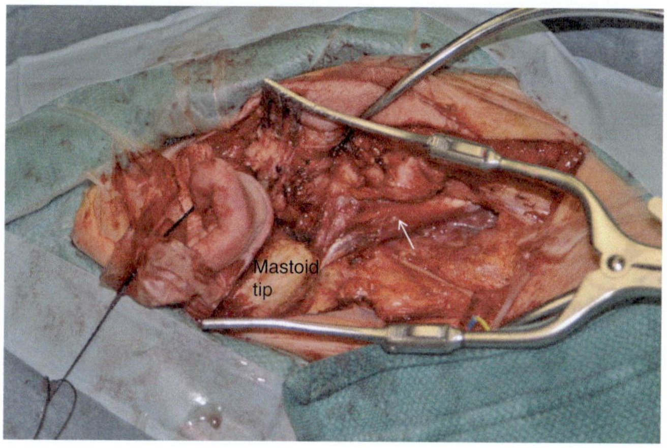

159. The main trunk of the facial nerve (*out of focus in this image*) was identified and, together with the parotid gland, was retracted superiorly. The internal jugular vein (*IJV*) and internal carotid artery (*ICA*) were identified in the neck and controlled with vessel loops. For this case, a mastoidectomy was performed to trace out the vertical segment of the facial nerve (*arrow*) to the stylomastoid foramen. Removal of this bone improves visualization of the hypoglossal foramen but is not absolutely necessary. The hypoglossal nerve was identified (*arrowhead*).

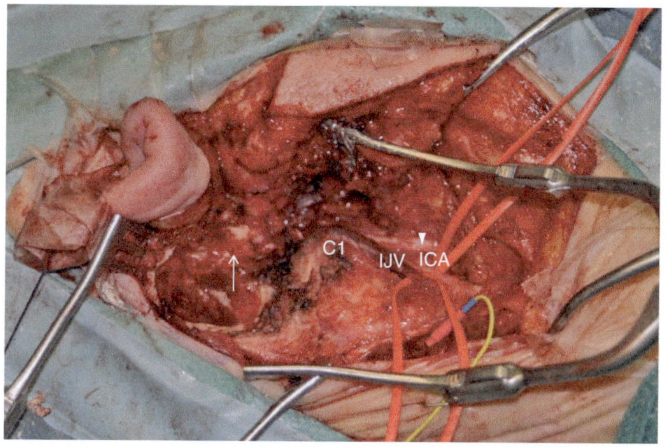

160. The internal jugular vein (*IJV*) and hypoglossal nerve (*arrowhead*) were directly anterior to the transverse process of C1. The hypoglossal nerve was then followed up to the skull base, the tumor was resected, and the incision was closed primarily.

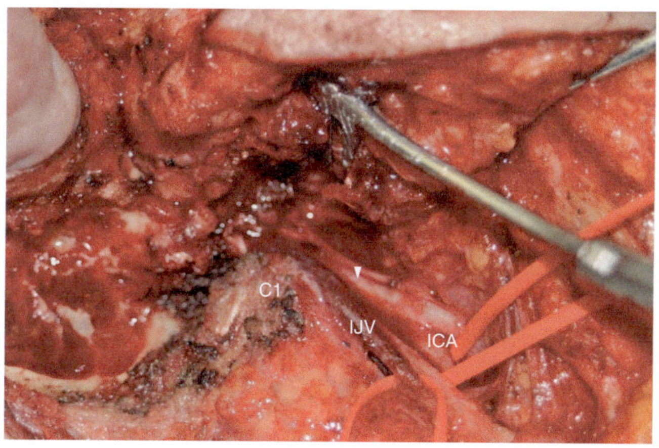

161. Case 3. A patient with a gigantic tumor of the right side of the head and neck. He had severe malnutrition and cachexia because he had been unable to swallow food for several months.

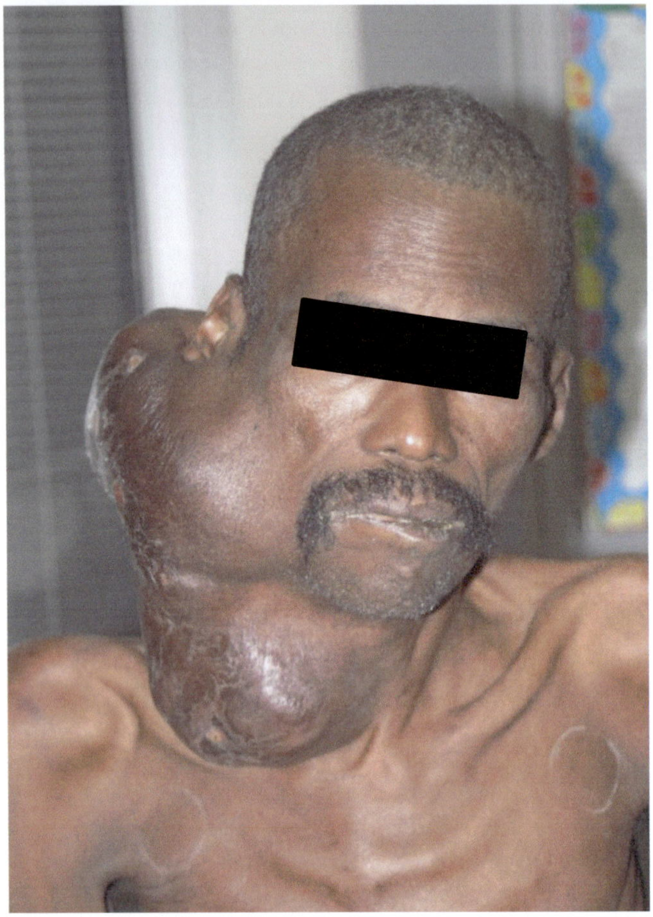

162. Axial CT demonstrated that the tumor involved the infratemporal fossa and eroded into the nasopharynx (*arrow*). There were large areas of necrosis. Because of malnutrition, the patient had developed disseminated intravascular coagulation. Urgent surgery was performed.

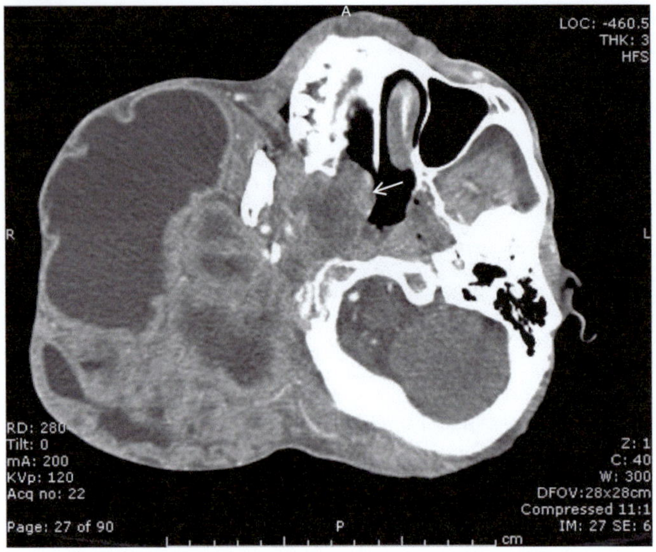

163. The patient was supine, and an incision was made across the posterior edge of the tumor. Significant bleeding was encountered because of his coagulopathy.

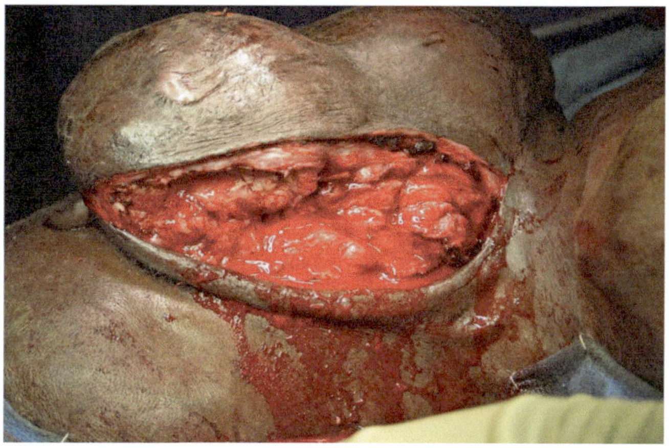

164. Dissection was carried out around the tumor with excision of the central area of skin.

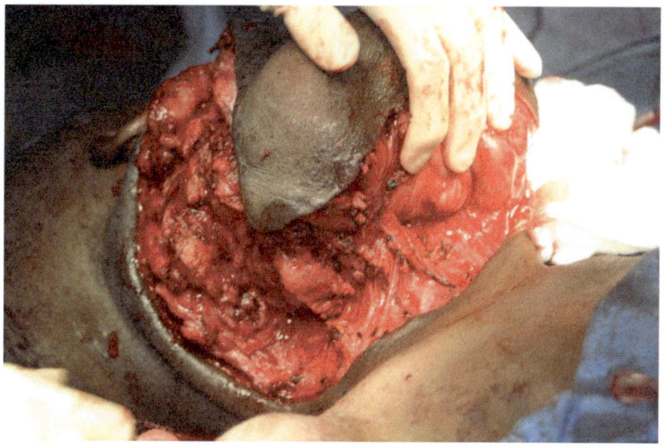

165. Skull base surgery is typically performed using a team-based approach. For most surgeries, this entails the surgeons trading off periodically. However, for very large and/or complex tumors such as this one, surgeons can operate together to maintain an ongoing discussion of how to proceed with the surgery. It has been our experience that two experienced surgeons working together helps in creating and maintaining an ideal management strategy in the face of unexpected intraoperative findings.

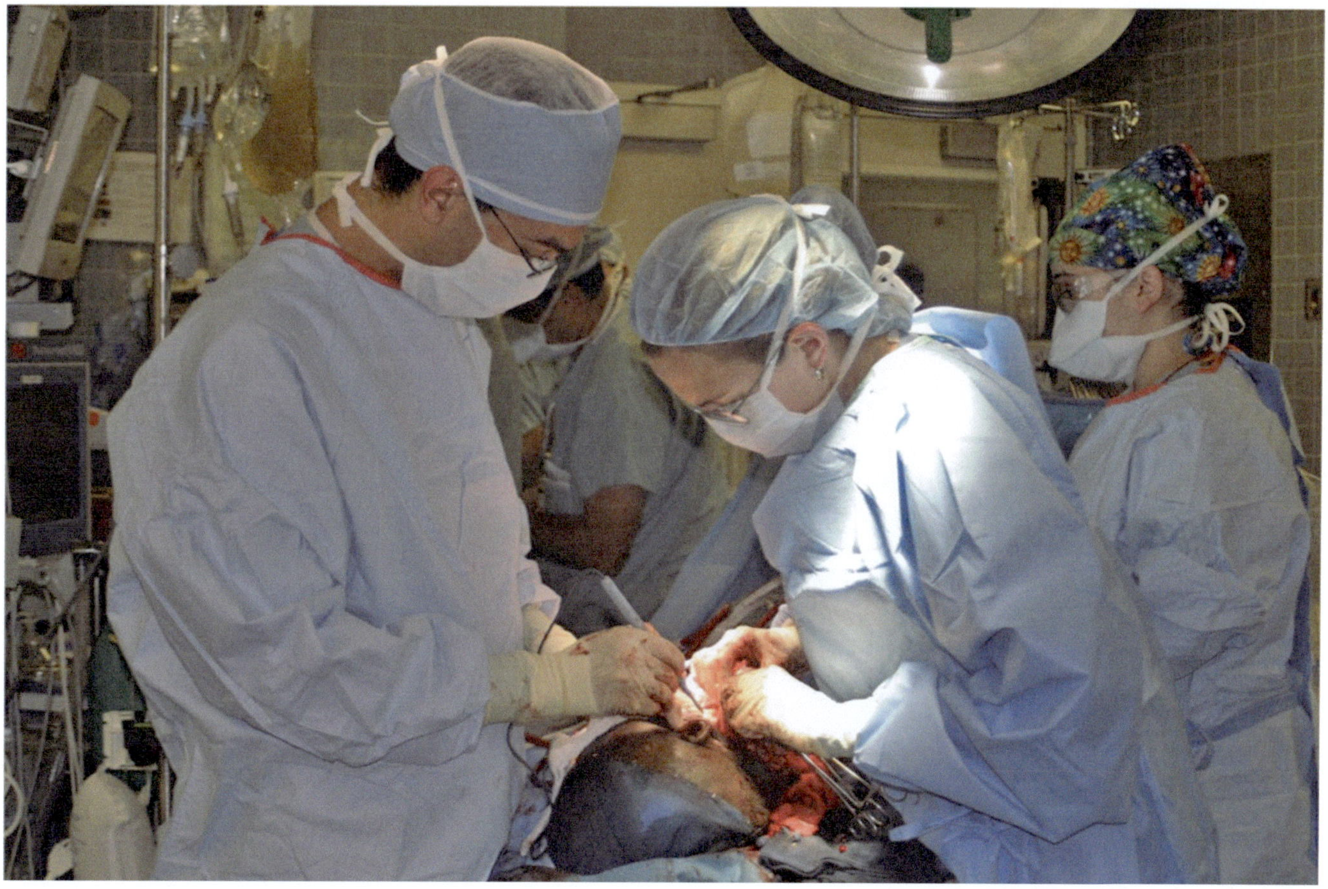

166. After resection of the majority of the tumor, only the deep portion within the parapharyngeal space and infratemporal fossa remained. The facial nerve was resected with the tumor.

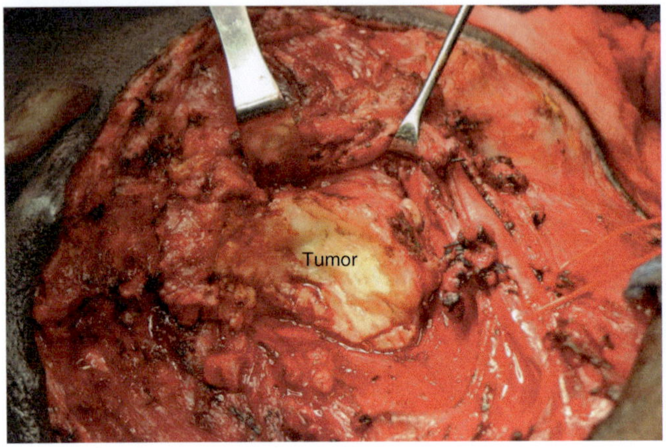

167. In this image, after total tumor removal, the internal carotid artery can be seen to be skeletonized (*arrowhead*), and the internal jugular vein was ligated (*arrow*). A plastic surgery team then reconstructed the defect with a free flap.

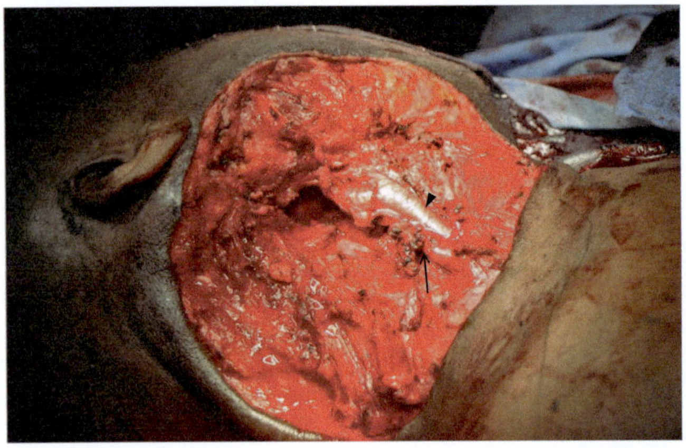

168. A happy patient. Two months later, the patient had recovered nicely and was ready for a facial reanimation procedure. Final pathology came back as carcinoma ex-pleomorphic adenoma.

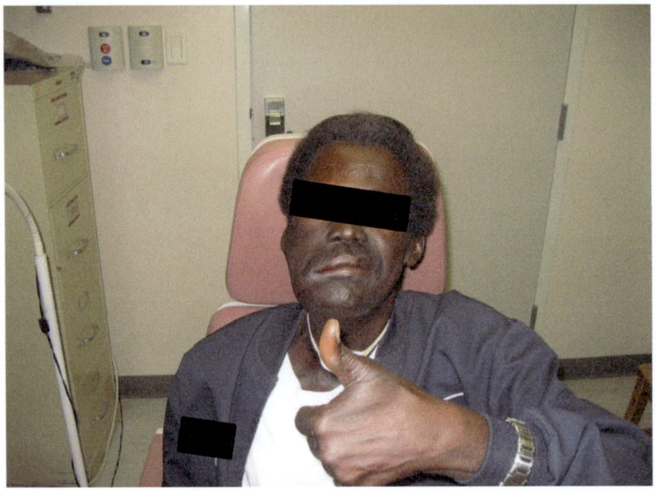

Temporal Bone Surgery for Infectious Disease

7

Simple Mastoidectomy for Acute Mastoiditis

- *Concept*
  - A simple mastoidectomy with myringotomy and placement of a pressure equalization tube drains purulence from both the mastoid and the middle ear.
- *Conditions treated*
  - Acute coalescent mastoiditis
  - Acute mastoiditis with a subperiosteal abscess
- *Risks*
  - Hearing loss
  - Facial nerve injury
- *Benefits*
  - While myringotomy and placement of a pressure equalization tube often are sufficient to treat acute mastoiditis, the addition of a mastoidectomy reduces the risk of an intracranial complication or facial nerve paralysis developing.
  - It is best to not give preoperative antibiotics when operating for acute mastoiditis because they can affect the culture results. The patient will often require long-term antibiotics, and it is best to use culture-specific antibiotic therapy. Immediately upon opening the wound, cultures are taken. Then, broad-spectrum antibiotics can be started. When the culture results are available, the antibiotic spectrum can be narrowed.
- *Additional notes*
  - The need for a mastoidectomy in acute mastoiditis is certainly debated. Overall, it probably decreases hospital length of stay, speeds recovery, and decreases the risk of developing the more serious complications of mastoiditis. For experienced surgeons, it is a short and low-risk operation. If there is a subperiosteal abscess or other complication such as facial nerve weakness, we will perform a mastoidectomy at the time of PE tube placement. In cases of noncoalescent mastoiditis and no other complications, a PE tube is generally adequate.

J.S. Oghalai, C.L.W. Driscoll, *Atlas of Neurotologic and Lateral Skull Base Surgery*,
DOI 10.1007/978-3-662-46694-0_7, © Springer-Verlag Berlin Heidelberg 2016

1. A subperiosteal abscess is illustrated. A standard postauricular incision is used, and cultures are taken immediately once the purulence is expressed.

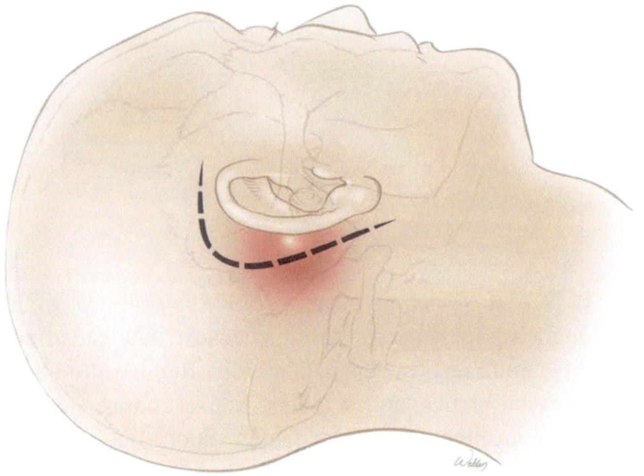

2. Elevation of the periosteum often reveals soft, inflamed mastoid cortex bone.

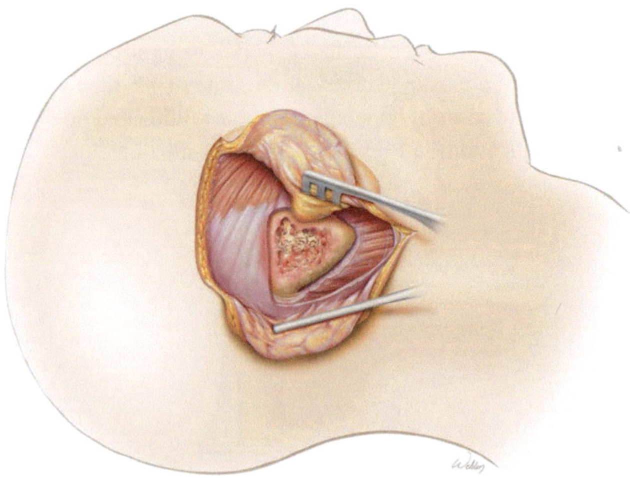

3. A simple mastoidectomy is performed with identification of the sigmoid sinus, the tegmen, the mastoid antrum, and the lateral semicircular canal. A bone pate collector can be used to collect bone dust for tissue culture if desired.

Only the antrum needs to be opened. There is no need to try and remove all inflamed granulation tissue from the aditus ad antrum, the facial recess, or even all the mastoid air cells.

After performing a mastoidectomy, the cavity is irrigated. The mastoid can be filled with ototopical antibiotic drops if desired.

The wound can be closed with a Penrose drain protruding from the mastoid cavity through the bottom of the incision if desired. The goal is to prevent reaccumulation of purulence within the mastoid.

A myringotomy with pressure equalization tube is then placed to drain the middle ear.

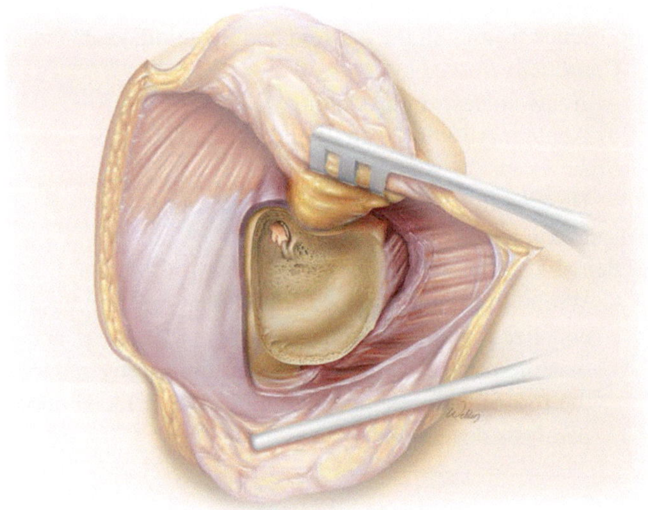

4. Case 1. Acute mastoiditis with a subperiosteal abscess. There is postauricular erythema and swelling.

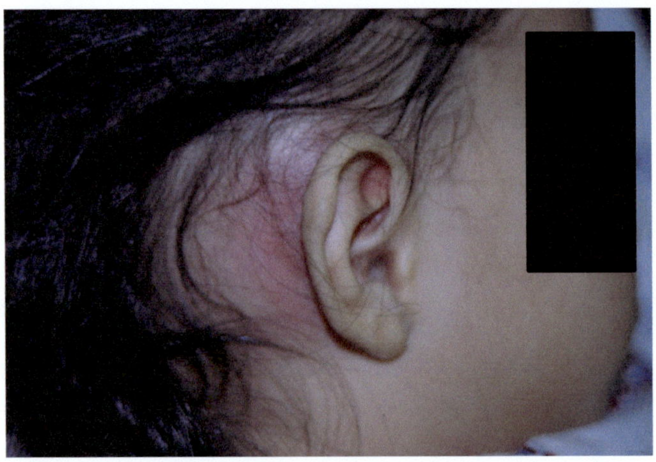

5. CT demonstrates erosion of the mastoid cortex (*arrows*).

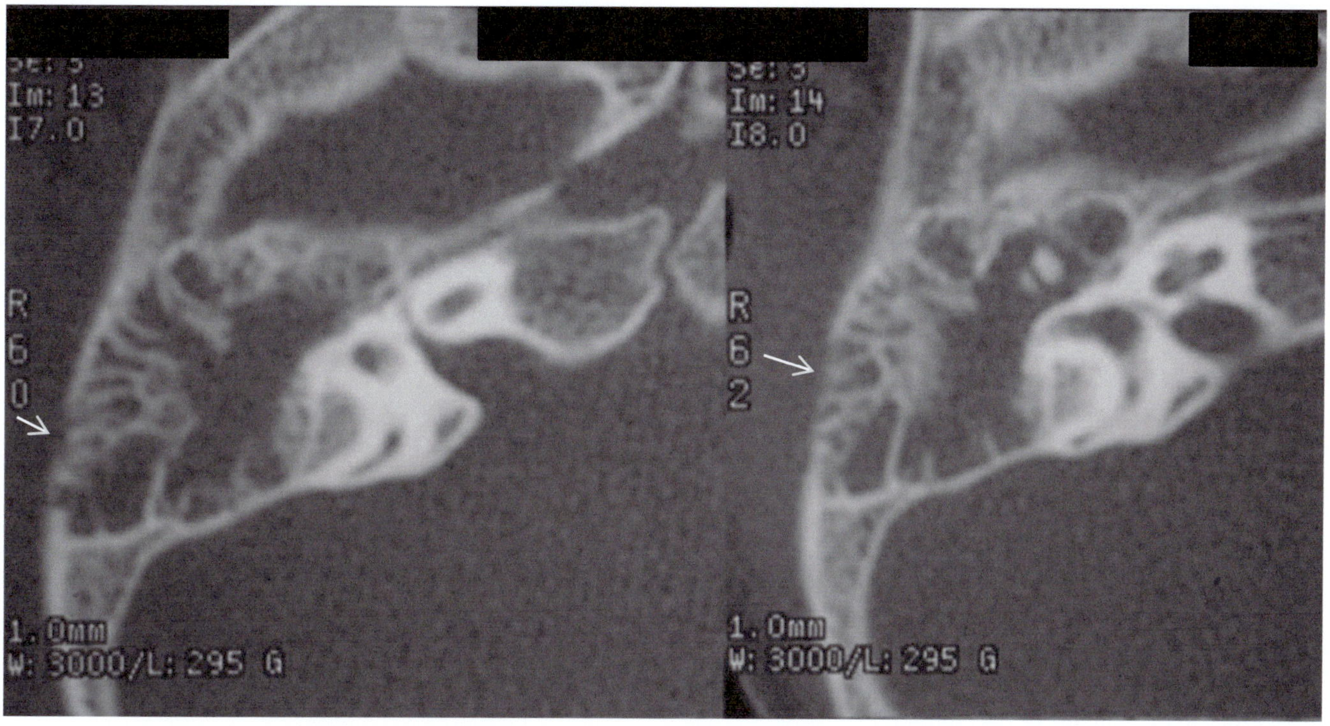

6. Case 2. Acute mastoiditis with a subperiosteal abscess in a baby.

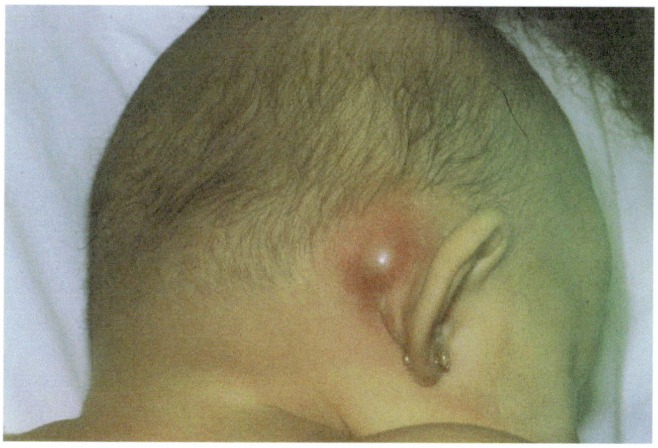

7. CT scan demonstrates erosion of the mastoid septae (*arrowhead*), the mastoid cortex (*arrow*), and a subperiosteal abscess (*asterisk*).

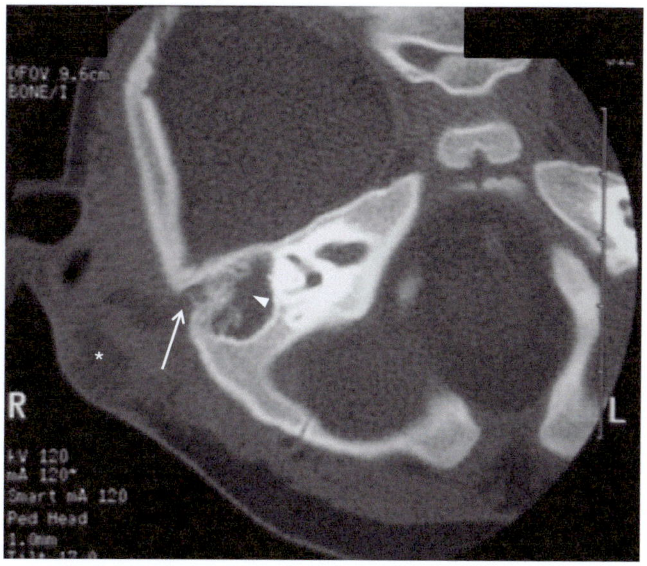

Retrolabyrinthine Craniotomy for Intracranial Complications of Acute Mastoiditis

- *Concept*
  - Perform a simple mastoidectomy, and then expose the posterior and/or middle fossa dura to address an intracranial complication.
- *Conditions treated*
  - Acute mastoiditis with an intracranial complication including sigmoid sinus thrombosis, an epidural abscess, or a subdural abscess
- *Risks*
  - Hearing loss
  - Facial nerve injury
  - Meningitis
  - CSF leak
- *Benefits*
  - The procedure not only drains the infectious etiology within the mastoid but also provides direct access to the intracranial sites of disease extension.
  - This is a hearing preservation approach.
- *Additional notes*
  - The management of an intracranial abscess that results from mastoiditis is also controversial. If the abscess is contiguous with the mastoid, we usually drain the intracranial component at the time of mastoidectomy. If it is not contiguous with the mastoid and the abscess is large, a separate approach will likely be required. However, a small intraparencymal abscess will likely not need surgical treatment and can usually be managed with intravenous antibiotics, close monitoring, and sequential imaging to verify that it is resolving.

8. Overview of the bone to be removed (*gray*).

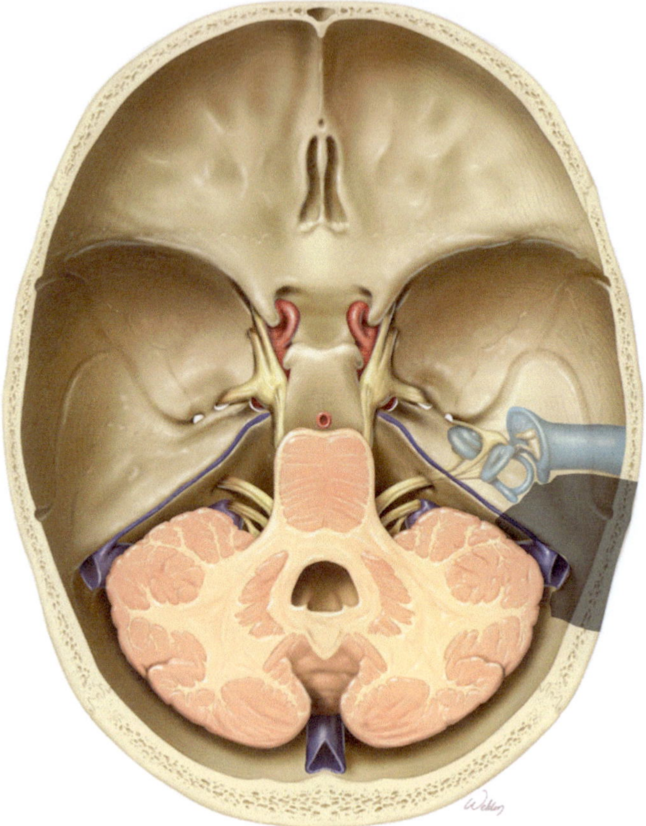

9. The retrolabyrinthine craniotomy begins with a standard postauricular incision.

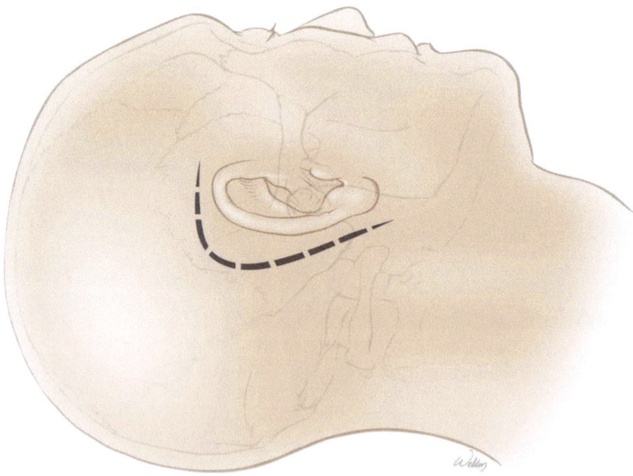

10. The periosteum is elevated off the mastoid cortex.

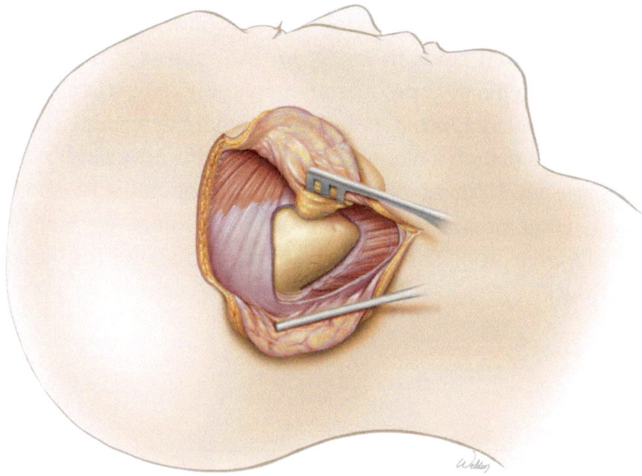

11. A simple mastoidectomy is performed with identification of the sigmoid sinus, the tegmen, the mastoid antrum, and the lateral semicircular canal.

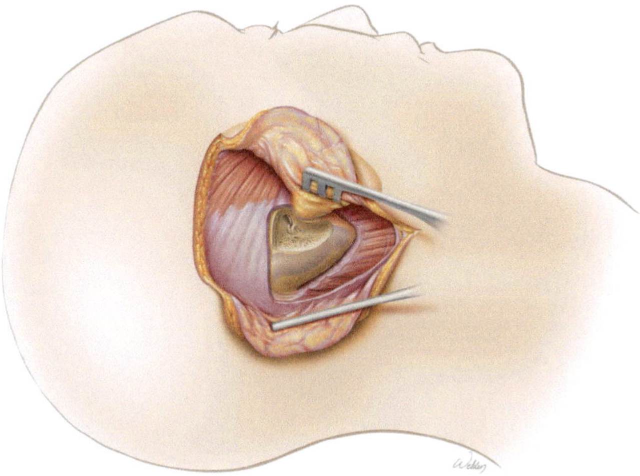

12. The retrosigmoid dura is identified and thinned with a large diamond burr. The bone is then removed.

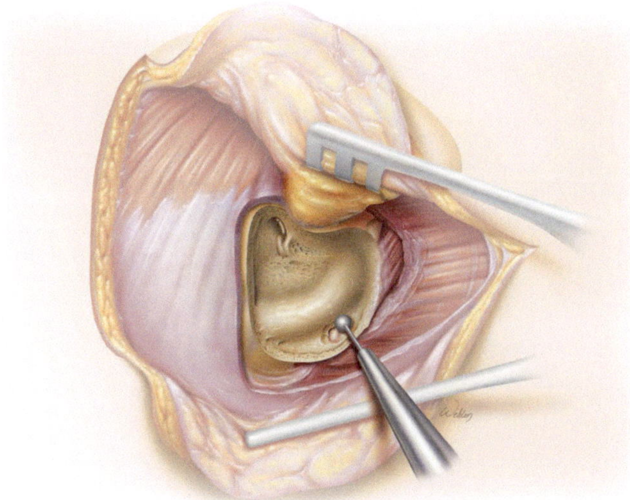

13. The bone over the sigmoid sinus is thinned and "egg shelled." A Joseph or Freer elevator is used to remove the bone fragments to visualize the sinus.

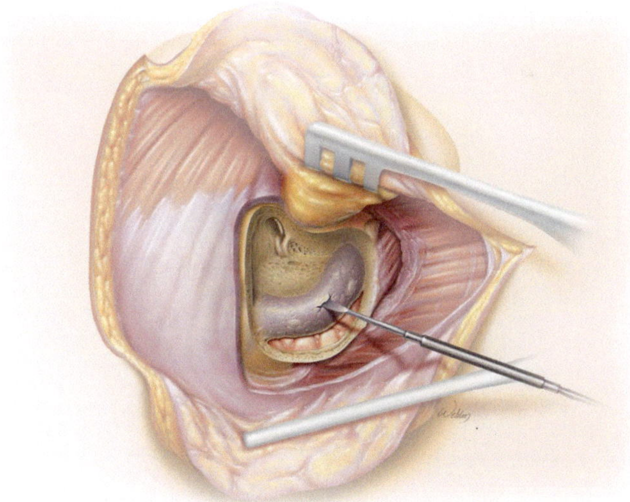

14. Malleable retractors are then used to retract the posterior and middle cranial fossa dura away from the bone. This bone is then removed down to the level of the labyrinth.

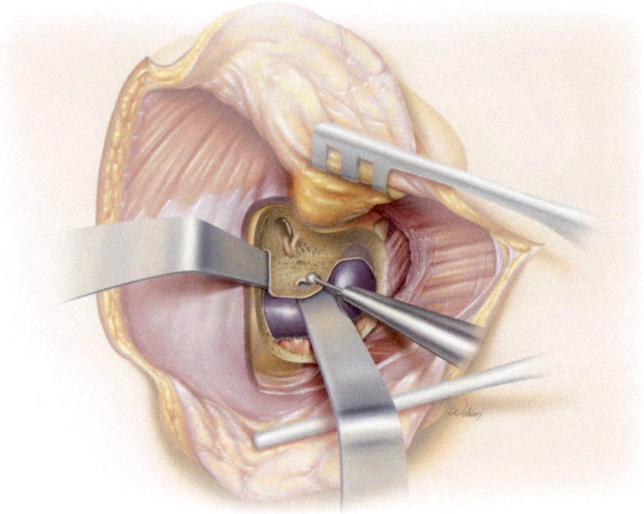

15. A completed retrolabyrinthine craniotomy provides access to the sigmoid sinus, the presigmoid posterior fossa dura, and the middle fossa dura superior to the mastoid.

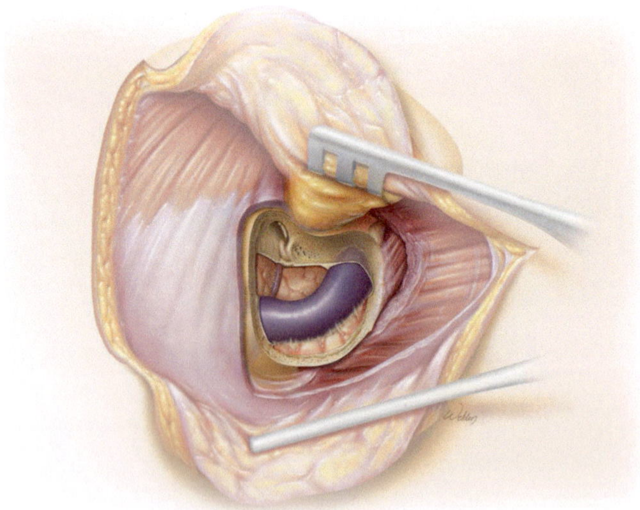

16. Representative illustration of a patient with sigmoid sinus thrombosis in which the lateral surface of the sigmoid sinus is distorted but intact.

The concept of making an exploratory opening into the sigmoid sinus to assess for thrombosis is not often used. Typically, preoperative imaging is sufficient to make this diagnosis. Palpation can help determine if the sinus is patent; a clot will feel firm and is not easily compressed. If there is a question intraoperatively about whether or not there is a clot in the sinus, a vascular Doppler probe should be brought in to assess for blood flow.

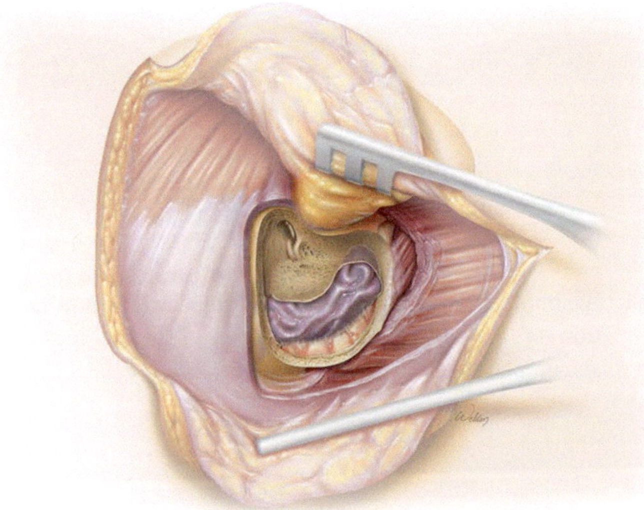

17. More commonly, however, the wall of the sigmoid sinus is disrupted when there is an infectious thrombosis (i.e., thrombophlebitis or an abscess within the sigmoid sinus). Simply exposing the sigmoid sinus reveals the problem.

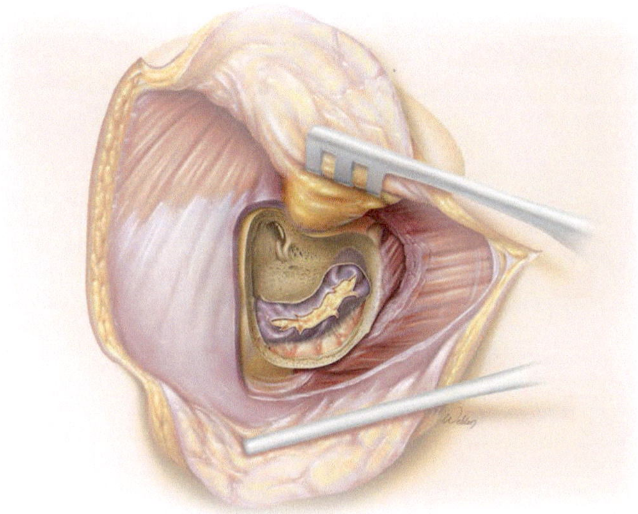

18. Gentle curettage of the abscess/clot/granulation tissue can be used to debride the sinus down to the medial wall. We typically do this with a Freer or duckbill elevator. In our experience, this usually won't bleed because both the proximal and distal sigmoid sinuses are occluded by the disease. However, this approach permits drainage of the abscess and necrotic tissue.

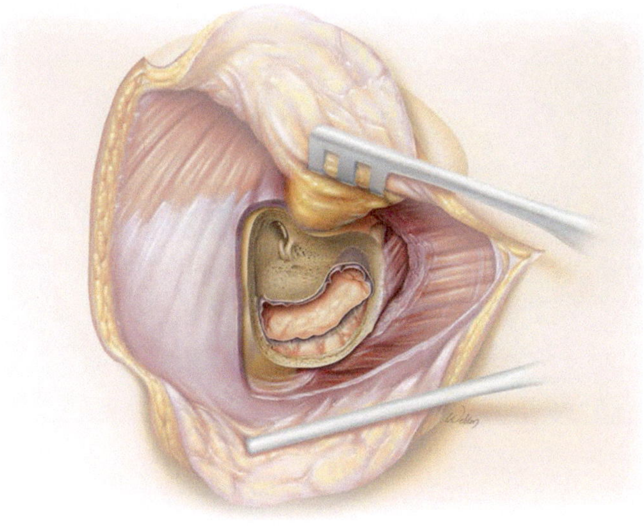

19. Representative illustration of a patient with an epidural abscess involving both the middle cranial fossa and the posterior cranial fossa. Removing the overlying bone reveals granulation tissue and necrotic material adherent to the dura, which can be curetted out.

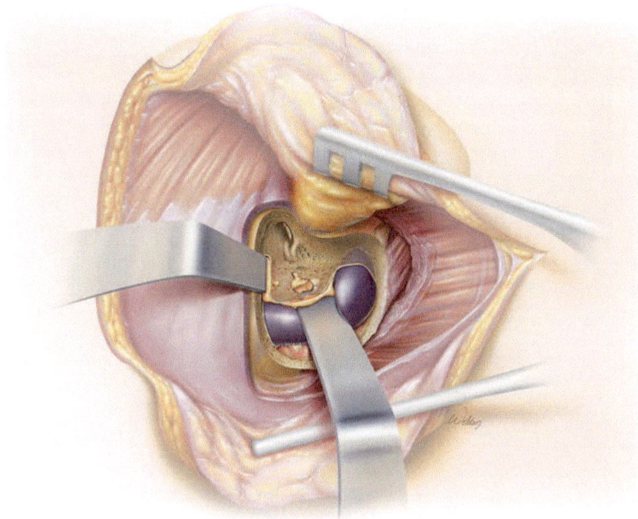

20. Representative illustrations of how to manage a posterior cranial fossa subdural abscess that lies directly under the presigmoid dura. This can be treated by incising the dura over the abscess. Alternatively, a retrosigmoid craniotomy could be performed.

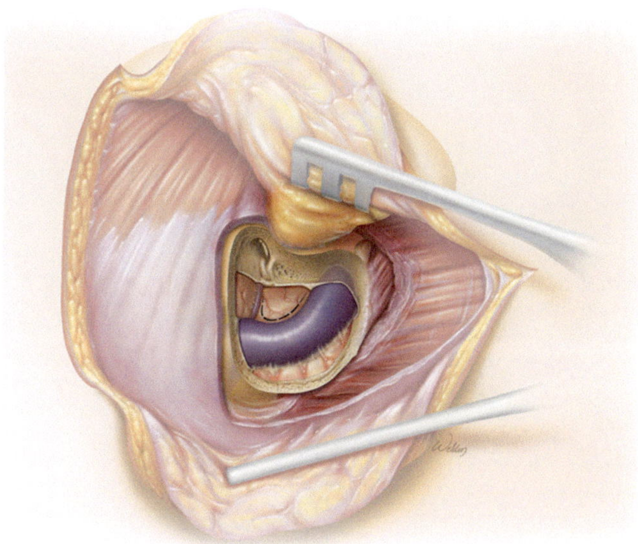

21. Opening the dura reveals the abscess wall.

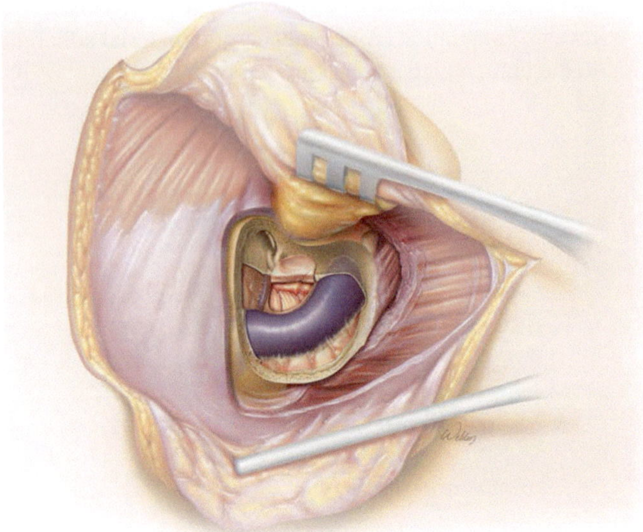

22. The abscess can be opened with a knife and the pus suctioned out. No attempt is made to dissect out the wall of the abscess. It will resolve with intravenous antibiotic therapy.

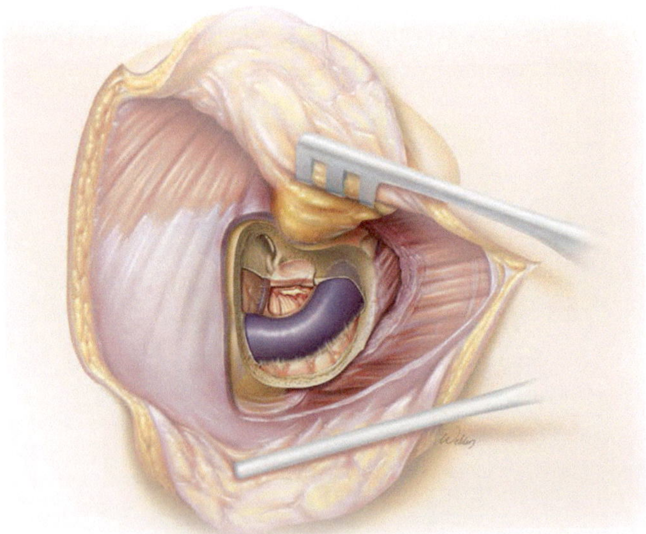

23. The dura should be closed in a watertight fashion to prevent CSF leak into the ear. Tisseal is helpful here.

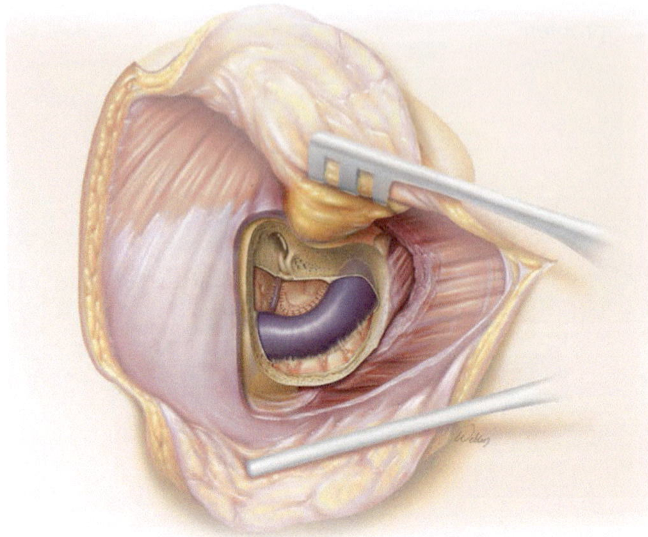

24. Case 1. A child presented with a protruding right ear. Axial CT with contrast demonstrated acute mastoiditis. There was erosion of the mastoid septae, and the wall of the sigmoid sinus was thickened (*arrows*). This child was very lethargic and in the ICU.

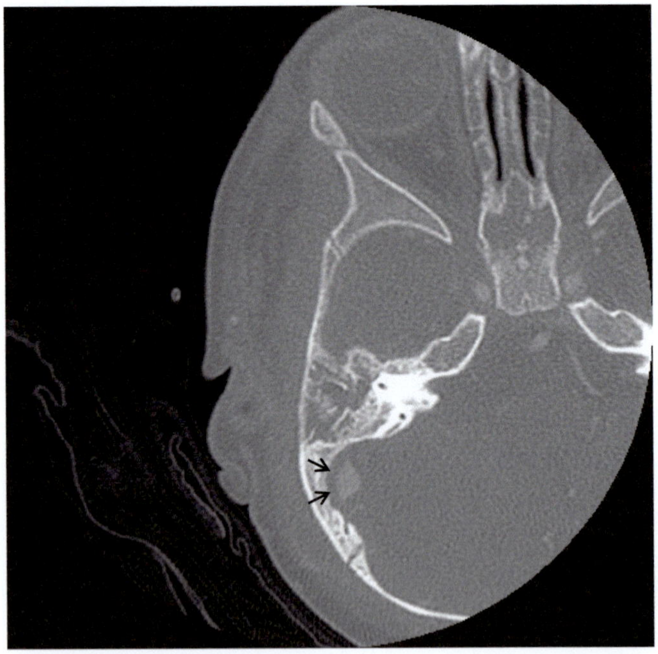

25. A lower cut demonstrates a filling defect (*arrowheads*) caused by thrombosis within the sigmoid sinus and jugular bulb.

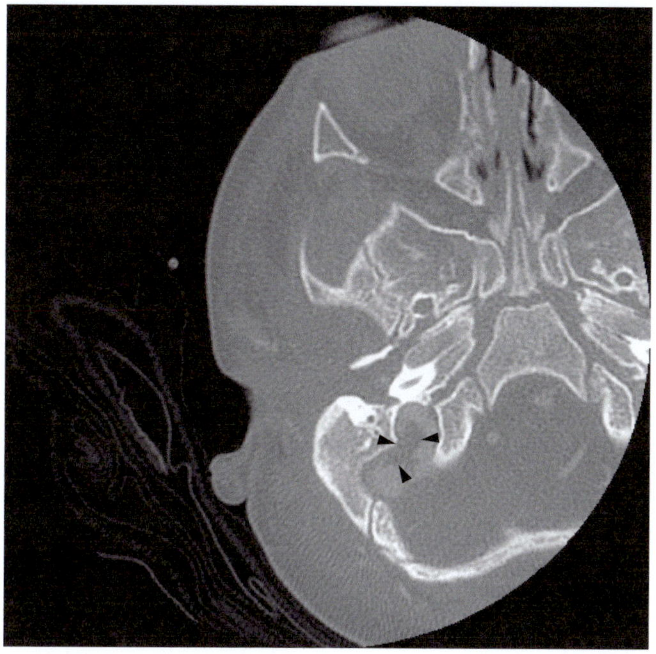

26. The thrombosis extended down into the neck. Note the filling defect within the right internal jugular vein (*black arrowhead*) compared to the normal left internal jugular vein (*white arrowhead*).

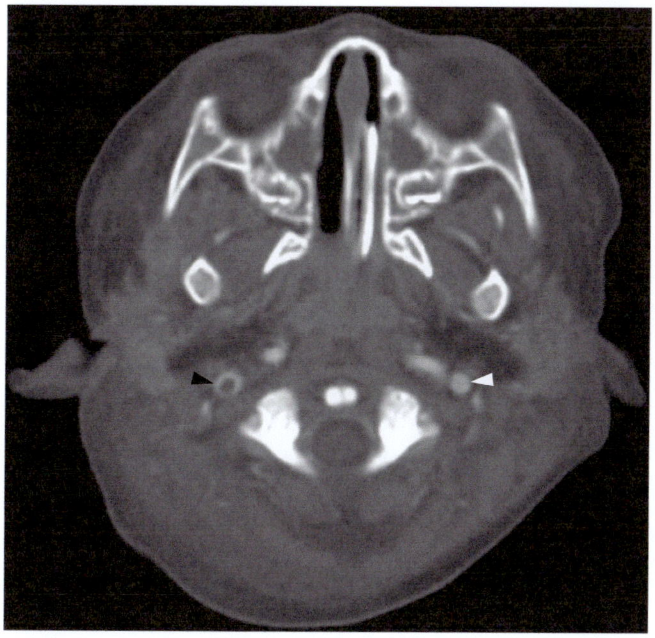

27. Coronal view better demonstrates the thrombosis within the jugular bulb and internal jugular vein (*arrowheads*).

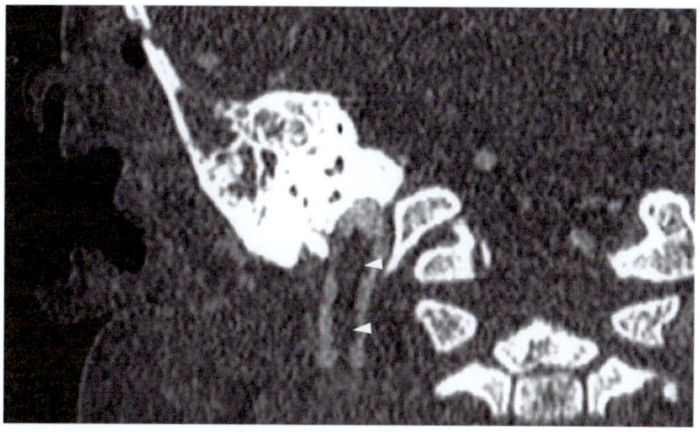

28. MRI with gadolinium demonstrates widespread enhancement of the soft tissues of the right side of the head consistent with inflammatory changes. There was also thickening of the sigmoid sinus wall and posterior fossa dura (*arrowheads*).

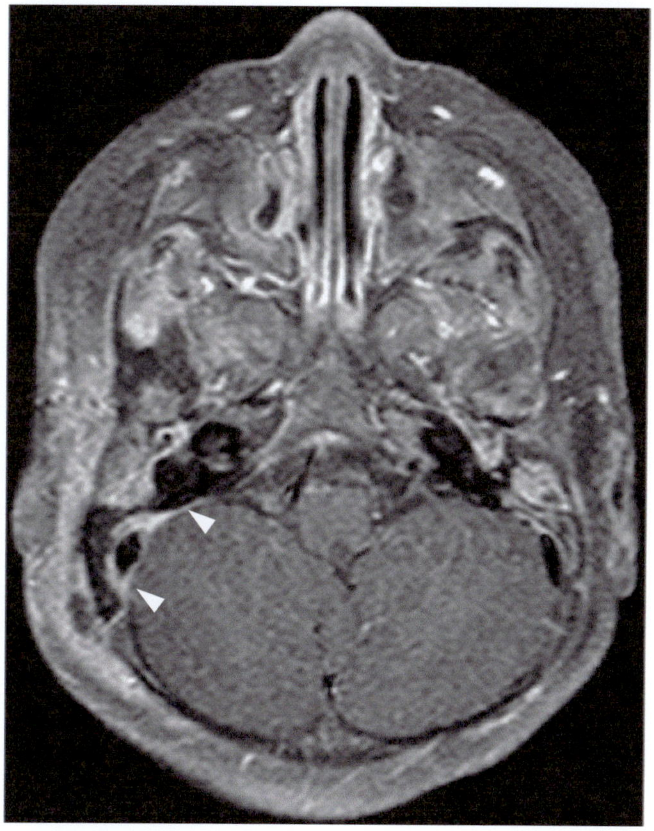

29. Coronal view demonstrates an epidural abscess along the temporal floor (*arrowhead*). Note the thickening of the dura with central lucency.

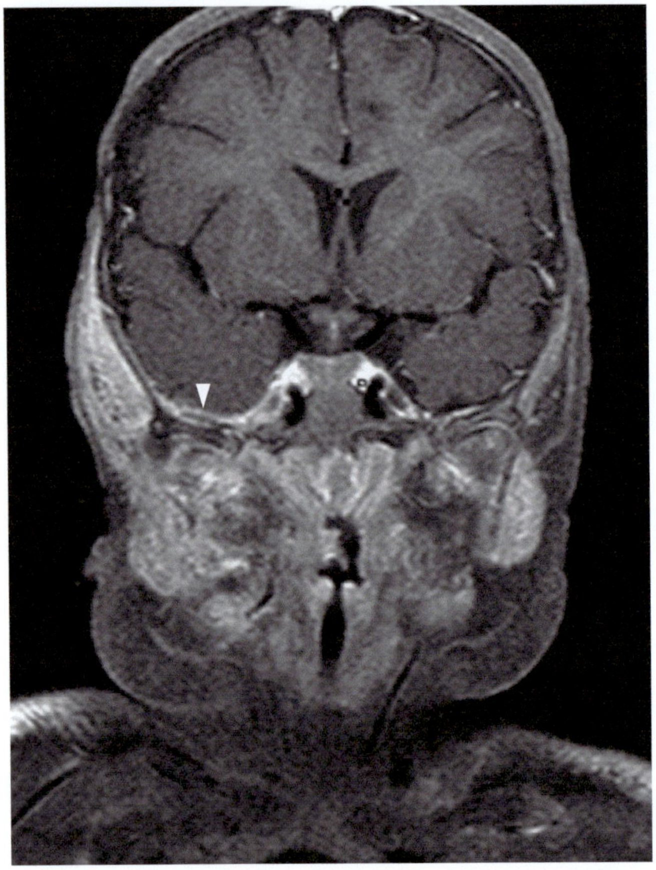

30. Treatment for this life-threatening infection requires surgical drainage. A standard cortical mastoidectomy was begun. The surgical goals were to debride the mastoid, drain the epidural abscess, and remove the thrombus from the sigmoid sinus.

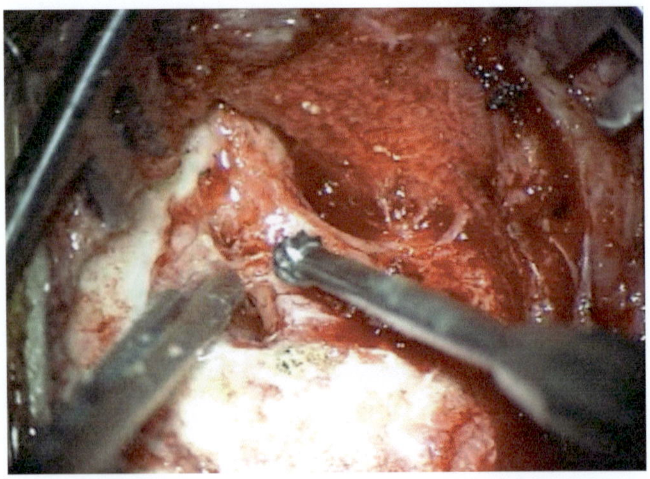

31. The mastoidectomy was completed and the bone over the lower half of the sigmoid sinus thinned.

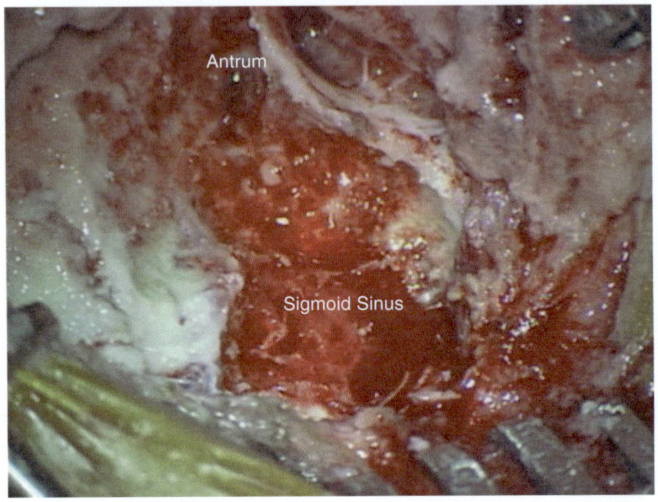

32. The posterior fossa dura and lateral aspect of the sigmoid sinus were dissected away from the overlying bone.

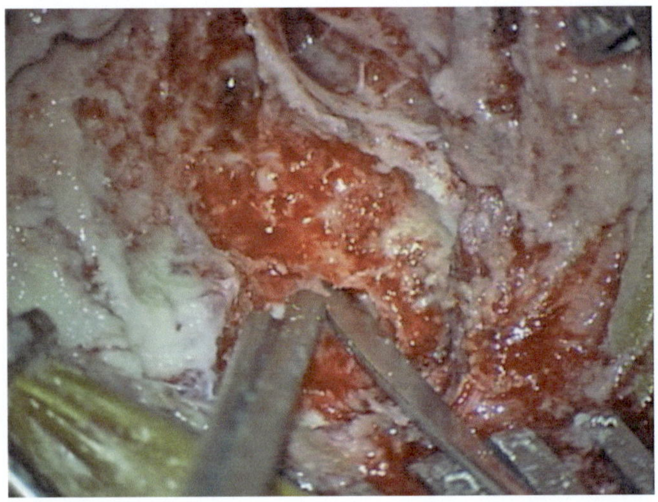

33. The tegmen was then removed to expose the middle fossa dura.

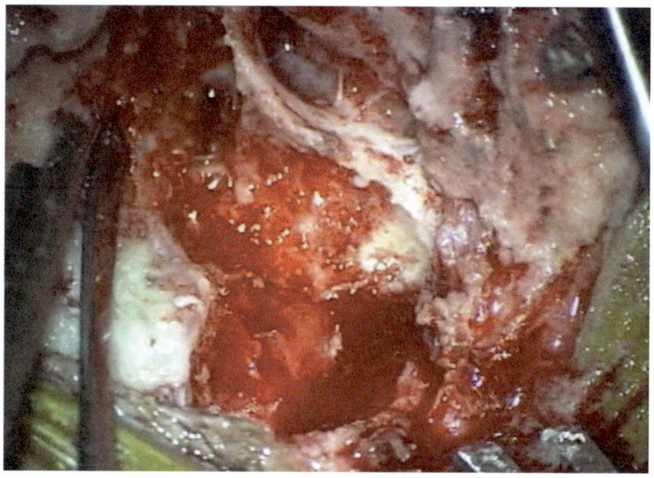

34. The area where the epidural abscess along the temporal floor was probed by sliding a dissector anteriorly between the dura and the bone. This drained the abscess.

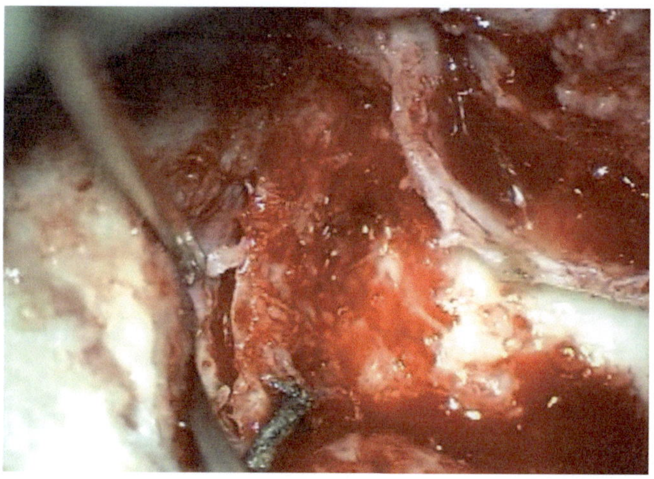

35. The granulations and inflammation along the posterior fossa dura were curetted away.

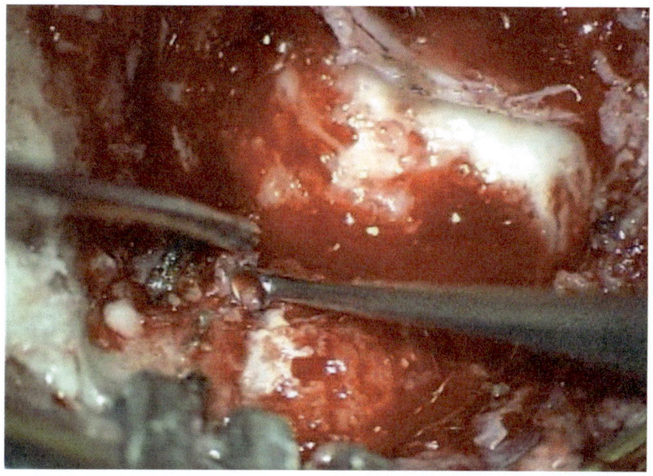

36. Looking inferiorly, the sigmoid sinus was retracted posteriorly away from the lateral bony wall and compressed superiorly.

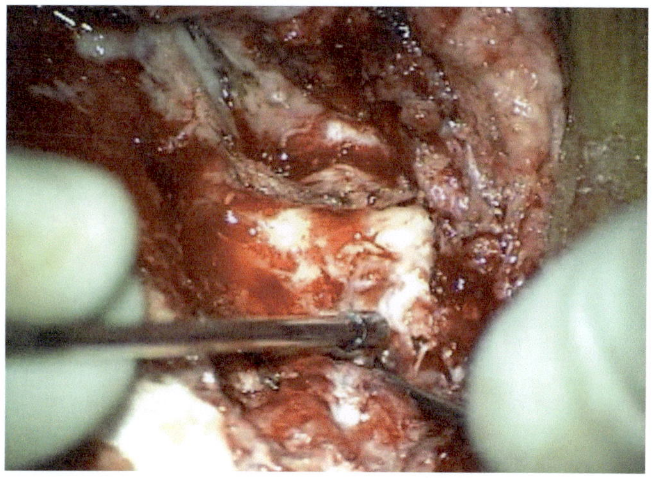

37. A small opening was made in the sinus, but because of the clot, no blood came out. A Fogarty catheter was placed through the opening and inserted past the area of the jugular bulb.

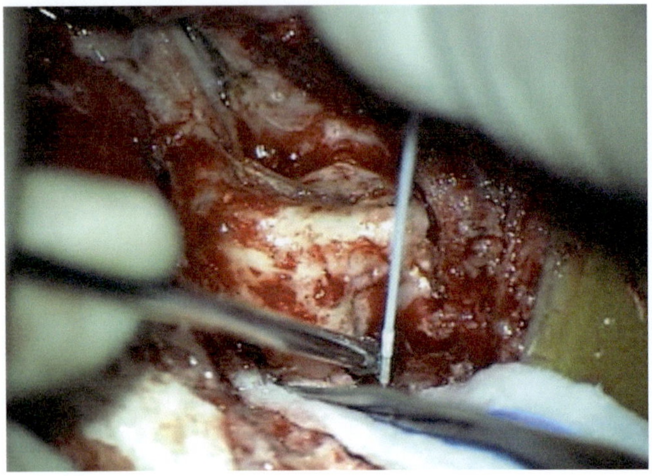

38. The balloon was then blown up and the catheter pulled back. Clots came out. Here, the balloon is visible just before it was removed from the sinus.

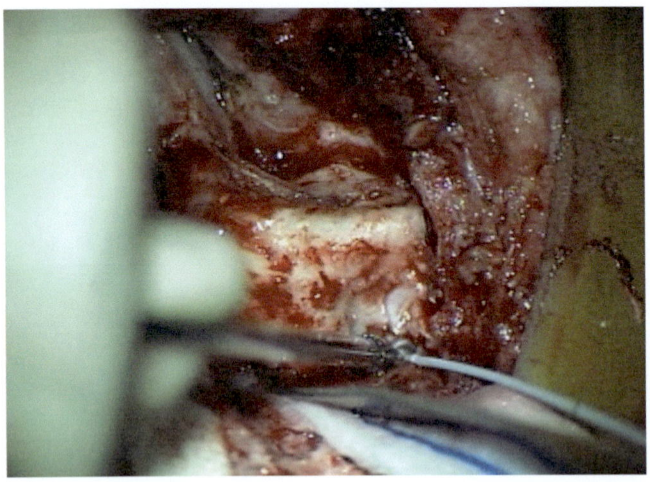

39. In this case, there was now a brisk flow of blood from the sinus, indicating good back flow.

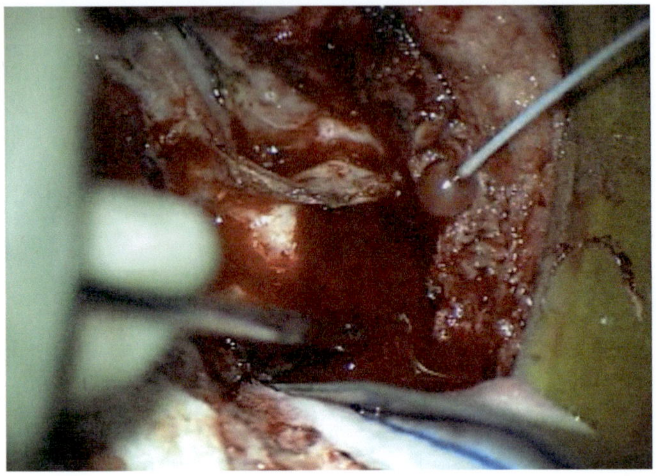

40. A piece of Surgicel was placed over the opening.

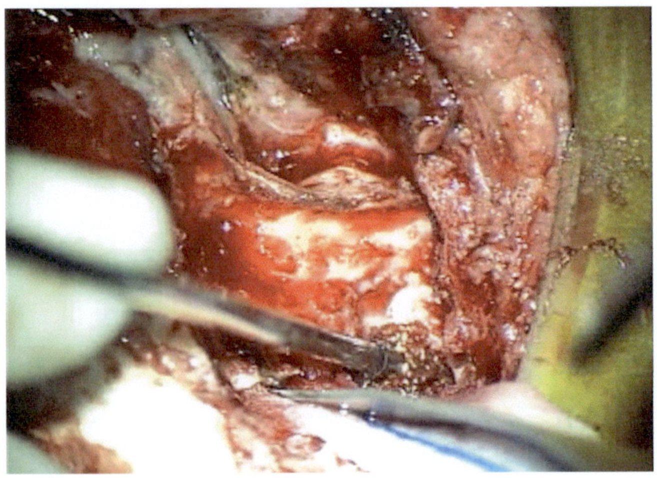

41. A cottonoid pledget was placed on top of the Surgicel and pressure applied to stop the bleeding.

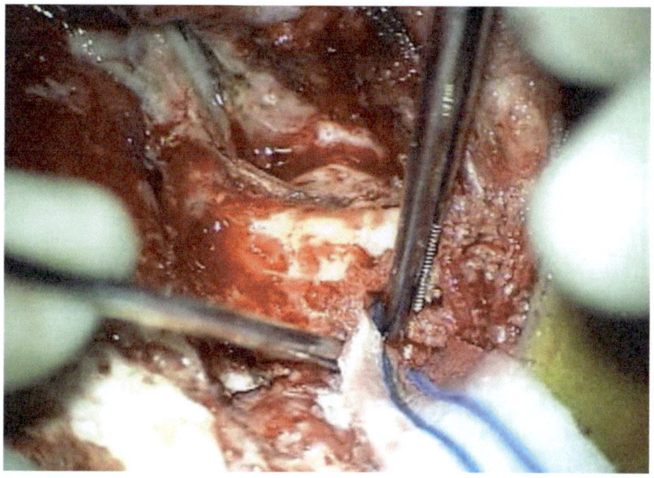

42. After 10 min, no further pressure was necessary, and the cottonoid could then be removed before closure. The Surgicel was left in place. The boy quickly improved postoperatively and was discharged in 10 days with no sequelae.

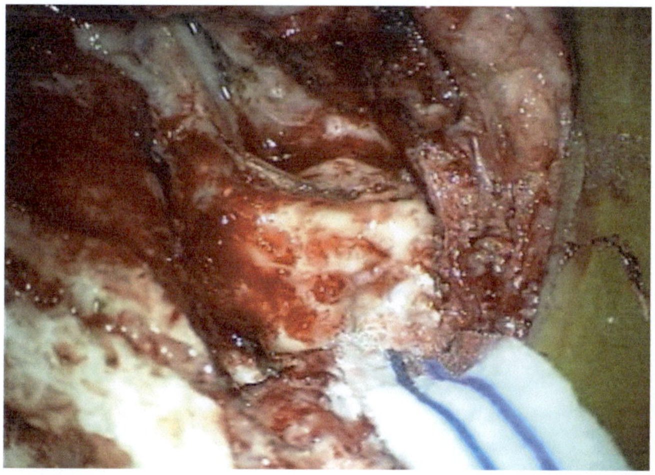

43. Case 2. The twin brother of the boy in Case 1, which our team was not consulted on. He had bilateral mastoiditis and thrombosis of both internal jugular veins (*arrowheads*). He was sicker than his brother and was comatose and on the ventilator.

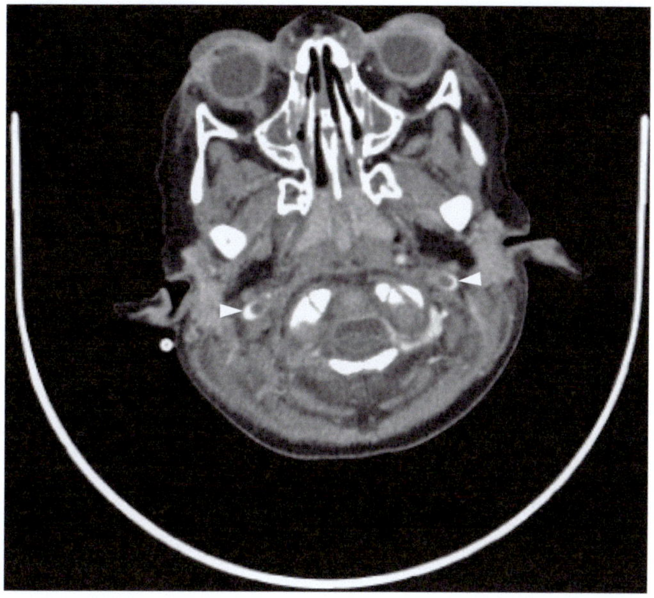

44. There was a thrombus within the right jugular bulb (*arrowhead*) but not the left.

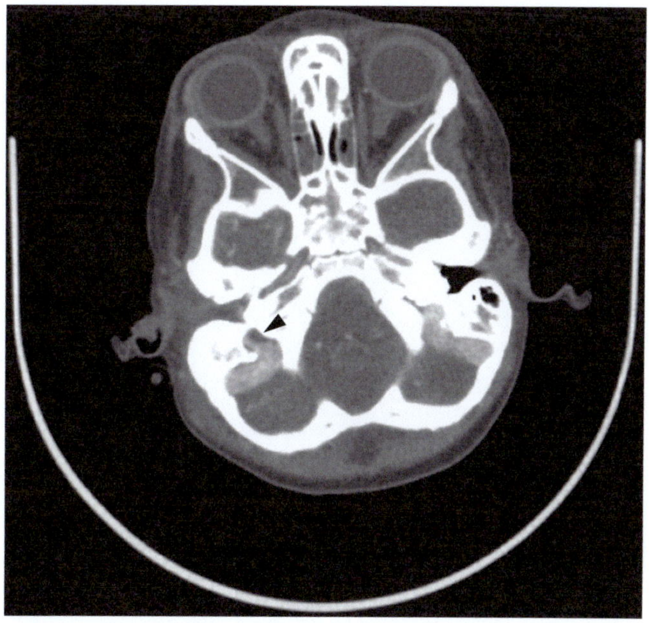

45. Because of the blockage of venous outflow, this patient developed otitic hydrocephalus. Note the enlarged lateral ventricles and effacement of the cortical sulci.

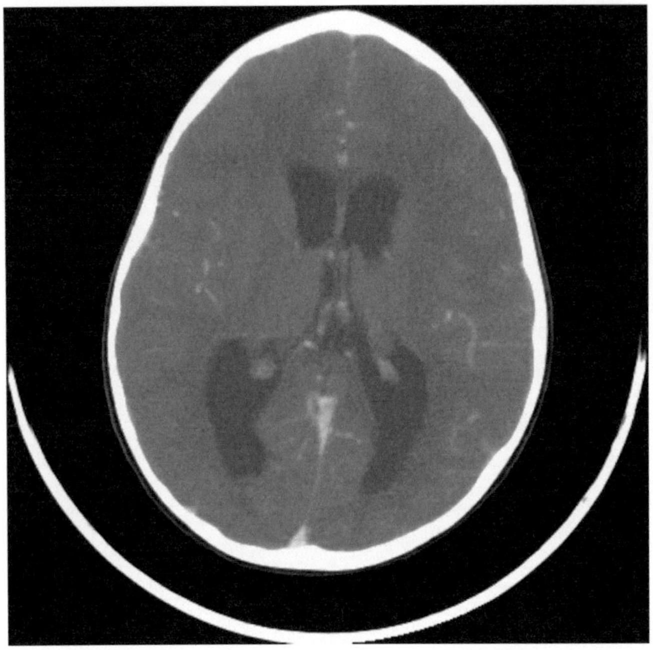

46. Within a couple of days, his elevated intracranial pressure eventually led to cerebral ischemia. Note the large areas of hypodensity indicating poor perfusion.

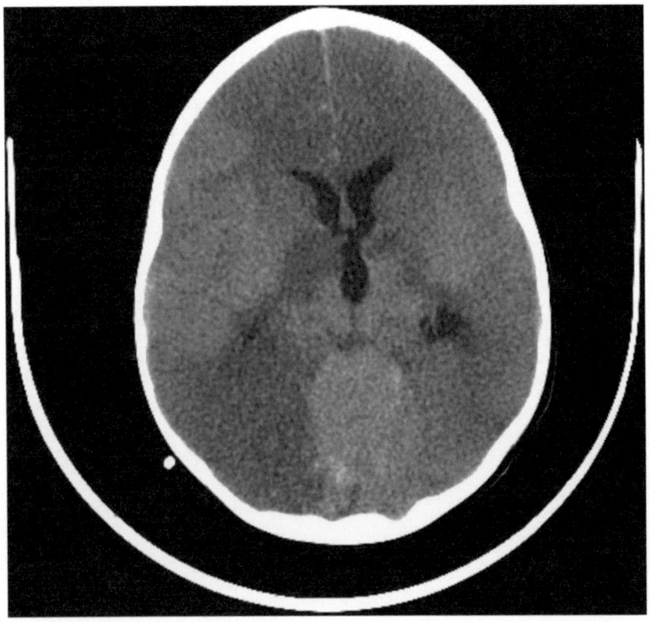

47. SPECT scan demonstrated no activity indicating brain death. This all occurred before our team was consulted. Based on this outcome, the ICU physicians consulted us to help with his brother (Case #1), whom we immediately took to surgery.

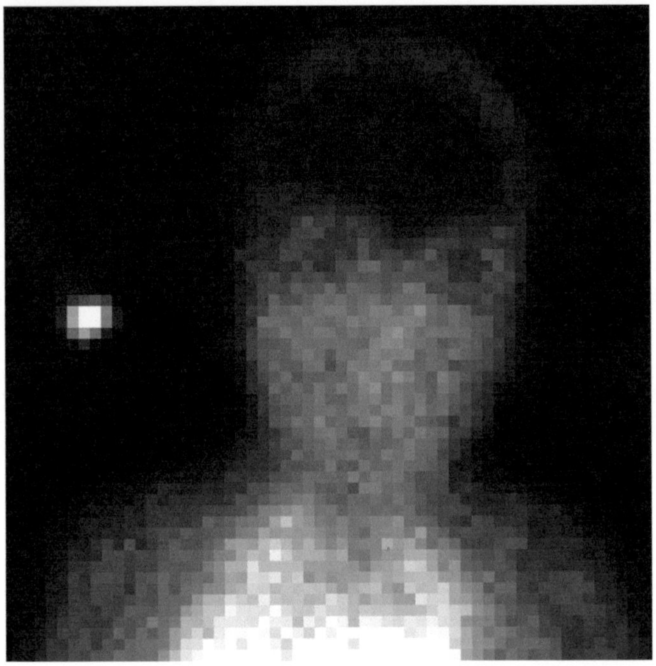

48. Case 3. Axial CT of an adult with acute mastoiditis. The loss of septae is obvious. Also, there was erosion of the inner table of the mastoid overlying the sigmoid sinus (*arrow*).

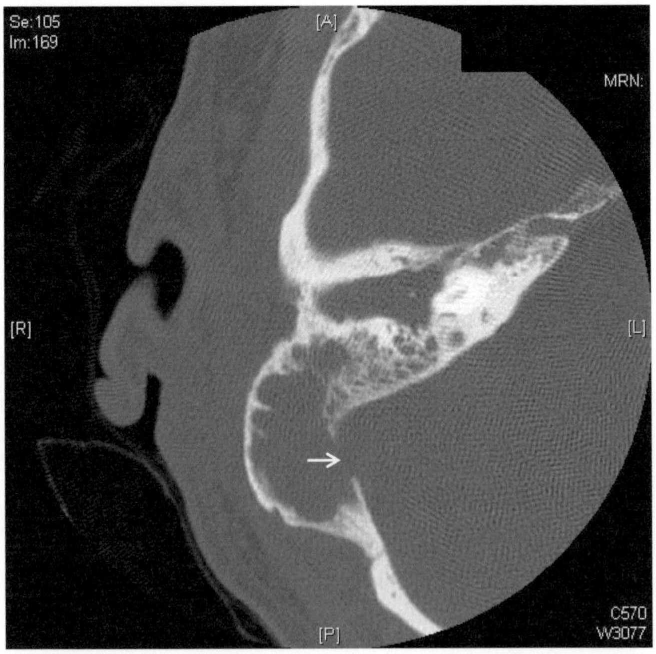

49. Axial MRI with gadolinium revealed inflammation of the dura and walls of the sigmoid sinus (*arrows*) as well as the abscess within the mastoid (*asterisk*).

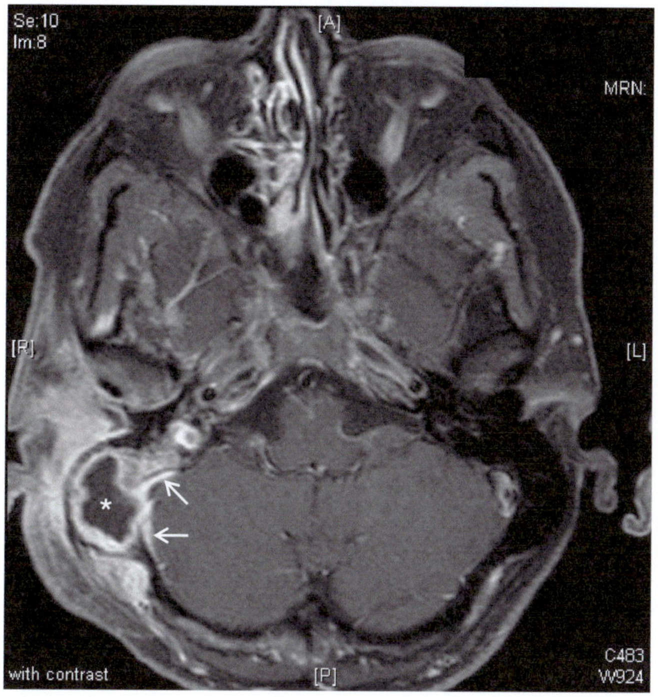

50. Case 4. Axial CT with contrast demonstrated right acute mastoiditis with a subperiosteal abscess (*asterisk*) and an epidural abscess that compresses the sigmoid sinus (*arrow*).

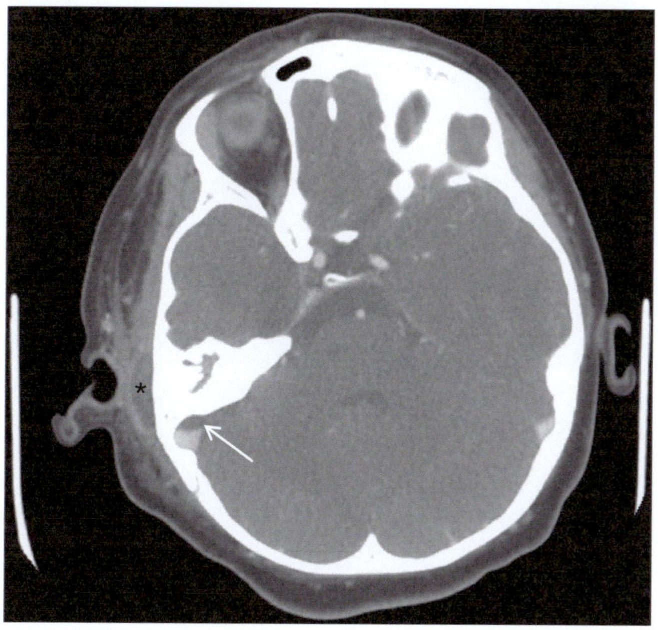

51. Axial MRI with gadolinium confirmed the epidural abscess (*arrow*).

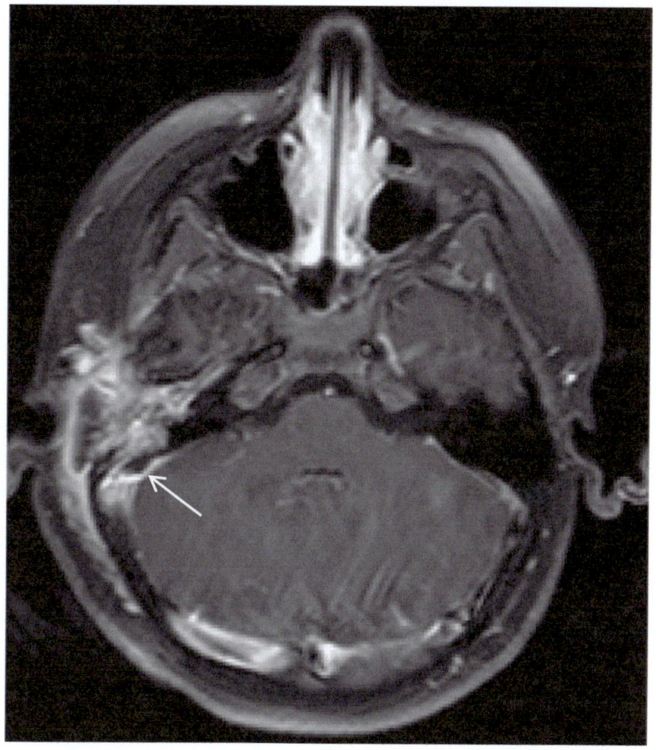

52. CT scan with bone windowing from the same patient demonstrated that there was no coalescence within the mastoid (i.e., there was no loss of septations). The bone overlying the posterior fossa also appeared intact. Thus, the epidural abscess likely occurred via hematogenous spread.

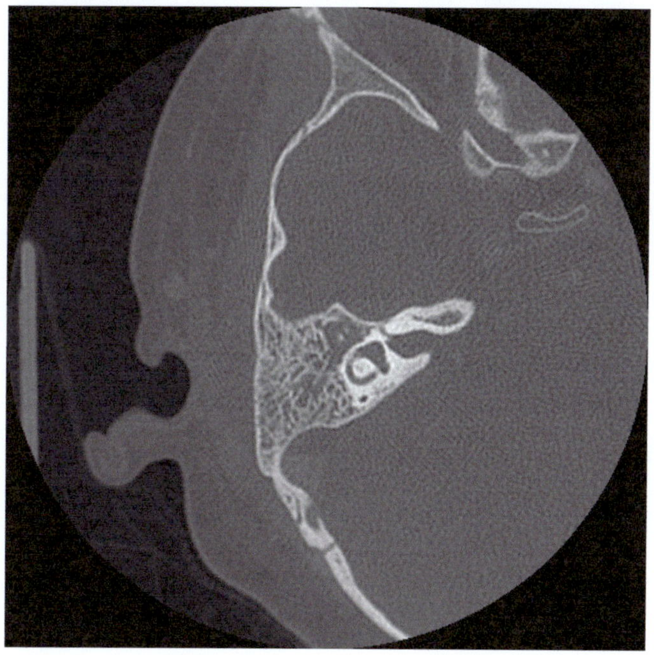

53. Post-op CT demonstrating the amount of bone removal after retrolabyrinthine craniotomy and drainage of the epidural abscess.

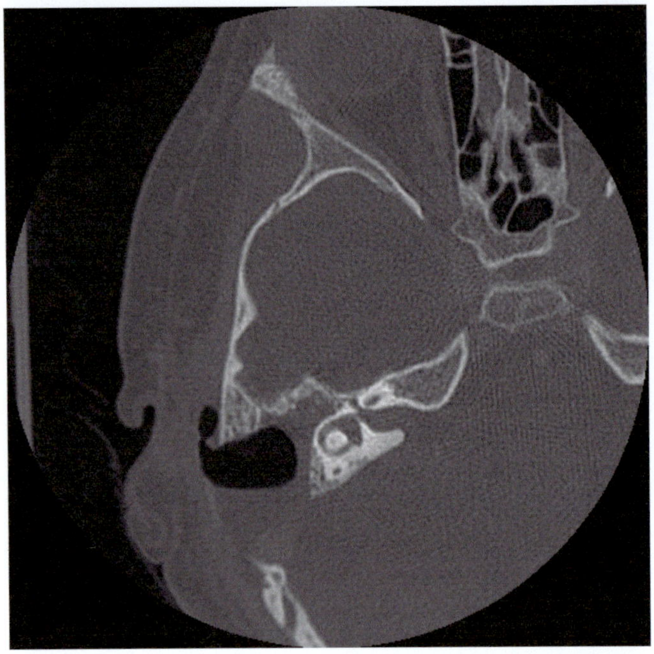

54. Case 5. CT demonstrating a large left subperiosteal abscess (*asterisk*) and sigmoid sinus thrombophlebitis (*arrow*).

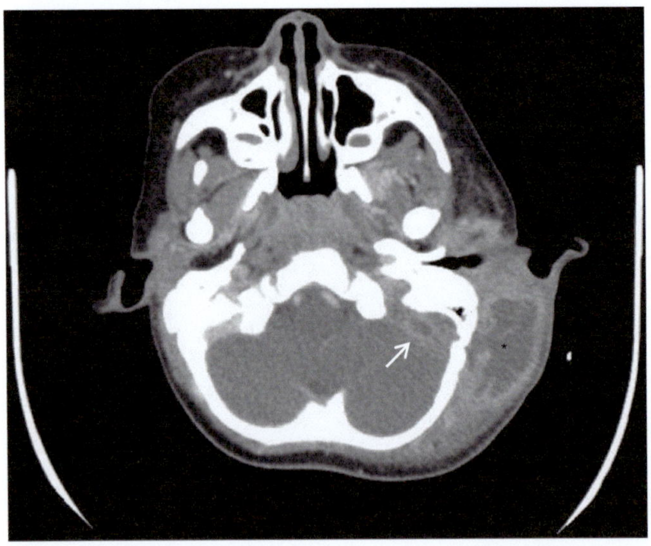

55. The bone-windowed CT demonstrated erosion of the bony cortex overlying the sigmoid sinus (*arrow*). This represents direct extension of the infection process. There was also coalescence of the mastoid air cells.

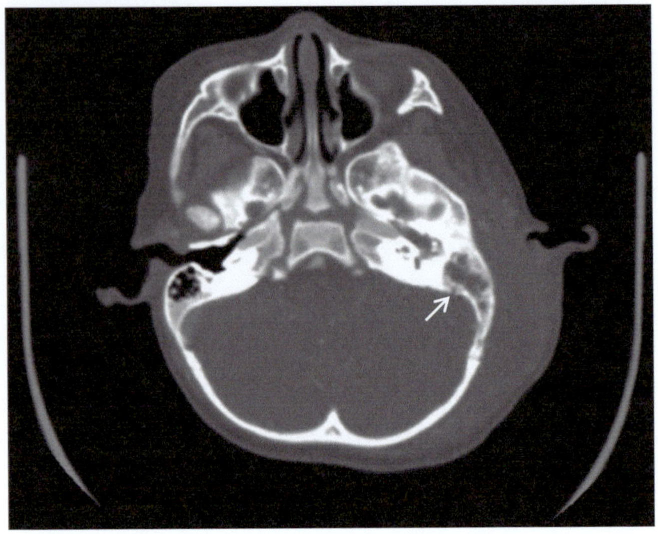

56. The MRV demonstrated occlusion of the left sigmoid sinus.

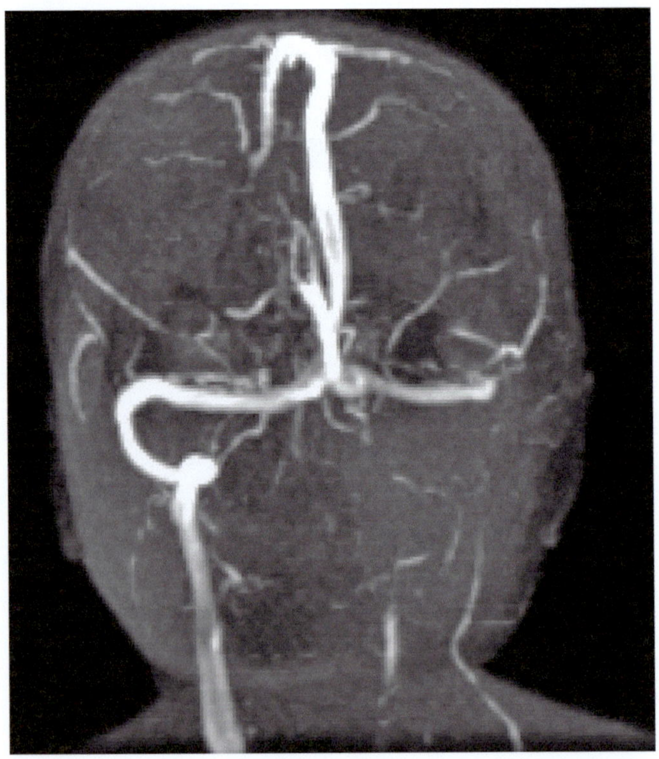

57. Surgical treatment was needed. The incision is drawn. Note the erythema and swelling behind the ear.

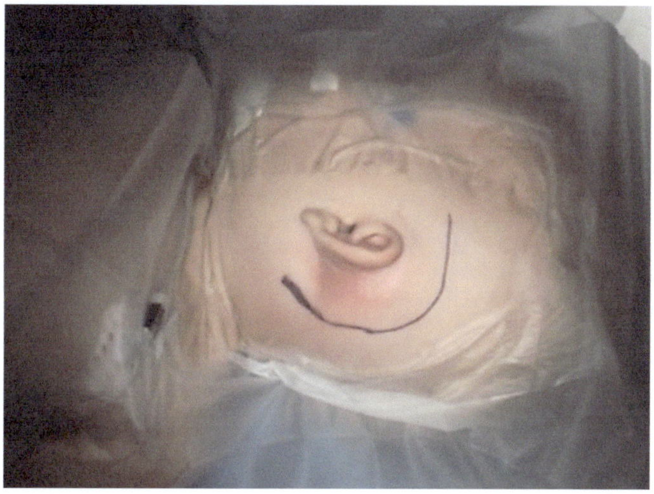

58. Immediately after making the incision, the subperiosteal abscess was drained and cultured.

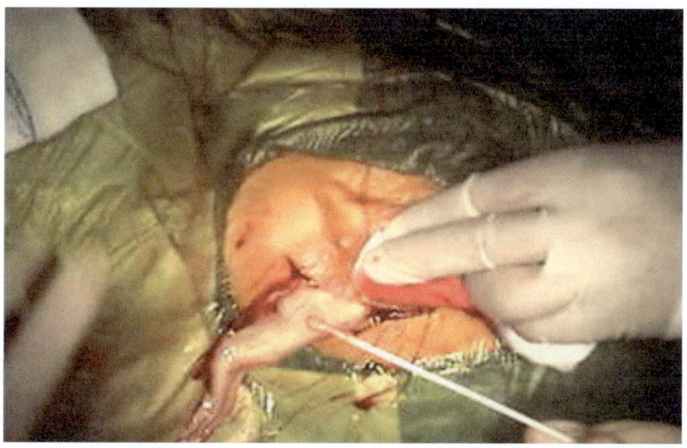

59. After cleaning away all the purulence, the cortex of the mastoid was noted to be eroded (*arrows*).

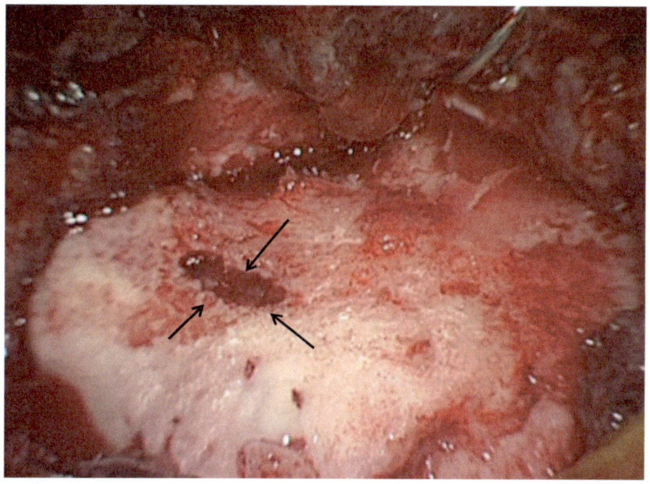

60. The sigmoid sinus was identified and the retrosigmoid dura exposed.

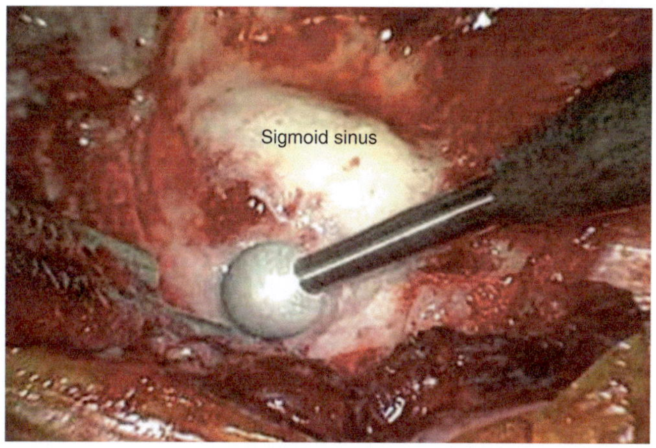

61. After completion of the mastoidectomy, the bone over the sigmoid sinus was thinned to allow inspection.

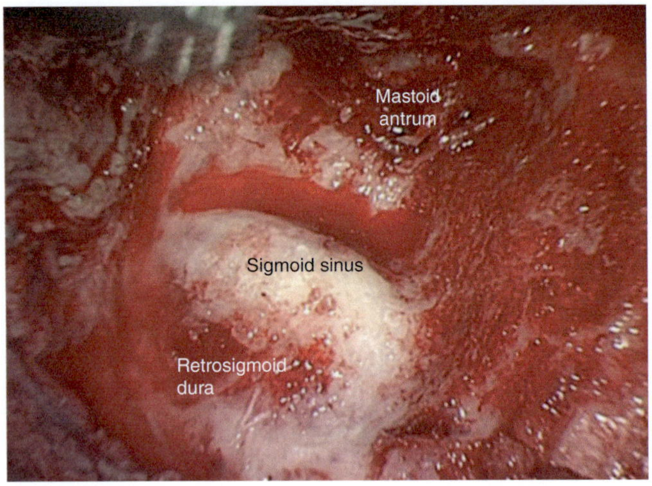

62. The bone over the sigmoid was gently dissected off. Note the yellowish material underneath. This was the abscess within the sigmoid sinus which was immediately visible. The lateral wall did not need to be opened as it was already destroyed by the disease. This is the most common presentation of sigmoid sinus thrombophlebitis in our experience.

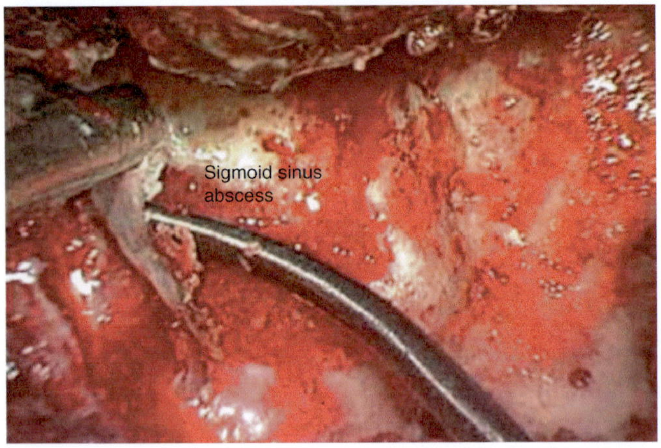

63. The disease was curetted out of the sigmoid sinus. No attempt was made to try to restore blood flow as the sinus was completely destroyed by the infection.

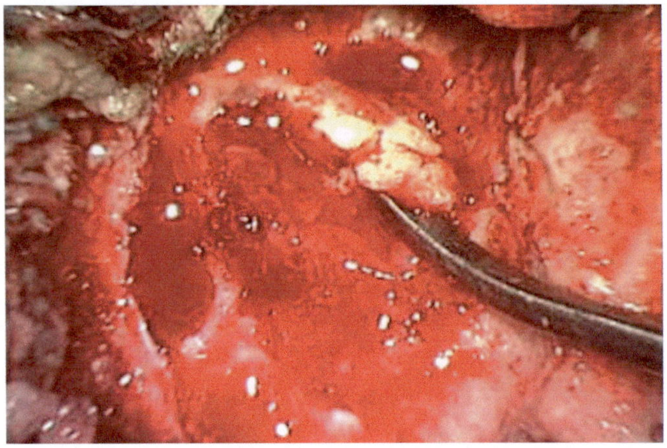

64. Post-op CT demonstrating the extent of bone removal.

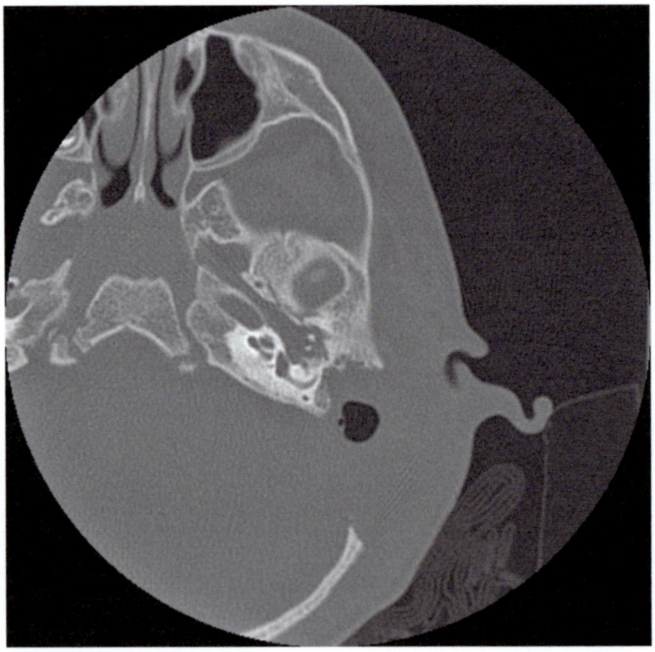

65. Post-op MRI demonstrating the persistent thickening and inflammation of the posterior fossa dura. This gradually resolved with long-term IV antibiotics.

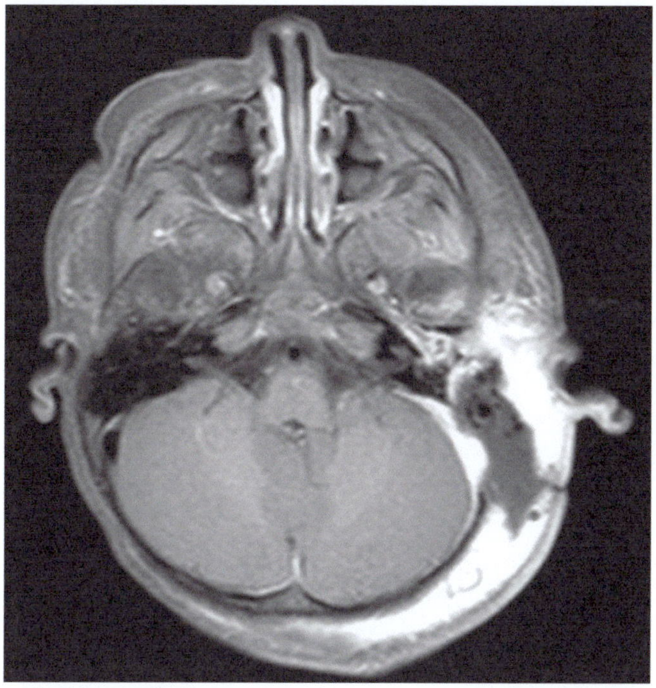

66. Case 6. Coronal CT of a patient with left mastoidits and an epidural abscess (*arrowhead*) in the middle cranial fossa that had eroded the skull to form a Luc's abscess (*arrow*) under the temporalis muscle.

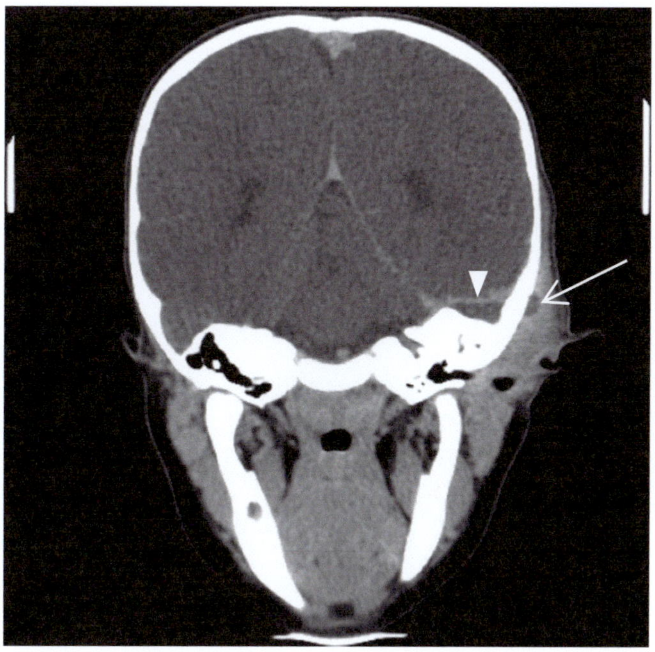

67. The epidural abscess also extended to the posterior fossa (*arrowhead*).

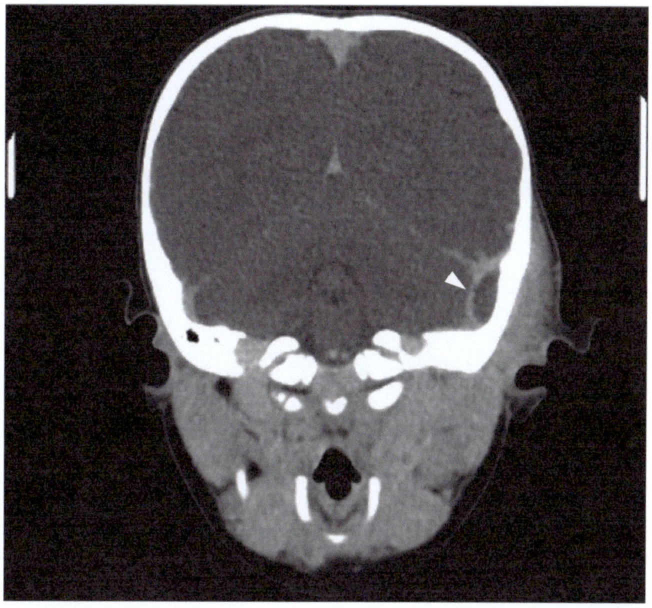

68. The Luc's abscess was drained and a small middle fossa craniectomy (*arrow*) performed to remove devitalized bone underneath it. A mastoidectomy was then performed. To finish the procedure, the mastoidectomy was extended into the retrolabyrinthine craniotomy in order to drain the middle and posterior cranial fossa abscesses (not shown).

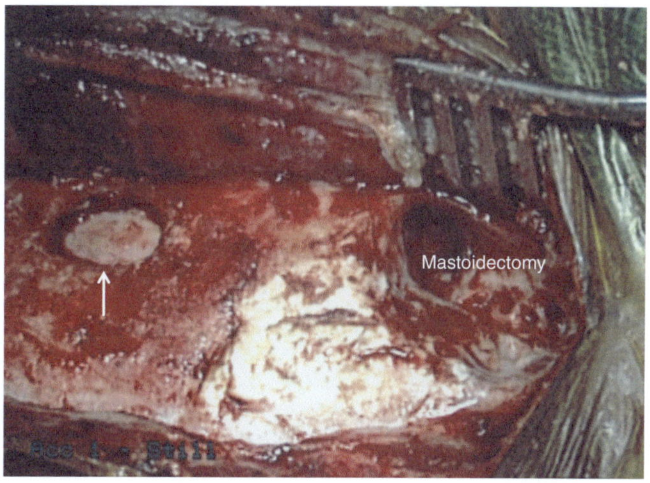

69. Case 7. Left coalescent mastoiditis with erosion of the inner table overlying the posterior cranial fossa (*arrow*).

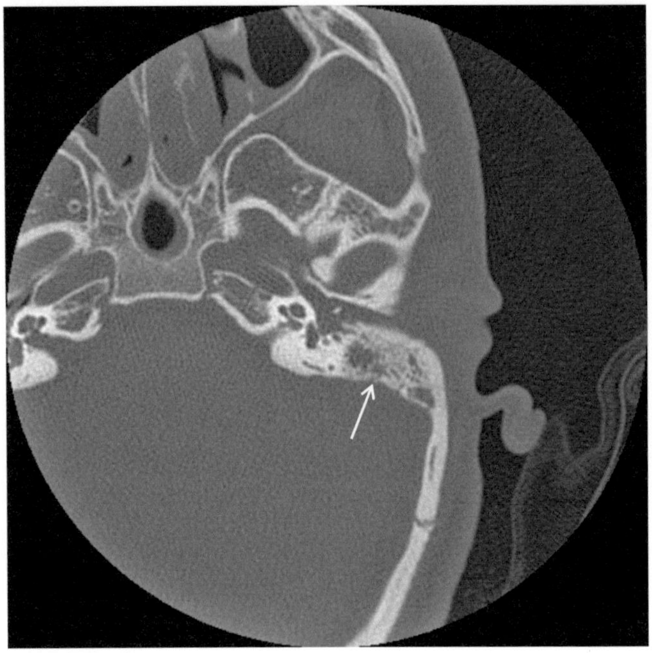

70. Axial MRI with gadolinium demonstrated thrombosis of the sigmoid and transverse sinuses (*arrows*).

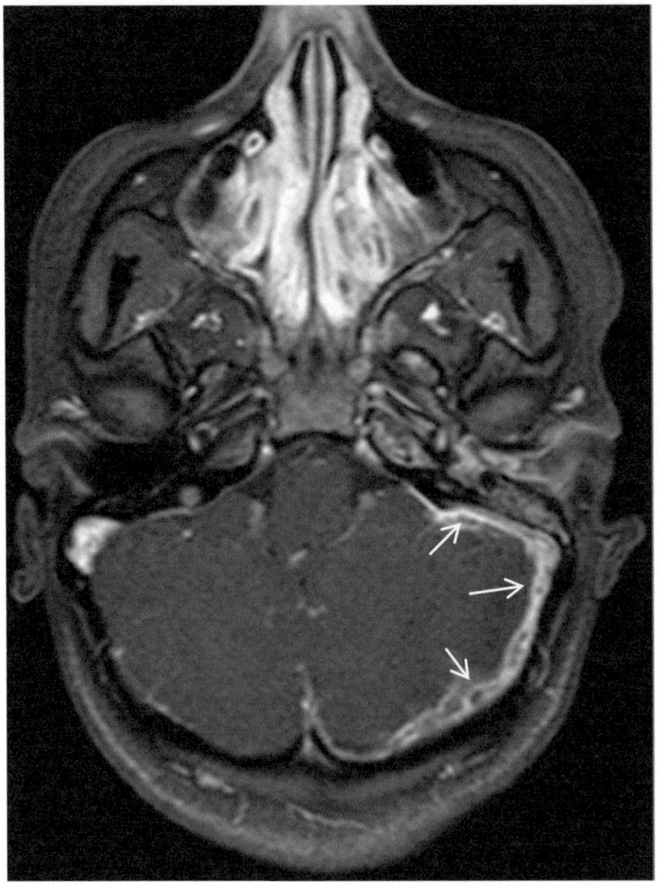

71. The venous occlusion was confirmed by MRV.

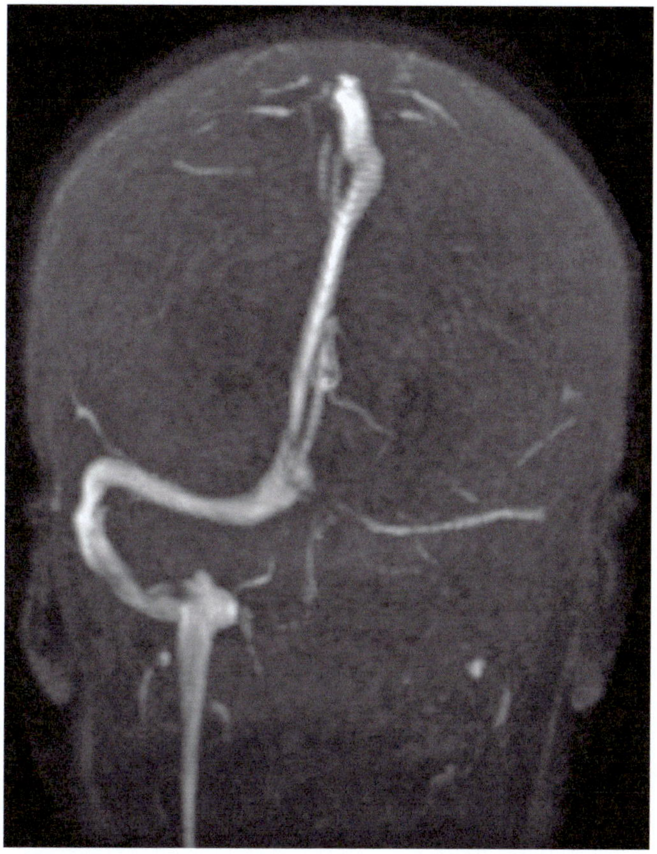

72. The patient also had a subdural abscess within the posterior fossa (*arrow*). There was compression of the cerebellum and enhancement of the cerebellar fovea.

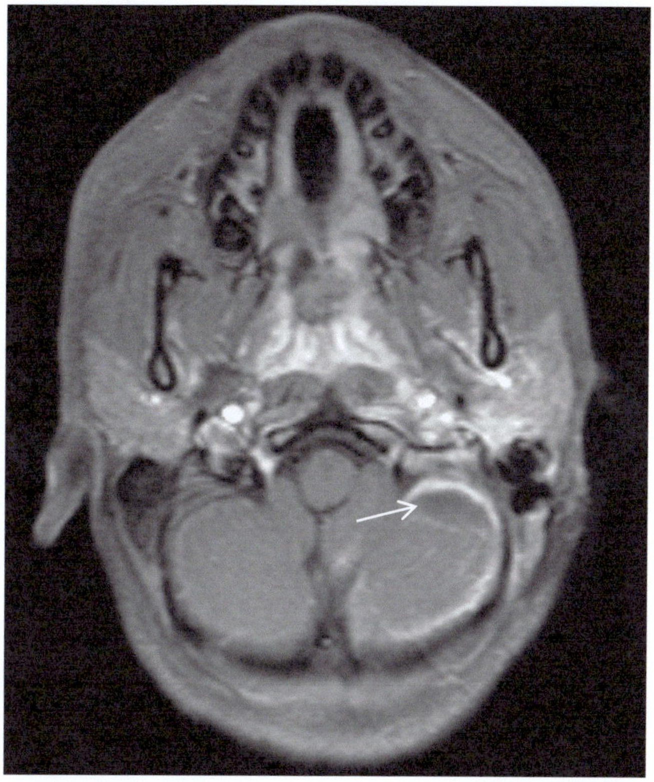

73. Coronal view of the subdural abscess (*arrow*).

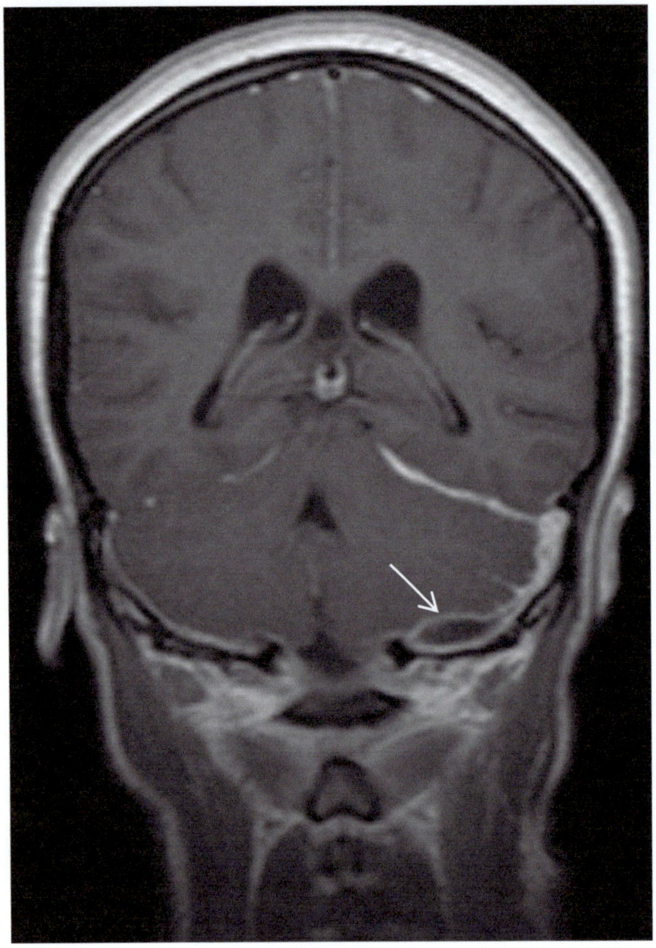

Subtotal (Circumferential) Petrosectomy for Acute Petrositis or Skull Base Osteomyelitis

- *Concept*
  - This procedure is performed for life-threatening infections of the temporal bone that have led to bone necrosis. Microbes can live within these areas that are protected from the patient's immune system and systemic antibiotics.
  - The goal is to debride as much temporal bone as possible while preserving hearing, balance, and facial nerve function.
  - Another key aspect of the procedure is to reconstruct the drilled-out defects with vascularized tissue. A vascularized muscle flap allows systemic antibiotics and the immune system to access residual areas of devitalized bone that could not be safely removed. Hyperbaric oxygen therapy is another adjunctive therapy to consider.
- *Conditions treated*
  - Recalcitrant skull base osteomyelitis
  - Acute petrous apicitis progressing on intravenous antibiotic therapy
- *Risks*
  - Injury to the temporal lobe such as contusion, edema, or stroke
  - Temporal lobe seizure
  - Anomic aphasia
  - Hearing loss
  - Facial nerve injury
  - Dry eye if the GSPN is transected
  - Meningitis
  - CSF leak
- *Benefits*
  - Preservation of the external auditory canal, otic capsule, and facial nerve
- *Additional notes*
  - This degree of bone removal should be tailored to the extent of disease. It is uncommon for the procedure to be performed in its entirety.

74. Overview of the bone to be removed (*gray*).

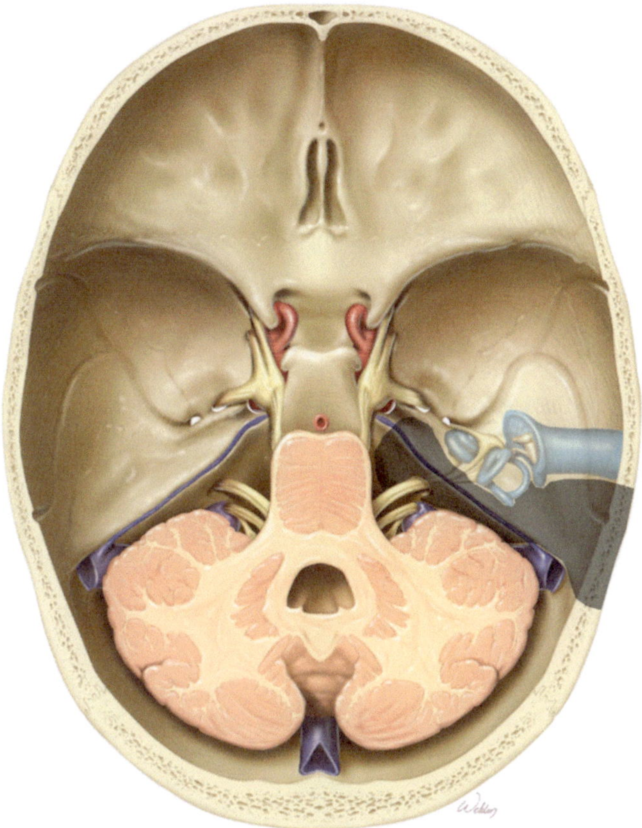

75. The incision for the circumferential petrosectomy should provide access from the temporalis muscle to the jugular foramen.

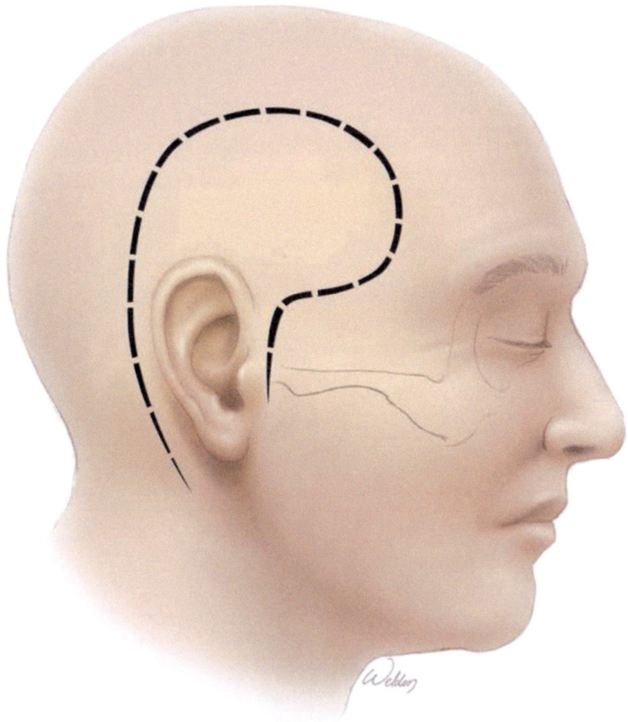

76. The skin and subcutaneous tissues are elevated off the temporalis muscle. The flap is retracted anterior-inferiorly, tethered at the ear canal.

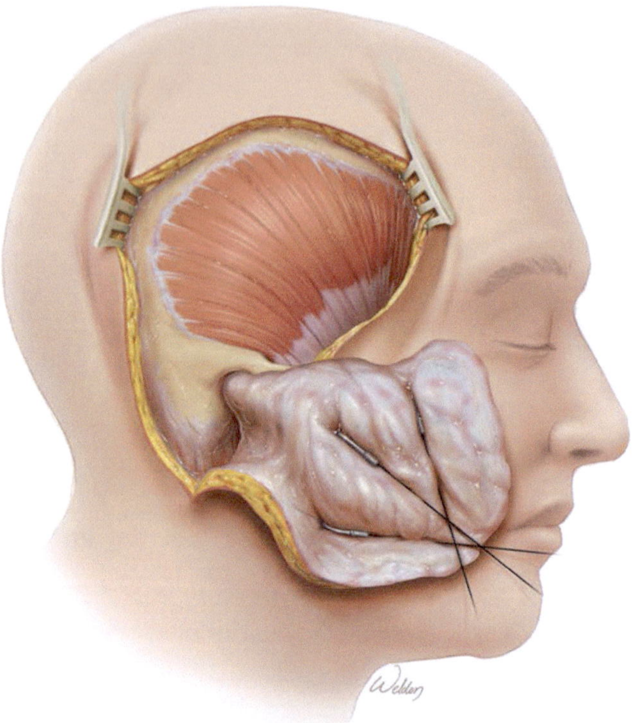

77. The temporalis muscle is then elevated off the skull as a separate flap. It is not left attached to the skin flap because it will be used for the reconstruction.

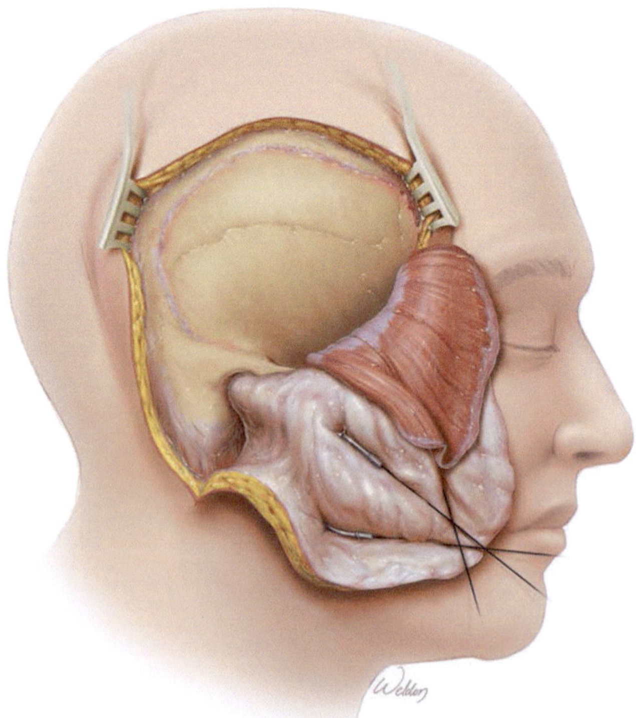

78. A mastoidectomy is performed identically to the initial stages of the translabyrinthine approach (Chap. 4). However, the semicircular canals are identified and skeletonized rather than removed. The sigmoid sinus, the posterior cranial fossa dura, and the middle cranial fossa dura are exposed.

While the aditus ad antrum is opened and the incus visualized, this opening should be left as small as possible to reduce the risk of postoperative adhesions forming to the incus that might produce conductive hearing loss.

The facial nerve is identified at the second genu and followed down to the stylomastoid foramen. The sigmoid sinus is then followed underneath the facial nerve to the jugular bulb. Finally, a fallopian bridge technique is used to dissect around the vertical segment of the facial nerve circumferentially while leaving it safely encased in bone. These procedures are identical to those described in the postauricular infratemporal fossa approach (Chap. 6).

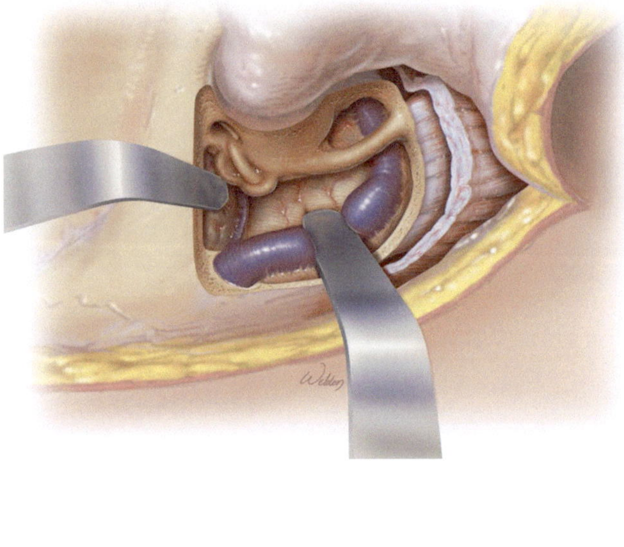

79. After dissecting the middle fossa dura away from the underside of the squamous portion of the temporal bone, a craniotome is then used to turn a bone flap. No burr holes are needed.

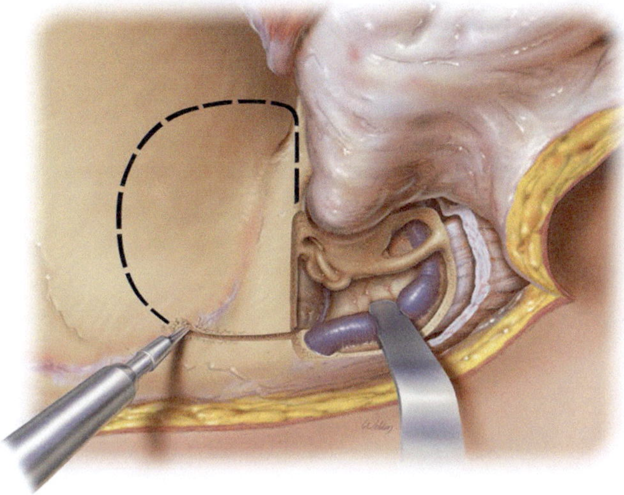

80. The surgeon moves his/her chair to the head of the bed and elevates the middle cranial fossa dura. Further removal of the bone of the petrous apex is performed as in a Kawase's triangle approach (Chap. 3).

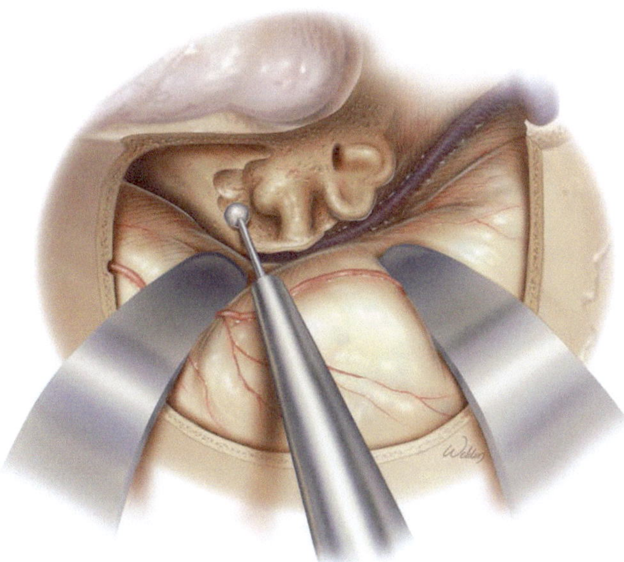

81. The anterior third of the temporalis muscle is left in place. The middle third is rotated into the petrous apex defect. The posterior third is rotated into the mastoid defect and sutured in place to the sternocleidomastoid muscle. These vascularized muscle flaps help to bring antibiotics and white blood cells to treat infection in residual bone. The craniotomy bone flap is plated back in place.

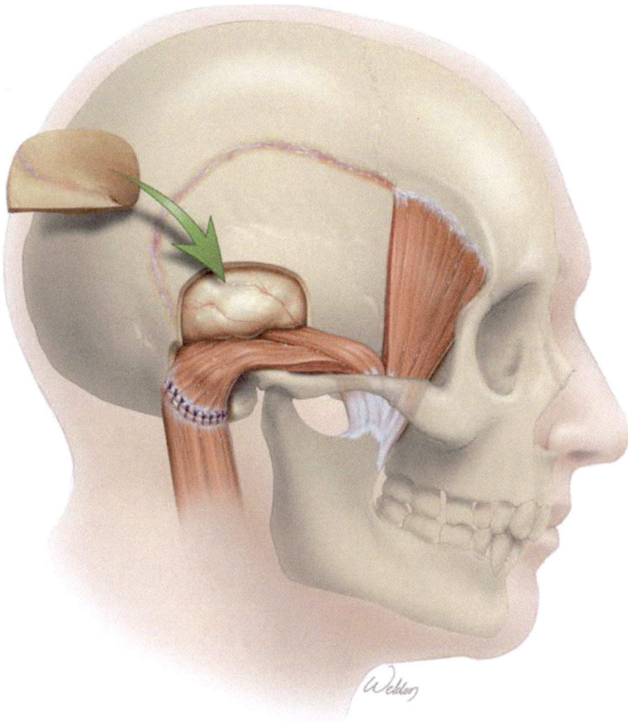

82. Case 1. A teenage boy presented with CN VI palsy. MRI demonstrated left acute petrositis. Note the inflammation of the petrous apex (*arrow*) as well as the narrowing of the internal carotid artery within the cavernous sinus (*arrowhead*).

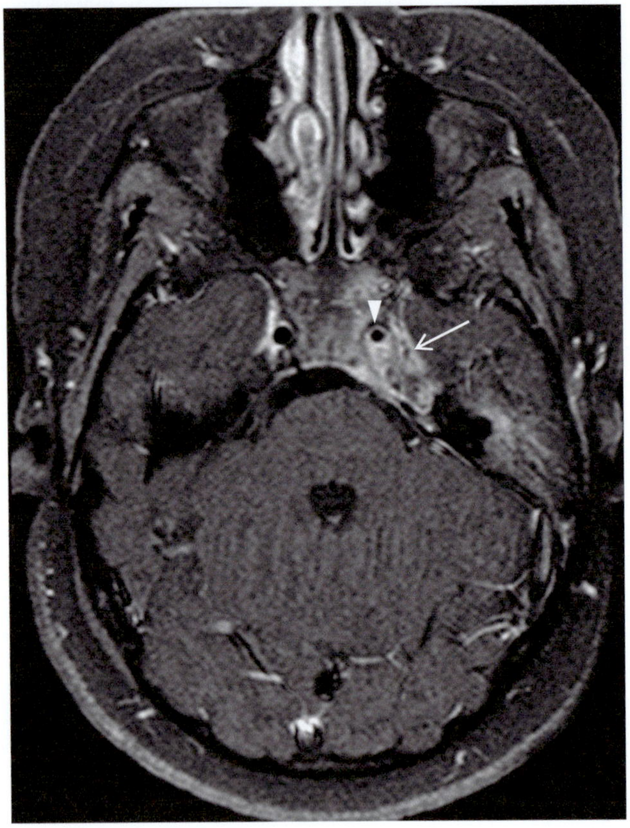

83. Coronal view again demonstrating enhancement of the left petrous apex.

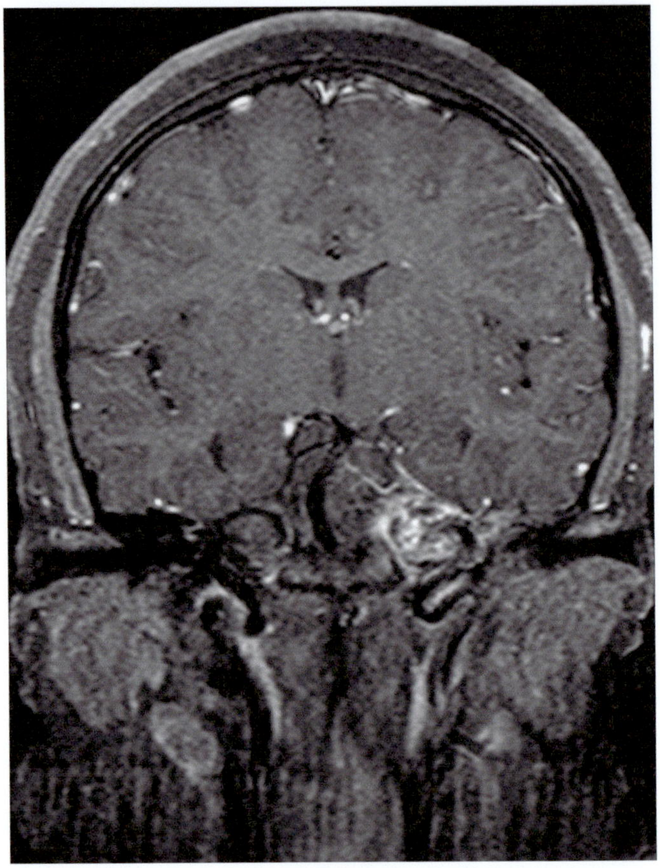

84. CT demonstrated coalescence of the petrous apex (*asterisk*).

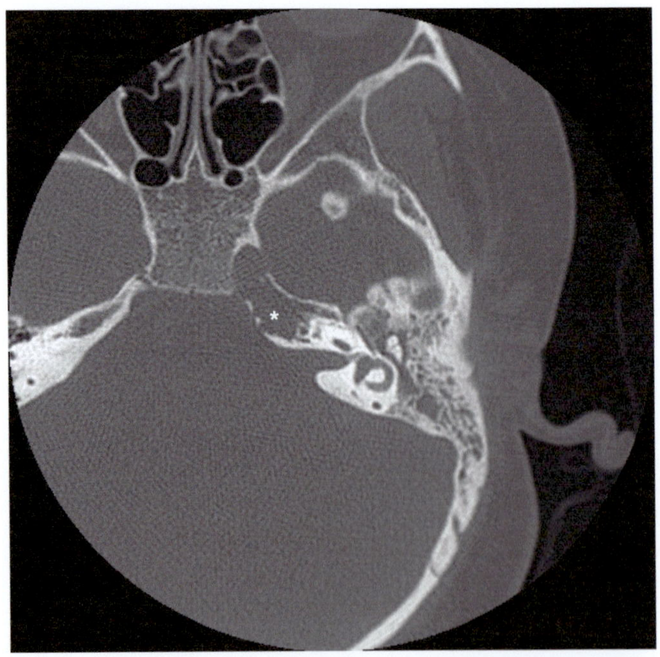

85. Post-op MRI. One week after circumferential petrosectomy, the inflammation of the petrous apex is dramatically improved, and the internal carotid artery has normal caliber (*arrowhead*). The temporalis muscle flap fills the mastoid defect.

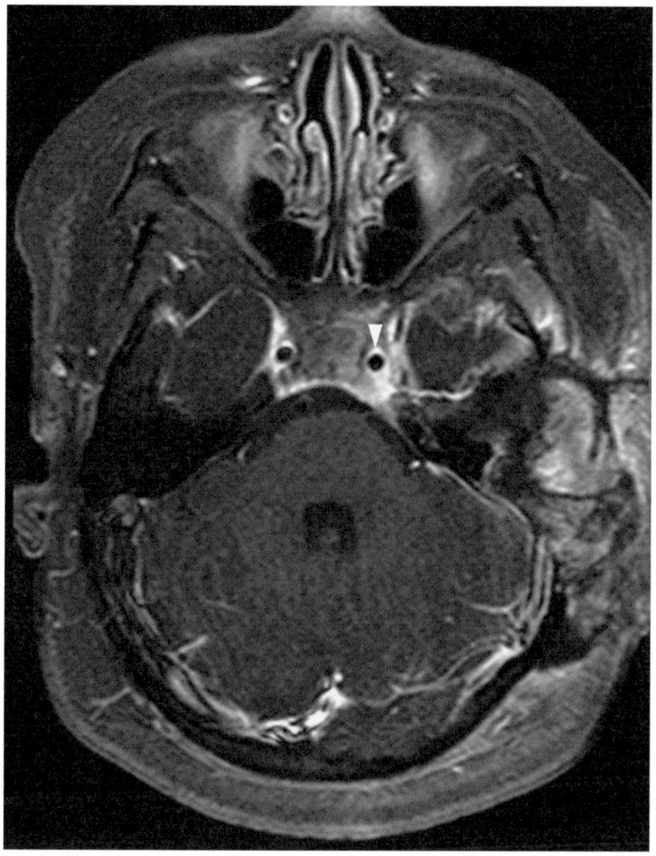

86. Post-op CT demonstrates the mastoidectomy and petrous apex debridement. In this case, the bone over the posterior fossa in the mastoid was not removed because there was little disease in that region.

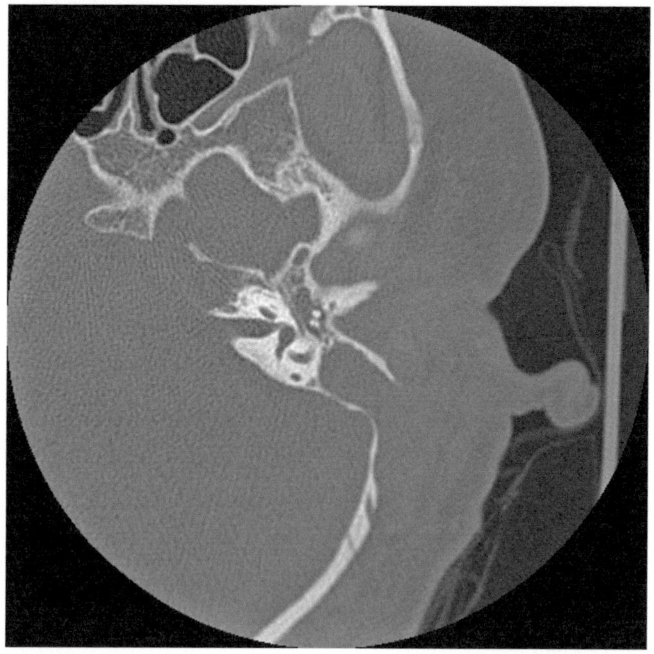

87. Case 2. Skull base osteomyelitis in an elderly diabetic. There is enhancement of the left petrous apex and clivus (*arrow*).

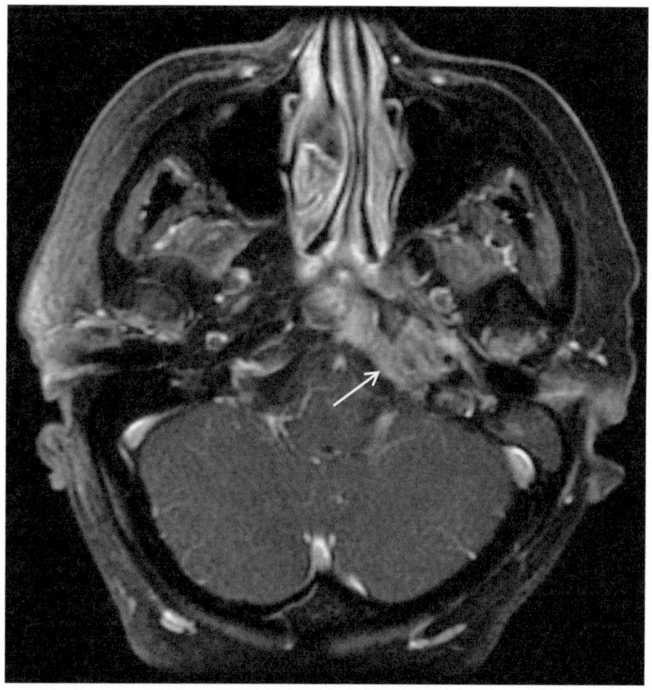

88. Coronal view demonstrated not only the petrous apex disease but also soft tissue inflammation within much of the soft tissues of the infratemporal fossa.

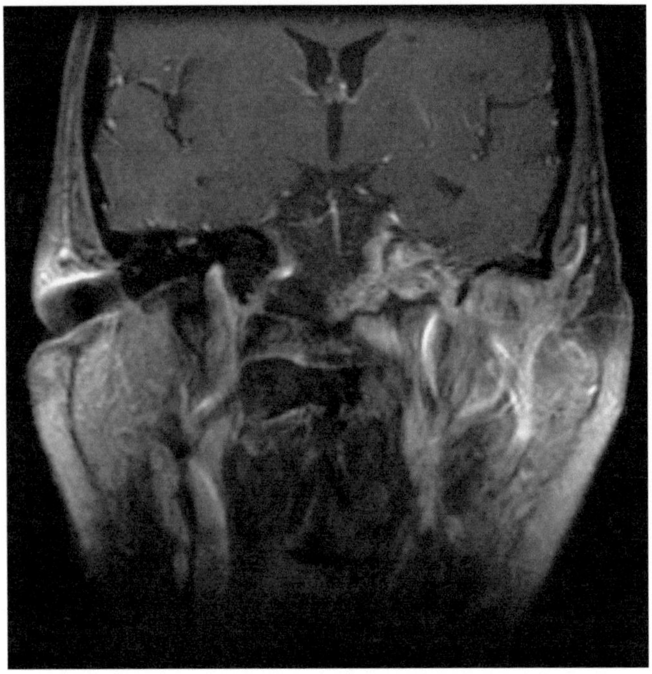

89. CT scan demonstrated no obvious changes other than low-density material within the middle ear and mastoid consistent with fluid.

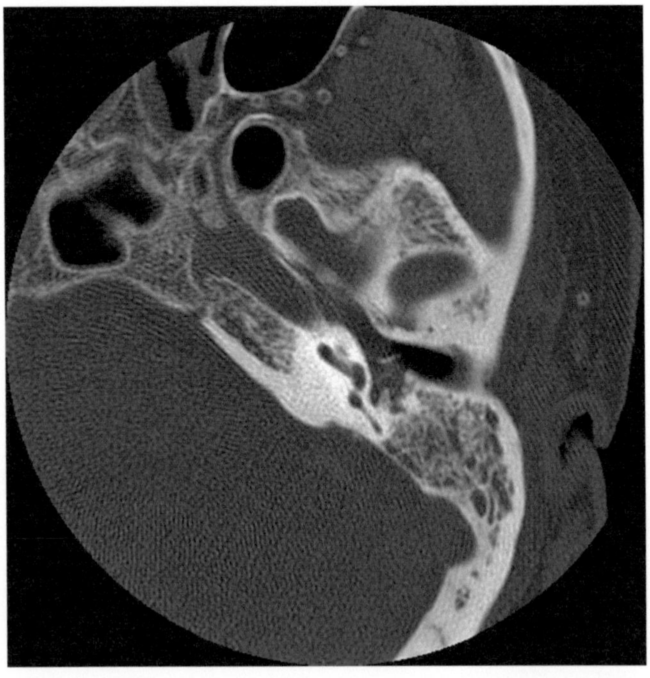

90. Technesium scan demonstrating uptake within the petrous apex consistent with osteomyelitis. This patient's disease did not improve with long-term IV antibiotics. After circumferential petrosectomy and another course of IV antibiotics, his disease resolved.

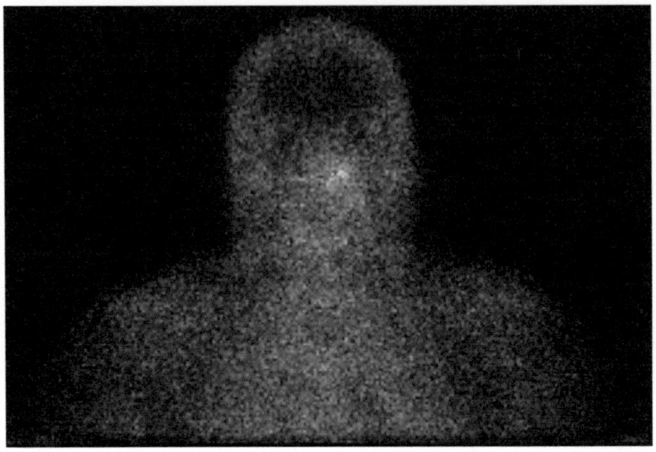

8 Temporal Bone Surgery for Encephaloceles, Superior Semicircular Canal Dehiscence, Neoplasia, and Lesions of the Petrous Apex

Repair of Temporal Lobe Encephalocele

- *Concept*
  - Defects in the bone of the temporal floor (the tegmen) are repaired.
- *Conditions treated*
  - CSF leak from the middle cranial fossa into the temporal bone
  - Temporal lobe meningocele or encephalocele
- *Risks*
  - Injury to the temporal lobe such as contusion, edema, or vascular compromise
  - Temporal lobe seizure
  - Aphasia
  - Hearing loss and dizziness if the labyrinth is violated
  - Facial nerve injury, typically if the geniculate ganglion is dehiscent and not recognized
  - Dry eye if the greater superficial petrosal nerve is transected
  - Recurrence of disease
  - Meningitis
- *Benefits*
  - Direct and wide exposure of the defect(s) or pathology.
  - Placing a vascularized muscle flap between the brain and the ear reduces the recurrence risk.
- *Additional notes*
  - Small defects (<1 cm^2), especially those located more lateral and posterior, can usually be repaired from below via a mastoidectomy. Most commonly, these are from iatrogenic injury. Typically, a cartilage graft can be squeezed through the bony opening and placed between the dura and the tegmen bone. The approach described here is for larger defects, multiple defects, and those located more anterior or medial.
  - In our opinion, patients with a chronic CSF leak preoperatively should be treated with lumbar subarachnoid drainage for 3–4 days postoperatively. This is because their CSF production has increased to compensate for the leak. Suddenly stopping the leak can lead to elevated intracranial pressure, which will predispose the repair to failure. This is not necessary for patients without a CSF leak or for those who are being treated for an acute-onset CSF leak.
  - If the amount of brain herniation into the mastoid and middle ear is relatively small, the entire procedure can be done through the middle fossa portion alone. A mastoidectomy may not be needed.
  - Spontaneous CSF leaks have become more common along with the rise in obesity. There are often multiple defects, and therefore, we repair all of these through a middle fossa craniotomy. This allows us to lay tissue and bone broadly across the floor. Even with some small solitary defects or encephaloceles, we often prefer to work from above. It is easier to be confident of graft placement and hemostasis. Working from below, pushing material up through a defect is less precise, and there is the potential to cause bleeding that cannot be seen.
  - Many patients use CPAP to treat obstructive sleep apnea, and deciding when to allow them to resume this is unclear. We know that the middle ear pressure is increased when using CPAP, thus there is a risk of pneumocephalus. The risks of oxygen desaturation and tension pneumocephalus must be assessed. While this varies on a patient-by-patient basis, it is nice when CPAP use can be held for at least 7 days after surgery. This typically requires a monitored bed in the hospital, however.

J.S. Oghalai, C.L.W. Driscoll, *Atlas of Neurotologic and Lateral Skull Base Surgery*,
DOI 10.1007/978-3-662-46694-0_8, © Springer-Verlag Berlin Heidelberg 2016

1. Normal coronal view of the temporal bone.

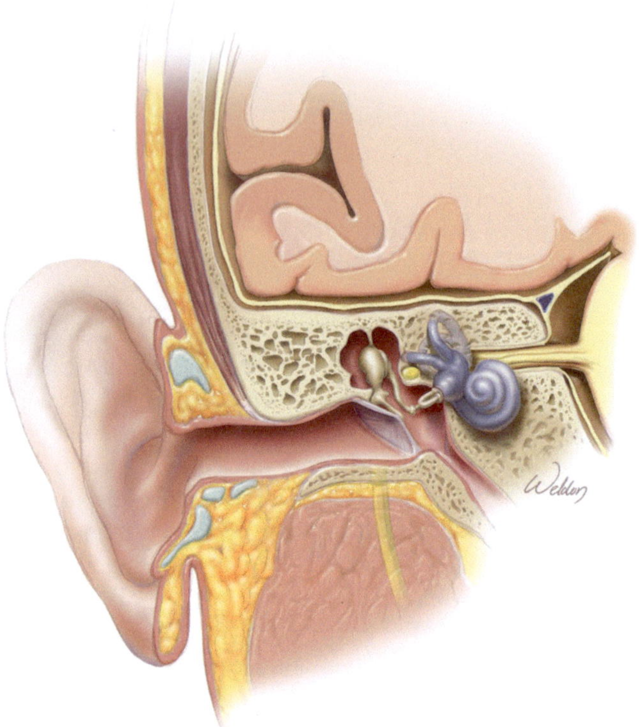

2. Proper postoperative appearance of a canal wall up mastoidectomy. Note that the tegmen (*black arrow*) and the posterior–superior ear canal are intact (*white arrow*).

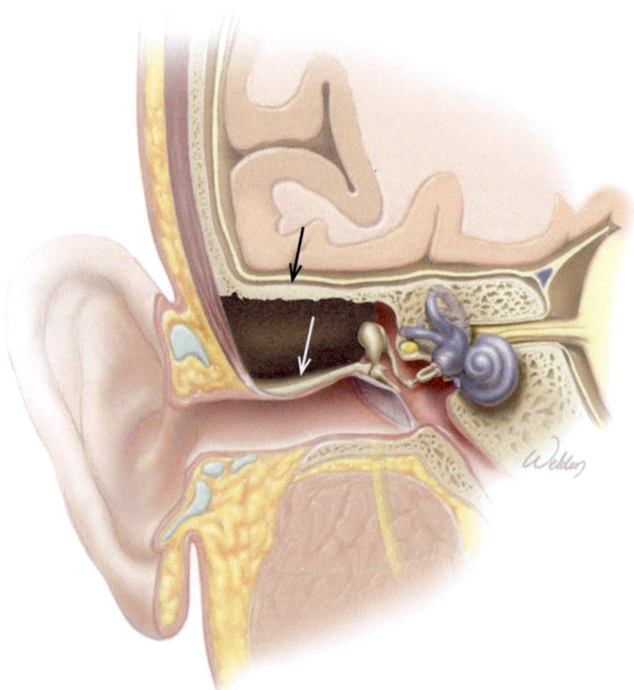

3. Proper postoperative appearance of a canal wall down mastoidectomy. In this case, the tegmen is intact, but the tympanic membrane lies across the horizontal and vertical portions of the facial nerve because the ear canal has been removed. There is also a large meatoplasty, and the ear canal slopes downward to promote healthy drainage.

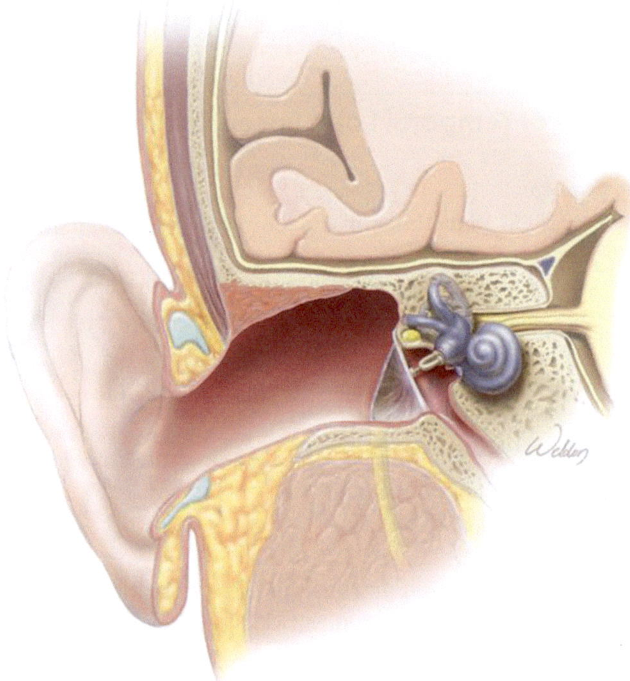

4. Inadvertent injury to the tegmen, and possibly also the dura, can lead to a temporal lobe encephalocele. This may not occur immediately after surgery but even years later. This image depicts an encephalocele into a canal wall up mastoidectomy.

   While CSF, or even brain, may be appreciated behind the tympanic membrane, often the only sign is a visible pulsing of the eardrum that synchronizes to the patient's heartbeat. This reflects transmitted brain pulsations to the middle ear and mastoid air space. It can be noted both with binocular microscopy and on tympanometry when the patient is sitting upright. This sign usually resolves when the patient is laid flat so that the brain does not exert as much downward pressure.

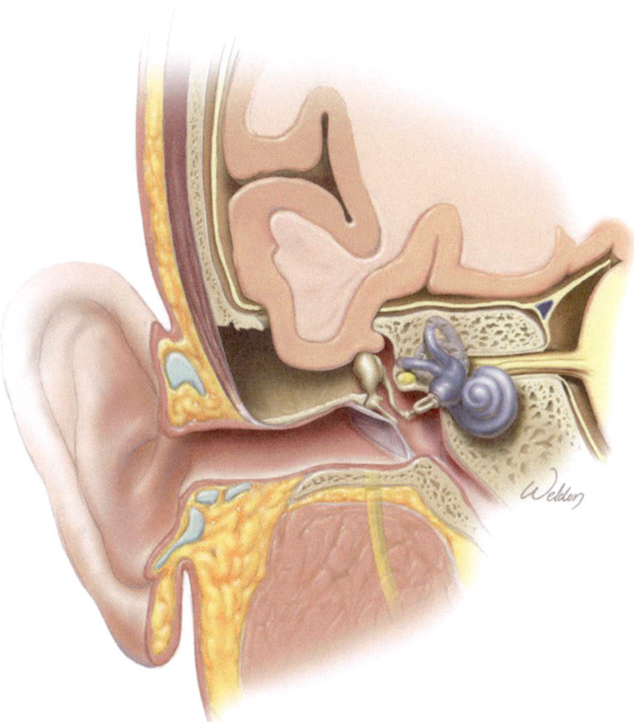

5. Treatment for an encephalocele is surgical. The incision is a standard postauricular incision that extends superiorly.

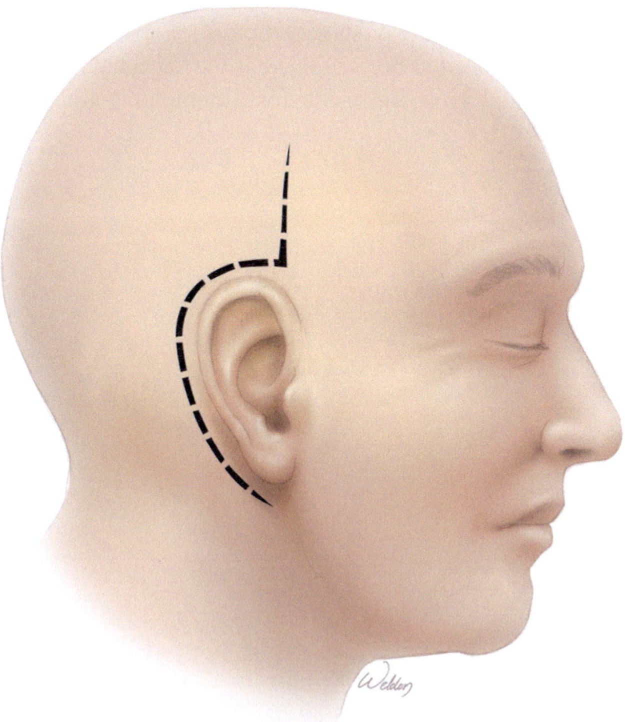

6. The temporalis is exposed superiorly and the sternocleidomastoid muscle attachment to the mastoid process exposed inferiorly. The periosteum over the mastoid process is elevated to the ear canal.

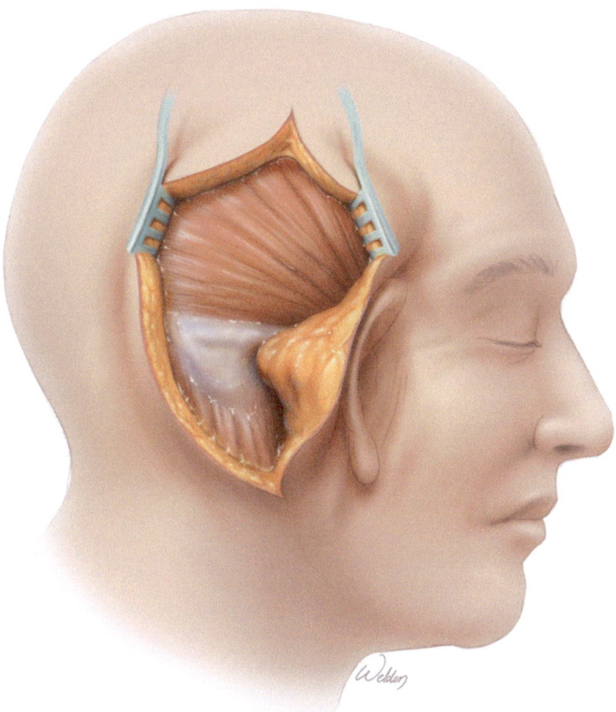

7. The temporalis muscle is then retracted off the skull anteriorly. A standard cortical mastoidectomy performed to expose the encephalocele (*asterisk*). For a small encephalocele, particularly those in patients that have never had mastoid surgery before, a mastoidectomy does not need to be performed as the encephalocele can be treated through a middle fossa craniotomy alone.

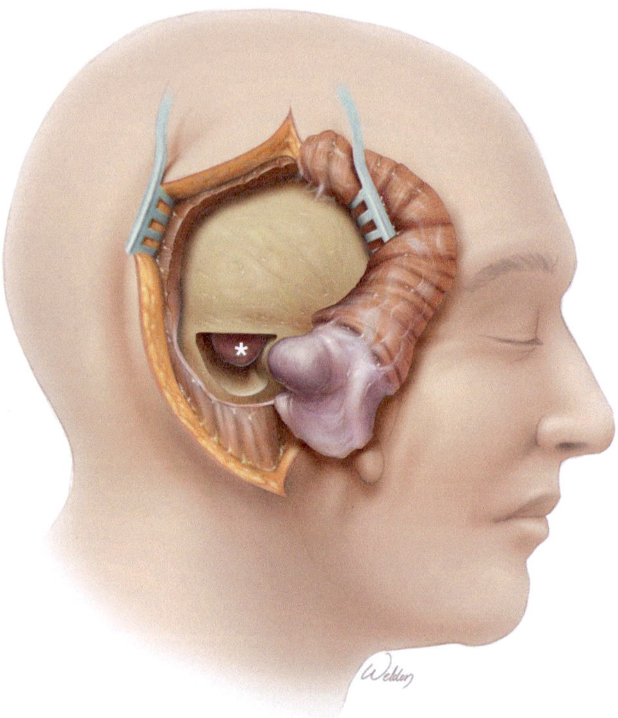

8. A middle fossa craniotomy is performed. This can be centered over the area of the encephalocele identified by preoperative imaging to allow it to be quite small. Details of this opening are given in Chap. 3.

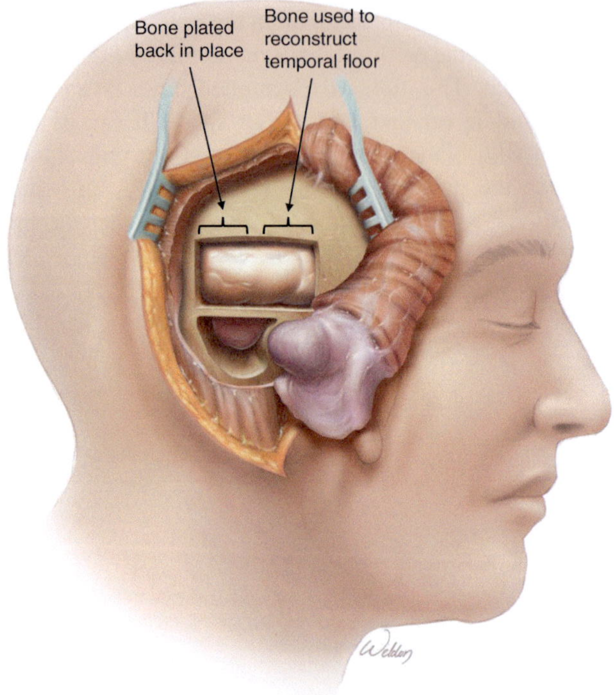

9. Extradural dissection with a periosteal elevator is performed to trace around the circumference of the dural defect.

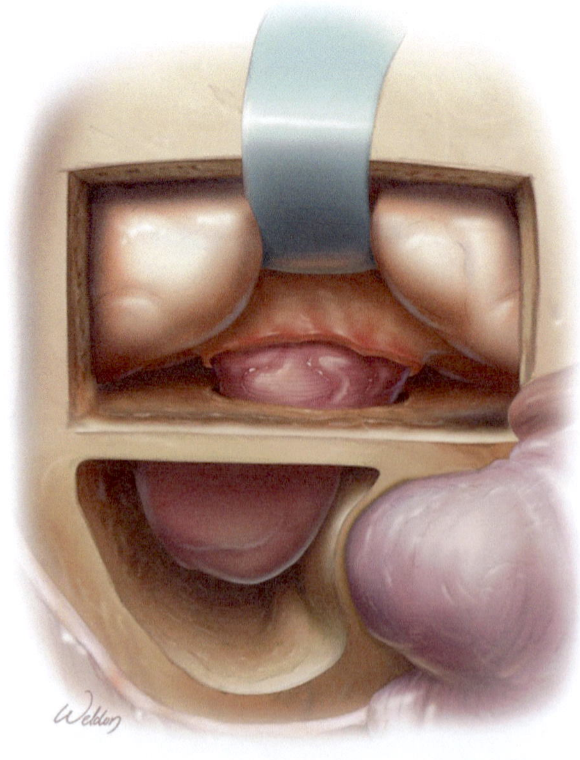

10. Large, plunging encephaloceles do not contain viable brain. A bipolar cautery is used to carefully divide the devitalized brain below from the healthy brain above. After this process, the healthy brain typically retracts up, and it is important not to lose track of any bleeding vessels when this happens. Meticulous hemostasis inside the dura is necessary.

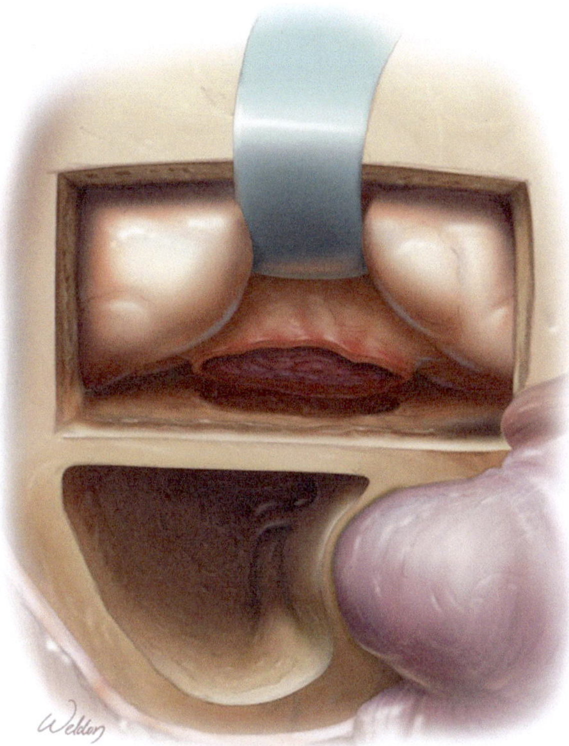

11. A three-layer closure is performed. The superior layer is a dural patch consisting of fascia, cadaveric dura, or artificial dura (i.e., Duragen). A larger piece than one expects to use is carefully inserted through the dural defect and the edges tucked up between the brain and the dura. Thus, the downward pressure of the brain when the patient is upright will help seal the defect. We usually cover this with a dural sealant as well (i.e., Tisseal or Duraseal).

The inferior layer is the bone graft. The bone flap removed during the craniectomy is cut and a portion of it used to bridge the bony defect in the tegmen. Usually, we cut the anterior half off and use it to reconstruct the tegmen. It is important to make sure it is laid on top of the medial edge of the defect for support. Sometimes, it is hard for the bone graft to stay in the appropriate location. In this case, it can be plated to the skull to prevent lateral migration.

Finally, the posterior half of the temporalis muscle is separated from the anterior half vertically and then rotated between the dural patch and the bone graft to form the middle layer. This should be sutured to a hole drilled in the skull or to the soft tissue around the ear canal to prevent the muscle from retracting out when the patient wakes up and begins to chew.

There are multiple ways to layer in your choice of tissues that are all likely to be successful. We like to put an intradural patch in those patients with multiple defects and very atrophic dura. An incision can be made over the lateral aspect of the temporal lobe and medial dissection performed intradurally. This allows us to place a large graft, essentially covering the whole floor.

Finally, the remaining bone flap is plated back to cover the craniotomy site. It is most important to cover the posterior portion of the defect as the temporalis muscle flap enters the middle fossa through the anterior portion and will provide adequate bulk to prevent trauma should the patient be bumped in the side of the head postoperatively.

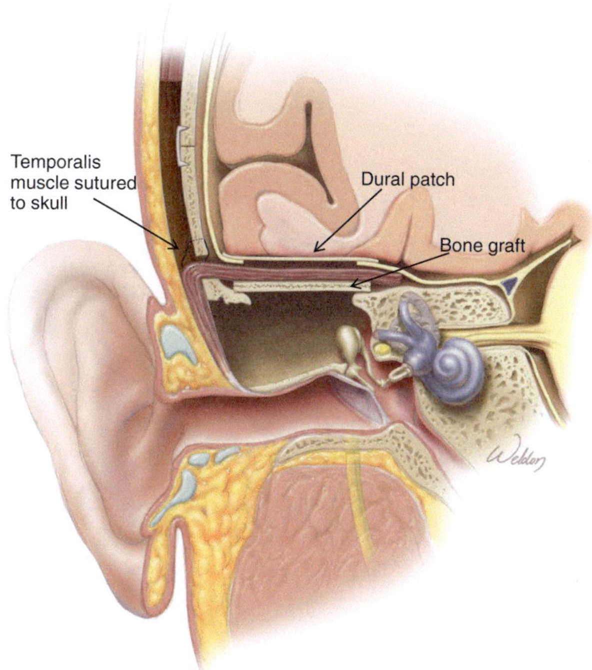

12. Diagram of a temporal lobe encephalocele into a canal wall down mastoidectomy. This is even more concerning than the canal wall up situation because the brain is directly exposed to the outside environment.

    In some cases, the skin of the cavity overlying the encephalocele is thick, and the repair can be done from above without violating the cavity. When this skin can be kept intact, the risk of post-op CSF leak is reduced, and the risk of infection may be less.

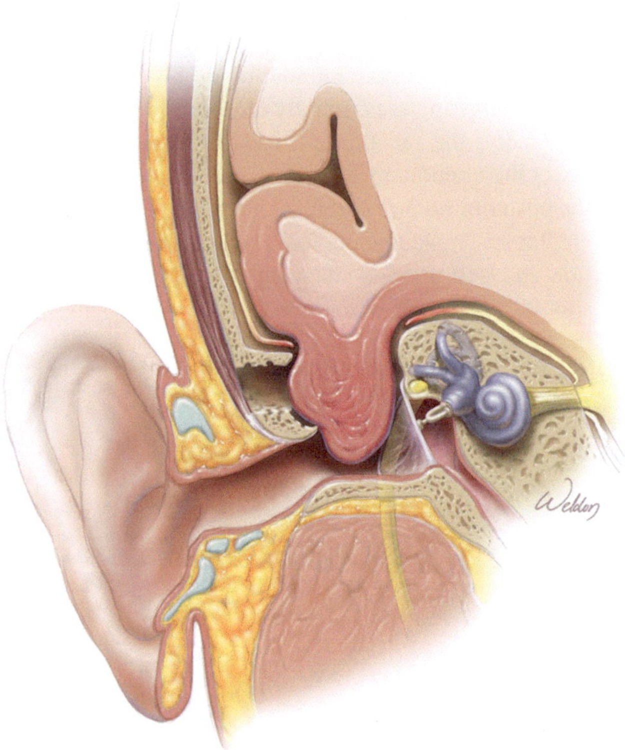

13. In other cases, the mastoid and middle fossa must both be opened up. The same incision can be used as for the canal wall up procedure.

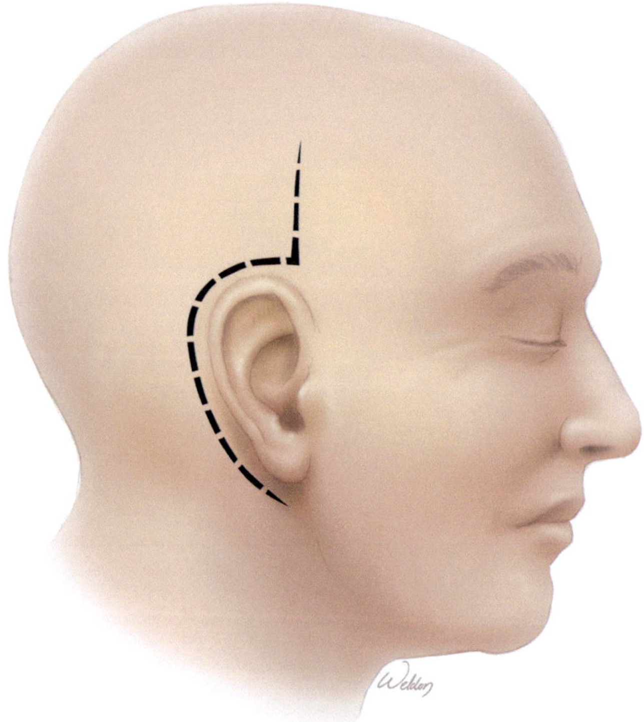

14. Exposure of the temporalis muscle.

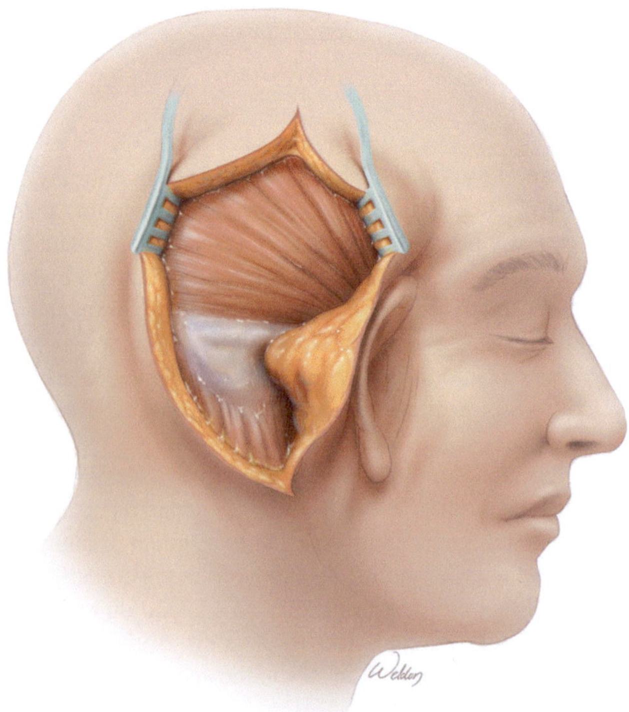

15. The mastoidectomy defect is opened. The facial ridge can be seen to be too high in this illustration (*arrow*). The anterior ear canal skin is left tethered to provide a vascular supply to the tympanic membrane.

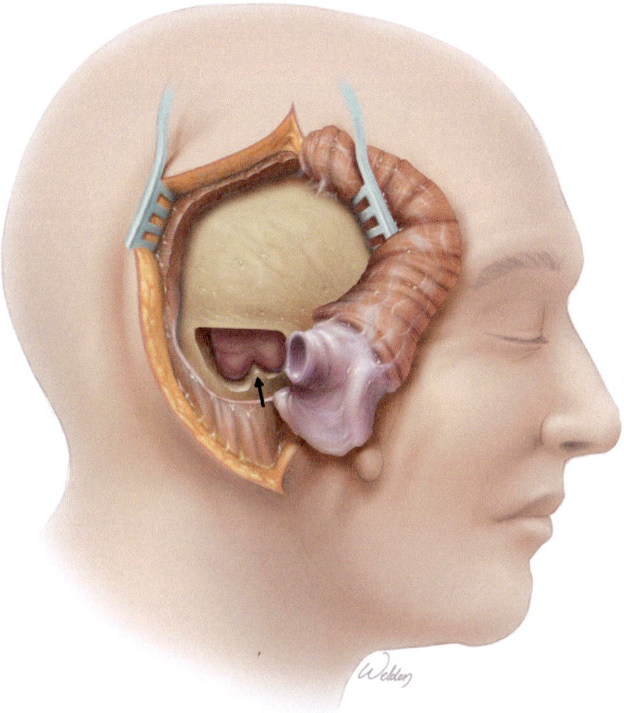

16. A middle fossa craniotomy is performed as described in Chap. 3.

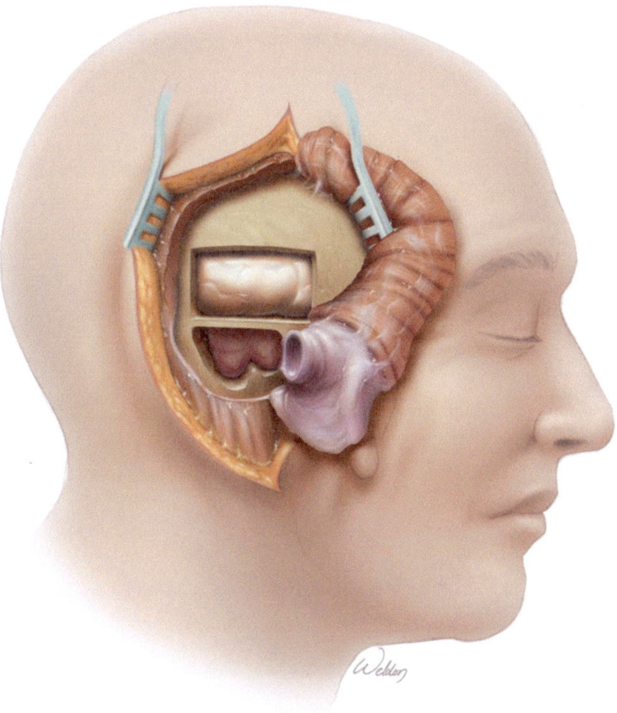

17. The dural defect is exposed circumferentially.

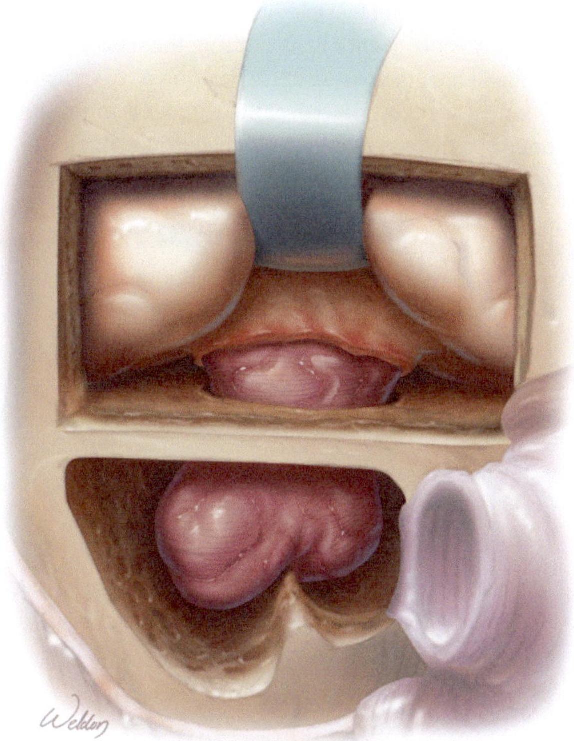

18. The encephalocele is divided and the facial ridge lowered.

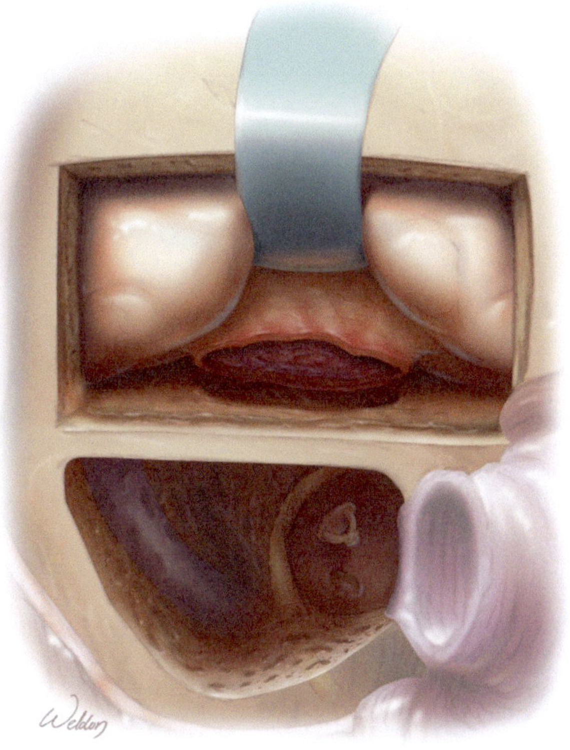

19. A three-layered closure is performed as described above. In this illustration, an alternative technique for suturing the tip of the temporalis muscle to the medial dura is shown (*arrow*). This technique, while challenging, is probably more secure than suturing the base of the muscle flap. Once the first stitch is tied down, it is impossible to get any more placed. Thus, two or three stitches should be thrown and then cinched down together using your assistant to help.

    The tympanic membrane may also need to be reconstructed using temporalis fascia and/or cartilage using routine otologic techniques. Ossicular chain reconstruction can be performed if desired (not shown).

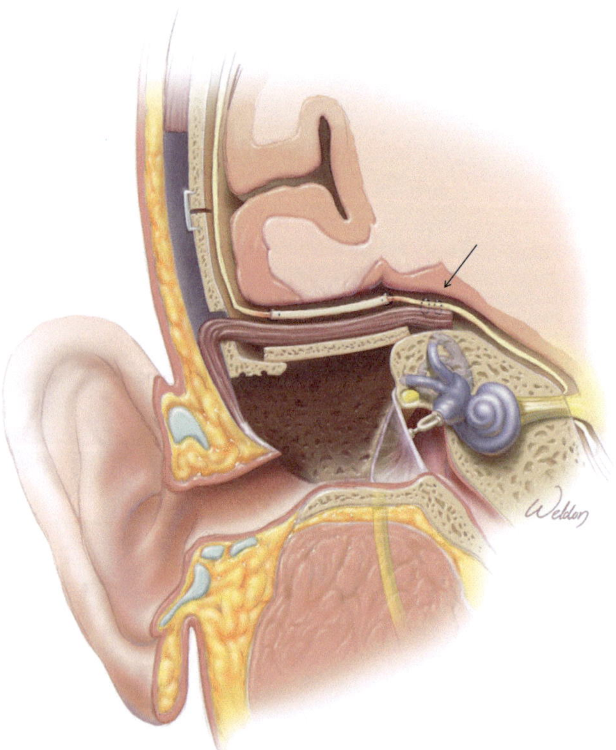

20. Case 1. Coronal CT of a patient with an idiopathic right temporal lobe encephalocele (*arrow*). She presented with CSF rhinorrhea and conductive hearing loss. Also, note the superior semicircular canal dehiscence (*arrowhead*), which is often found in patients with this condition.

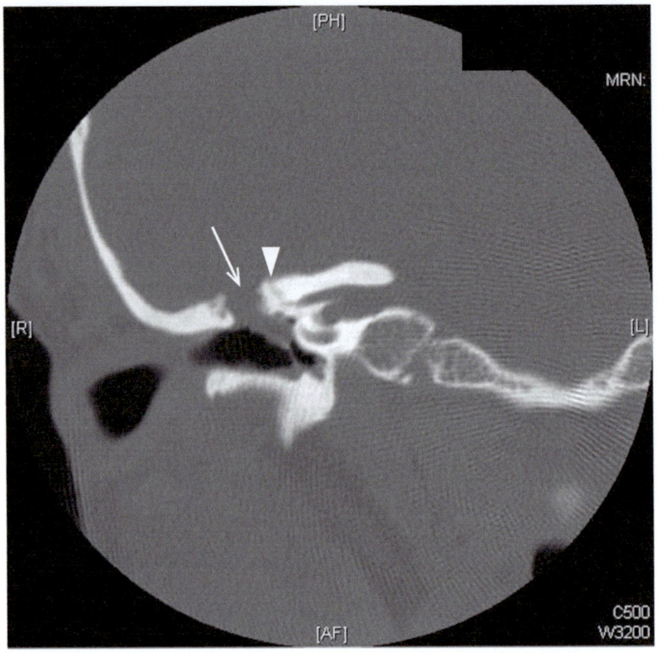

21. Coronal MRI demonstrates a very small encephalocele (*arrow*) on the left side.

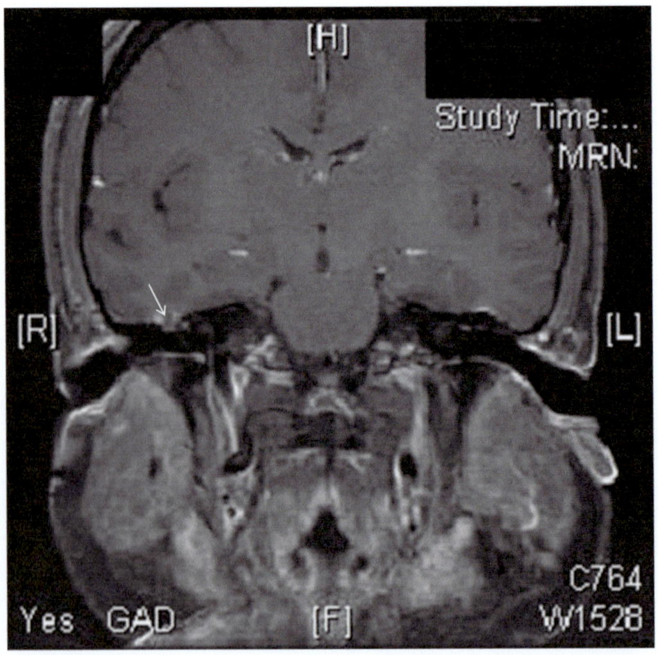

22. Only a middle fossa craniotomy was needed to reduce the encephalocele and repair this small skull base defect. Here, the surgeon is sitting at the head of the patient, and the temporal lobe is retracted by the malleable retractor in an extradural fashion. However, the small encephalocele is visible to the left of the retractor (*asterisk*). The defect in the temporal floor is clearly seen (*arrow*).

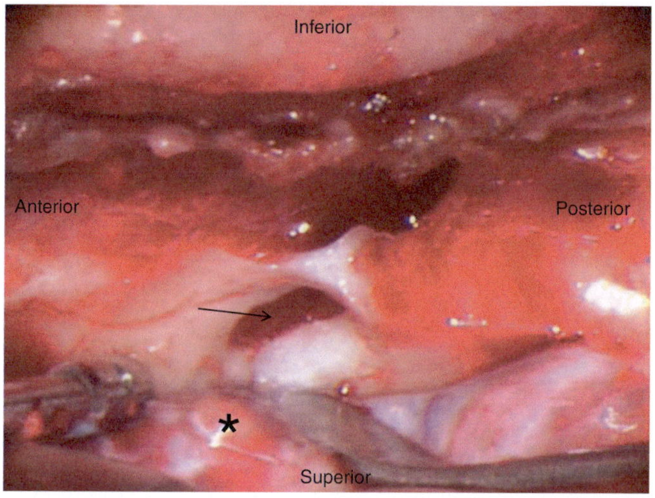

23. The encephalocele was reduced and the dura closed with a suture.

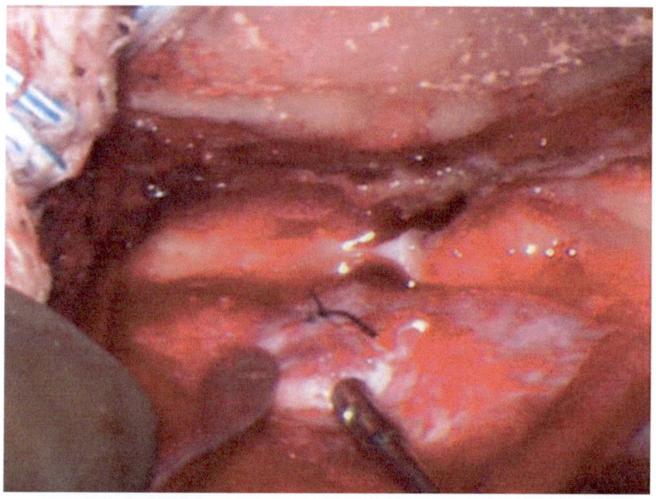

24. A bone graft was inset to cover the defect. This was the anterior half of the bone flap harvested during the craniotomy.

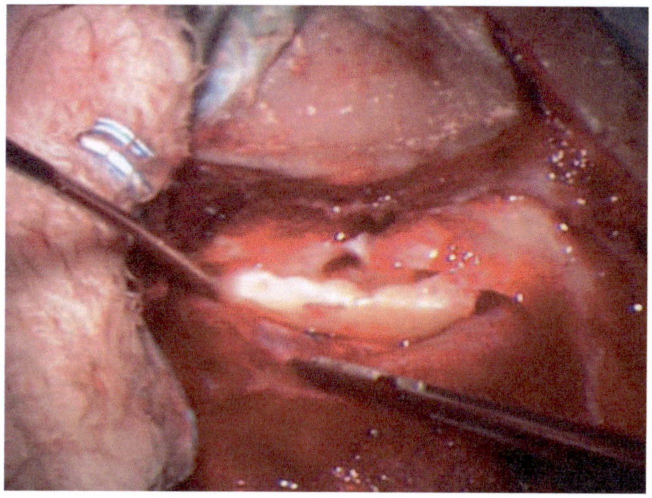

25. The posterior half of the temporalis muscle was then swung in between the bone and the dura (edges outlined by *arrows*) and the posterior half of the bone flap plated. The temporalis muscle bulk protects the anterior half of the craniotomy site where there is no bone. The temporalis muscle was sutured to the bone flap to hold it in position.

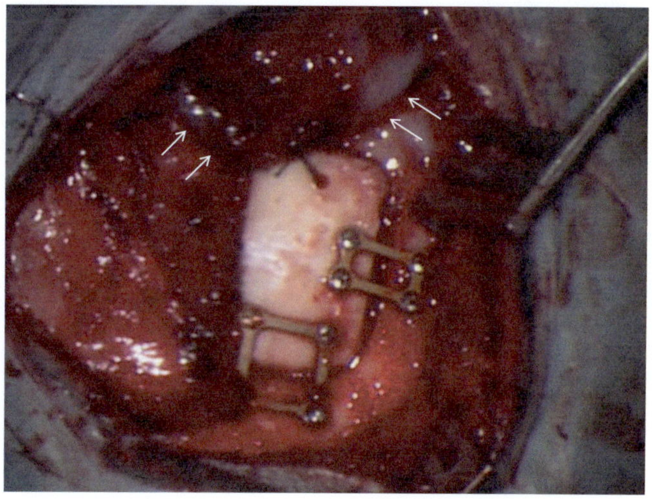

26. Case 2. Coronal CT scan demonstrates a larger left temporal lobe encephalocele (*arrow*).

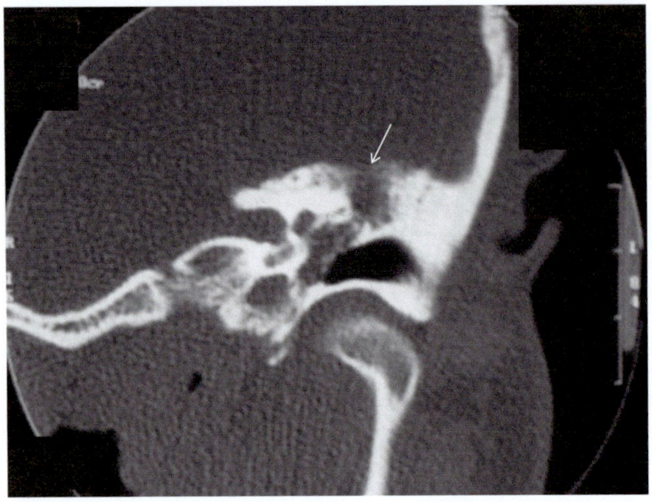

27. T2 coronal MRI demonstrates CSF penetration into the mastoid cavity (*arrow*).

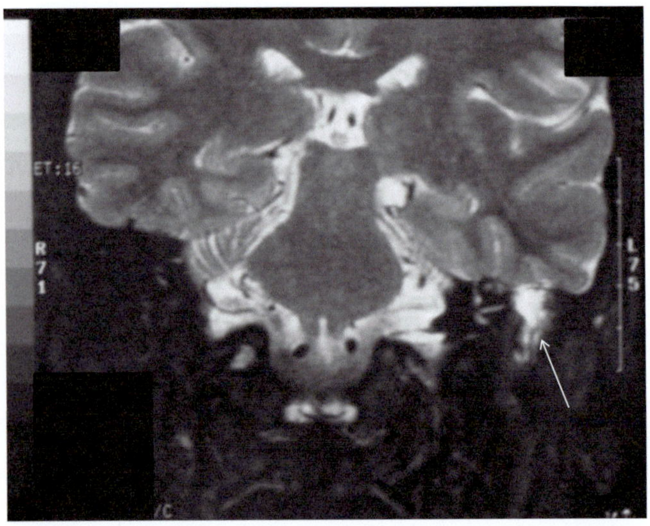

28. A mastoidectomy and middle fossa craniotomy were performed. The encephalocele was identified and resected using the bipolar to cauterize across the neck of the devitalized brain at the level of the tegmen and then dividing it with a microscissors. This revealed the defect in the temporal floor (tegmen; *arrow*).

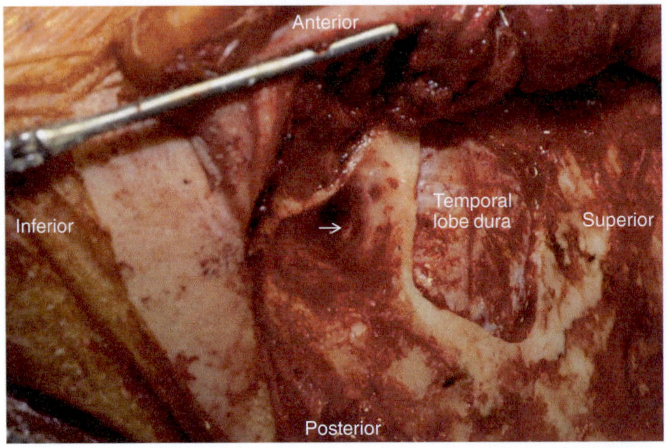

29. The temporal lobe was elevated and a bone graft inset to cover the defect.

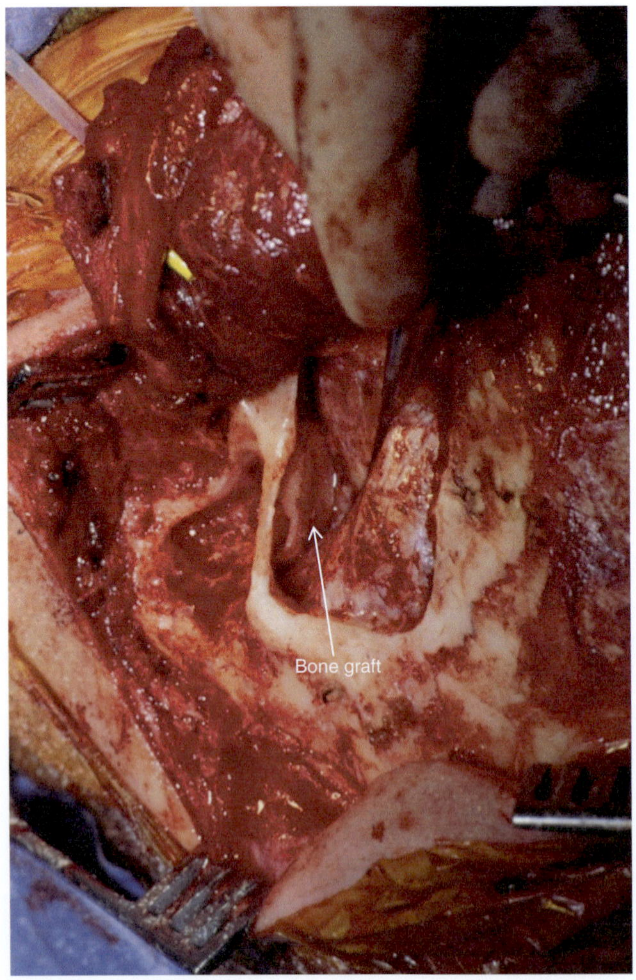

30. Because of the size of the defect and because the bone graft did not remain in a stable position, a titanium plate was used to fix the bone graft securely.

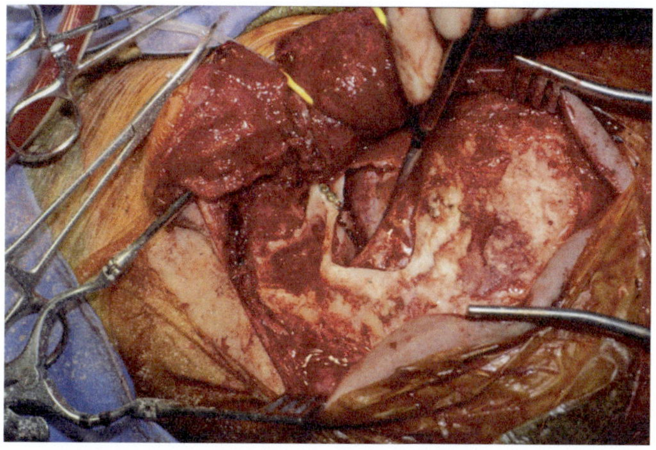

31. The posterior third of the temporalis muscle was then separated from the anterior portion of the muscle for use as a vascularized flap. It is being held up by the forceps.

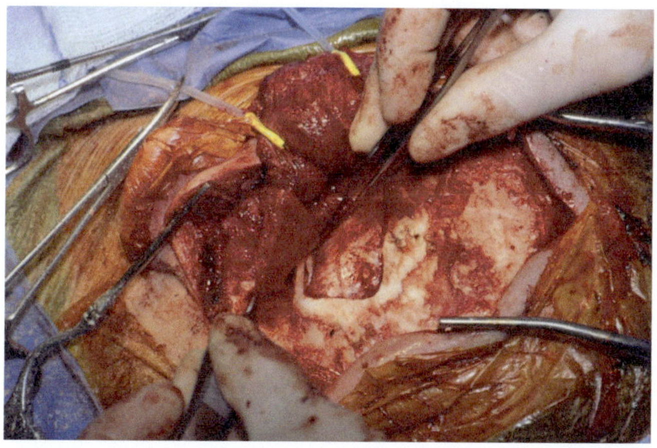

32. After insetting the flap through the inferior aspect of the craniectomy, the remaining bone was plated back. Because we needed a larger bone graft than typical, we used a piece of mesh in this case to cover most of the defect.

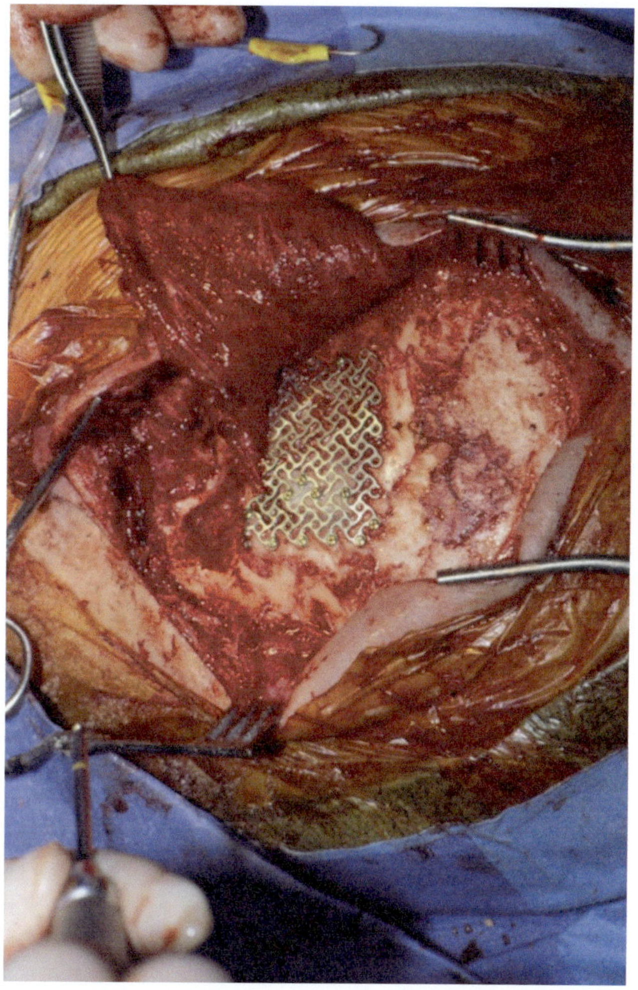

33. Case 3. A large meningocele protruding into the left mastoid (*arrows*). This patient presented with recurrent meningitis. The inflammation of the mastoid can be noted at the enhancement within the mastoid air cells on this coronal T1 MRI with gadolinium.

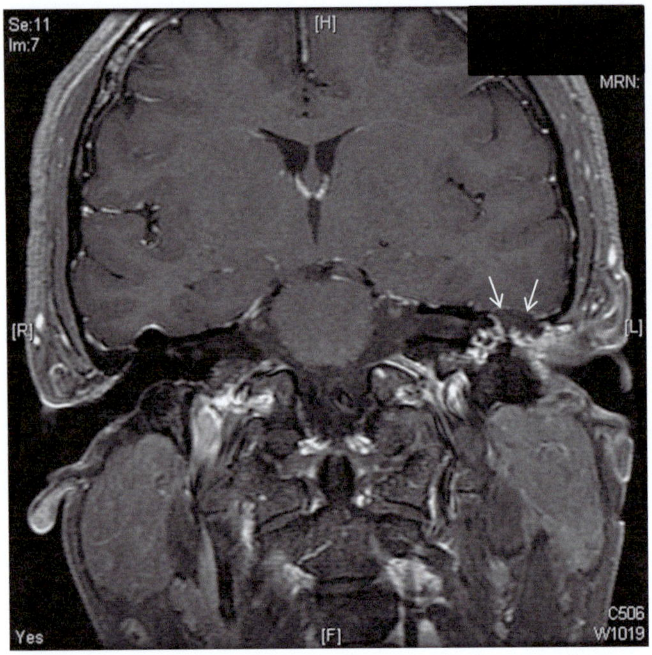

34. Axial view of the same patient demonstrating the large circular meningocele in the mastoid antrum (*arrows*). Surgical repair was performed using only a middle fossa approach.

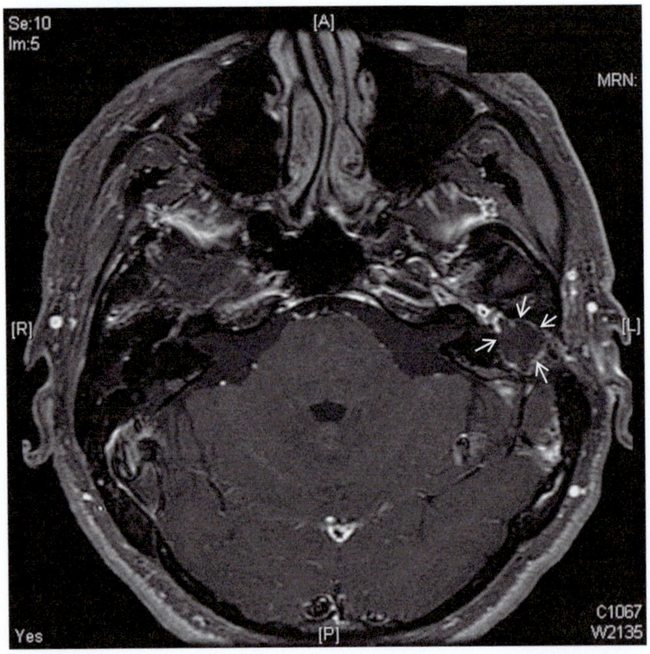

35. Case 4. A patient presenting with CSF rhinorrhea. Axial T2 MRI demonstrated that the mastoid, middle ear, and petrous apex were filled with fluid.

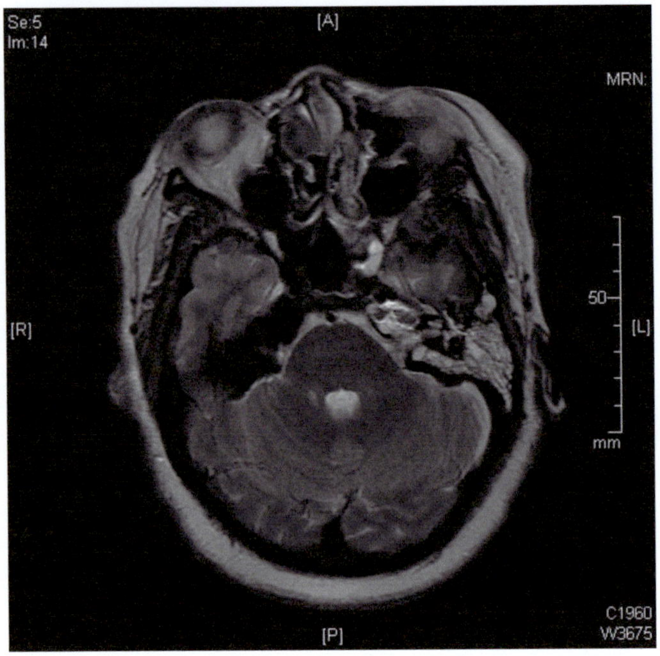

36. Coronal T1 MRI with gadolinium from the same patient demonstrates that the left temporal lobe was lower than the right temporal lobe. Also, the lining of the dura was inflamed (*arrows*).

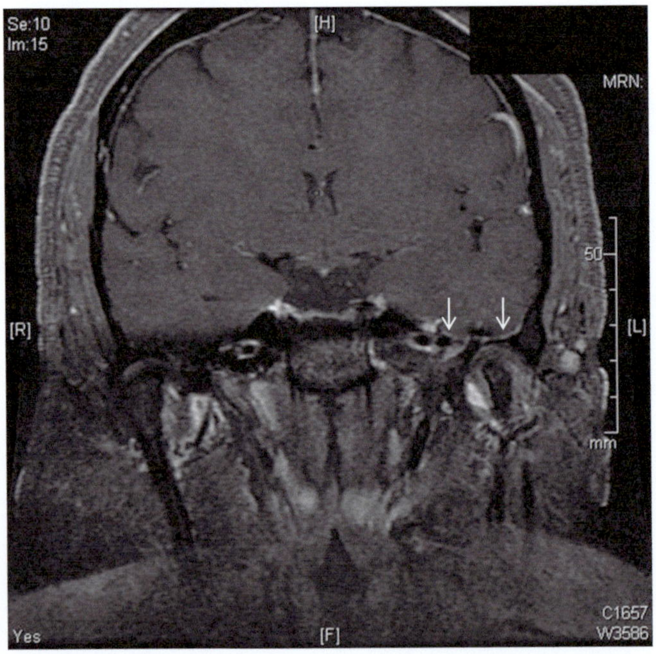

37. Sagittal T1 MRI from the same patient demonstrates flattening of the pituitary gland (*arrow*). This "empty sella" sign suggests the patient has intracranial hypertension and is often found in patients with idiopathic spontaneous temporal lobe encephalocele or CSF leak. A neuro-ophthalmology consult should be obtained to look for ocular manifestations of increased intracranial pressure.

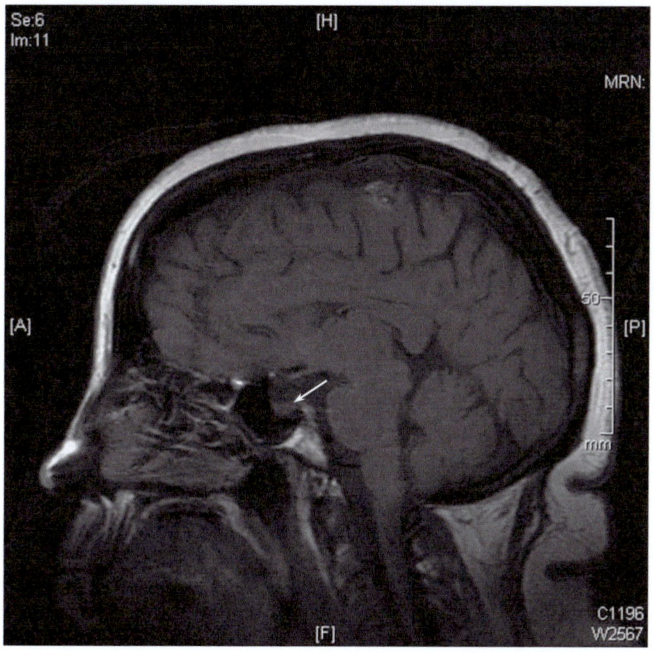

38. Case 5. Intraoperative photos from a patient with a right temporal lobe encephalocele into the middle ear causing conductive hearing loss. Because it was relatively small, only the middle fossa portion of the procedure needed to be performed. After performing a craniotomy, the temporal lobe dura was retracted superiorly by a malleable. The herniated brain is seen (*arrows*).

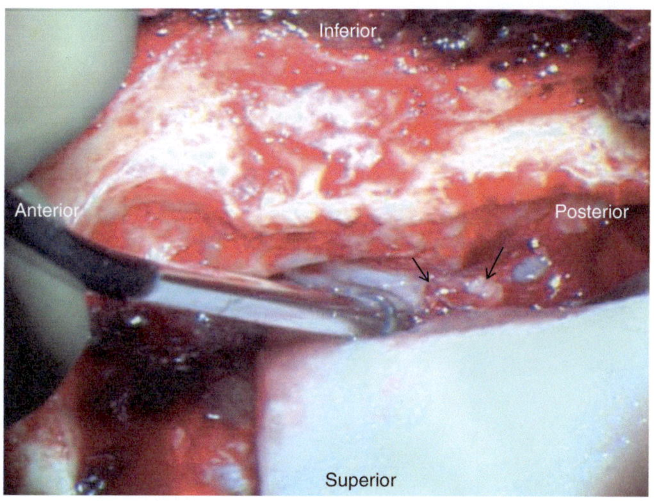

39. The encephalocele was divided at its neck and dissection continued medially. This patient also had superior semicircular canal dehiscence (the groove at the dome of the arcuate eminence; *arrows*).

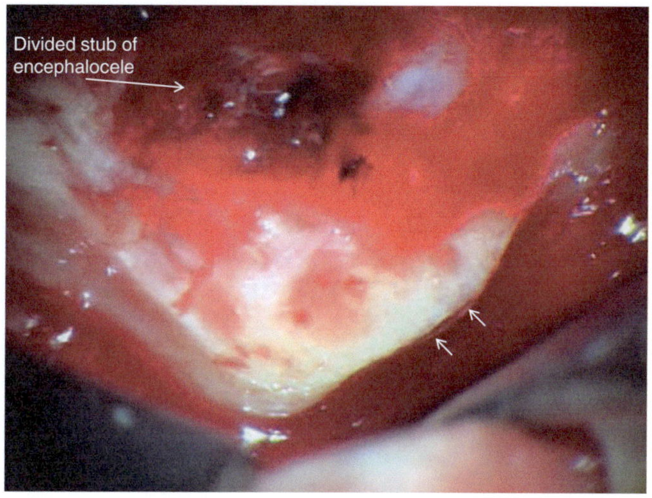

40. The encephalocele was microdissected out of the middle ear.

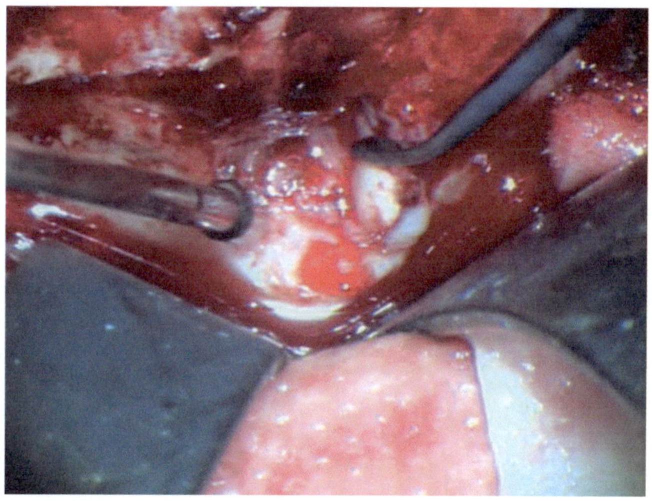

41. Removal of the encephalocele. Note that several patches of missing bone were connected together to improve access.

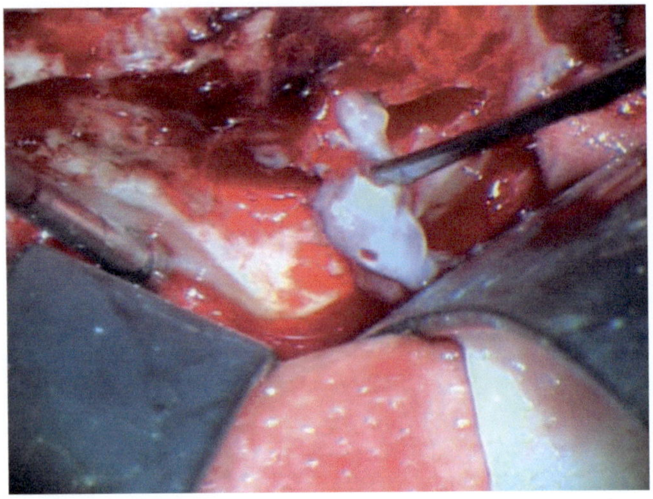

42. After removal of the encephalocele.

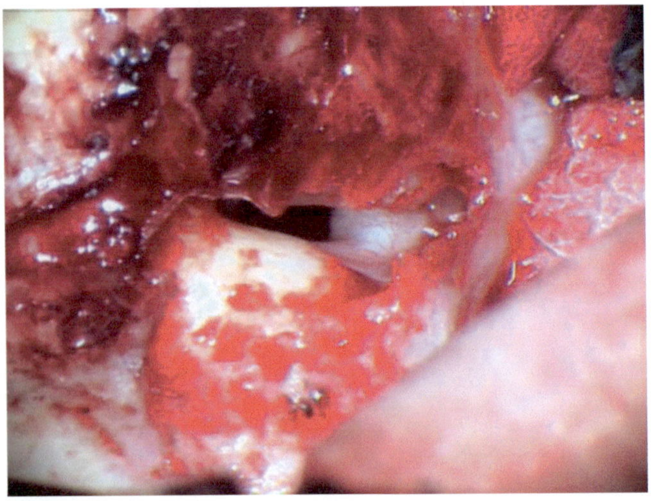

43. A piece of the bone flap was plated in place. Some pieces of Gelfoam were placed under the bone flap to help seal around the edges.

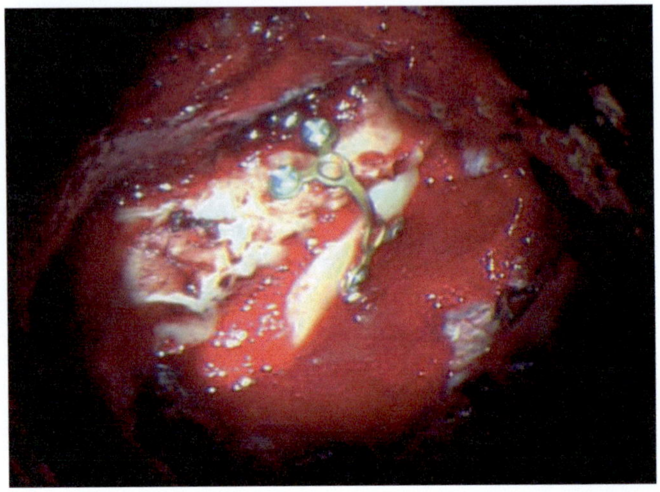

44. Case 6. A small right idiopathic temporal lobe encephalocele removed via the middle fossa approach. The craniotomy has been performed, the dura of the temporal lobe elevated, and the encephalocele truncated at its neck. The defect filled with the encephalocele is visible (*arrow*).

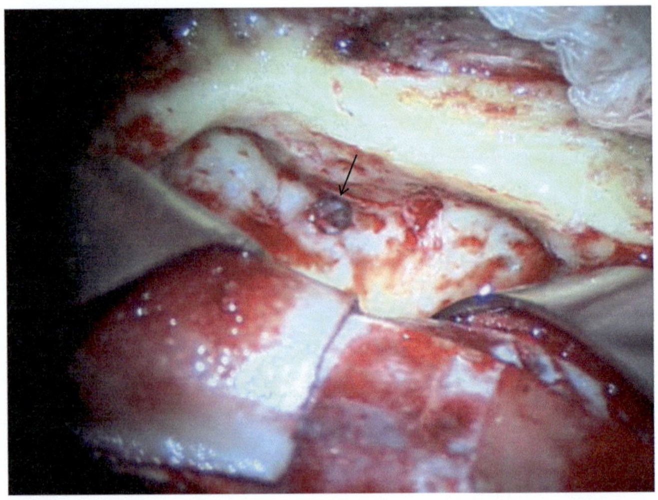

45. Microdissecting the encephalocele off the ossicular chain with a Rosen needle. The bony sheath covering the horizontal facial nerve is seen (*FN*).

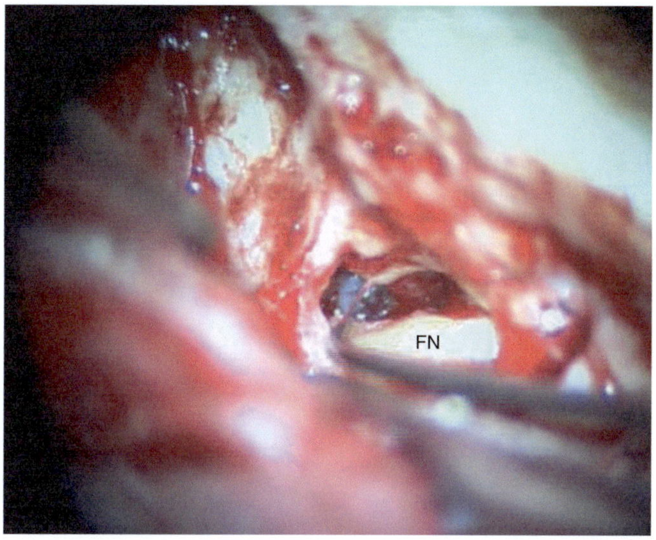

46. After removing the encephalocele, the stapedial tendon (*arrow*) and the incudostapedial joint (*arrowhead*) are visible.

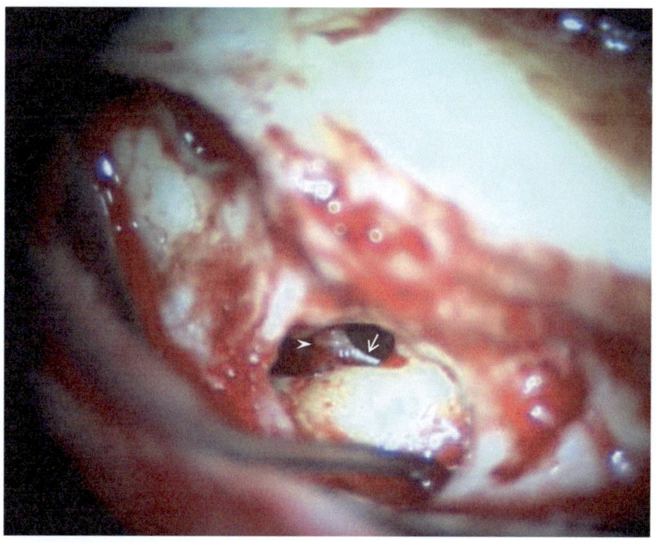

Repair of Superior Semicircular Canal Dehiscence

- *Concept*
  - Erosion of the bone of the temporal floor into the superior semicircular canal. This creates a "third window" whereby loud sounds evoke vertigo when the sound pressure wave passes through the vestibular system.
- *Conditions treated*
  - Superior semicircular canal dehiscence
- *Risks*
  - Injury to the temporal lobe such as contusion, edema, or vascular compromise
  - Temporal lobe seizure
  - Aphasia
  - Hearing loss and dizziness
  - Facial nerve injury, typically if the geniculate ganglion is dehiscent and not recognized
  - Dry eye if the greater superficial petrosal nerve is transected
  - Recurrence
  - CSF leak
- *Benefits*
  - Direct view of the dehiscence of the superior semicircular canal
- *Additional notes*
  - Superior semicircular canal dehiscence can be treated by resurfacing (rebuilding the tegmen), plugging both limbs of the canal, or a combination of both. Current literature suggests that the recurrence risk is lowest when canal plugging is performed, although there is likely to be a higher risk of sensorineural hearing loss. We prefer to perform both techniques in combination.
  - It is also possible to repair this defect via a transmastoid approach, although at the time of writing this atlas, the authors have not had extensive experience with this technique.
  - Most fistulas are located on the most superior aspect of the canal, and thus the middle fossa approach provides the best access, and it is probably the most reliable way to achieve a good repair. For fistulas located along the superior petrosal sinus, we may use a transmastoid approach.

47. The incision. This is the same incision used for a temporal lobe encephalocele, but since only a middle fossa craniotomy is needed, the inferior extent is shortened.

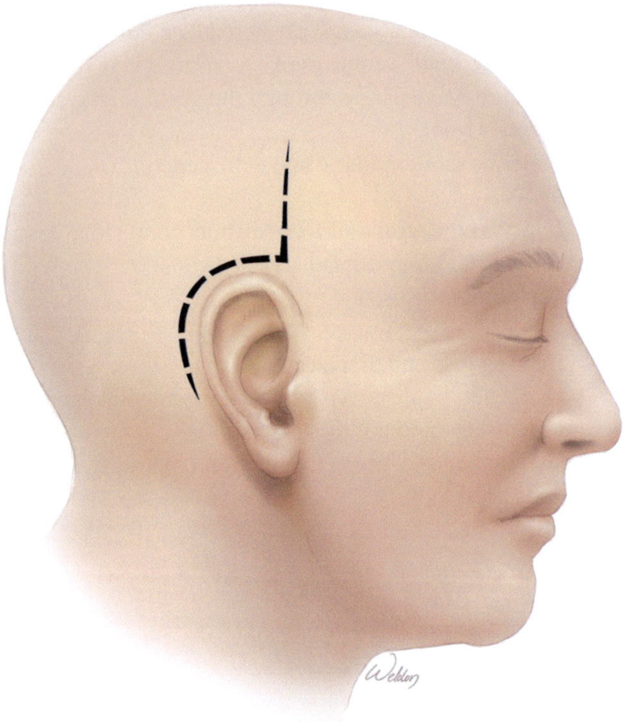

48. The temporalis muscle is reflected off the skull and a standard middle fossa craniotomy opening performed (fully described in Chap. 3). The surgeon sits at the top of the patient's head. The external auditory canal (*EAC*) and the burr holes (*BH*) are shown.

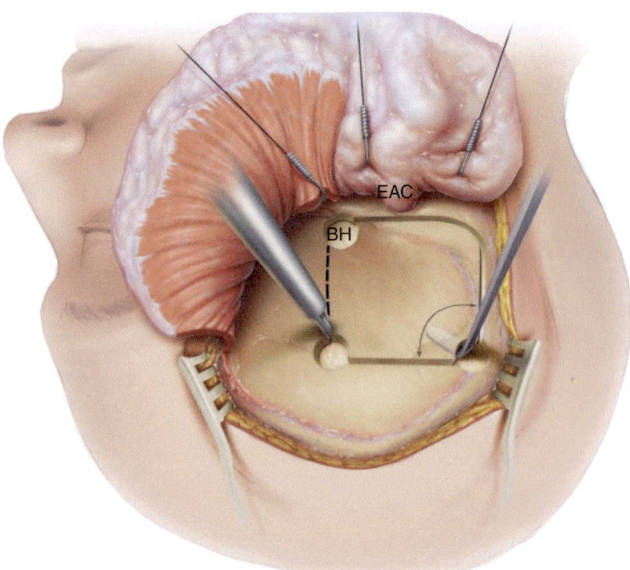

49. The dura is elevated off the temporal floor to the petrous ridge. A right superior semicircular canal dehiscence is shown. This is then plugged and/or resurfaced as described below.

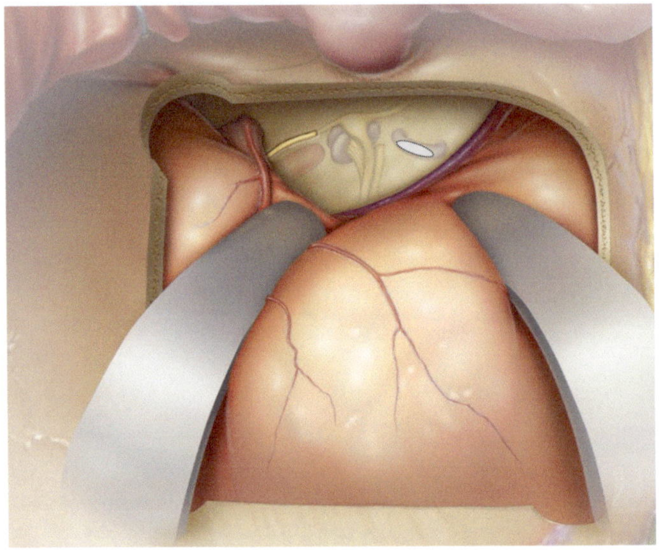

50. Case 1. A patient with symptomatic left semicircular canal dehiscence is undergoing repair. In this case, a linear skin incision with vertical division of the temporalis muscle was performed. A bone flap was then turned and removed.

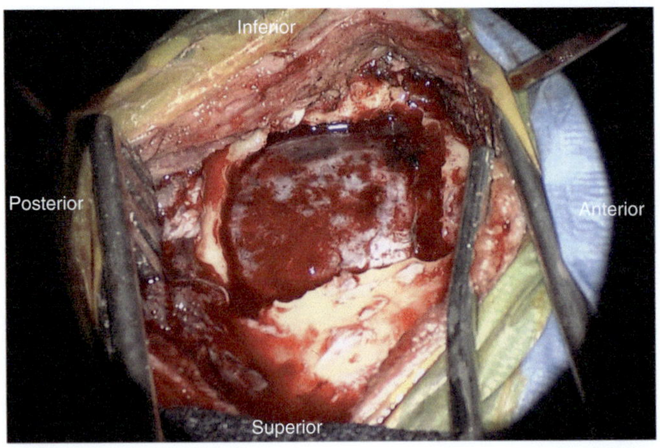

51. Elevation of the temporal dura from the tegmen was performed with a Joseph elevator. Identify the superior petrosal sinus first as this will orient you to the expected location of the fistula. Before elevating across the fistula, we dissect anteriorly across the geniculate region and greater superficial petrosal nerve and then come across the arcuate eminence and fistula. This allows the surgeon to keep the suction deeper in the dissection toward the petrous apex and well away from the fistula.

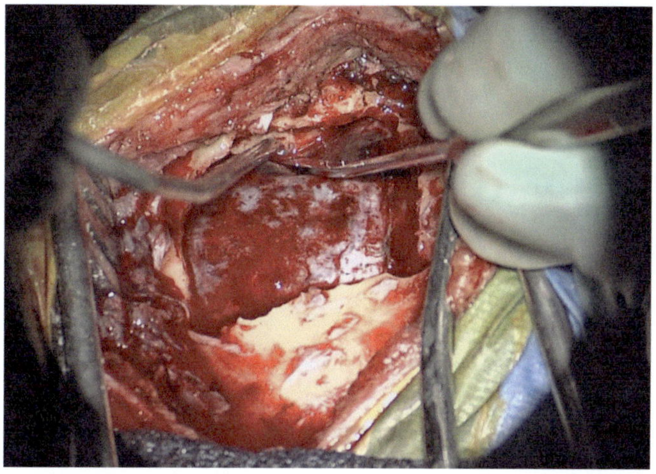

52. Malleable retractors can be used to help expose the floor. Note the cottonoid in the left side of the craniotomy. This is lying over a piece of Surgicel and is used to control venous bleeding from the junction of the transverse and sigmoid sinuses.

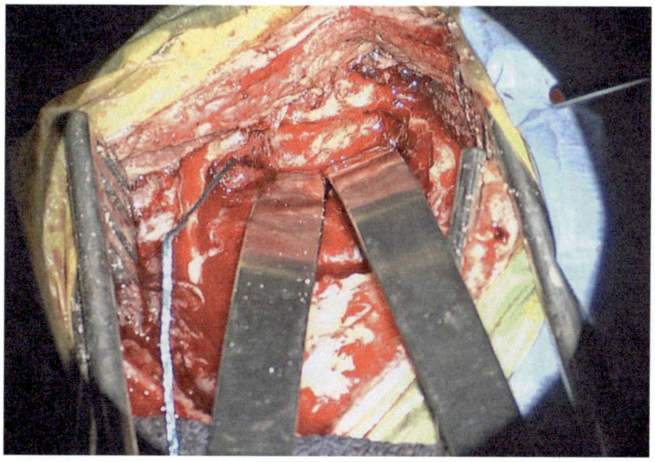

53. The arcuate eminence is the upward bulging of the superior semicircular canal, and the dehiscence can be seen at its vertex (*Rosen needle is pointing to it*). When operating for semicircular canal dehiscence, no further exposure is needed. Resurfacing and/or plugging of the canal can then be performed.

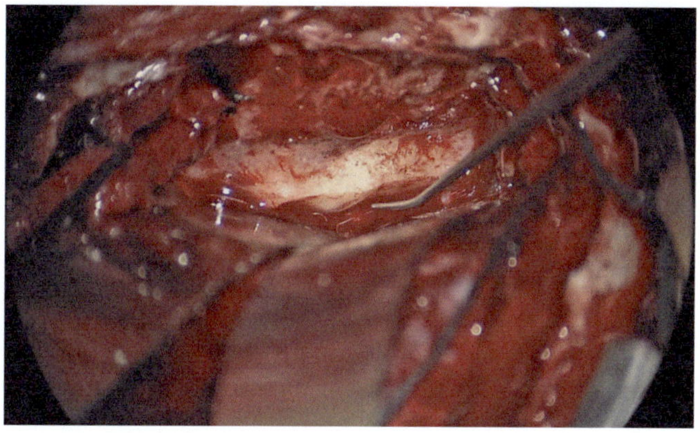

54. We took a small piece of temporalis fascia (*held by the Rosen needle*) and gently inserted it into the anterior limb of the dehiscent semicircular canal. Another piece was inserted into the posterior limb. This plugging of the canal has the potential to disrupt the membranous labyrinth and potentially create sensorineural hearing loss. Thus, plugging should be performed very gently.

Another option to repair the fistula after exposure is to initially occlude the canal with bone wax (slowly and carefully). Once this is done, the inner ear should be protected, and additional layers of fascia and bone can be placed to provide additional levels of barrier.

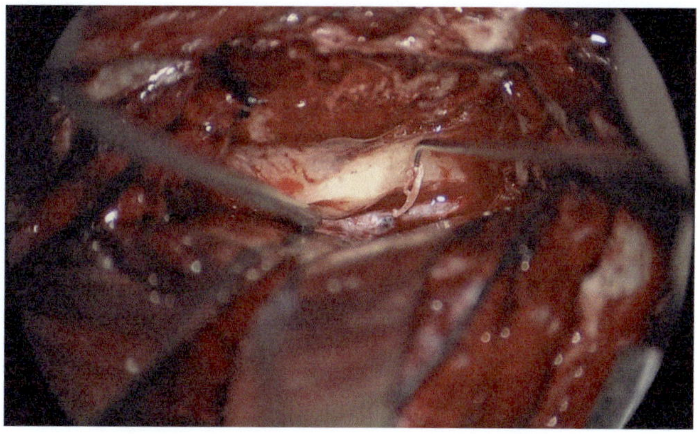

55. After plugging, the back ends of the two pieces of fascia can be seen filling the dehiscence (*arrow*).

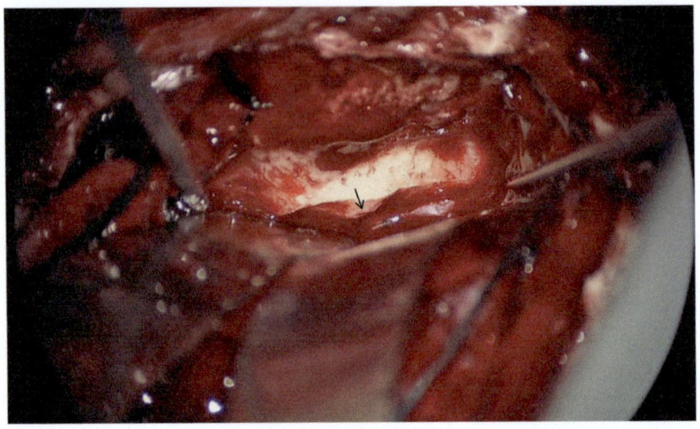

56. While a bone graft can be used to resurface the tegmen as in the repair of an encephalocele, this small defect does not require as much structural integrity. In this example, we used a hydroxyapatite bone paste instead of a bone graft to cover the defect in an effort to minimize the risk of symptom recurrence.

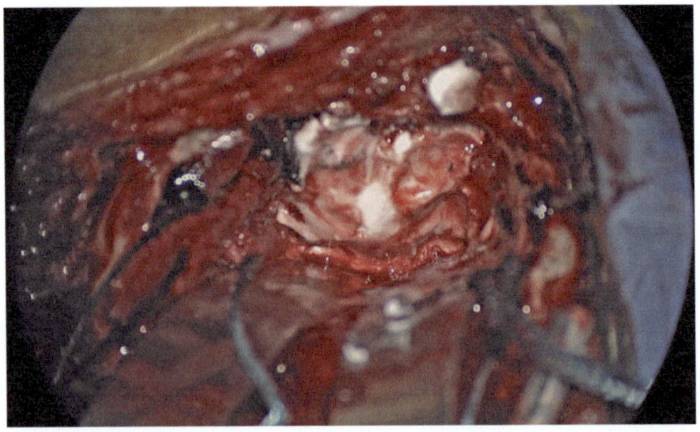

Temporal Bone Resection

- *Concept*
  - A lateral temporal bone resection is used to resect tumors of the ear canal and mastoid that do not penetrate medial to the tympanic membrane.
  - A total temporal bone resection is reserved for tumors that invade medial to the tympanic membrane.
- *Conditions treated*
  - Skin cancer involving the ear canal
  - Parotid malignancies that involve the temporal bone
  - Skull base osteomyleitis refractory to more conservative management techniques such as long-term intravenous antibiotics, mastoidectomy, and circumferential petrosectomy
  - Osteoradionecrosis of the temporal bone refractory to local care
  - Huge tumors of the skull base
- *Risks*
  - Hearing loss
  - Facial nerve injury
  - Taste disturbance
  - Malocclusion
  - Chronic temporomandibular joint pain
- *Benefits*
  - Permits complete resection of tumors limited to the ear canal.
  - Closure of the ear canal with temporalis muscle vascularized flap reconstruction permits radiation to the area without chronic otorrhea due to osteoradionecrosis.
  - A total temporal bone resection with facial nerve sacrifice provides tremendous access to the largest of skull base tumors. Most of the side and bottom of the head can be accessed with this approach.
- *Additional notes*
  - Patients undergoing a temporal bone resection commonly require postoperative XRT. Thus, it is important to plan for this. Leaving the patient with a mastoid bowl is often regretted because after radiation, chronic inflammation, osteoradionecrosis, and otorrhea frequently develop. Hearing can be rehabilitated with a bone-conducting device when the inner ear is preserved.
  - Instead, we close the ear canal and Eustachian tube and usually rotate a pedicled temporalis flap into the defect.
  - Hearing can be rehabilitated with a bone-conducting device when the inner ear is preserved.

57. A *sleeve resection* is rarely performed and is reserved only for tumors of the cartilaginous canal (*dotted lines*). If the cancer extends into the bony ear canal, a lateral temporal bone resection is indicated.

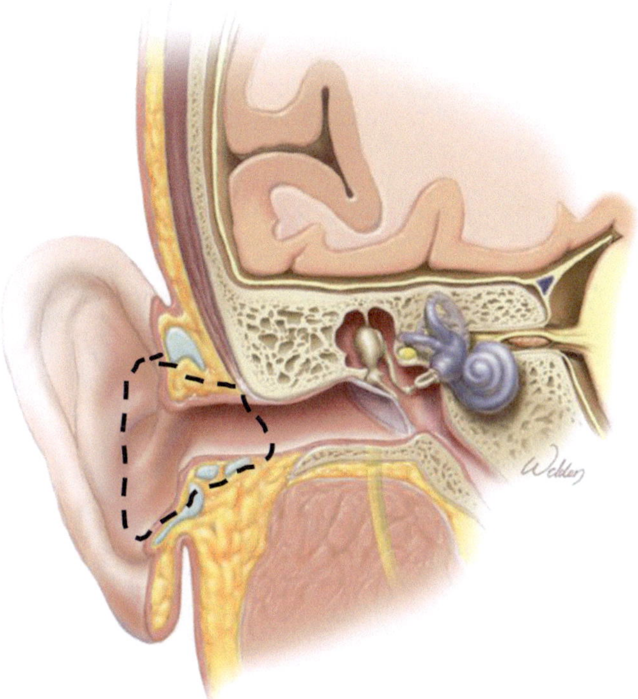

58. A *lateral temporal bone resection* is for tumors of the ear canal and/or mastoid that do not extend medial to the tympanic membrane. Overview of the bone to be removed (*gray*). The facial nerve may be resected or spared depending on its degree of involvement.

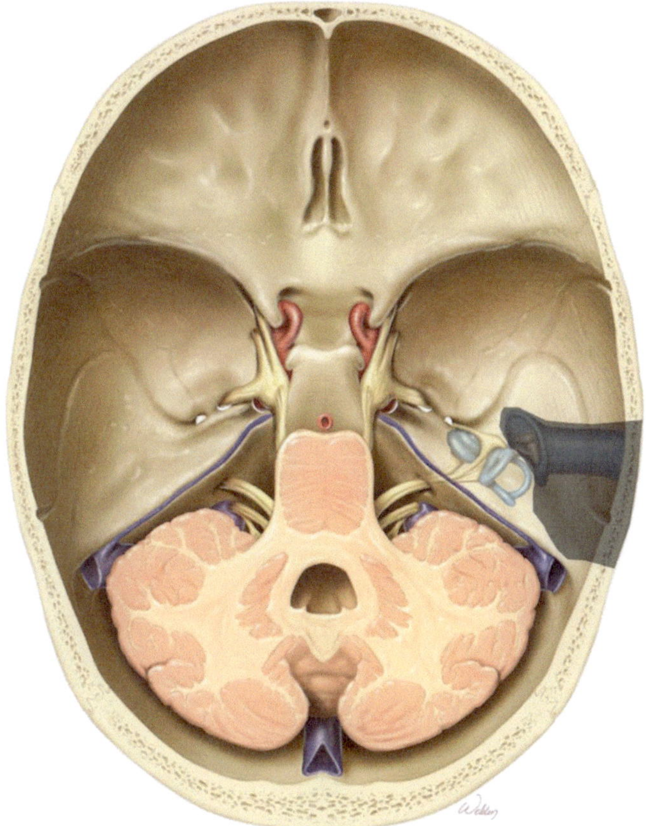

59. A *total temporal bone resection* is for tumors of the ear canal and/or mastoid that do extend medial to the tympanic membrane. Overview of the bone to be removed (*gray*). This procedure is the same as a transcochlear approach, although the dura does not need to be opened unless it is involved with tumor. The facial nerve may be resected or spared depending on its degree of involvement.

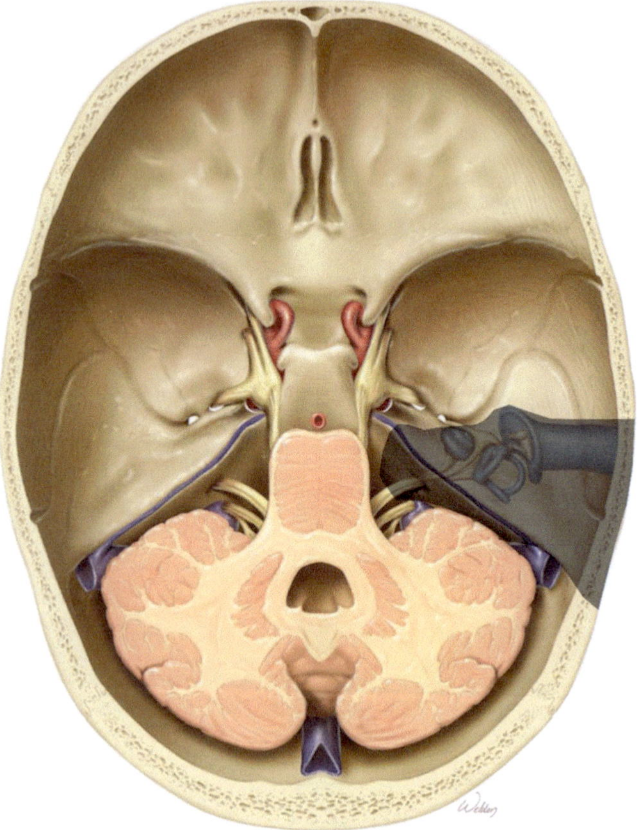

60. The surgical procedure for a lateral temporal bone resection for a small tumor confined to the bony ear canal is depicted in these illustrations. There is a post-auricular incision. Also, a separate skin incision courses around the ear canal meatus lateral to the tumor.

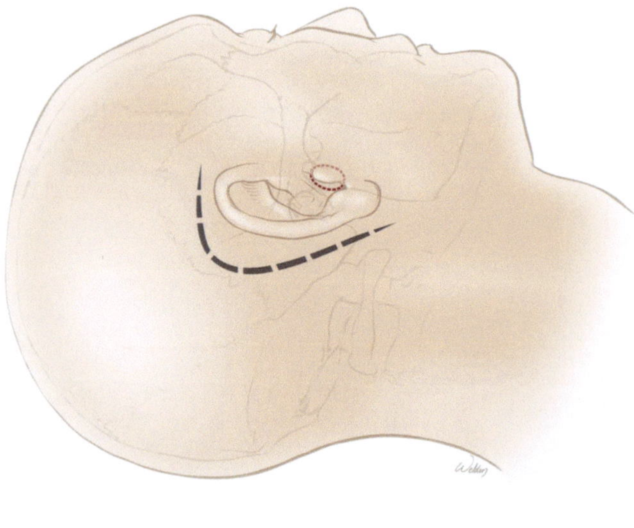

61. The pinna is elevated in a subperiosteal fashion. The ear canal is completely separated from the pinna using the previously made cut at the meatus. The ear canal skin can be sutured closed to separate the operative field from the tumor inside the ear canal.

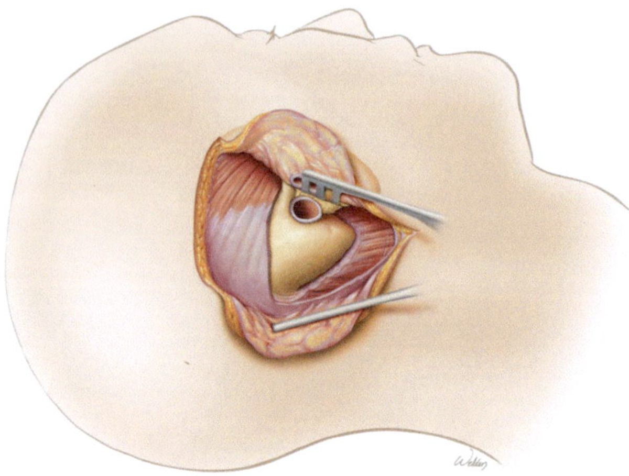

62. A standard canal wall up mastoidectomy is then drilled.

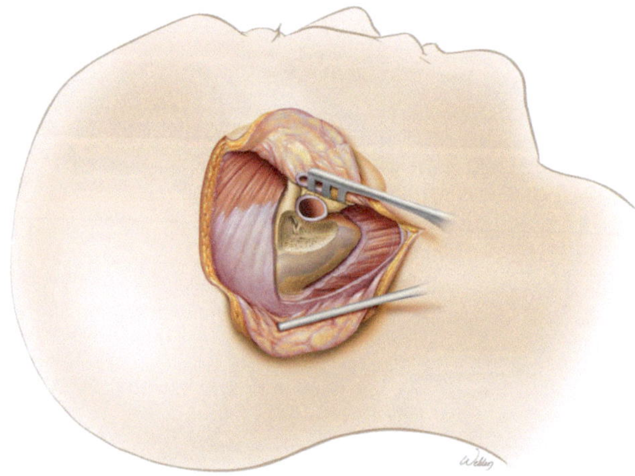

63. Then, an extended facial recess approach is performed. This means that the facial recess is opened, the chorda tympani nerve sectioned (*Ch*), and the facial nerve (*F*) traced out inferiorly. The incudostapedial joint should be divided through the facial recess as shown using a sickle knife or small Beaver blade (the #5910 works well). Then, drilling is continued to create troughs superior and inferior to the ear canal. The anterior border for each trough is the temporomandibular joint (*TMJ*). The goal is to drill around the ear canal, leaving a bony margin around it that will be removed with the tumor.

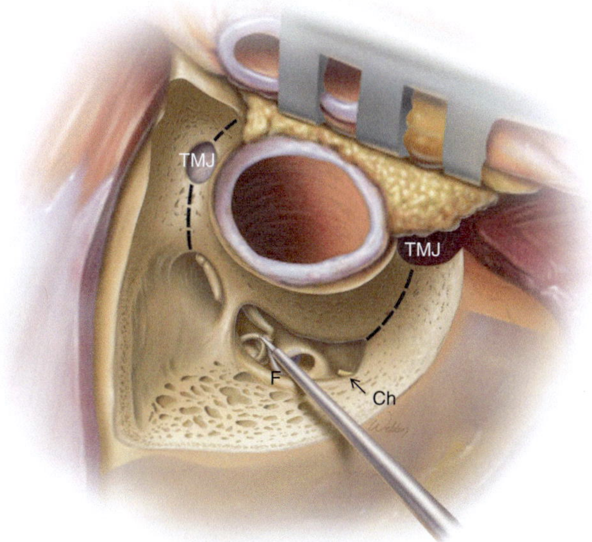

64. The incus is removed and the tensor tympani tendon (*TT*) divided. The soft tissues of the parotid, TMJ, and infratemporal fossa are dissected free of the anterior ear canal bone. By staying close to the ear canal bone, the facial nerve will not be at risk, and so this can be done with a knife, bovie, and/or bipolar cautery. Finally, the surgeon gently pushes the ear canal forward with his/her thumb to crack the remaining bone at the anterior lip. This takes only minimal pressure if adequate drilling was performed. The specimen is then removed *en bloc*.

To plug the Eustachian tube, first the mucosa inside the Eustachian tube must be denuded and/or inverted. Then, a piece of temporalis muscle is inserted into the Eustachian tube to help it to scar shut. Finally, several pea-sized pieces of bone wax are pressed into the Eustachian tube using a ½ inch cottonoid pledget to create a smooth contour as shown.

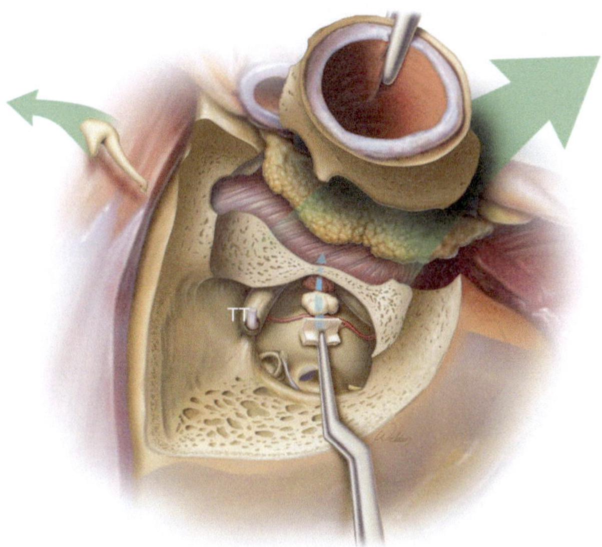

65. The external ear canal must be closed off. The cartilage of the ear canal is removed, permitting the skin edges to be everted out of the ear canal. The ear canal is then closed with interrupted sutures (*1*). The subcutaneous tissues on the medial side of the ear canal are closed with interrupted sutures (*2*). A flap of periosteum can also be used to provide a three-layer closure of the ear canal (*3*).

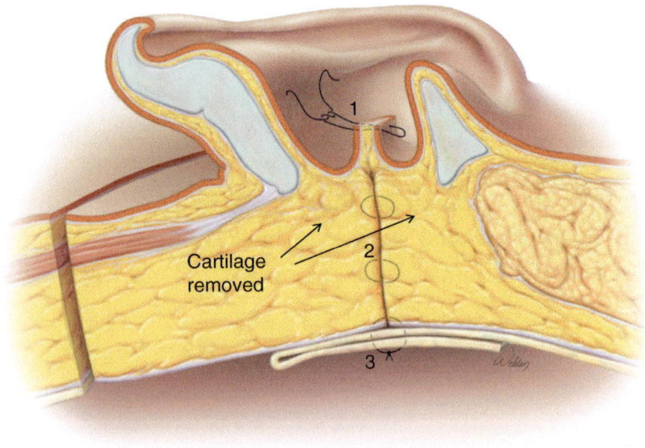

66. Case 1. A large fungating SCCA of the ear. A total auriculectomy was performed together with a lateral temporal bone resection and total parotidectomy. A vascularized myocutaneous flap was used for reconstruction.

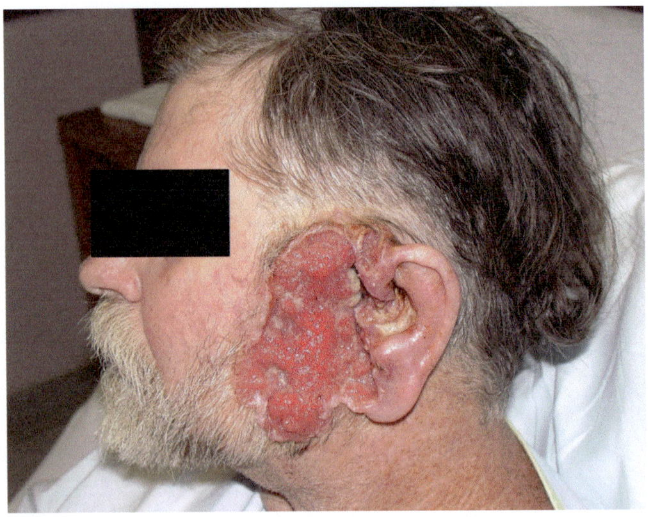

67. Case 2. A patient with chronic left otorrhea refractory to otic antimicrobial drops. Biopsy of a mass deep within the left ear canal revealed a SCCA. The patient had profound sensorineural hearing loss in that ear but normal facial nerve function.

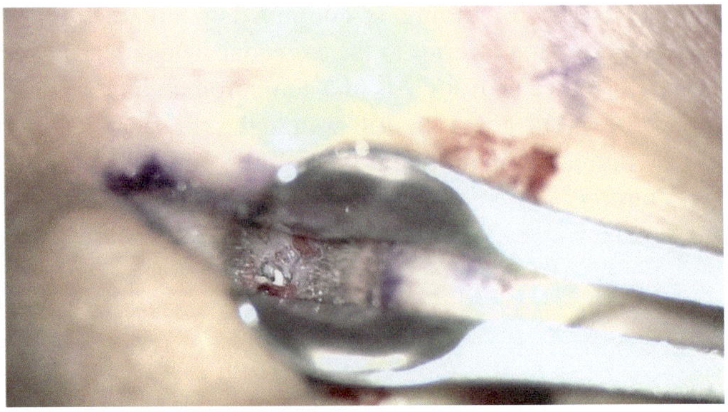

68. Axial CT demonstrated extensive bone erosion of the left temporal bone. An MRI could not be performed because the patient had a pacemaker.

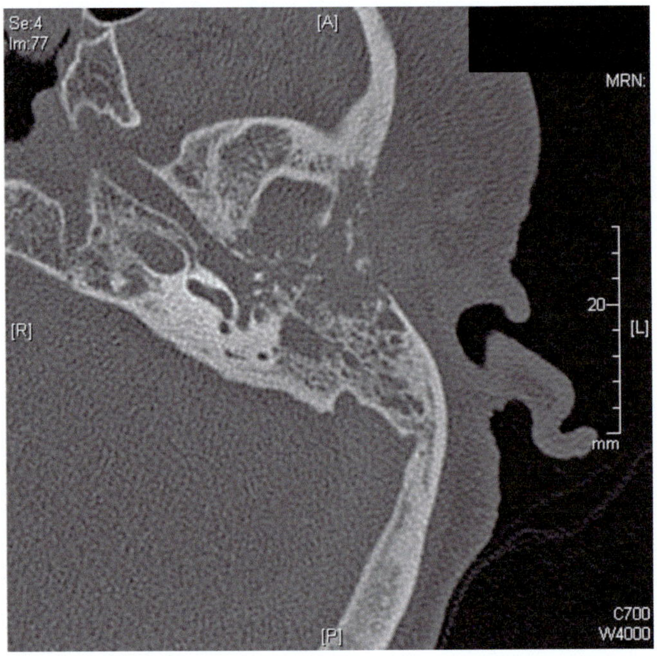

69. The coronal CT image demonstrated that the tumor eroded the tegmen (*arrow*). There was also invasion through the otic capsule bone into the superior semicircular canal (not shown).

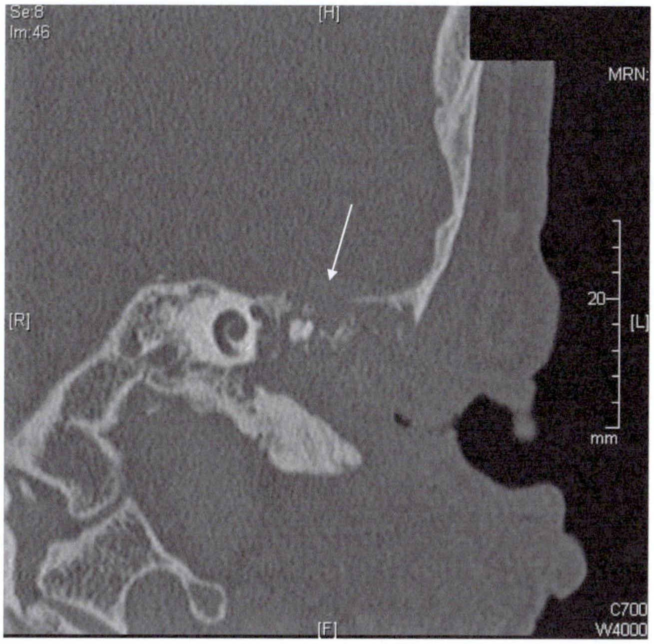

70. CT with contrast demonstrated enhancement consistent with tumor extension into the middle cranial fossa (*arrows*).

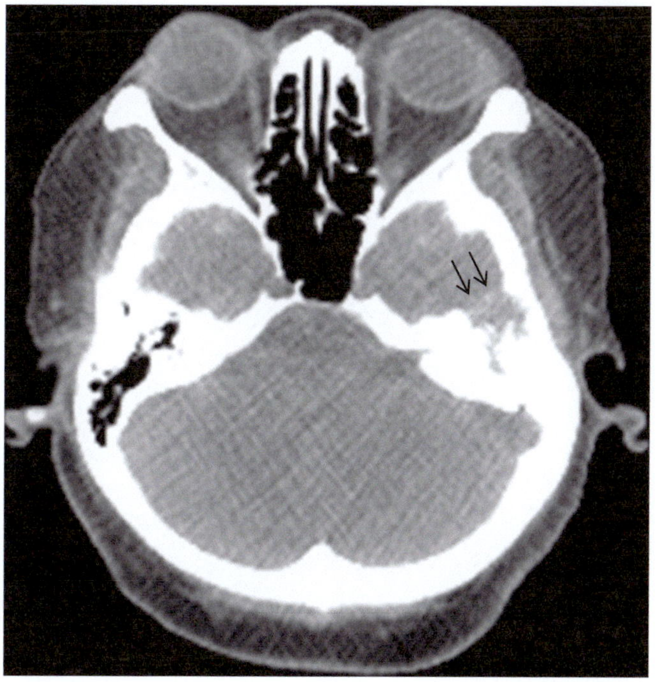

71. Surgical resection was indicated. Because the pinna was uninvolved, the lateral incision was the meatus of the ear canal (*purple circle*).

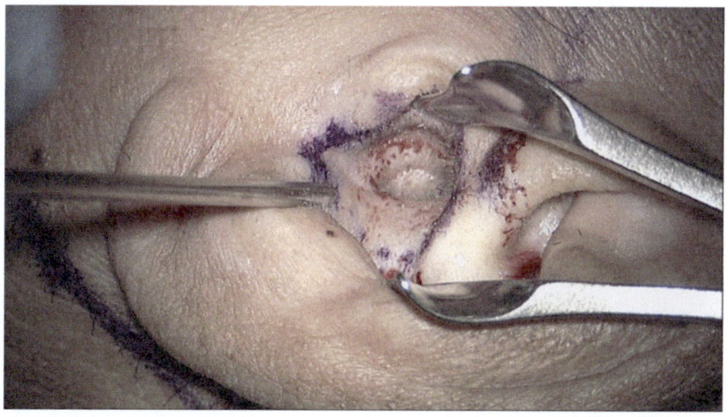

72. The skin incision was outlined. This was designed to access not only to the mastoid and temporalis muscle but also to the middle cranial fossa. The tape at the back of the head was used to prevent hair from getting into the wound during surgical preparation.

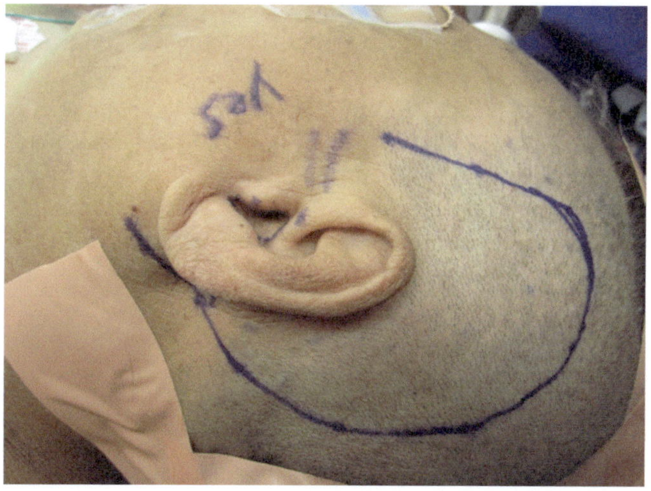

73. The skin incision was made, the ear canal transected laterally at the marked site, and the skin flap elevated to the parotid gland (under the gauze). As shown here, the temporalis muscle is being elevated as a separate flap for use in reconstruction. In order to increase the length of the flap, the periosteum over the mastoid (*P*) was left attached to the temporalis muscle.

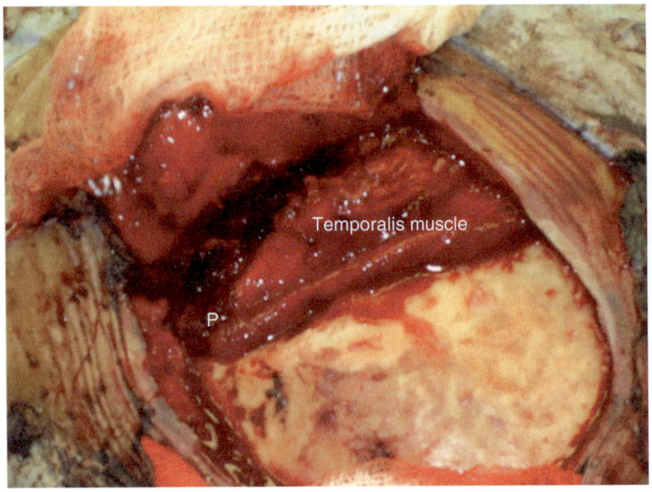

74. A standard canal wall up mastoidectomy was performed. The tumor extending from the ear canal superiorly through the attic and zygomatic air cells into the middle cranial fossa was divided. This allowed the resection to be performed in three steps. First, the temporal bone resection was performed. Second, the rest of the temporal bone was drilled out to remove the tumor invading into the inner ear. Third, the tumor invading the middle cranial fossa was resected. While conceptually it would be ideal to remove the tumor en bloc, in practice skull base surgery can rarely be performed this way because of the damage it would cause to the normal surrounding structures. Removing a portion of the tumor often provides the necessary exposure to be able to safely remove the rest of the tumor.

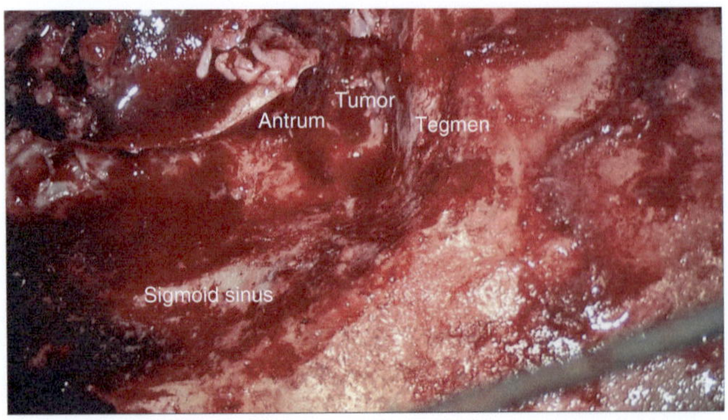

75. The extended facial recess was performed and the trough inferior to the ear canal drilled as shown.

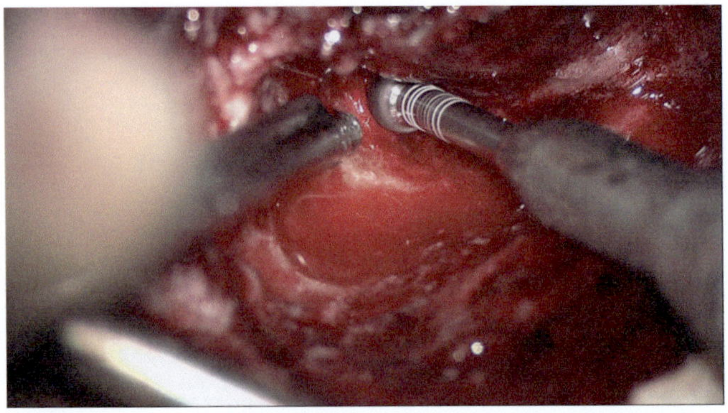

76. After completion of both troughs, the soft tissues anterior to the ear canal (i.e., the parotid gland) were divided with a 15 blade scalpel. Care must be taken to prevent injury to the frontal branch of the facial nerve in this region. This is done by dissecting close to the anterior side of the tragal cartilage and bony ear canal.

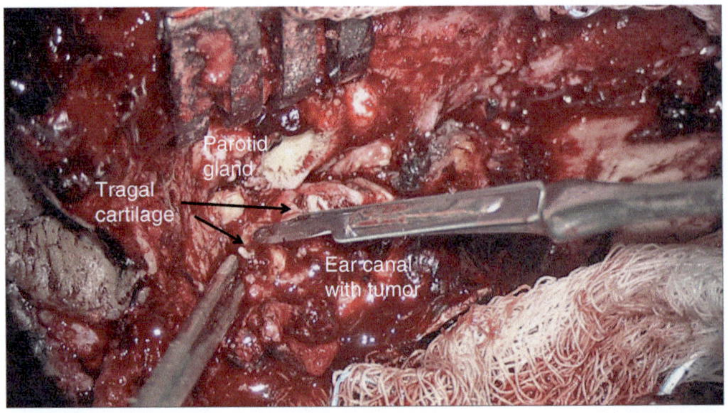

77. An Allis clamp was used to control the specimen while the deep tissues anterior to the ear canal were divided to remove the specimen. A chisel can be used to make the vertical split in the anterior bony ear canal. However, in practice, if appropriate drilling has been performed, the bone usually just cracks free with gentle manipulation. This completed the lateral temporal bone resection.

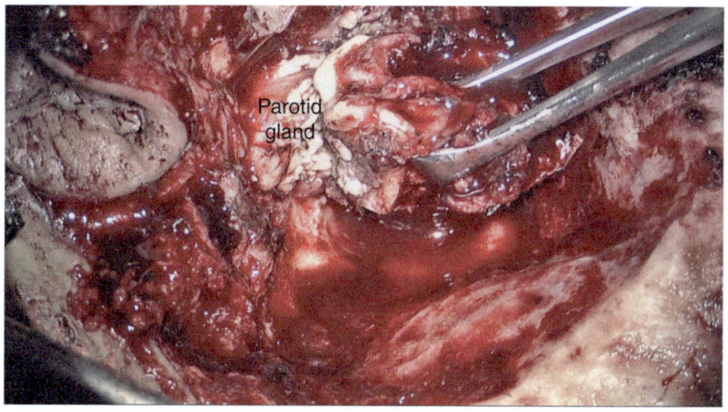

78. Then, the rest of the temporal bone was removed to address the tumor invasion into the inner ear. The lateral and superior semicircular canals were drilled away, revealing obvious tumor within the ampulla of the superior canal (*arrow*). The ridge of bone in the center of the image is the horizontal portion of the facial nerve (*asterisks*). The tumor was found to extend into the vestibule.

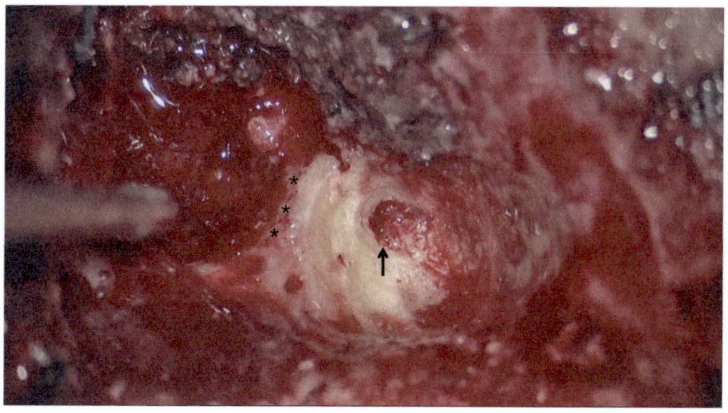

79. A transcochlear approach was then performed to remove all tumor within the vestibule and potentially the cochlea. The horizontal facial nerve was left within its fallopian canal, and as shown here, a crabtree dissector demonstrates the fallopian bridge. Also shown is the cochlea in midresection after being opened (*arrow*).

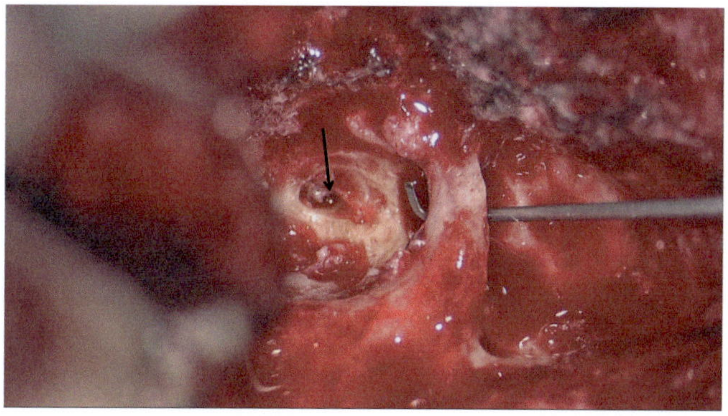

80. The internal structures of the cochlea were then dissected. As seen, one cochlear turn is being removed. The basilar membrane (*BM*) is the darker-appearing region between the white osseous spiral lamina (*OSL*) and the gray spiral ligament (*SL*). After removing the semicircular canals, vestibule, and cochlea, the total temporal bone resection was complete.

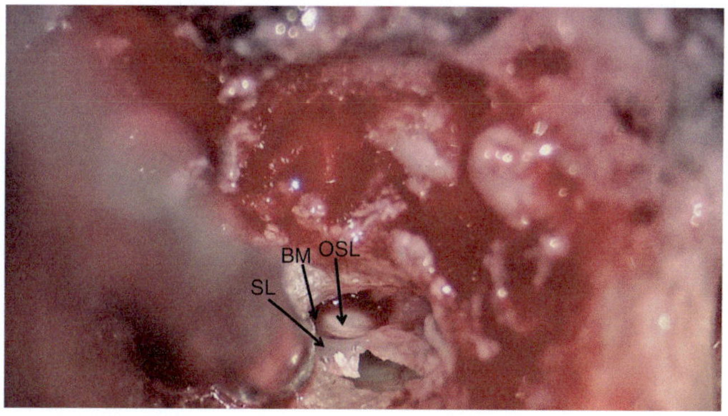

81. Finally, attention was turned to the middle fossa component of the tumor. There was frank invasion of the middle fossa dura. This was excised by first opening the lateral dura using a 15 blade scalpel, leaving a margin of ~3–4 mm. The forceps were used to retract the edge of the tumor. The course of the facial nerve is outlined (*dotted lines*).

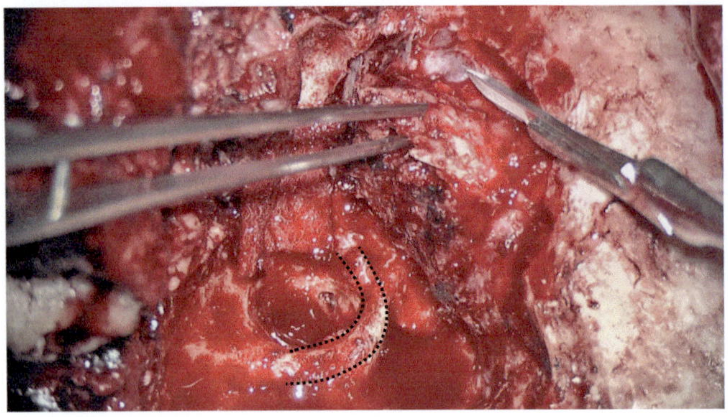

82. Once a small opening in the dura was made, a Penfield 4 elevator was used to carefully separate the dura from the underlying temporal lobe.

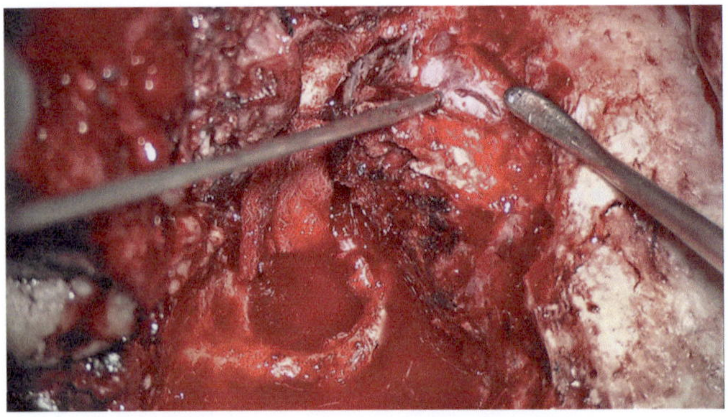

83. The Penfield has been inserted, allowing the assistant to cut on top of it with a knife. Alternatively, it can be removed, and the surgeon can cut the dura with a scissors, holding the dura up off the brain with either a Cushings forceps or a dural hook.

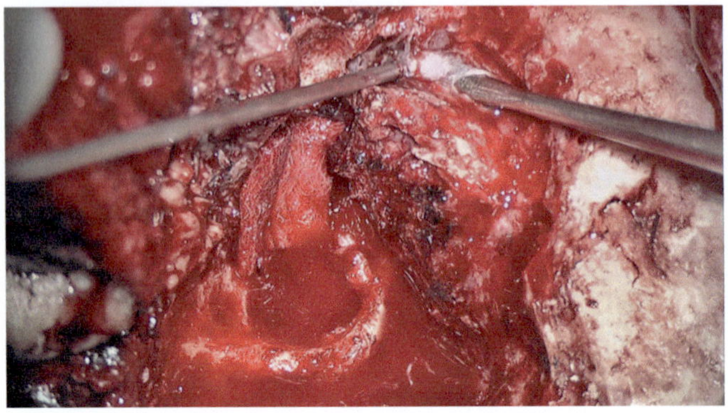

84. Working around the tumor. The inner surface of the dura is not involved with tumor and the brain looks healthy. Clearly, the dura is an excellent barrier to direct tumor extension.

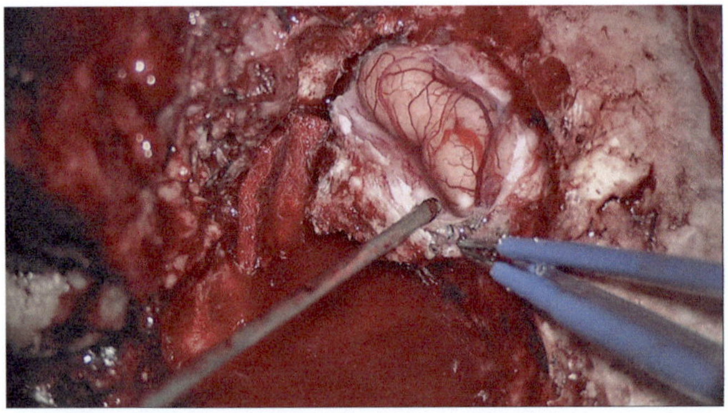

85. A Telfa strip is used to protect the brain while continuing the dural resection medially.

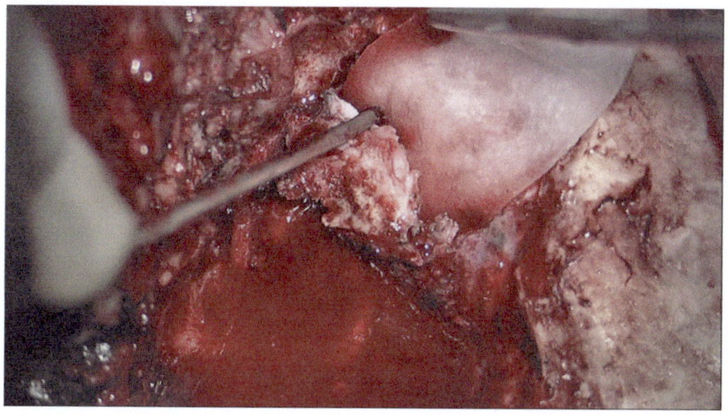

86. The dura is held only at the most medial aspect at this point.

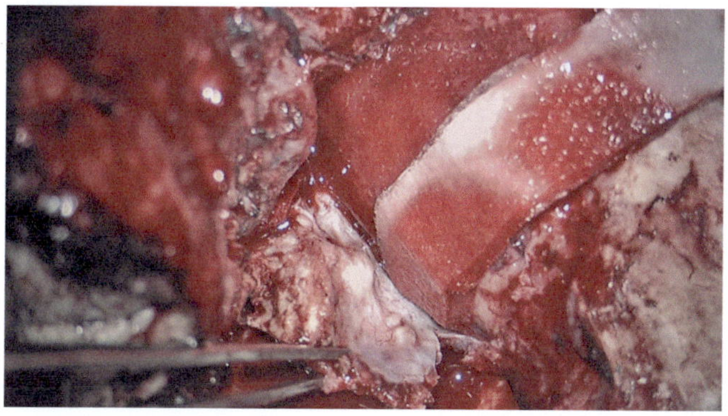

87. Complete dural resection. A piece of Surgicel (*S*) was placed on a small bleeding vessel attached to the temporal lobe. This is safer than attempting to cauterize the vessel and potentially damaging the patient's left temporal lobe. Note the large vein on the undersurface of the brain (*V*). This is a branch of the vein of Labbé. Damaging it could cause a large venous infarct, which would produce severe neurological defects and possibly death. Dural margins consisting of a circumferential rim of an additional 1–2 mm were then taken, and frozen section revealed them to be free of tumor.

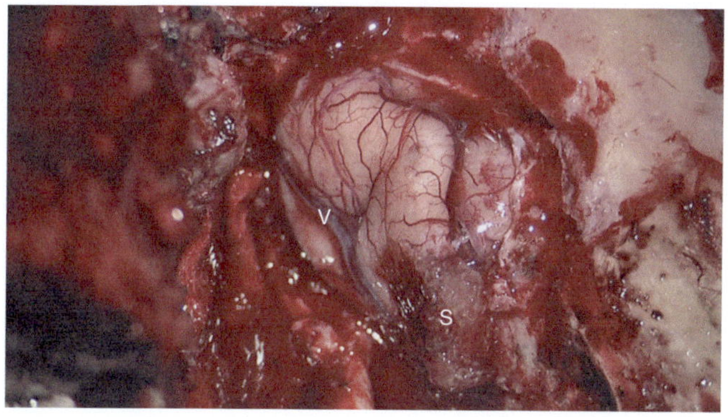

88. An artificial dural graft (Duragen) was placed over the defect.

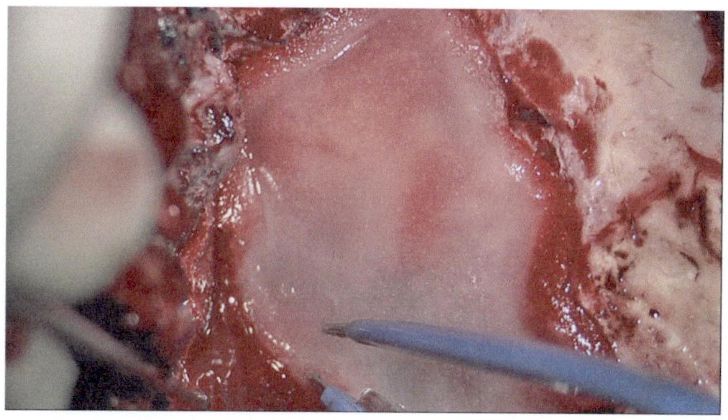

89. The edges of the graft were then tucked under the edges of the normal dura to provide a good seal.

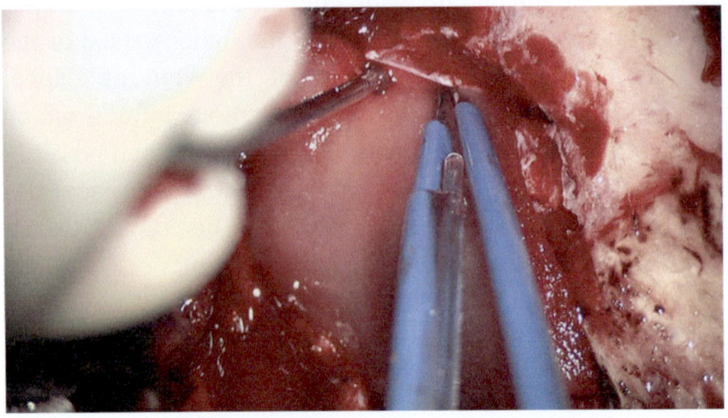

90. After completion of the dural patch.

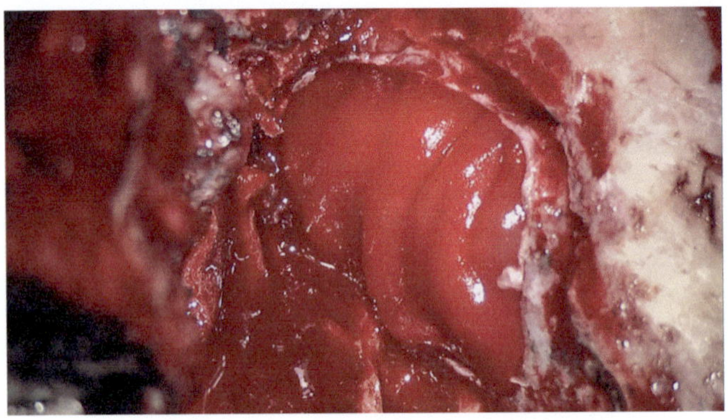

91. Tisseal was then applied over this to provide an additional level of protection against CSF leak.

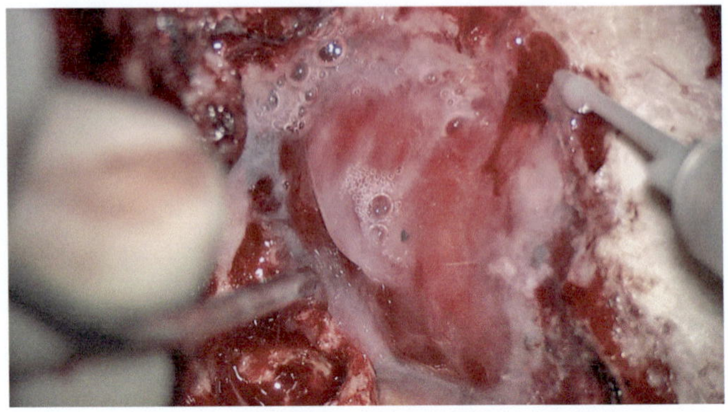

92. The temporalis muscle was then rotated into the large defect. Since the ear was closed off and the muscle flap was filling the mastoid cavity, no bone was needed to reconstruct the defect in the temporal floor. Stitches were placed to tie the flap to the sternocleidomastoid and occipital musculature. These stitches hold the temporalis muscle flap in place. One would not want the patient to wake up, start to clench his/her jaw, and have the flap retract out of the mastoid.

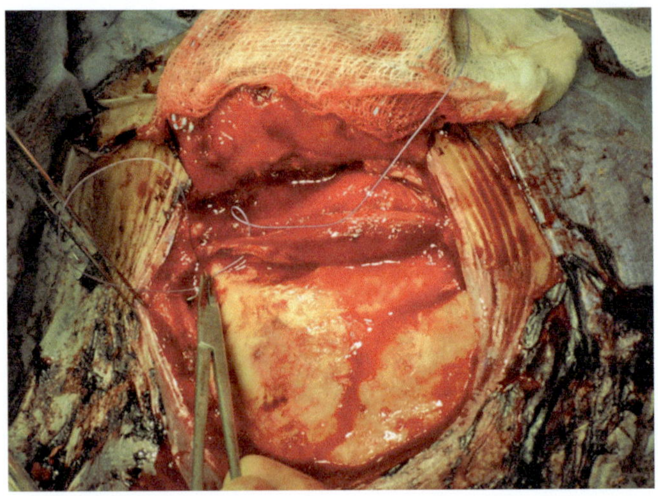

93. Post-op axial CT demonstrating the extent of the temporal bone resection. A drain can be noted (*arrow*).

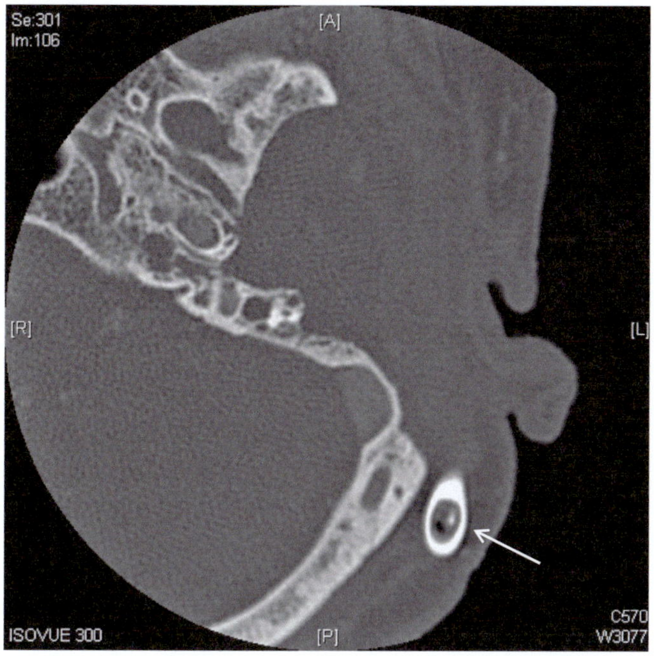

94. Post-op coronal CT. The facial nerve within its fallopian canal bridge (*arrow*) and the large tegmen defect can be seen. A drain was in the subcutaneous space to prevent hematoma formation along the side of the head where the temporalis flap was harvested.

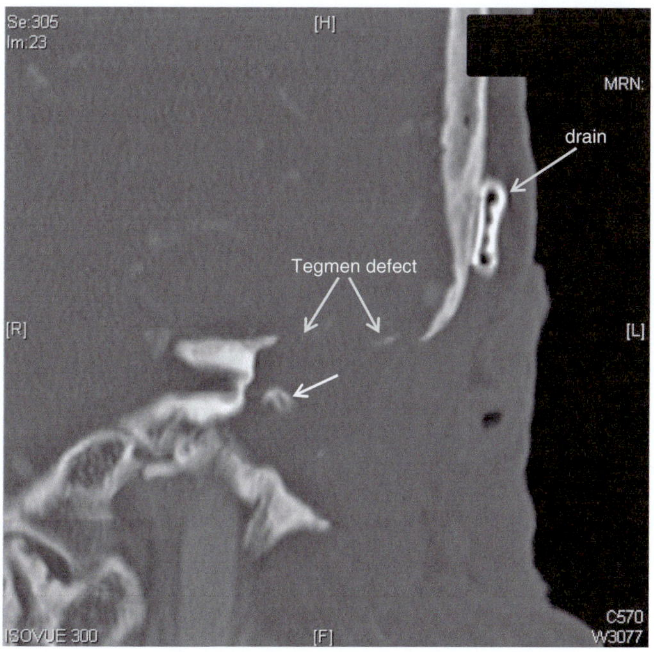

95. Case 3. A multiply recurrent BCCA of the left pinna that invaded the temporal bone. A previous skin graft was included in the planned resection. This patient could not have an MRI because of an implantable defibrillator. The CT scan (not shown) simply demonstrated erosion of the mastoid in the region of the tumor.

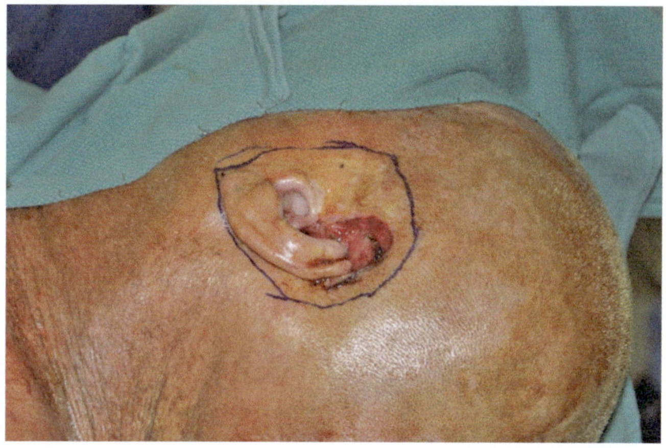

96. The skin and soft tissues were cut down to the bone and resected.

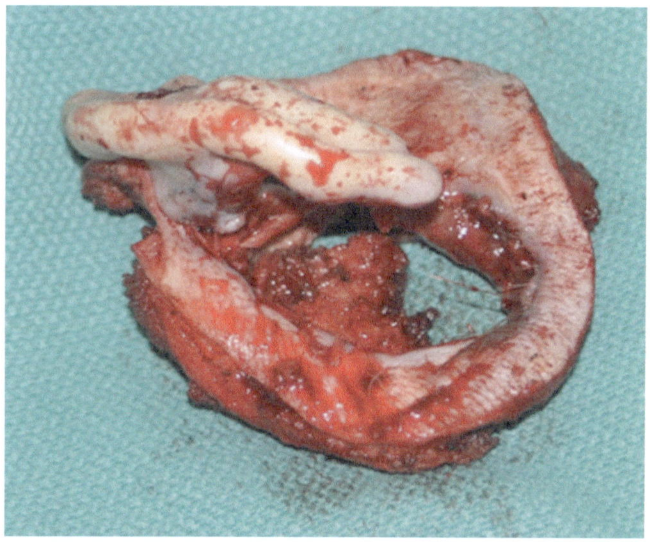

97. After resecting the specimen, a large area of bone erosion was obvious.

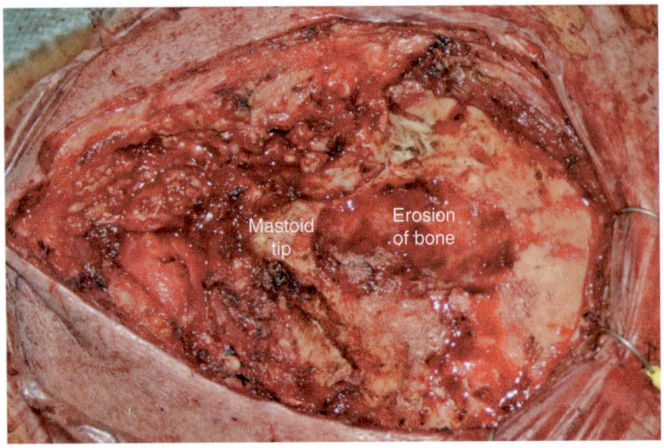

98. A lateral temporal bone resection was performed and the tumor found to infiltrate the dura at three different positions. The disease within two positions, the middle fossa dura and presigmoid posterior fossa dura, could be safely resected. The vein of Labbé was visible along the lateral surface of the temporal lobe. The third disease focus (*arrowheads*) was the lateral surface of the sigmoid sinus at the area where it turns to form the transverse sinus. When initially removing the disease in the posterior fossa dura, we had considered resecting this portion of the sinus to remove the entire disease burden and even made an opening in the dura posterior to the sigmoid sinus in preparation for this. However, after removing the tumor in the middle fossa dura, we changed our mind when we found that the vein of Labbé entered the sigmoid-transverse sinus junction in this area. We felt that resection was not worth the risk of a venous infarct, and instead we cauterized this area well with the bipolar.

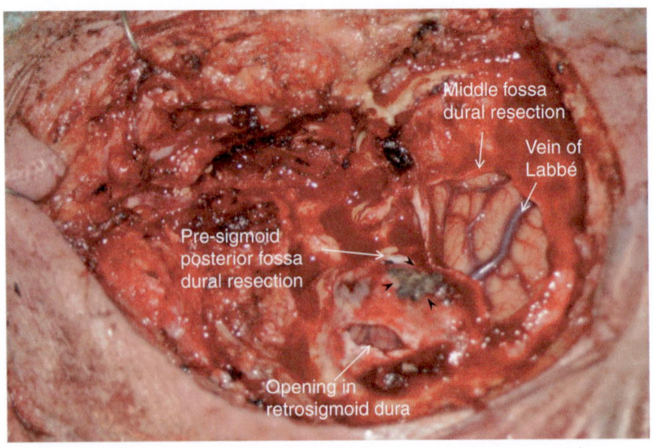

99. A view from sitting at the head of the patient looking inferiorly demonstrated the insertion of the vein of Labbé at the transverse-sigmoid junction.

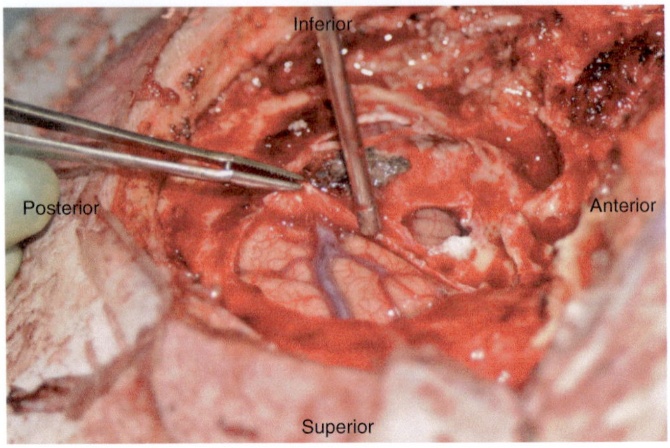

100. Free-flap reconstruction was performed. Because the patient had chronic obstructive pulmonary disease, we also performed a planned tracheotomy.

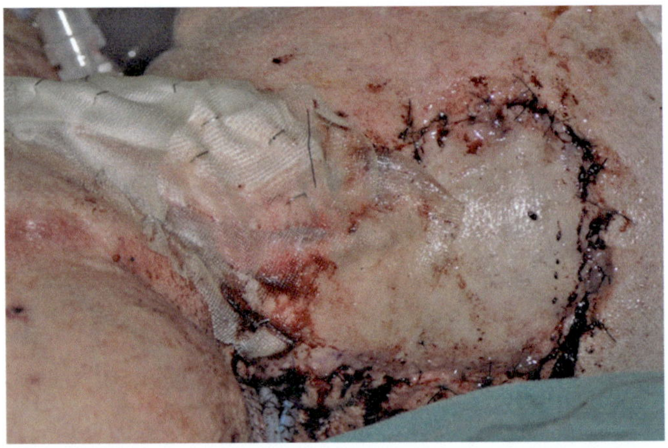

101. Case 4. This patient had an exophytic SCCA of the pinna that extended down into the ear canal. Preoperative CT demonstrated cervical lymphadenopathy, and so temporal bone resection, superficial parotidectomy, and upper neck dissection were planned.

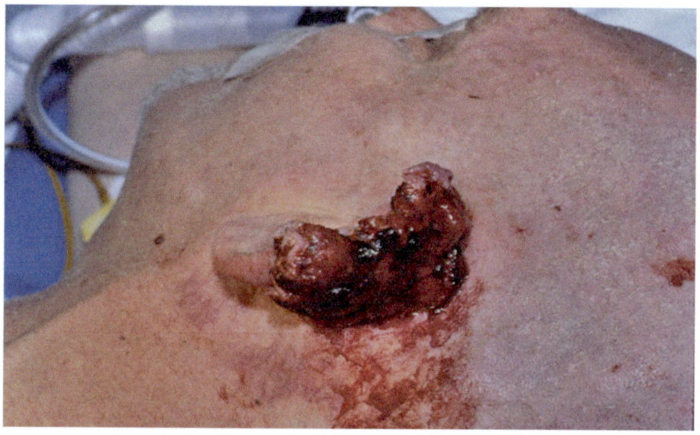

102. The flaps were elevated and the specimen isolated. Very large exposure was performed because a pedicled trapezius myocutaneous flap was planned to be used for reconstruction.

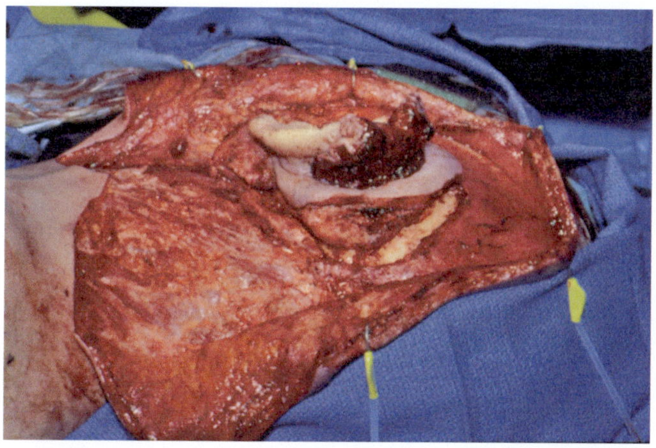

103. The facial nerve was identified at the stylomastoid foramen and a superficial parotidectomy performed first.

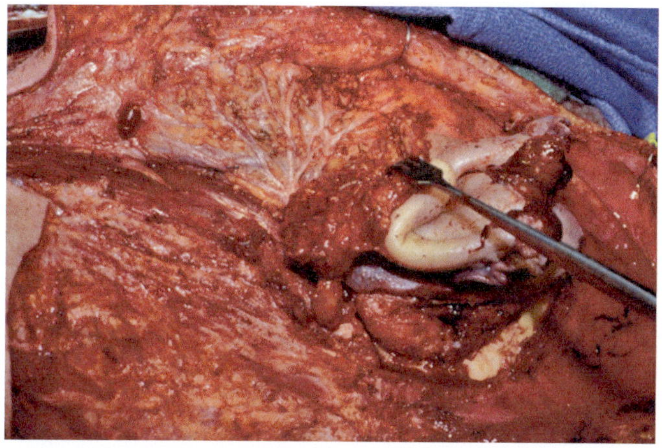

104. The temporal bone resection was then performed. The facial nerve within the vertical segment (*arrow*) was delineated and connected up to the previously identified extracranial facial nerve.

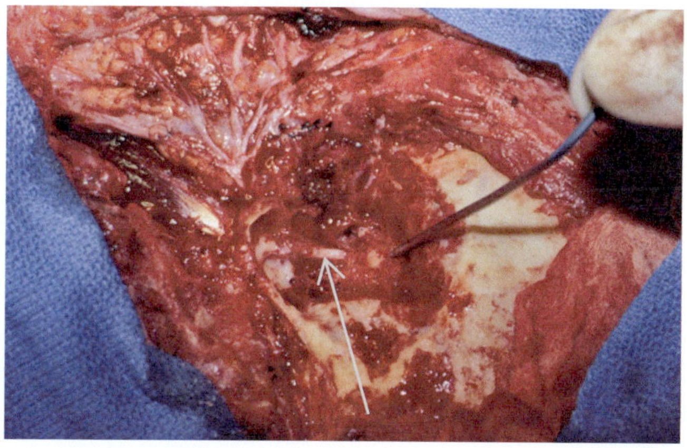

105. Case 5. How to close off an ear. This example is not from a temporal bone resection but from a congenital CSF leak through the inner ear. Nevertheless, the steps are the same. In this image, the Eustachian tube is visible (*arrow*). The canal wall was drilled away and the cavity smoothed to have no sharp edges.

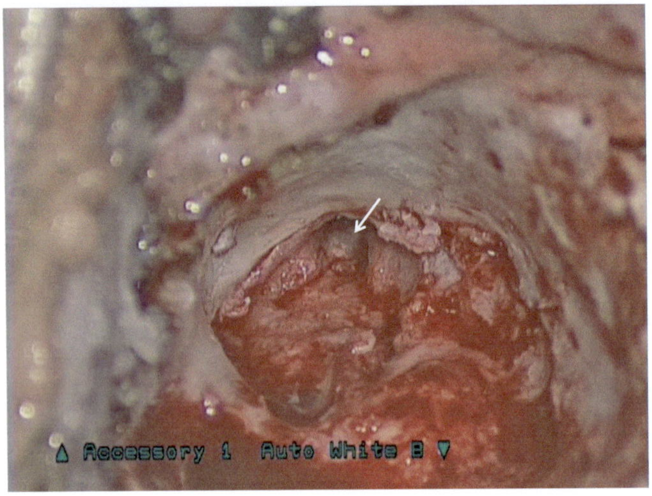

106. The Eustachian tube must be securely plugged. First, the middle ear mucosa around its opening was elevated up off the bone and pushed down into the Eustachian tube. The goal is for the cut edges to seal to each other within the lumen of the Eustachian tube.

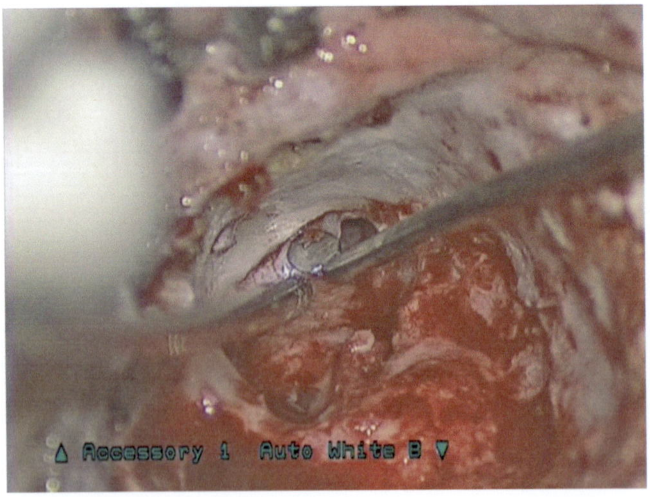

107. Next, the Eustachian tube was plugged with a piece of muscle to help it scar shut. This is most commonly a free plug of temporalis muscle (not shown). In this case, a pedicled tensor tympani flap was used. The thin bone covering the lateral surface of the tensor tympani muscle was drilled away with a small diamond burr, and the tensor tympani muscle (*arrow*) was rotated down into the Eustachian tube. Since its anterior surface maintains a blood supply, this creates a small vascularized muscle flap. This approach probably improves healing and the formation of a tight seal.

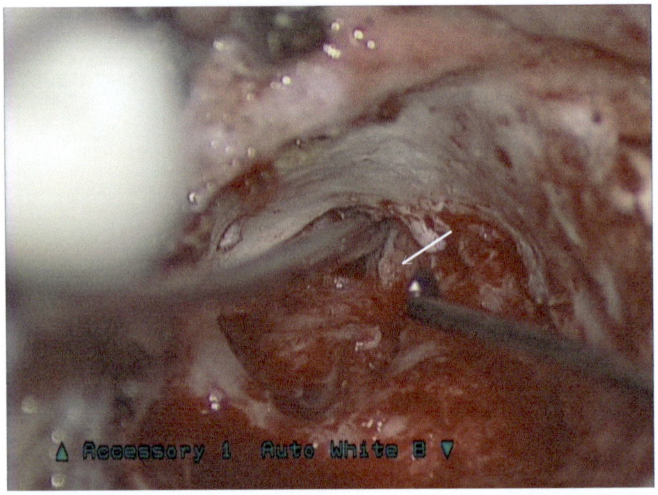

108. A plug of bone wax was placed at the orifice of the Eustachian tube with an elevator.

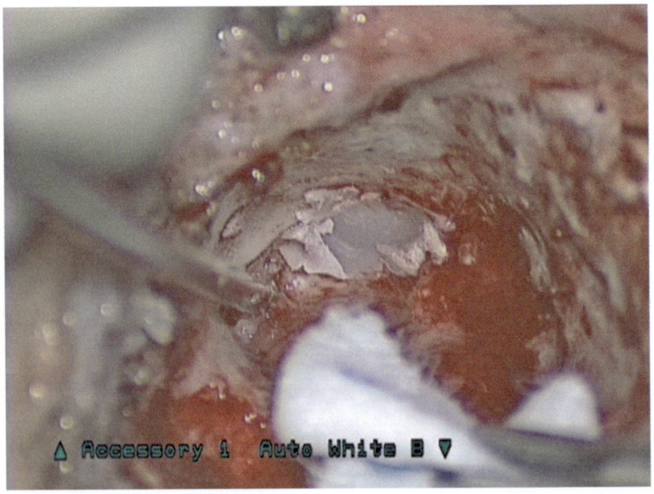

109. This wax was pressed into the Eustachian tube with a cottonoid patty.

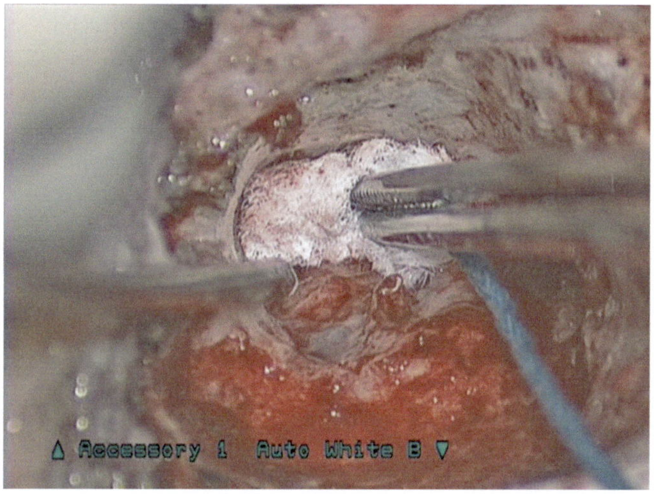

110. After repeating this process three or four times, a watertight seal is achieved.

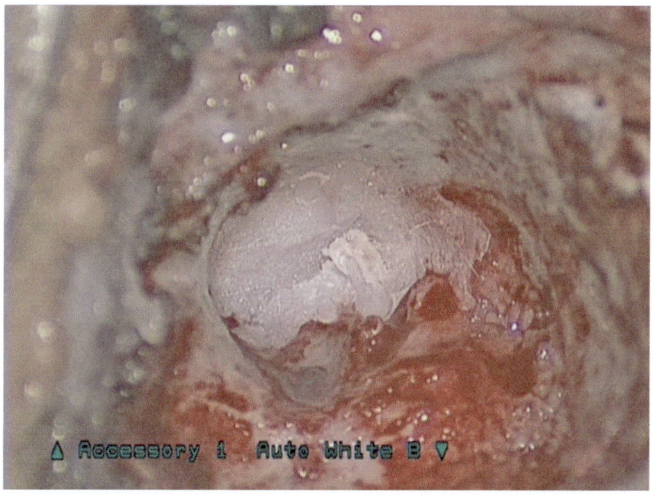

111. Next, the skin of the ear canal is dissected away from the tragal and conchal cartilages from behind and stitches placed in the superior and inferior free edges. These stitches are passed through the meatus and elevated as shown in the picture. This everts the skin edges.

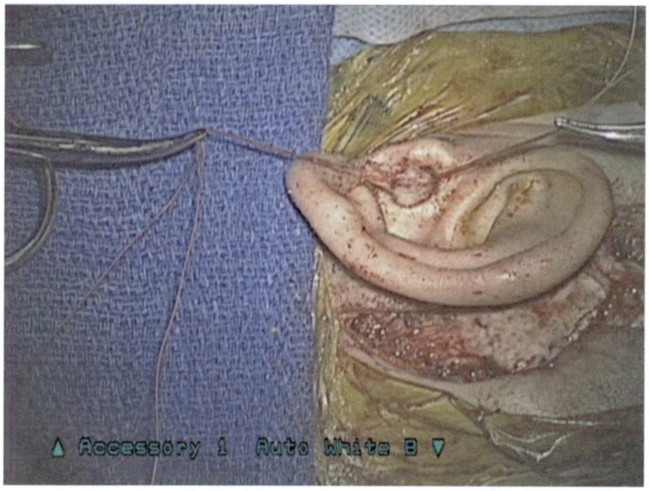

112. 5-0 plain gut sutures were used in an interrupted fashion to suture the skin closed. A horizontal mattress suture was also placed deep to the incision to provide additional closure strength and help prevent CSF from leaking out the ear canal.

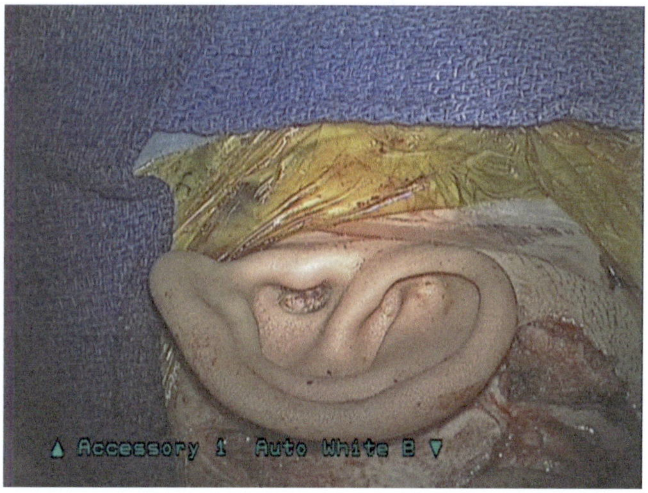

113. Lastly, the periosteum was reflected over the back side of the ear canal and stitched closed. Thus, a multilayer, watertight seal is achieved.

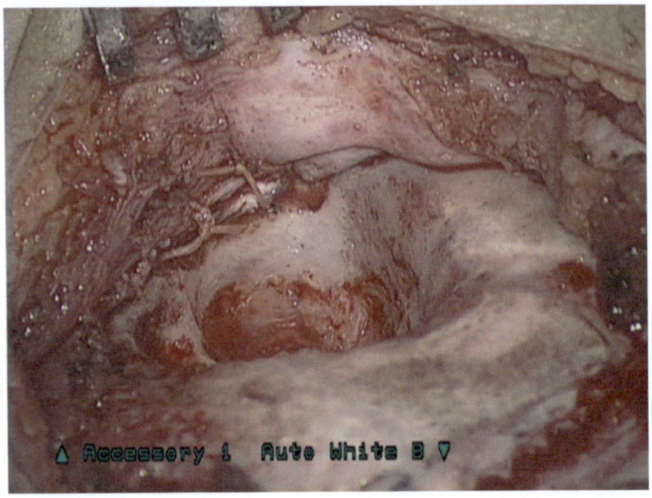

Drainage of Petrous Apex Lesions

- *Concept*
  - An expansive cystic lesion within the petrous apex is treated by drainage to prevent further enlargement. The most common techniques include the infracochlear, infralabyrinthine, and endoscopic transphenoidal approaches. Tumors of the petrous apex require resection rather than drainage, and the techniques are in the middle fossa, posterior fossa, and infratemporal fossa chapters.
- *Conditions treated*
  - Cholesterol granuloma
  - Cholesteatoma
- *Risks*
  - Scarring of the drainage pathway leading to recurrence
  - Hearing loss
  - Vertigo
  - Facial nerve injury
  - Taste disturbance
- *Benefits*
  - Hearing preservation
  - Outpatient procedure
- *Additional notes*
  - The majority of cholesterol granulomas do not need treatment, but the larger and progressively expansile lesions may need removal or drainage. Determining when these lesions are symptomatic is at times difficult. For lesions completely contained within the anterior petrous apex bone, growth demonstrated by serial imaging is a reasonable way to demonstrate the need for treatment. Hearing loss, impingement upon the internal auditory canal and/or otic capsule, or brainstem compression are generally indications for immediate treatment.
  - Conventional wisdom states that a drainage pathway needs to be created as part of the surgery. However, for some lesions, we have approached through the middle fossa and have been able to remove all or virtually all the lining and certainly all the contents. Packing with a fat graft has prevented recurrence.
  - For very large lesions, we combine the middle fossa exposure with a retrofacial and retrolabyrinthine dissection to create a very wide pathway for drainage. The middle fossa exposure allows us to thoroughly clean out the contents of the cholesterol granuloma that is often multiloculated and contains thick debris that will not simply drain through a small opening. If simple drainage is the goal, we also consider a transnasal endoscopic approach.

114. The infracochlear approach to the petrous apex is the most common technique used to access and drain the petrous apex. The inferior ear canal is then drilled down to visualize the hypotympanum. A coronal illustration demonstrating the amount of inferior canal wall bone that needs to be removed is shown here (*gray region*).

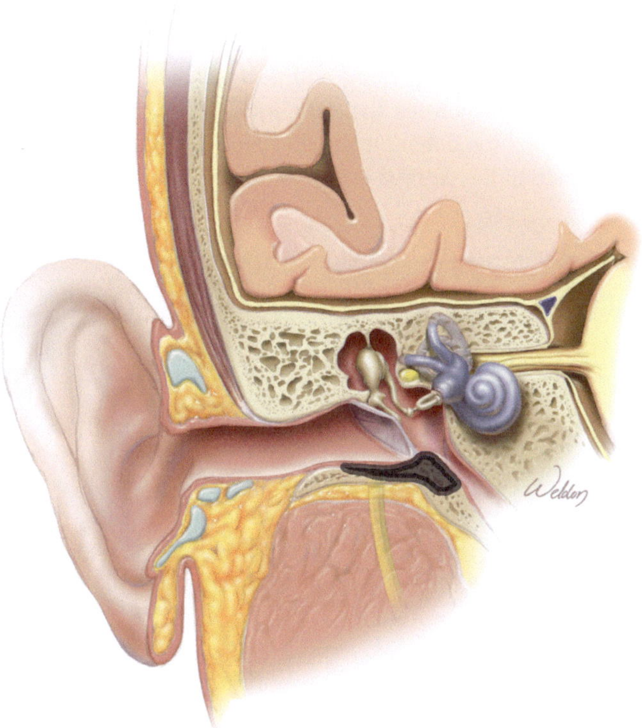

115. To perform the infracochlear approach, a standard postauricular incision is made.

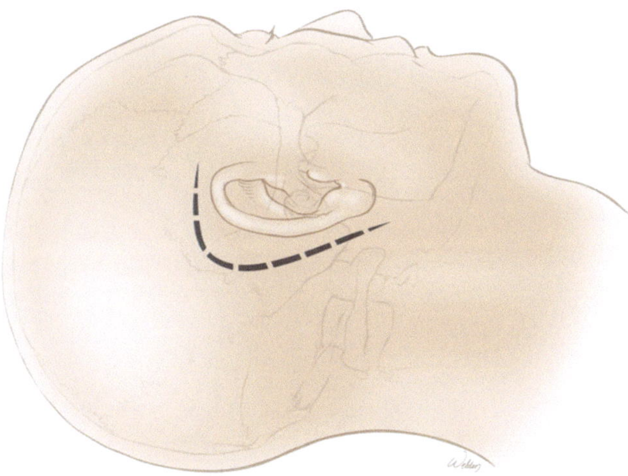

116. The soft tissues are elevated off the mastoid cortex to reach the ear canal. A tympanomeatal flap is made as when performing a tympanoplasty. This flap should be extended around the inferior aspect of the ear canal and elevated to visualize the cochlear promontory.

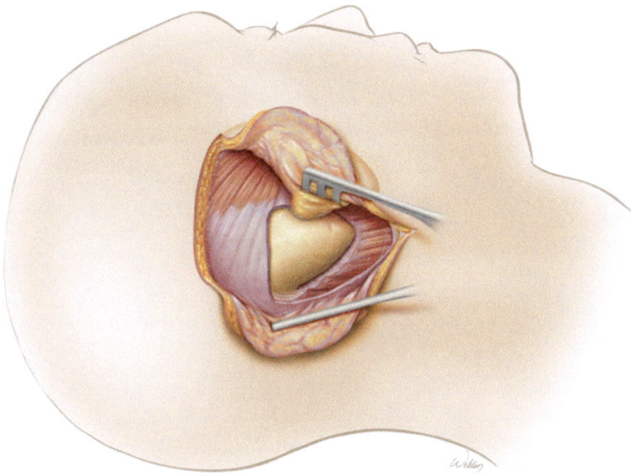

117. The inferior ear canal bone is then drilled away to expose the hypotympanum. The stapes and round window are shown for orientation. The internal carotid artery (*ICA*) and jugular bulb (*JB*) should be skeletonized, leaving a thin layer of bone over them. The space between these structures and the cochlea is then drilled to reach the petrous apex (*dotted line*).

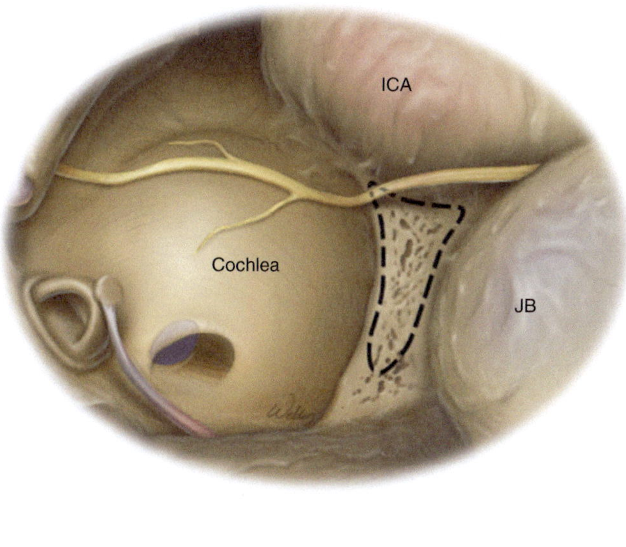

118. Axial CT of a temporal bone. This example demonstrates a normal petrous apex that is extremely well aerated (*asterisk*). The infracochlear approach to the petrous apex (*arrow*) involves going through the space between the internal carotid artery (*ICA*) and the jugular bulb (*JB*).

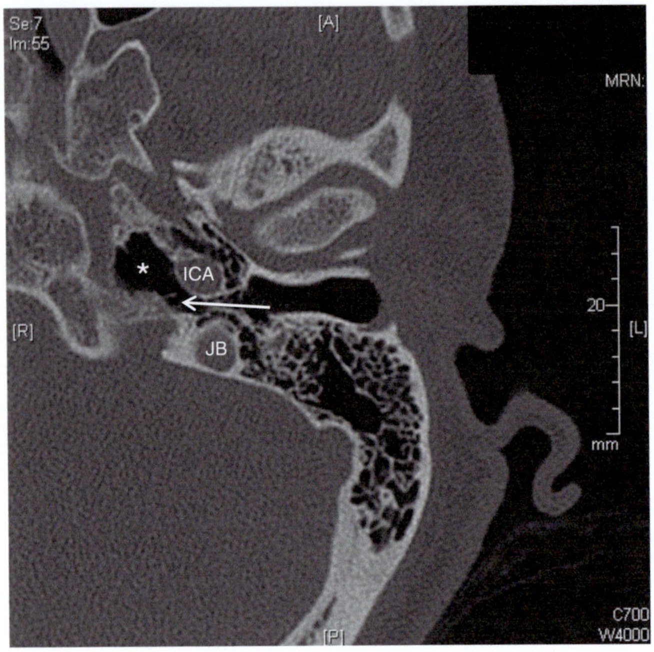

119. Coronal CT from the same patient. To open this tract to the petrous apex (*arrow*), the solid bone of the inferior ear canal needs to be drilled down (*region within dotted line*). The cochlea, which lies directly above the infracochlear air cells, must be respected.

This approach is done through a standard postauricular approach for a tympanoplasty. The ear canal is opened and the skin elevated off the posterior and inferior ear canal. After raising a tympanomeatal flap, the inferior ear canal bone is drilled away to expose the hypotympanum. The space between the jugular bulb, internal carotid artery, and cochlea is drilled open to access the petrous apex. Pre-op CT is helpful in verifying that the potential space is large enough to open this route to the petrous apex.

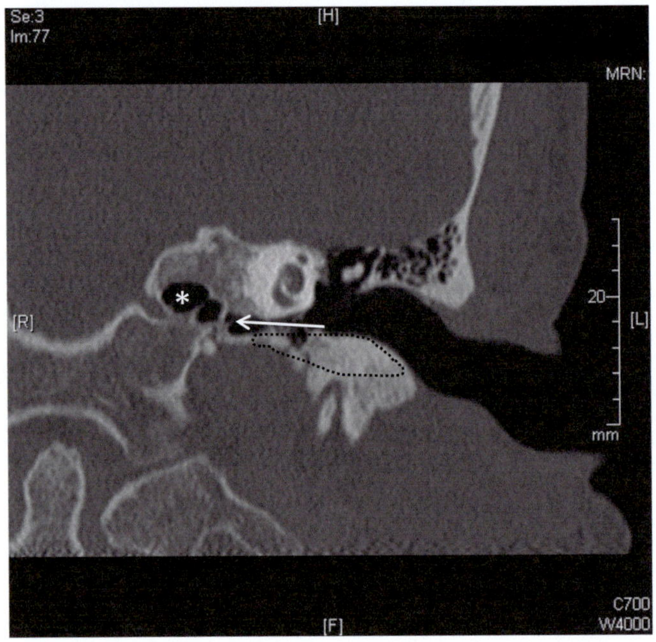

120. Case 1. Right petrous apex cholesterol granuloma. It is bright on this axial T1 MRI. No gadolinium was given, and fat suppression techniques were not used.

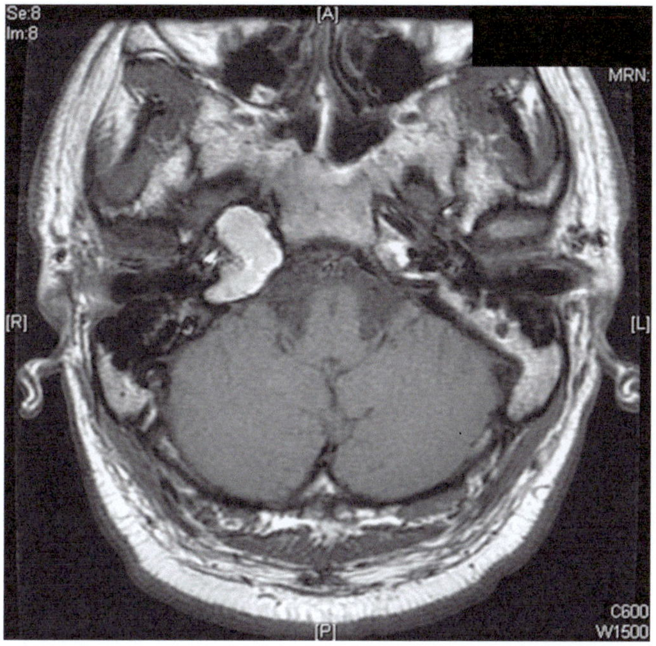

121. In this image, gadolinium was given and fat suppression techniques applied. The fat suppression can make the cholesterol granuloma less bright, but it is still brighter than brain signal intensity.

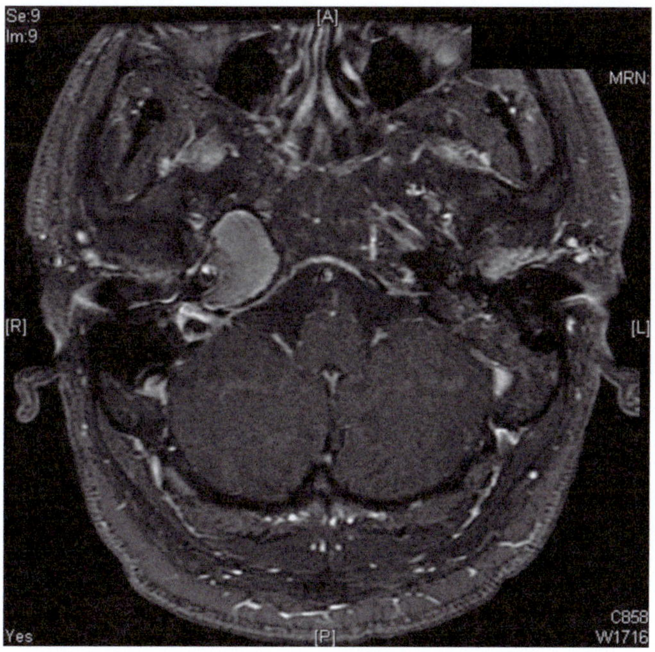

122. T2 MRI demonstrates that there are some bright and some dark areas within the cyst.

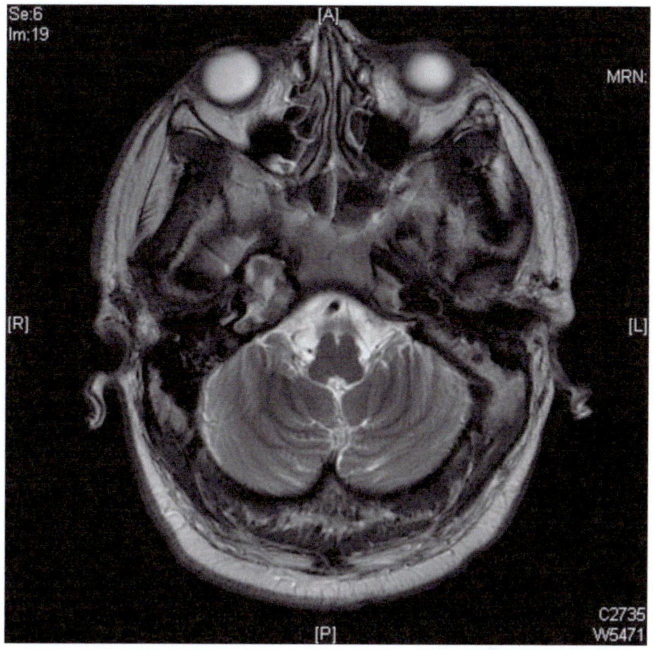

123. Axial CT scan demonstrates that the cyst had eroded bone throughout the petrous apex and into the sphenoid wing. The borders were smooth and sharp in contrast to what is usually seen with a malignant lesion. The edge of the petrous apex had not expanded medially into the posterior fossa, and the lesion was entirely confined within the bone. Thus, there was no brain compression caused by this cyst. However, this cyst demonstrated progressive growth on serial imaging, and so surgical drainage was recommended.

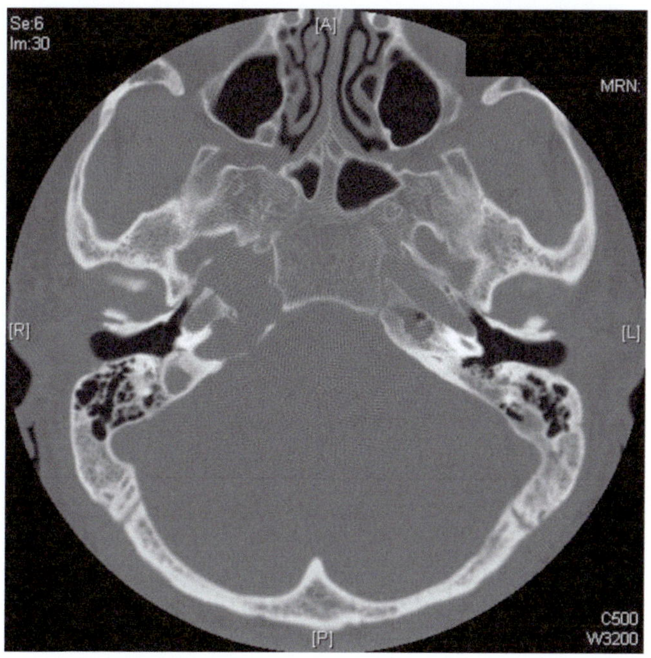

124. An infracochlear approach was performed. A postauricular incision was used, the pinna was reflected anteriorly, and the ear canal was entered. Note the excellent exposure of the inferior ear canal (*arrowheads*). The mastoid and tympanic membrane (*TM*) are visible.

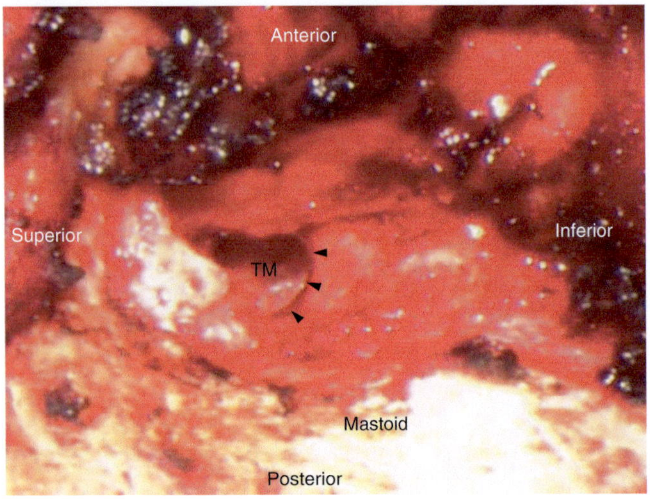

125. The inferior ear canal skin was elevated and pushed anterosuperiorly. The inferior ear canal bone was then drilled away with a diamond burr. Thus, the ear canal is oval rather than round.

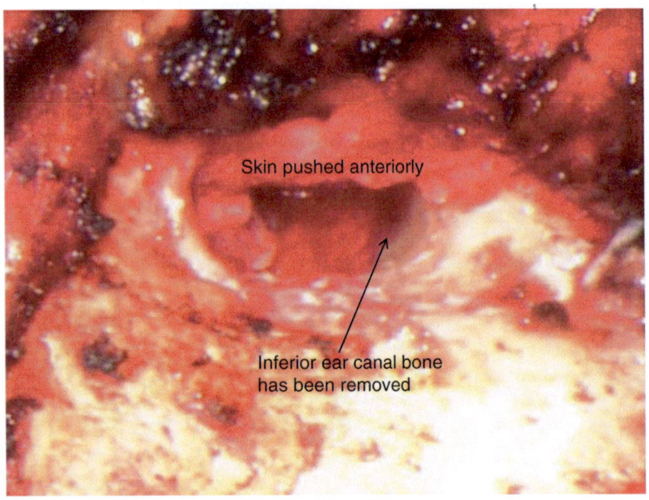

126. After drilling away the inferior tympanic annulus, the jugular bulb (*JB*) and promontory of the cochlea (*C*) are visible.

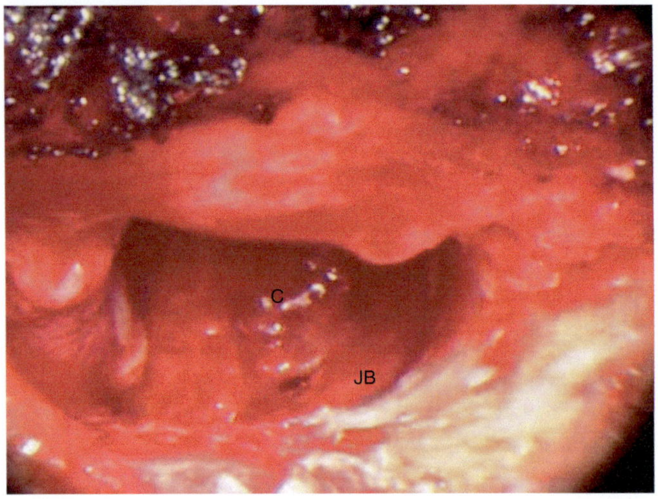

127. The cochlea (*C*) and the jugular bulb (*JB*) are now better exposed. Also, the area of the internal carotid artery (*ICA*) can be noted. Also, the cyst capsule of the cholesterol granuloma (*CG*) is poking through the thinned bone.

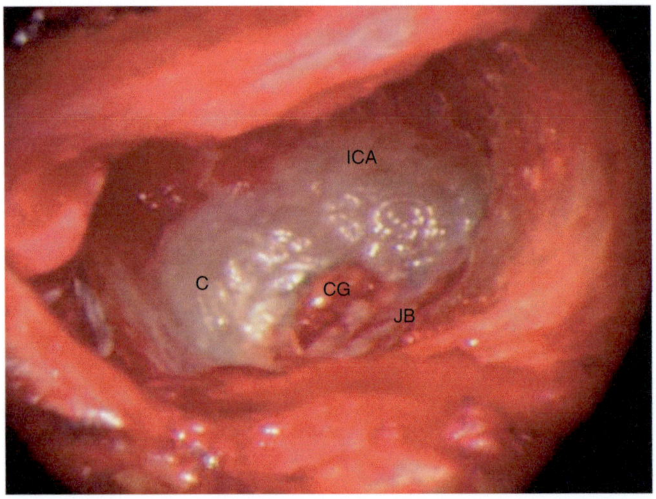

128. The cyst is popped open and cholesterol granuloma fluid released.

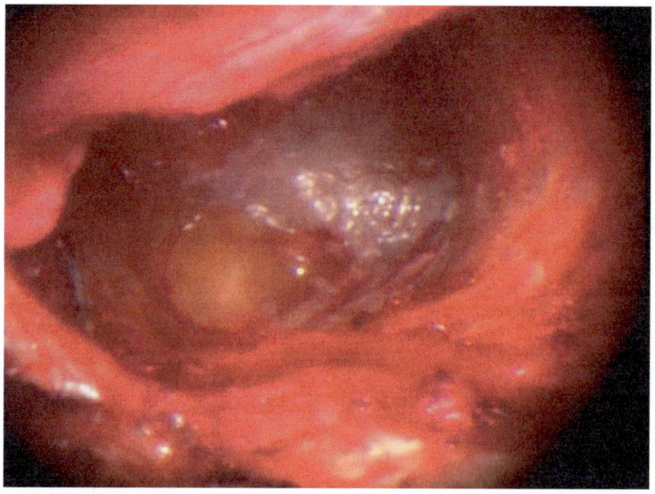

129. The cyst wall is widely marsupialized for maximum drainage.

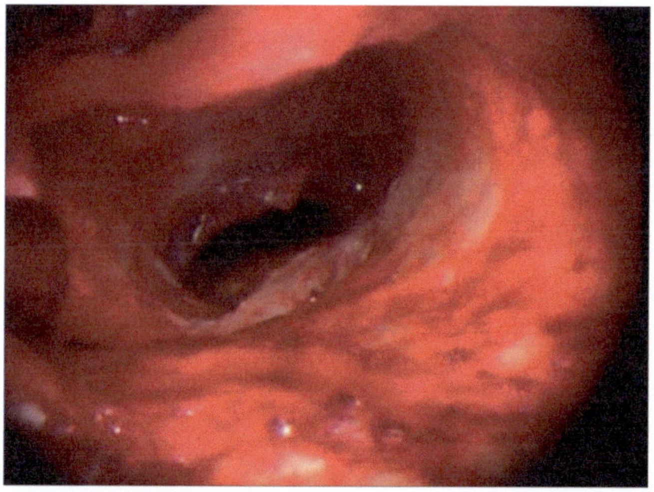

130. A sheet of silastic is folded and inserted into the cyst to help maintain patency of the drainage pathway.

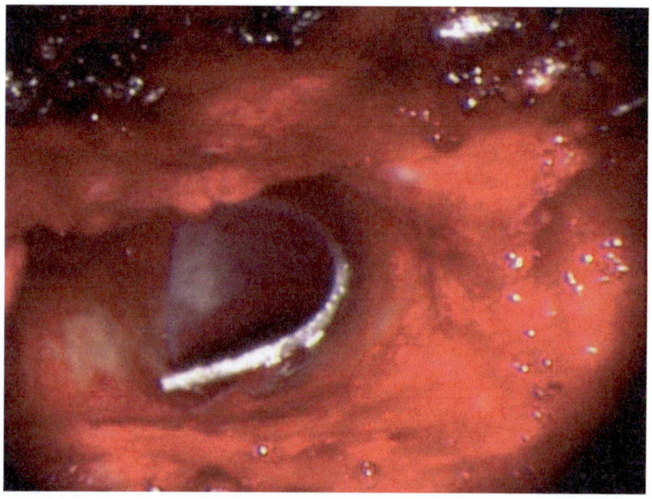

131. A piece of temporalis fascia is laid down to graft the inferior tympanic membrane, which must now be made bigger than it was before. The tympanic membrane is then lowered down on top of it to complete the reconstruction.

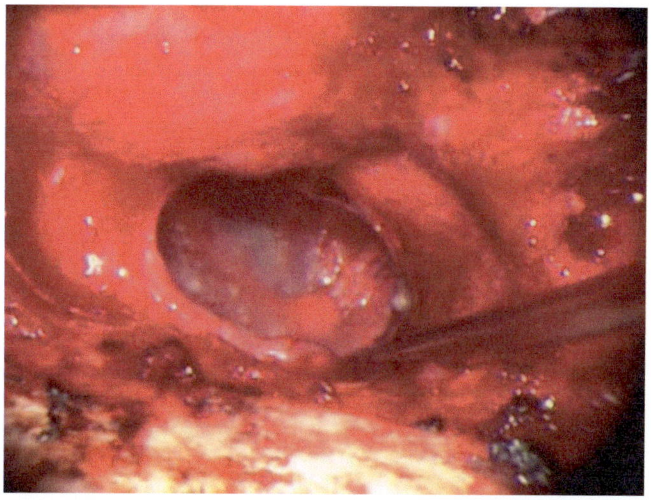

132. Case 2. Another patient with a right petrous apex cholesterol granuloma. It is bright on T1 MRI.

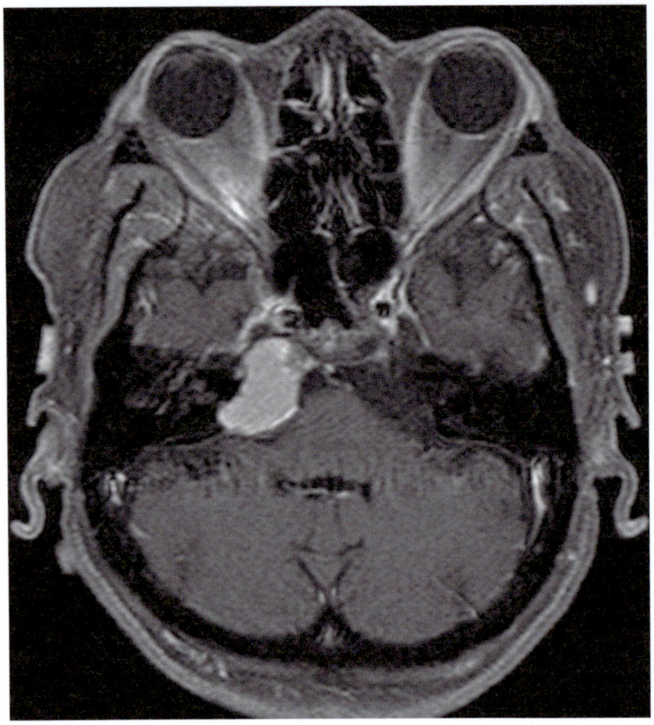

133. The lesion is also bright on T2 MRI. There is distention of the medial bony margin with evidence of mild brainstem compression.

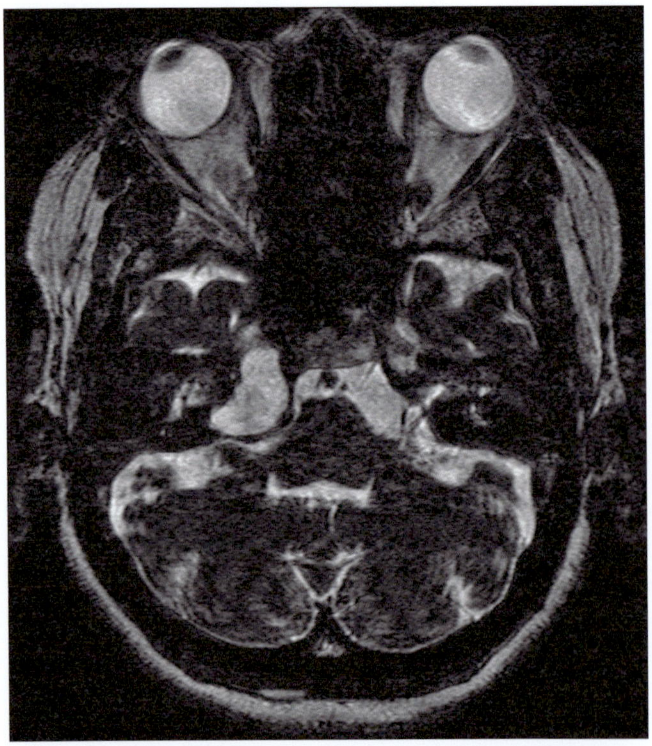

134. CT demonstrates the smooth, expansile margins of the cyst wall.

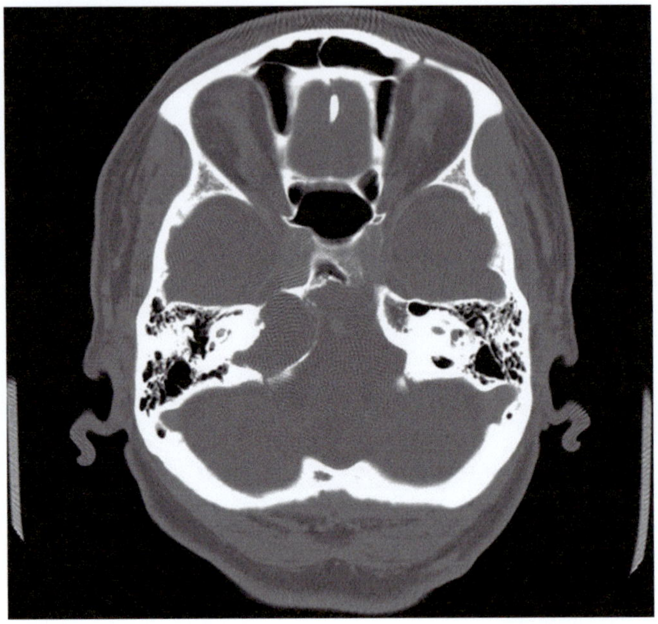

135. Case 3. A left bilobed cholesterol granuloma that is bright on T1 MRI.

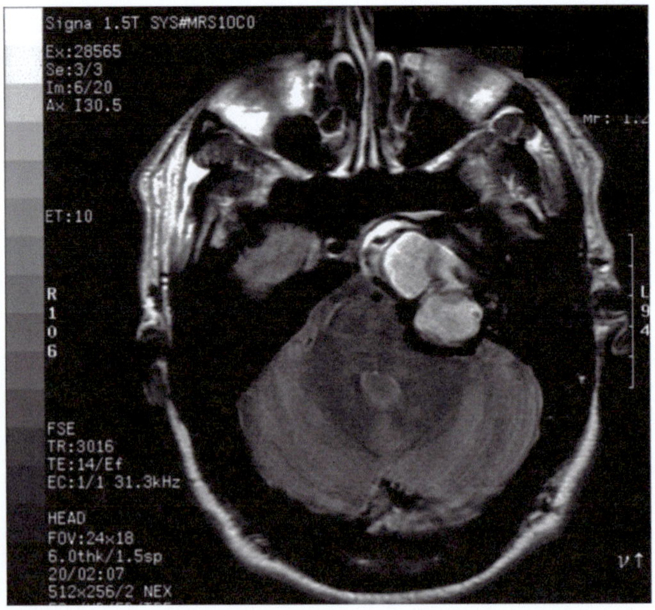

136. With T1 MRI with fat suppression techniques and gadolinium, the bright signal intensity is lacking except at the edge. This is an example of why one must be careful when interpreting MRI scans. It is important to look at the unenhanced images as well as the enhanced images.

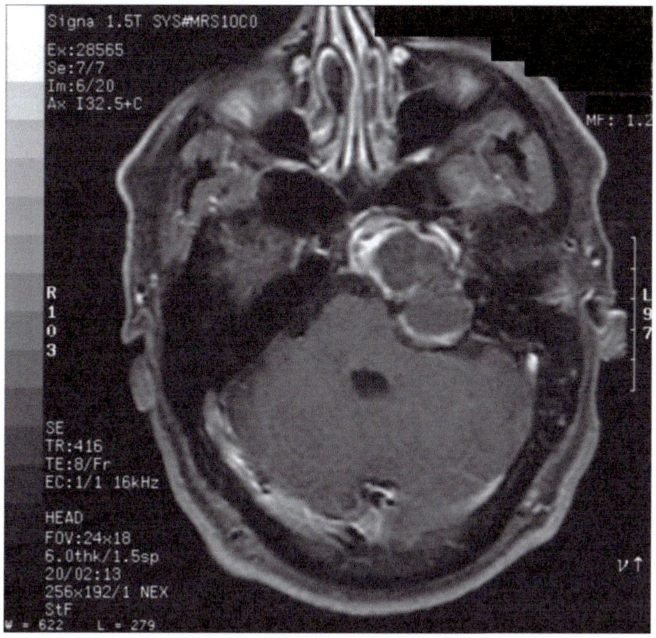

137. The cyst is bright on T2 MRI.

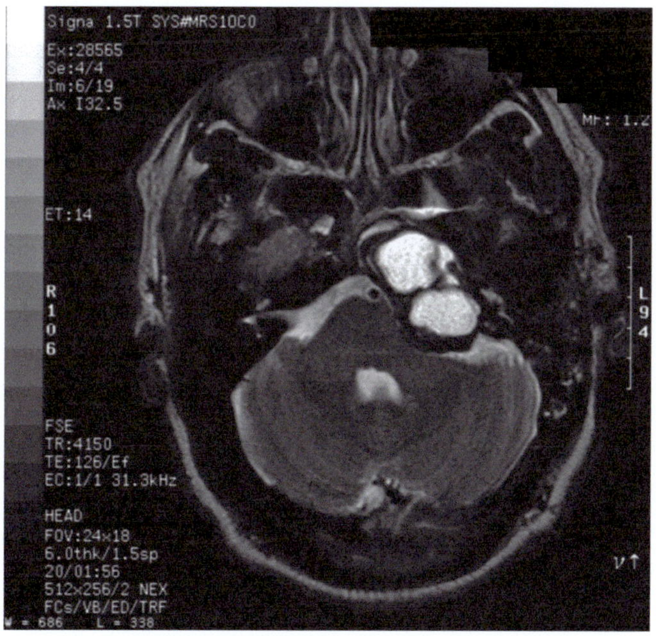

138. Axial CT demonstrates the smooth margins of the cyst. It has pushed the internal carotid artery laterally (*asterisk*) and is pushing into the sphenoid sinus (*arrow*). Because it is so easily accessible from an anterior approach, this cyst would be best drained using the endoscopic transphenoidal technique.

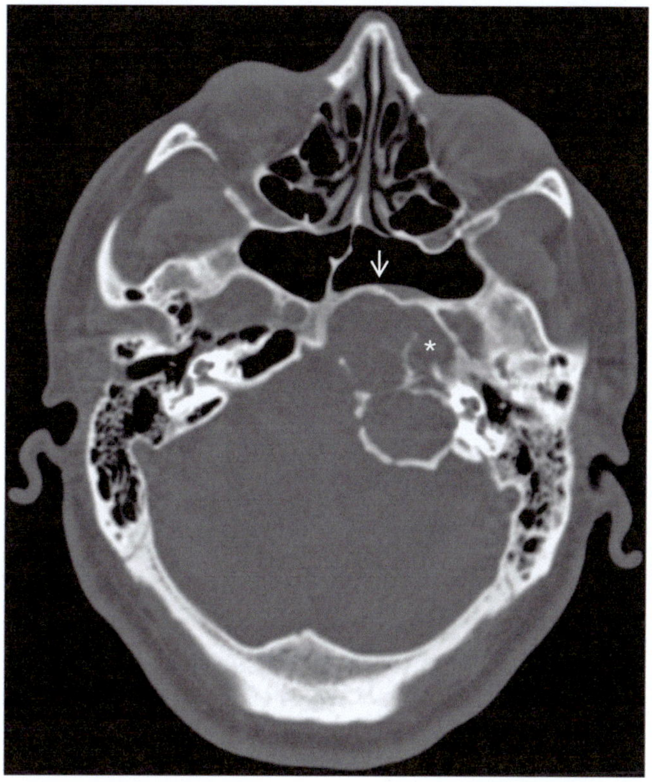

139. Coronal CT of the same patient demonstrating that the cyst has pushed superiorly to compress the temporal lobe.

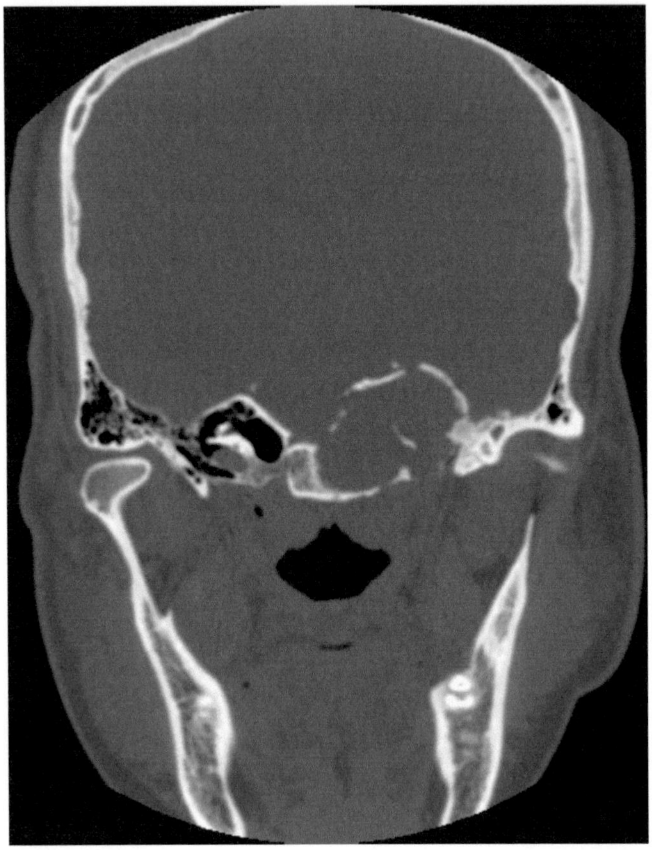

9 Facial Nerve Surgery

- *Concept*
  - *Nerve decompression* is performed when the facial nerve is intact but inflamed. In this situation, the pressure within the fallopian canal increases above that of the mean arterial blood pressure, and the nerve becomes ischemic. This can lead to permanent facial nerve paresis or paralysis. Decompression treats this condition by removing the bony sheath covering the facial nerve. By achieving adequate decompression (i.e., at least 90° and more typically ~180° of the nerve's circumference), a nerve that is inflamed and edematous can swell without having the pressure within the fallopian canal increase.
  - When the facial nerve is transected, *primary nerve repair* or *interpositional nerve grafting* are the preferred reconstructive options.
  - When the proximal end of the facial nerve is not accessible, facial reanimation can be achieved by connecting the distal end of the facial nerve to either CN V (*trigeminal–facial anastomosis*) or CN XII (*hypoglossal–facial anastomosis*).
- *Conditions treated*
  - Facial nerve palsy due to Bell's palsy with >90 % nerve degeneration diagnosed by ENoG can be treated by decompression.
  - Facial nerve palsy due to trauma such as a temporal bone fracture can be treated by decompression (if it is intact) or nerve repair or interpositional nerve grafting (if it is transected).
  - Facial nerve paralysis after resection of an invasive tumor.
  - Iatrogenic injury to the facial nerve.
  - Nerve decompression may be performed for facial nerve palsy due to compression by a cholesteatoma.
- *Risks*
  - Poor facial function. Once the facial nerve has been divided, none of the reconstruction techniques provide better than a House–Brackmann grade 4/6 function.
  - Hearing loss
- *Benefits*
  - Repair of the facial nerve provides dynamic motion to the face as opposed to static procedures that provide symmetry at rest but obvious asymmetry with motion.

J.S. Oghalai, C.L.W. Driscoll, *Atlas of Neurotologic and Lateral Skull Base Surgery*,
DOI 10.1007/978-3-662-46694-0_9,

1. Illustration of the approach for facial nerve decompression in the mastoid. A postauricular incision is made.

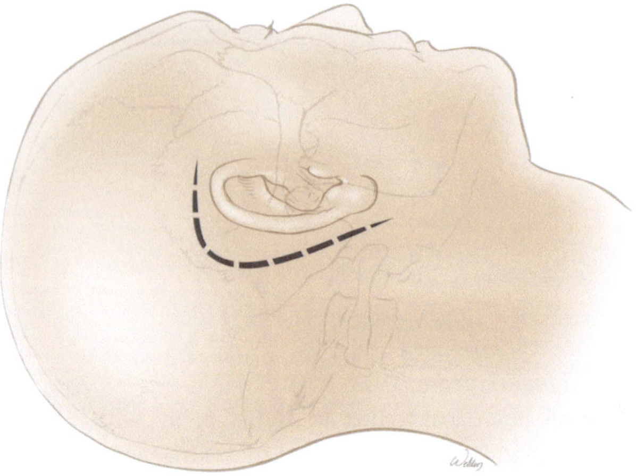

2. The soft tissues are reflected off the mastoid cortex.

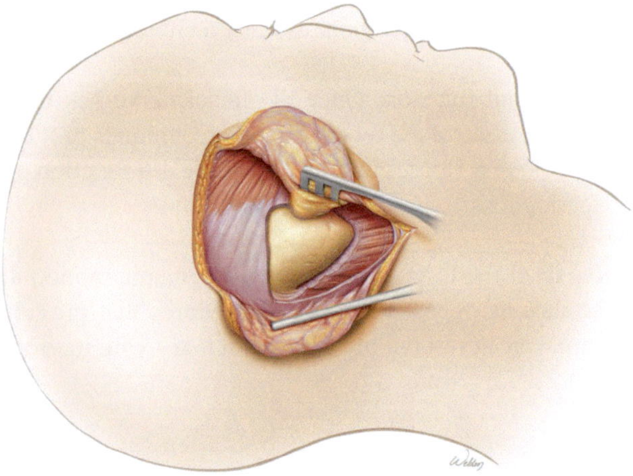

3. A simple cortical mastoidectomy is performed. The ear canal is thinned.

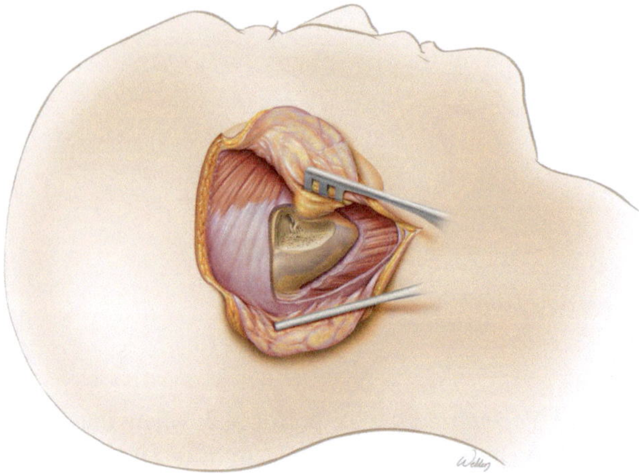

4. A facial recess approach is then drilled (fully described in Chap. 10).

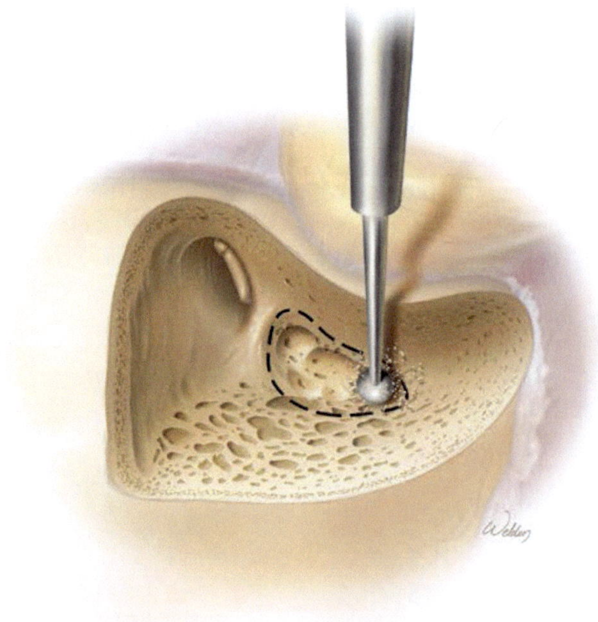

5. The facial nerve can be found just inferior to the second genu, which is a highly consistent location. It is at the same depth in the mastoid as the lateral semicircular canal. The vertical segment can then be traced inferiorly to the stylomastoid foramen. By carefully thinning and removing the bone over the facial nerve epineurium (shown in the cases below), decompression is performed.

   In order to access and decompress the horizontal segment of the facial nerve, the incudostapedial joint is separated, the incus and incudal buttress is removed, and the head of the malleus is clipped. This permits visualization of the horizontal facial nerve all the way to the geniculate ganglion (shown in the cases below).

   In order to decompress the labyrinthine segment of the facial nerve, a middle fossa approach or translabyrinthine approach is used depending on whether a hearing preservation or nonhearing preservation strategy is desired.

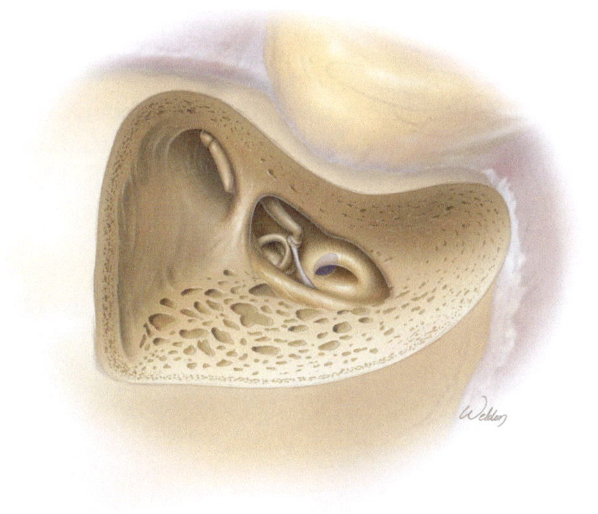

6. Case 1. Facial nerve decompression. Axial CT scan of a patient who sustained a left longitudinal temporal bone fracture and developed delayed-onset total facial nerve paralysis. The fracture line (*arrows*) went from the mastoid cortex to near the geniculate ganglion. Presumably, the facial nerve sustained a stretch injury in this location. ENoG testing revealed >90 % degeneration, and a total facial nerve decompression was performed. There is blood within the mastoid air cells. The labyrinthine portion of the facial nerve is visible (*arrowhead*). Decompression in this setting is controversial but may result in the best chance of satisfactory recovery. In addition, nerve repair can be performed if the nerve is found to have been transected.

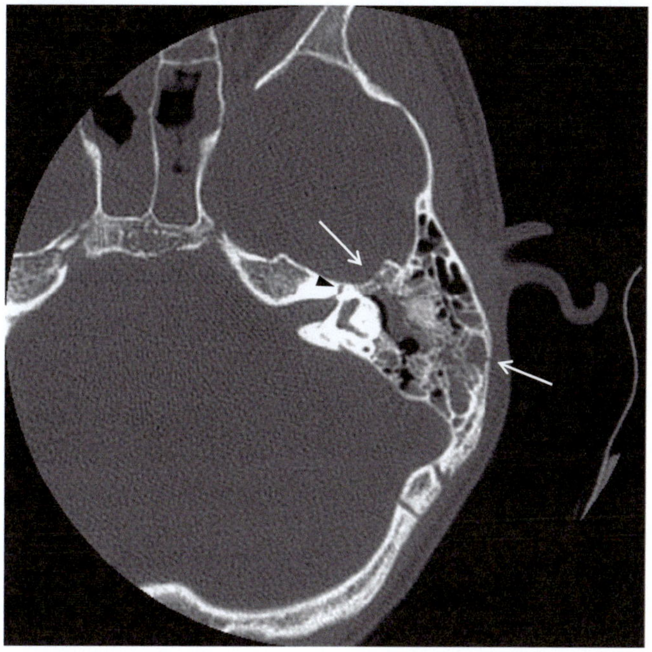

7. First, a standard canal wall up mastoidectomy was performed to decompress the horizontal and vertical segments of the facial nerve. The incudostapedial joint was divided, the incus removed, and the head of the malleus clipped. When approached through the mastoid, there is no way to access the horizontal segment without doing this. Often, the ossicular chain is already disrupted due to the fracture; if not, this portion of the nerve may be decompressed along with the geniculate ganglion and labyrinthine section through a middle fossa approach. The vertical segment of the facial nerve (*arrow*) is visible through the bone just inferior to the lateral semicircular canal (*LSCC*).

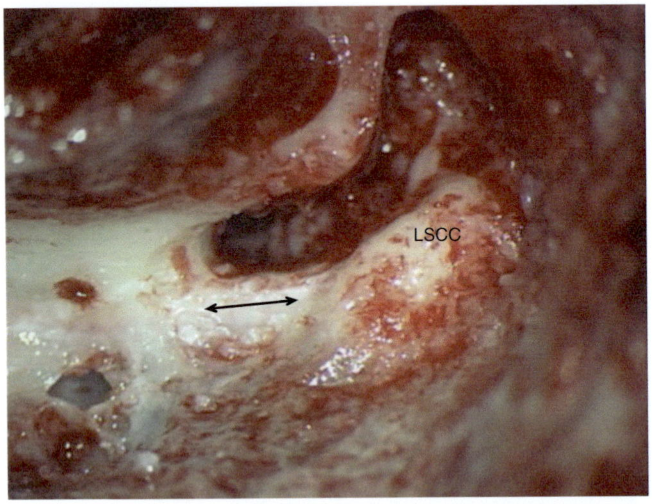

8. The bone overlying the horizontal segment of the facial nerve (*arrow*) was carefully thinned with the drill.

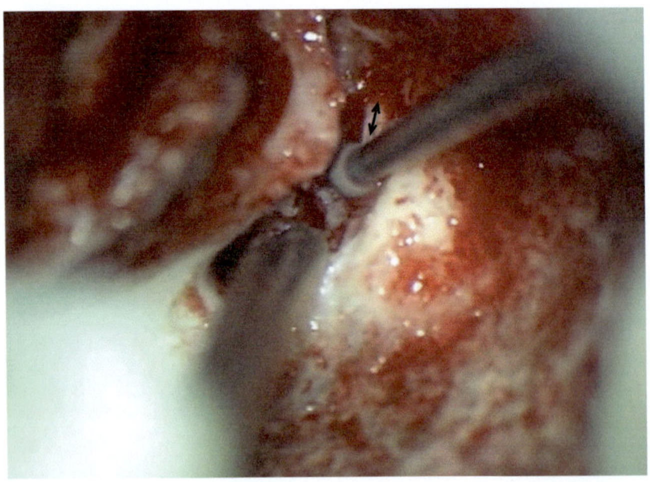

9. The facial nerve was followed through the second genu.

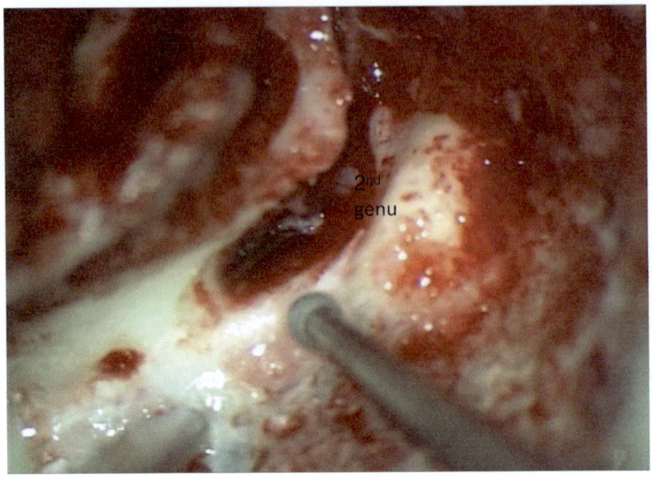

10. The vertical segment was followed inferiorly. This can be continued all the way to the stylomastoid foramen if desired. In this case, we did not because the injury was limited to the region near the geniculate ganglion.

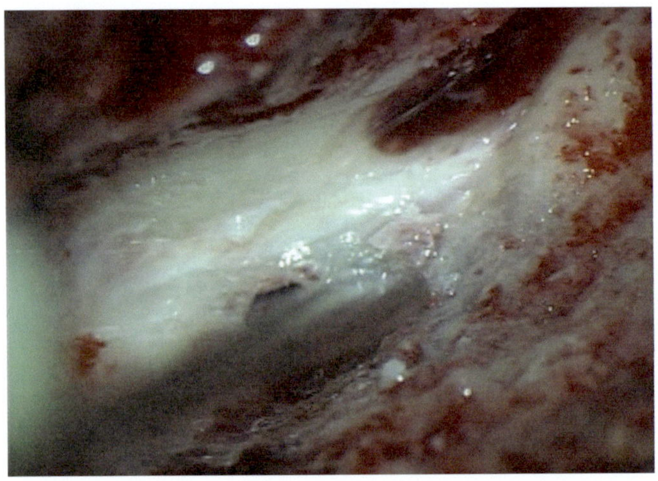

11. Once the bone overlying the nerve was thinned, it was removed manually (rather than with the drill) to minimize trauma to the nerve.

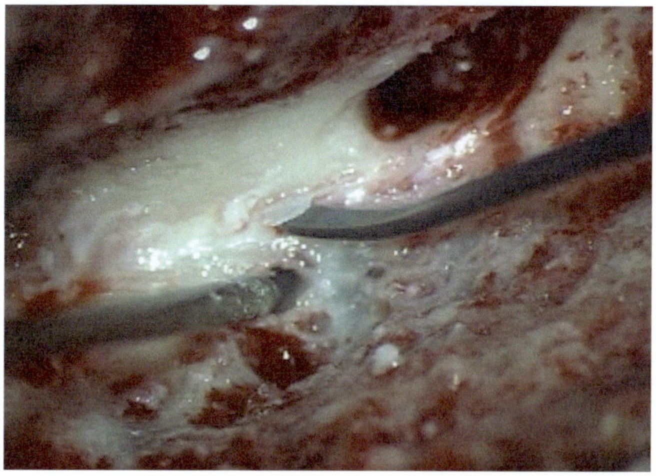

12. The remaining thin fragments of bone over the horizontal segment were also picked away manually.

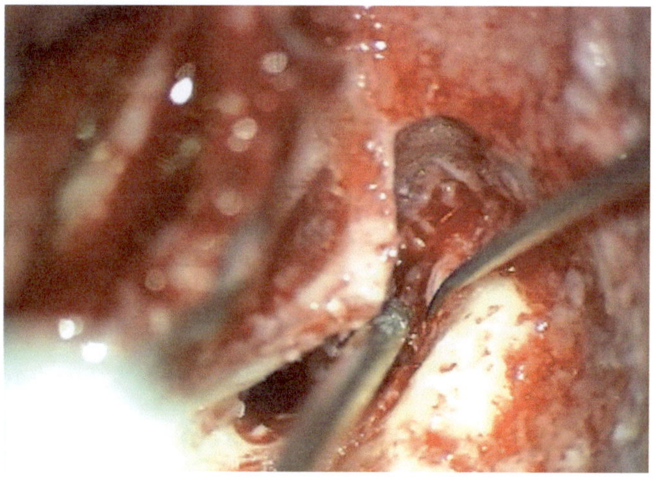

13. A middle fossa craniotomy was then performed. Note that viewing angle has changed because the surgeon has moved to the head of the bed. The malleable retractors were positioned within the extradural space, and the drilled-out mastoidectomy is visible.

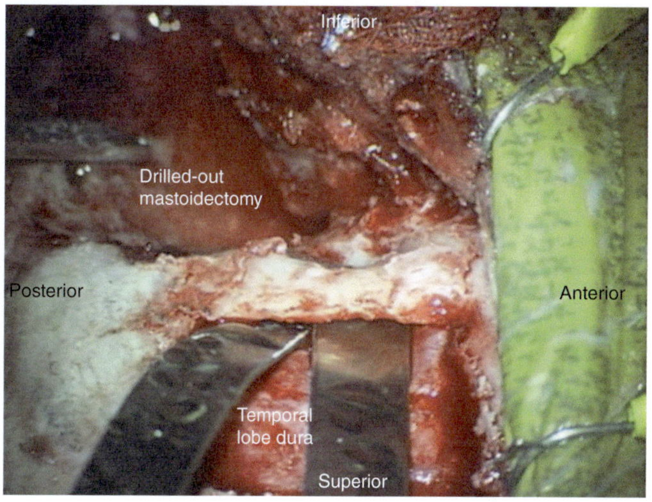

14. The temporal lobe dura was retracted to expose the floor of the middle cranial fossa.

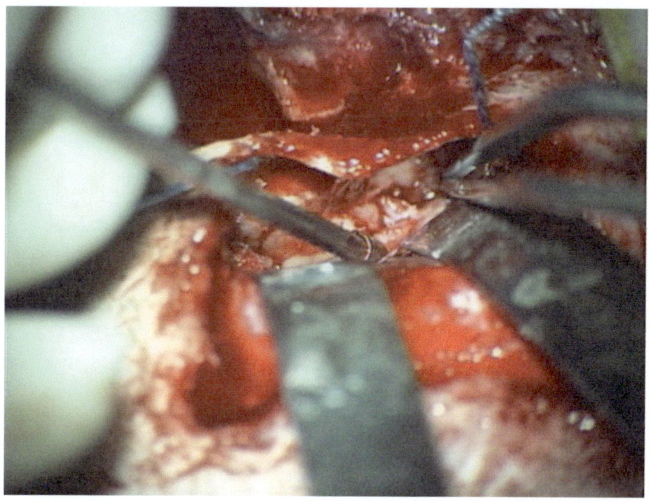

15. The geniculate ganglion (*GG*) was found to be dehiscent and quite swollen. The greater superficial petrosal nerve (*GSPN*) branched off anteriorly and was adherent to the dura as is typical.

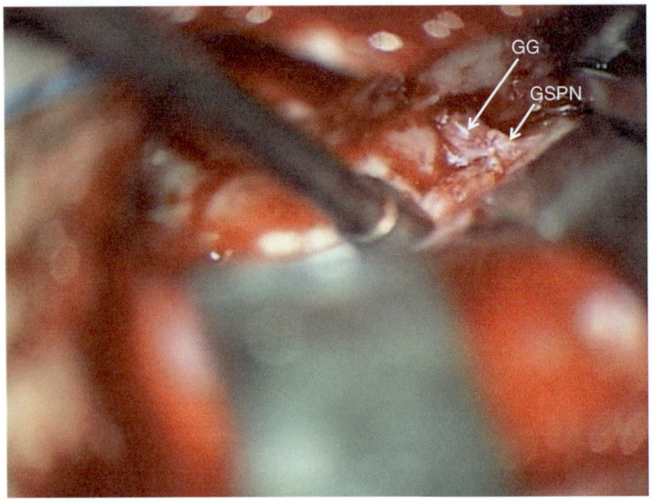

16. Drilling commenced medial to the geniculate ganglion (*GG*).

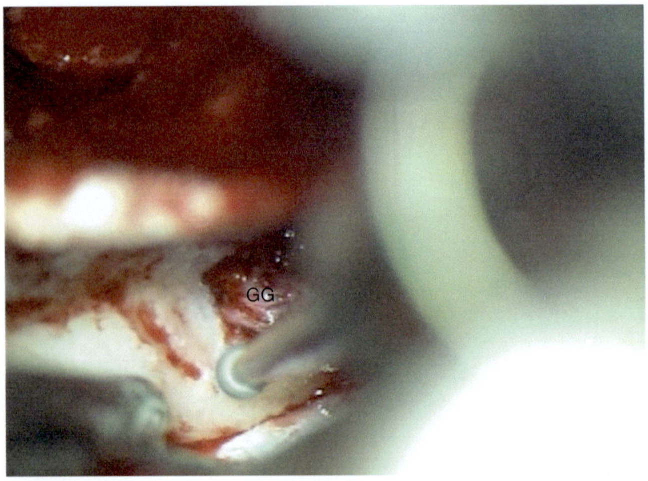

17. After separating the GSPN from the dura for a short distance.

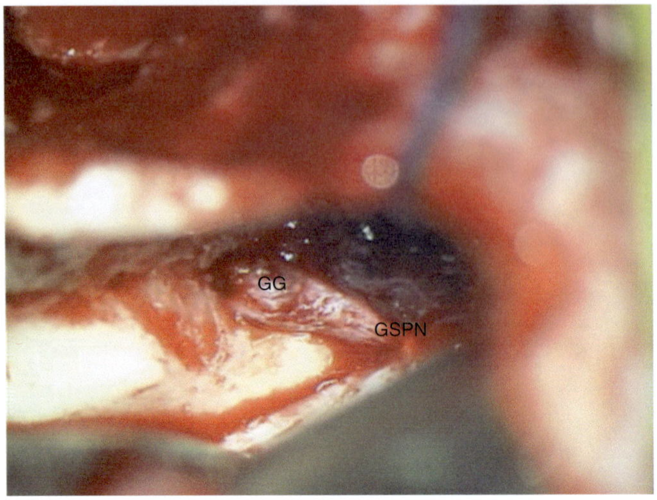

18. Further drilling demonstrates the beginnings of the horizontal segment (*HS*) and the labyrinthine segment (*LS*) of the facial nerve.

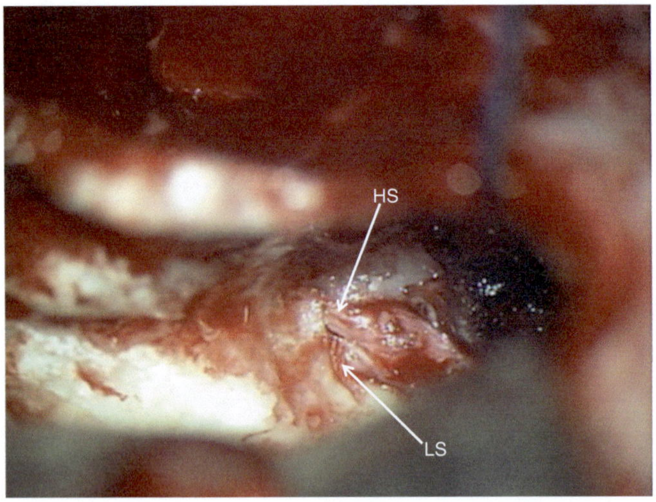

19. The anterior horizontal segment was gently mobilized to verify that the decompressed region seen here connected up to the decompressed region within the middle ear and mastoid.

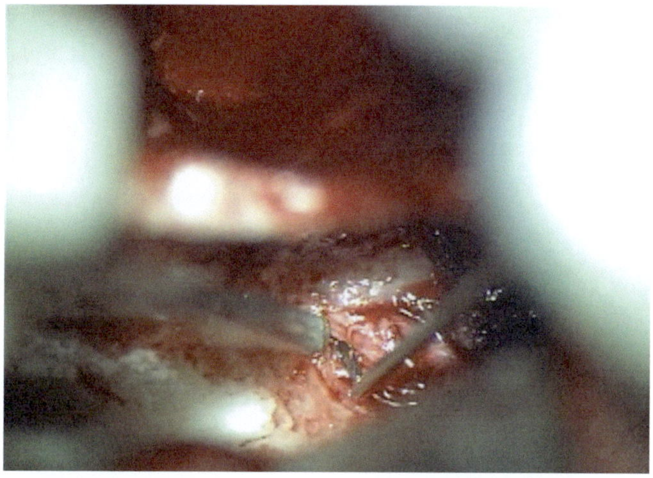

20. The labyrinthine segment of the facial nerve (*LS*) was now decompressed to the fundus of the internal auditory canal. Note that the nerve dives inward at a steep angle, and so the deep portion is out of focus with the geniculate ganglion. This angle is critical to recognize when decompressing the labyrinthine portion of the facial nerve. This is particularly important if the nerve is decompressed in the opposite direction (from the internal auditory canal to the geniculate) because it would be easy to drill into the nerve as it ascends superiorly. This angle can be appreciated by studying coronal CT images. The labyrinthine segment cannot be widely decompressed due to the proximity of the cochlea and superior vestibular nerve. Decompressing the lateral portion of the internal auditory canal can help with orientation and allow for maximal decompression of the labyrinthine segment.

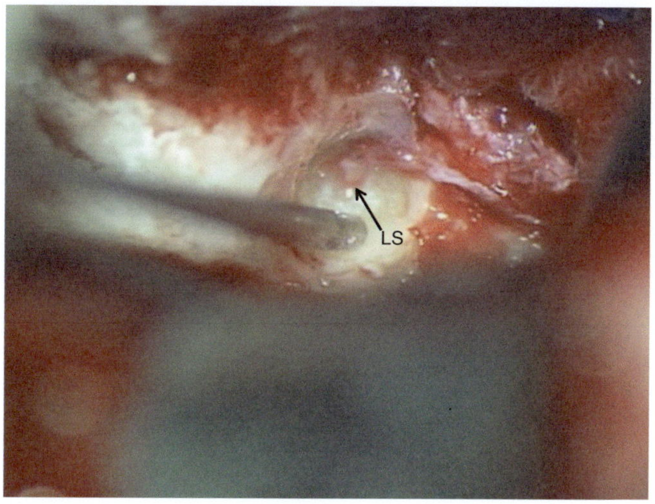

21. Postoperative axial CT demonstrating excellent decompression of the geniculate ganglion. The labyrinthine segment of the facial nerve was only decompressed along its superior aspect, which can not be appreciated in this image.

The surgical approach used in this case is illustrative of what it takes to reach all segments of the intratemporal facial nerve. Clearly accessing the descending (mastoid) segment is most straightforward and is associated with essentially no morbidity. Decompression of the tympanic segment cannot be reasonably accomplished without removing the incus, and thus, hearing is likely to be permanently compromised. Some have stated that the geniculate can be adequately decompressed through the transmastoid approach. We do not subscribe to that theory and prefer the middle fossa approach. This extradural procedure carries little risk of complications, but it is an intracranial procedure, and therefore, the risks are nontrivial. The scientific evidence behind the value of decompression is limited, and the risk/benefit should be carefully considered. Further complicating decision-making in patients who have suffered trauma is the other injuries they may have sustained including brain injuries and the potential for negative side effects from undergoing a surgical procedure.

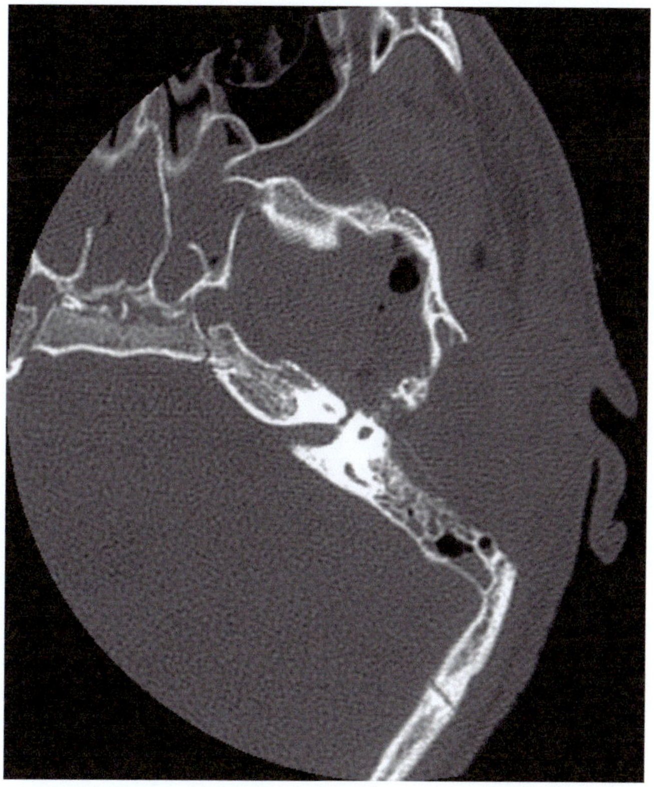

22. Case 2. Intraoperative image of a patient whose left facial nerve was decompressed along the vertical segment (*VS*) to the stylomastoid foramen (*SMF*). The lateral semicircular canal (*LSCC*) and parotid gland are visible. While only a 90–180° decompression is needed to treat trauma-induced neural edema, this decompression was more extensive (360°) because it was performed as part of a jugular foramen tumor resection. This image clearly shows the course of the vertical portion of the facial nerve and how it turns to exit the stylomastoid foramen.

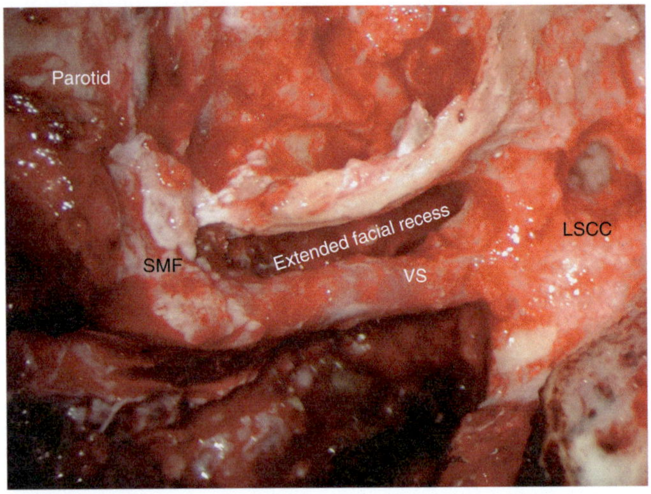

23. Case 3. Axial CT demonstrating a gunshot wound through the left ear canal that caused a comminuted fracture of the temporal bone. The bullet (*asterisk*) lodged in the cerebellum.

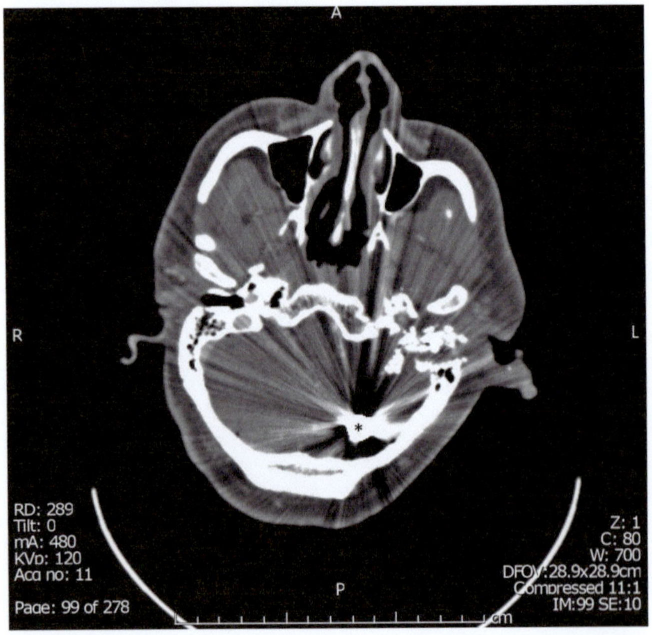

24. Bone windowing demonstrates the severity of the injury. With this type of injury, it is reasonable (and correct in this case) to assume that the entire vertical segment of the facial nerve has been destroyed.

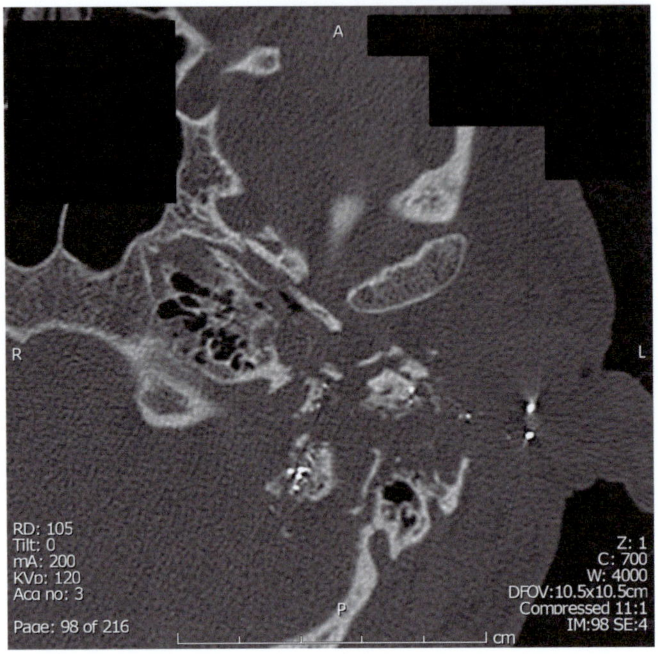

25. CT angiography demonstrates patency of the internal carotid artery. Also, the supratentorial brain appears healthy. We ended up obliterating the ear and using an interpositional graft from the horizontal segment of the facial nerve to the pes anserinus using a greater auricular nerve graft.

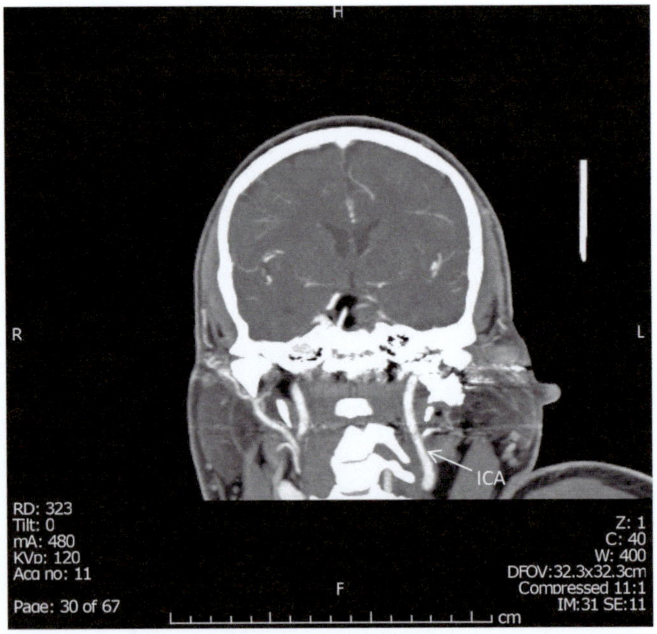

26. Case 4. Axial CT of a patient with a geniculate hemangioma (*arrows*). Note its expansive, partially calcified nature characteristic of this type of tumor.

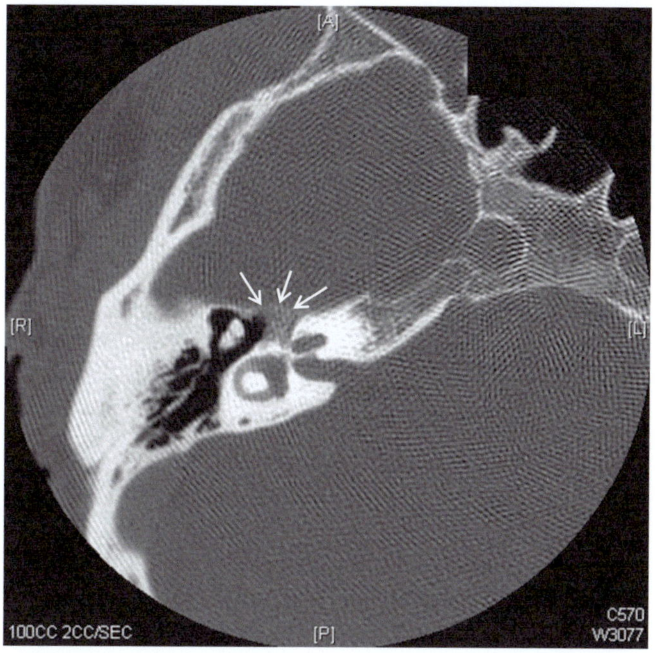

27. Coronal CT demonstrating the tumor extent (*arrows*). This patient had partial facial paralysis (House–Brackmann grade 4) and underwent surgical resection in an effort to prevent complete facial palsy.

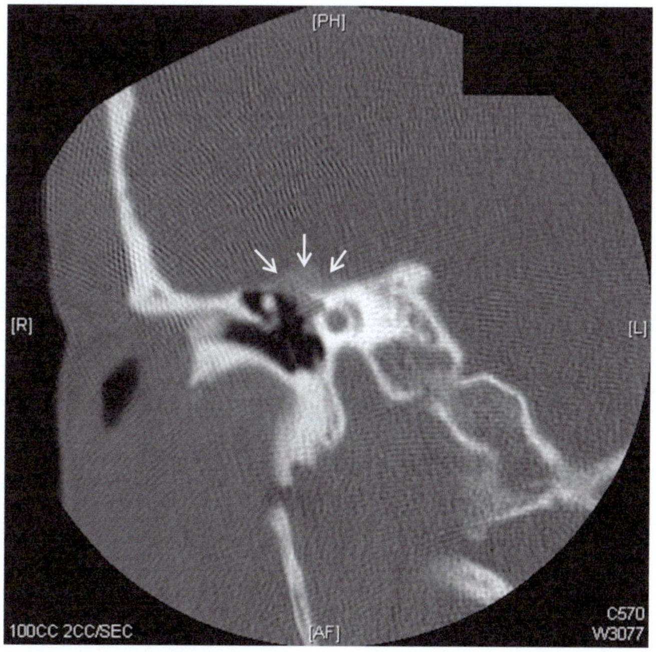

28. Postoperative coronal CT after surgical resection of this tumor. Note the dehiscence in the area of the geniculate ganglion (*arrow*). The tumor could be removed off the nerve, although some involved fibers were resected with the tumor. Postoperatively, the patient had a total facial paralysis that recovered to the preoperative baseline within 8 months.

Geniculate hemangiomas involve the facial nerve in two distinct patterns that cannot be predicted based on imaging. Some tumors completely involve the nerve and cannot be resected with nerve preservation. Wide decompression of the geniculate ganglion can result in improved facial nerve function, and unless the nerve function was very poor, we would not resect the tumor in its entirety. Other tumors are largely or completely outside the nerve and can be resected with excellent nerve preservation. Therefore, even in patients with excellent facial nerve function, we will offer exploration and tumor resection. Sometimes, a subtotal resection ends up being performed due to our efforts to spare the facial nerve.

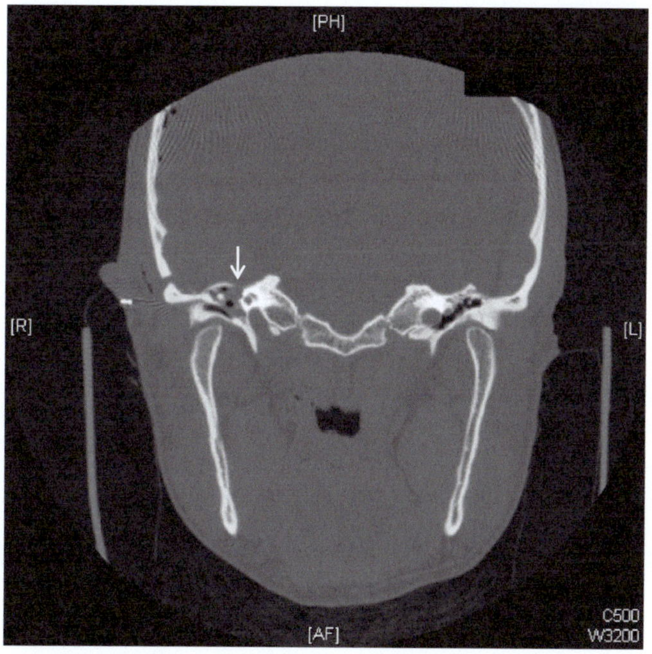

29. Case 5. Axial CT of a patient with a right cholesteatoma that grew into the anterior epitympanic region and compressed the facial nerve. She presented with a draining ear and a partial facial palsy that recovered after a course of antibiotics. Note the bone destruction around the lateral aspect of the geniculate ganglion (*arrow*) that was caused by the cholesteatoma.

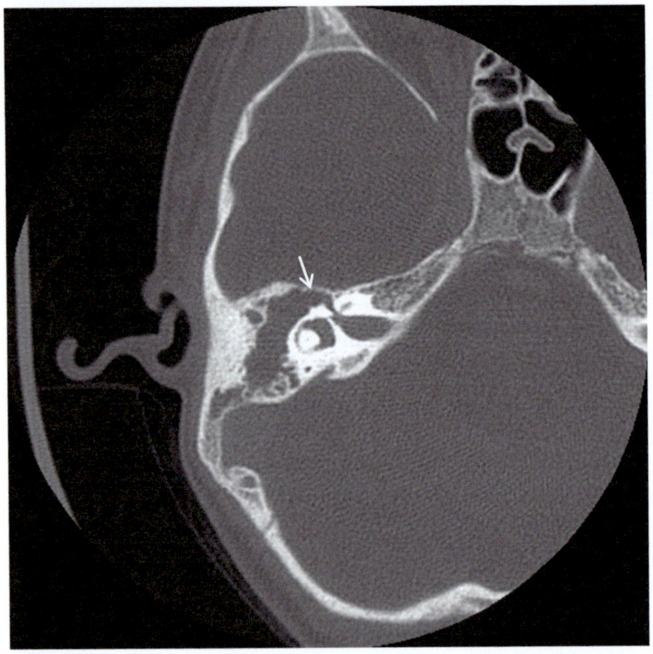

30. The left ear demonstrated the normal bony anatomy lateral to the geniculate ganglion (*arrow*).

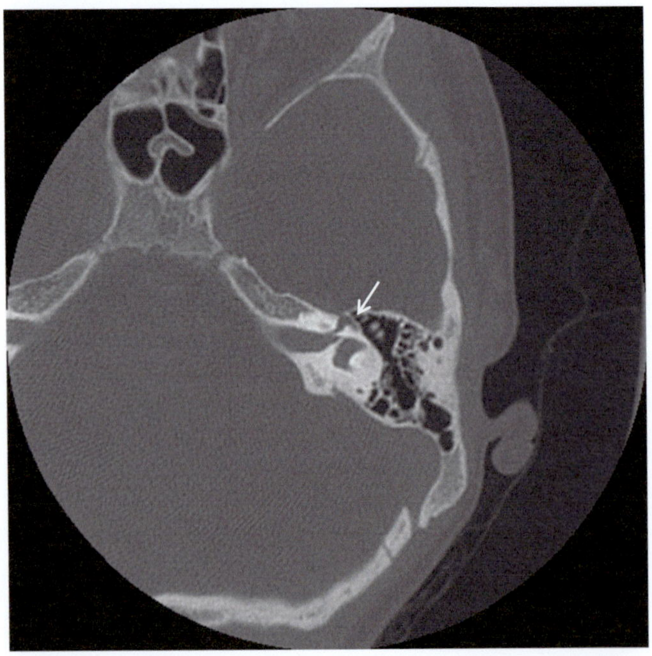

31. Axial T1 MRI with gadolinium demonstrates the right ear disease to be nonenhancing (*arrow*).

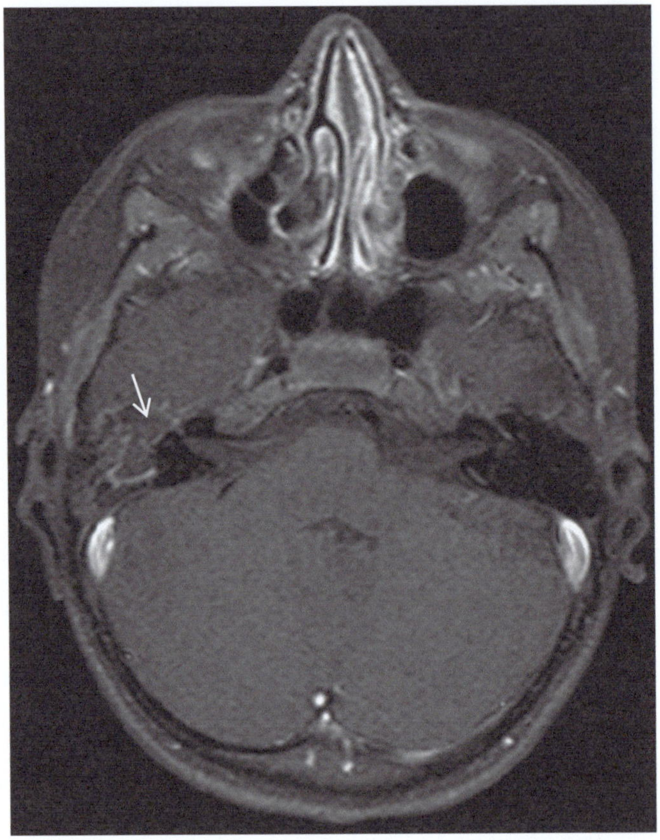

32. Intraoperative view after a canal wall up mastoidectomy was performed. The incus and head of the malleus were removed. This view is just anterior to the lateral semicircular canal (*LSCC*). Cholesteatoma matrix lines the anterior epitympanic air cell region and can be seen to dive medially at the level of the geniculate ganglion.

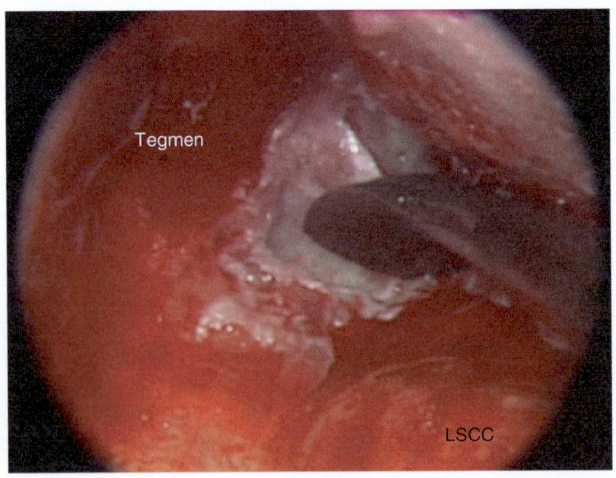

33. The depth of the pocket can be appreciated after insertion of the duckbill elevator.

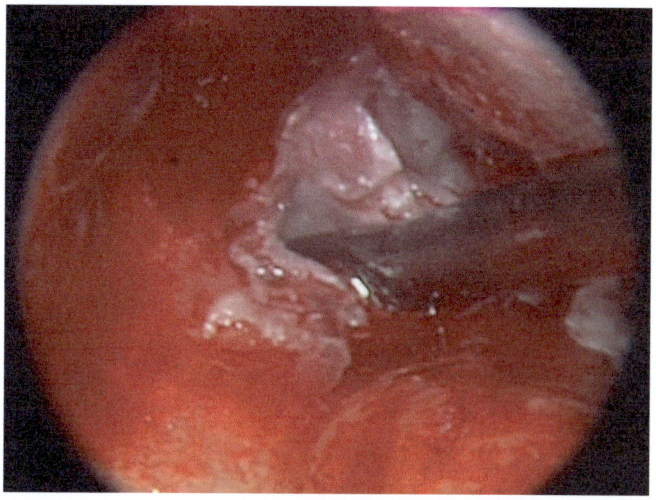

34. After carefully microdissecting the matrix out of this pocket, the dehiscent geniculate ganglion (*GG*) can clearly be seen. The horizontal facial nerve (*FN*) and lateral semicircular canal (*LSCC*) are also visible.

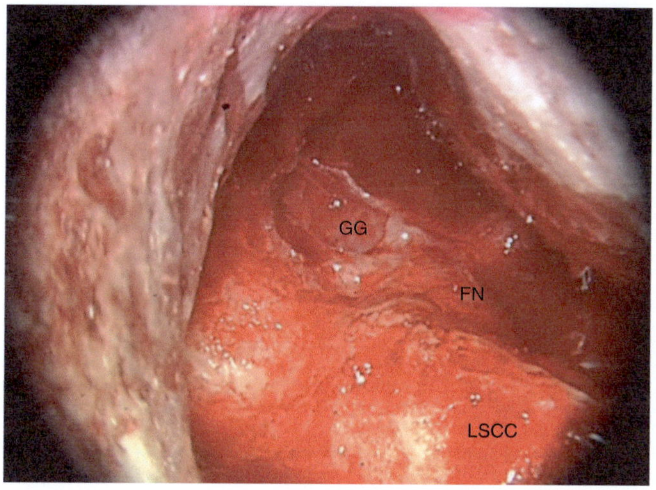

35. Case 6. A right-sided facial nerve schwannoma extending into the temporal bone caused complete facial paralysis. First, it was exposed along the vertical segment.

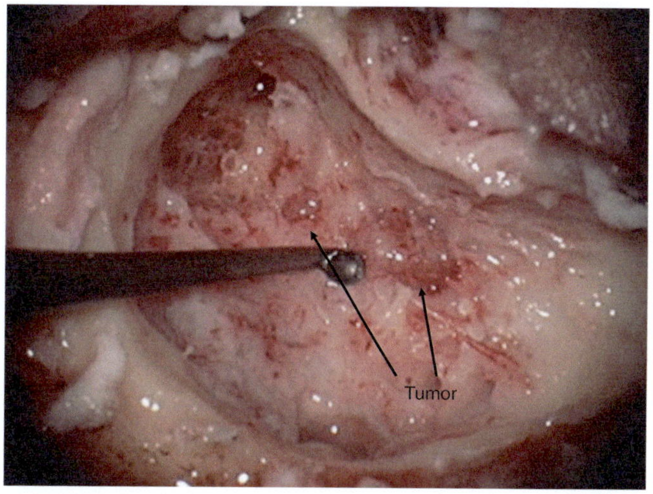

36. A canal wall up mastoidectomy was performed, the incus removed, and the head of the malleus clipped. The proximal margin was just distal to the geniculate ganglion. The stapes and round window (*RW*) can be noted.

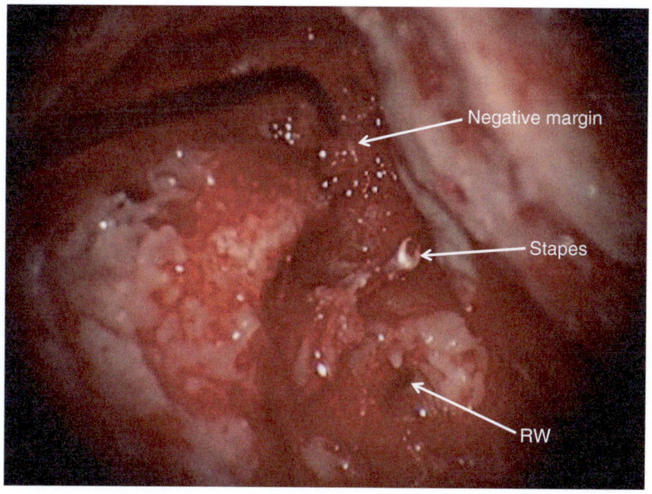

37. A sural nerve interposition graft was placed from the proximal margin to the main trunk of the facial nerve just distal to the stylomastoid foramen. In this view of the distal anastomosis, the technique of using multiple interrupted sutures to bring the epineurium of the graft and the facial nerve trunk together circumferentially can be seen. We usually use 8-0 or 9-0 nylon.

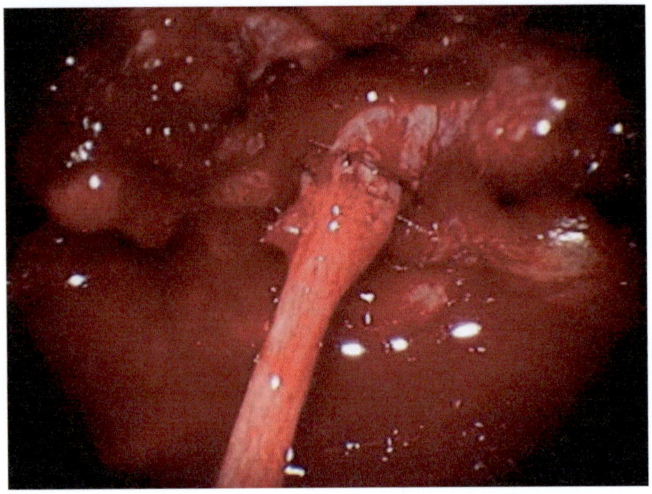

38. Case 7. A patient had a mucoepidermoid carcinoma of the left parotid gland that invaded the main trunk of the facial nerve. The tumor and facial nerve were resected, and a sural nerve graft was placed from the second genu (*arrowhead*) to the upper and lower divisions of the facial nerve.

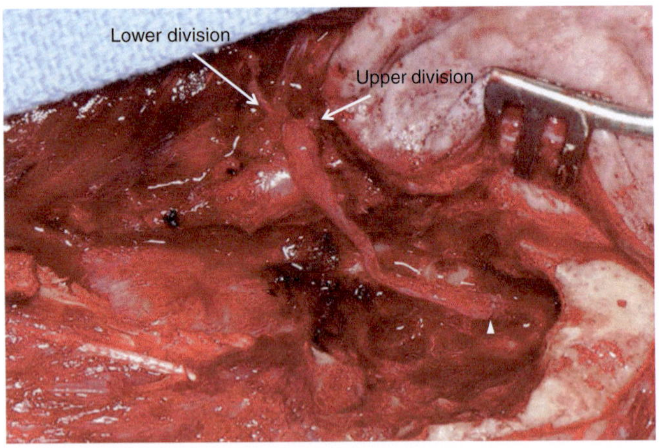

39. Case 8. Greater auricular nerve graft harvest (*arrowheads*). A standard parotid incision has been made on the right side of the face and neck. The nerve is visible just lateral to the sternocleidomastoid muscle (SCM). When it is possible to use it, the greater auricular nerve is ideal for grafting the facial nerve. Not only is it in close proximity, it is also close in size to the facial nerve.

The downside of using the greater auricular nerve is that it may not be long enough to reach from the proximal facial nerve all the way out to terminal branches. Also, invasive malignancies may infiltrate into the nerve. Lastly, the surgeon needs to think ahead when starting the case to plan on harvesting the nerve before dissecting down to the parotid gland. If the nerve is accidentally cut during the initial process of raising the skin flap, the residual nerve may be too short.

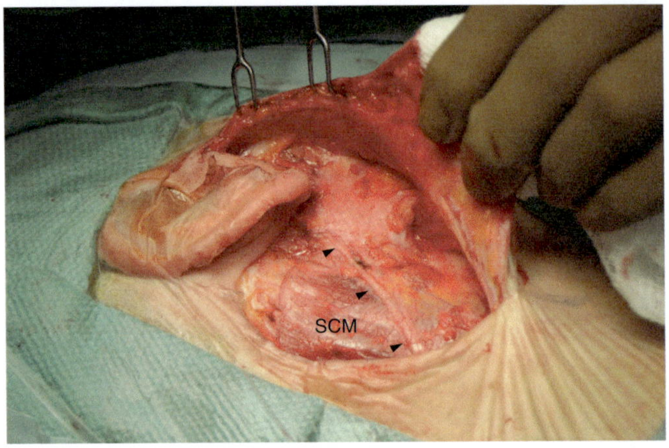

40. Case 9. Sural nerve graft harvest. The lateral aspect of the right ankle and leg were prepped out. The incision started posterior to the lateral malleolus of the ankle. Dissection was performed to identify the small saphenous vein and the sural nerve, which run together.

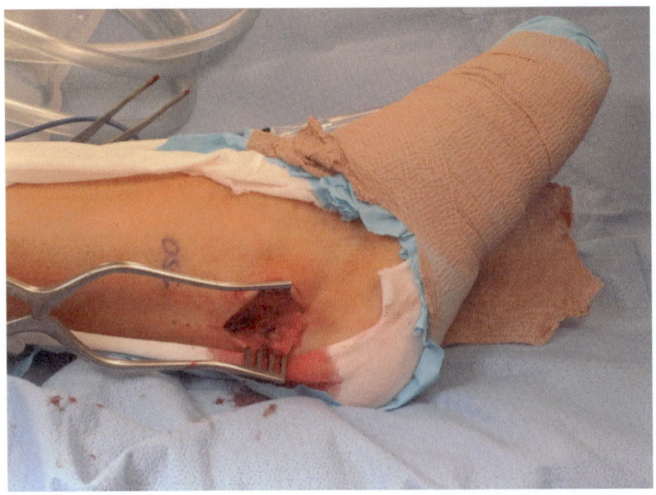

41. Dissection was carried superiorly to trace out as much of the sural nerve (*arrowheads*) as was necessary.

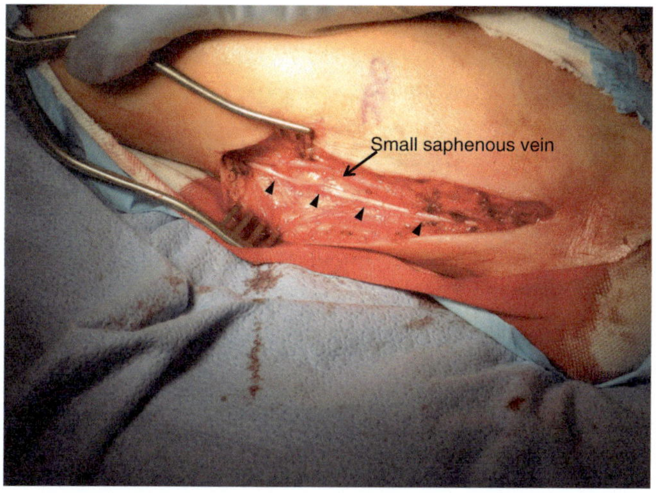

42. As shown here, compared to the greater auricular nerve, a much longer graft can be harvested from the sural nerve, and there is no risk of it being involved with tumor in patients with malignancies. The downside of using a sural nerve graft is the side effect of numbness along the lateral aspect of the foot. Also, the size of the graft may be large and not an ideal match for the facial nerve.

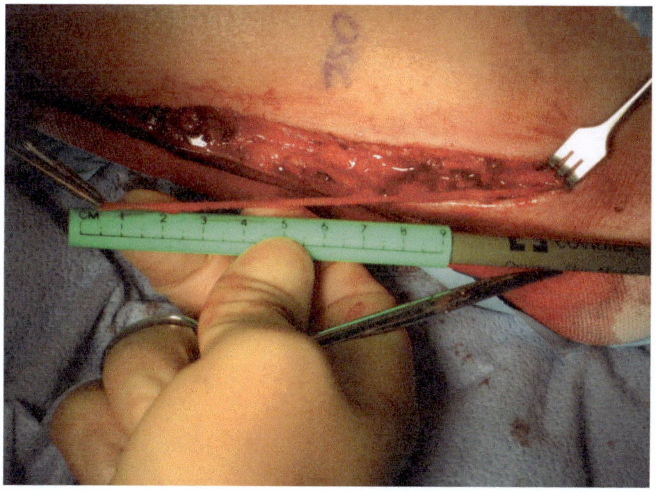

43. The trigeminal–facial nerve anastamosis. CN V supplies motor innervation to the muscles of mastication. In this procedure, the branches to the masseter muscle are identified and dissected out. Shown here is the normal anatomy of the nerves to the masseter muscle.

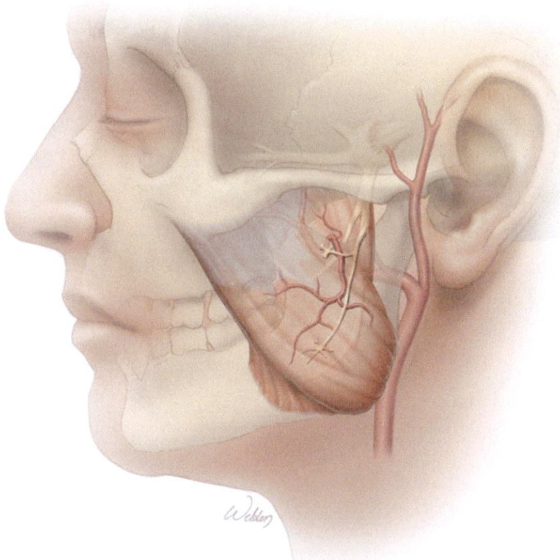

44. The largest branch can be sutured to the main trunk of the facial nerve. As shown here, some surgeons divide the zygomatic branch in order to reduce hyperkinesis that can occur with nerve transposition operations like this. Alternatively, the nerve can be left intact and Botox used as needed.

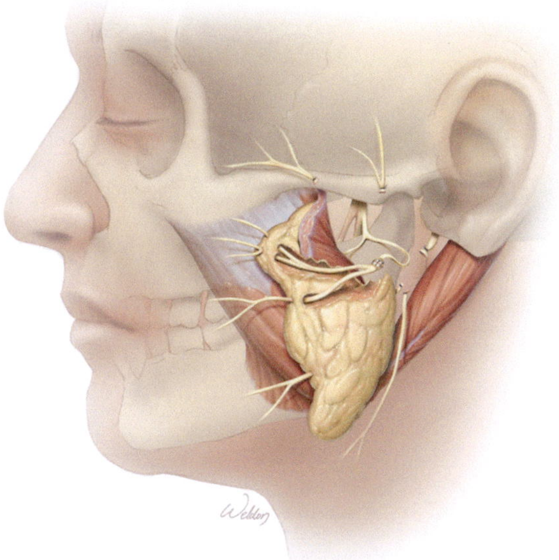

45. The hypoglossal–facial nerve anastomosis. The normal courses of the facial nerve and the hypoglossal nerve (*XII*) are shown. Not that the hypoglossal nerve is easily found just medial to the digastric muscle. There are many small veins in this region that can be safely divided to find the nerve. The retromandibular vein (*arrowhead*) occasionally needs to be divided for adequate exposure.

A direct XII-VII anastomosis is performed by dissecting the hypoglossal nerve as far out as possible toward the tongue and then bringing it up and suturing it to the main trunk of the facial nerve (*top inset*). Contraindications to this procedure include loss of function of other lower cranial nerves such as IX or X. The additional loss of CN XII can lead to dysphagia. As long as the other cranial nerves are fine, this procedure has little to no effect on speech or swallowing after a period of compensation.

An alternative approach is to perform a XII-VII jump graft anastomosis (*bottom inset*). CN XII is sectioned in half, and a greater auricular nerve graft is sutured from the cut portion to the main trunk of the facial nerve. This preserves much of the function of the tongue, has nearly as good facial function results as a direct transfer, and has less hyperkinesis than a direct graft.

If there is adequate length of the facial nerve, then a direct end-to-side anastomosis can be made. If the facial nerve can be harvested up to the tympanic segment, it can usually reach the hypoglossal nerve. The facial nerve will need to be mobilized to the pes anserinus. The digastric may need to be divided, and the hypoglossal nerve needs to be traced and mobilized superiorly as far as possible. A tension-free environment needs to be achieved.

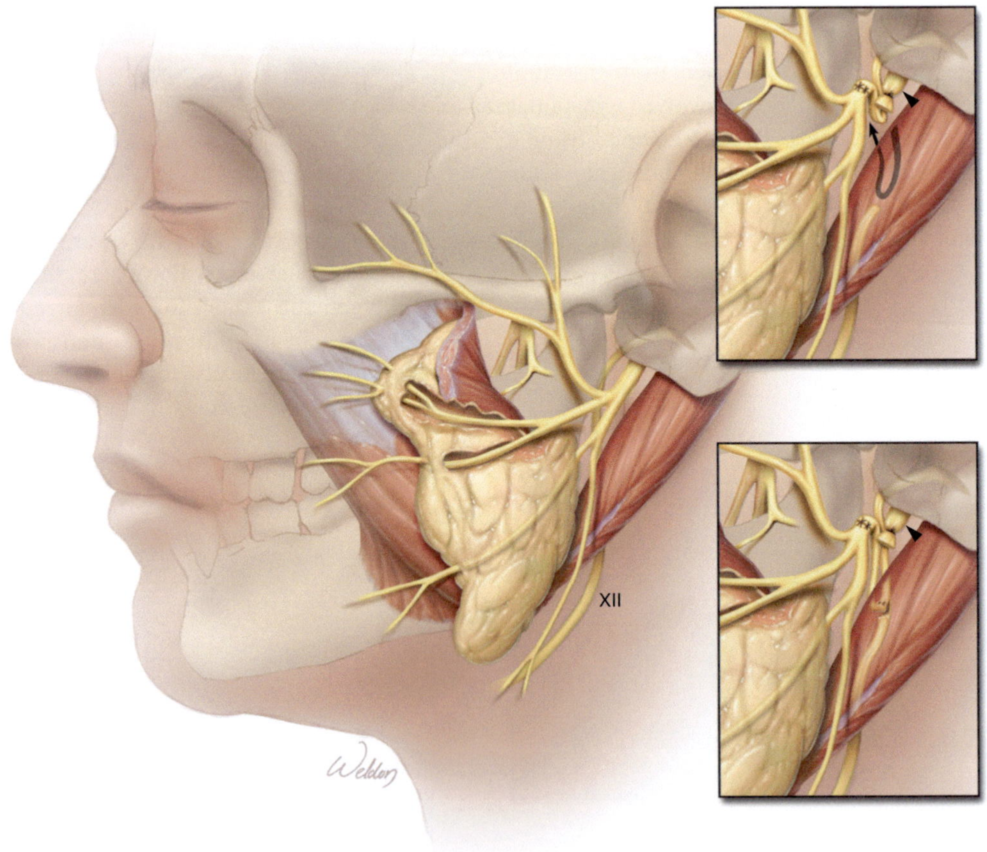

46. Case 10. Skin incision on a patient undergoing a left XII-VII jump graft anastomosis after a neurosurgical resection of a brainstem arteriovenous malformation led to complete facial palsy.

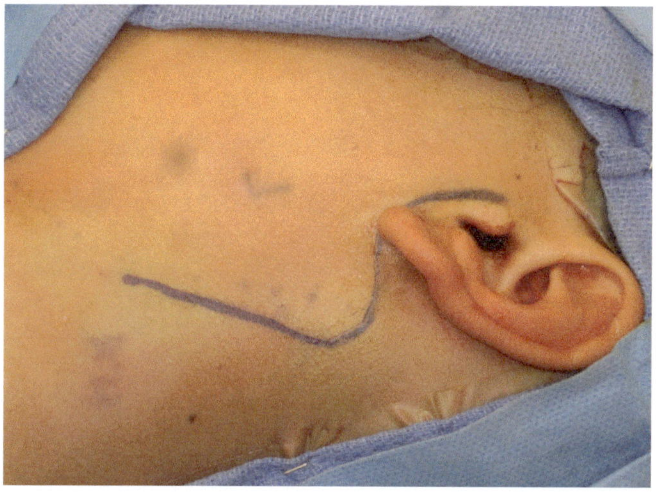

47. The greater auricular nerve (*arrow*) was identified on the lateral border of the sternocleidomastoid muscle. The nerve should be handled gently to limit trauma that might negatively impact regeneration.

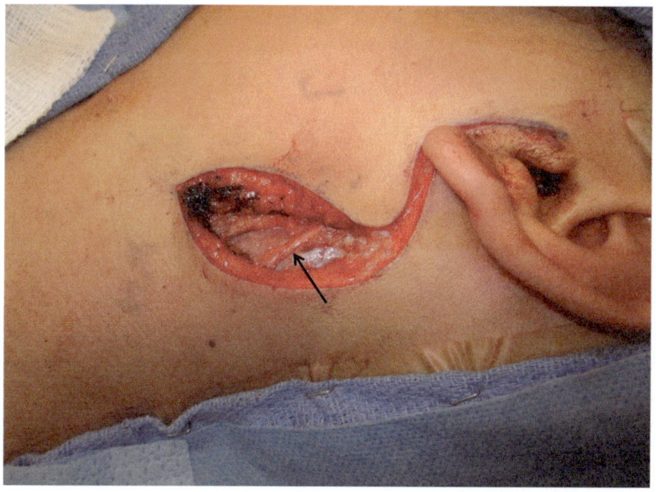

48. The greater auricular nerve was cut distally and dissected out medially. The facial nerve was identified and traced to the pes anserinus. The hypoglossal nerve was identified inferior to the digastric muscle (*DM*).

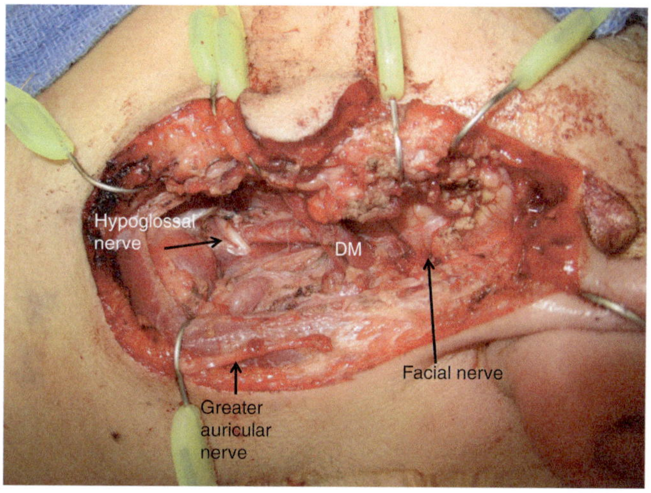

49. The microscope was brought in, making the main trunk of the facial nerve and the pes anserinus clearly visible. The upper division (*UD*) and lower division (*LD*) of the facial nerve can be seen.

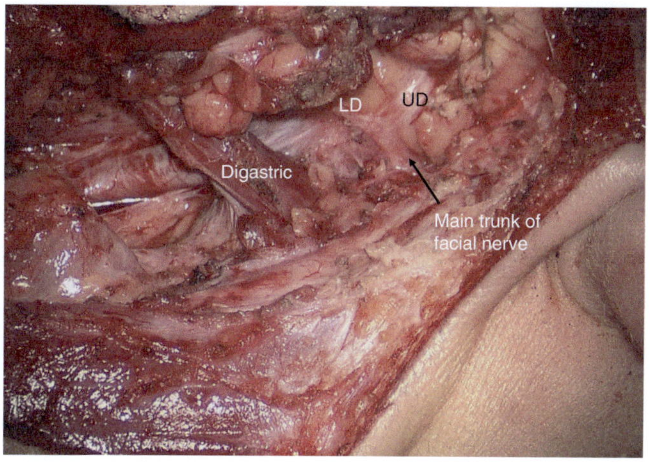

50. The epineurium and surrounding tissue around the main trunk of the facial nerve was gently grasped with a Cushing forceps and the medial aspect of the nerve dissected free from the underlying tissues.

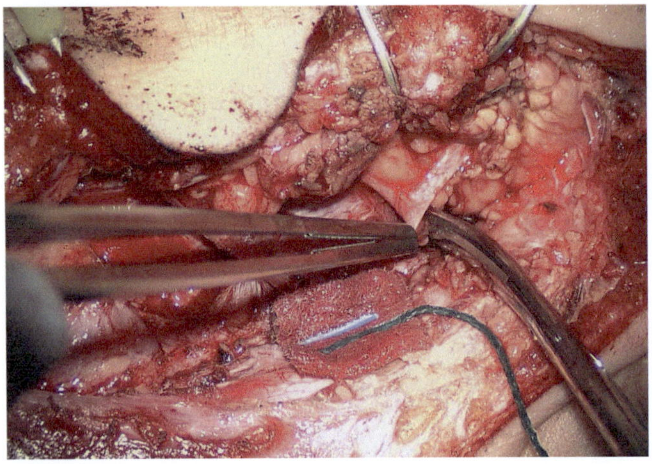

51. The main trunk of the facial nerve was cut as close to the stylomastoid foramen as possible, and the undersides of the upper and lower divisions were dissected free.

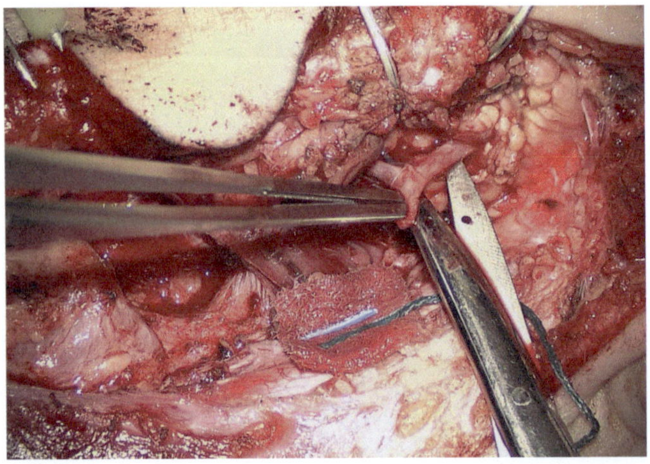

52. After harvesting the greater auricular nerve graft, the first stitch was placed on the bottom (medial aspect) of the anastomosis. We use interrupted stitches placed within the epineurium. The green plastic sheet under the nerves improves the visualization during this process.

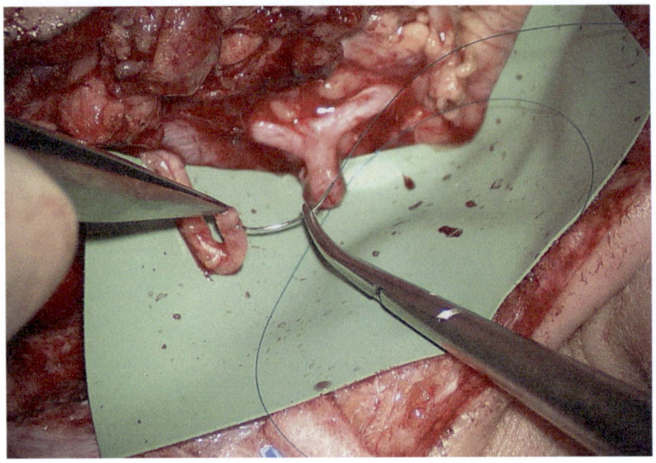

53. After completion of the anastomosis between the greater auricular nerve graft and the main trunk of the facial nerve.

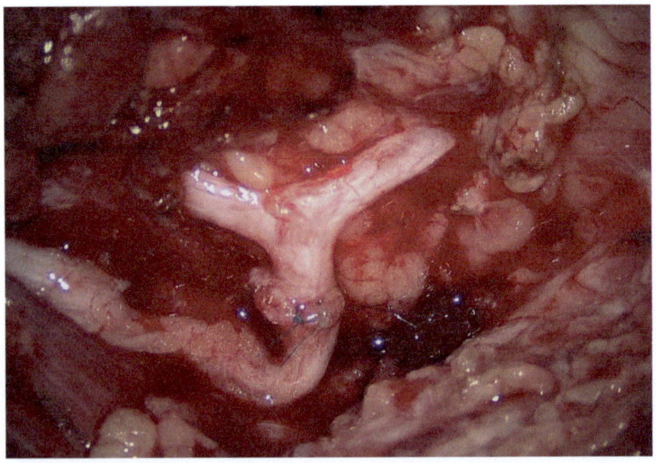

54. The greater auricular nerve graft (*arrowheads*) was tunneled medial to the digastric muscle to reach the hypoglossal nerve. A cut was made into the hypoglossal nerve (*arrow*) to divide about 50 % of the diameter of the nerve with an 11 blade scalpel.

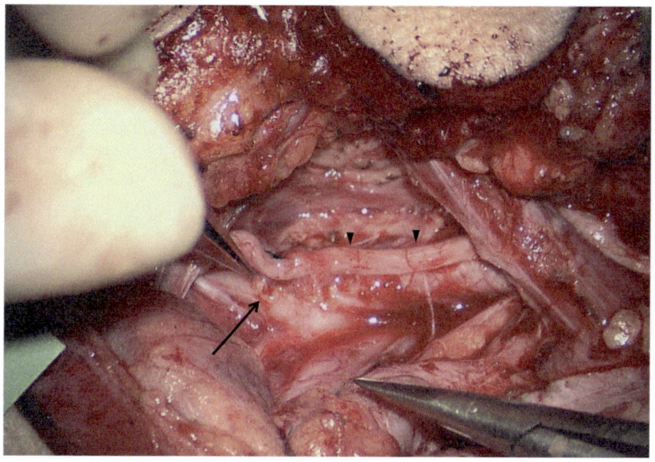

55. The greater auricular nerve graft was curved around and an anastomosis made to the cut proximal end of the hypoglossal nerve.

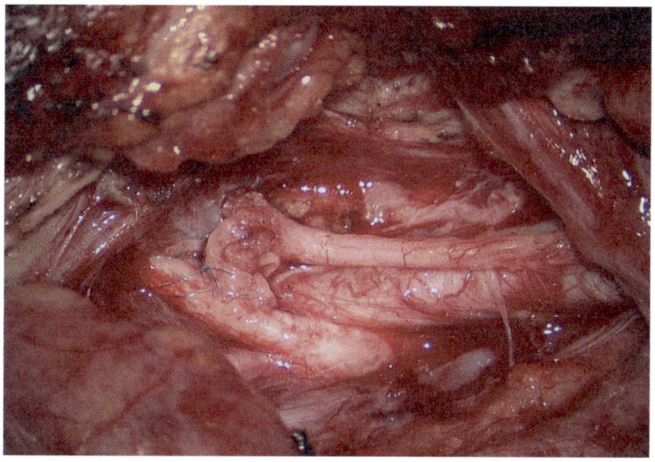

56. Overview of the entire field after the procedure. Careful closing must be performed so as not to disrupt either anastomosis.

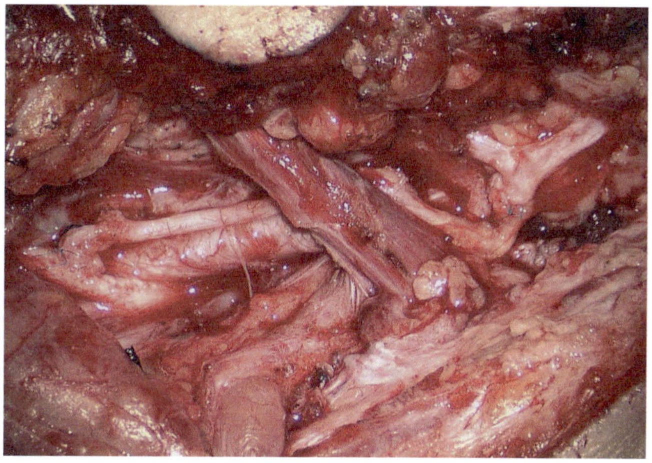

10 Cochlear Implantation

- *Concept*
  - Most hearing loss is due to cochlear dysfunction. A cochlear implant performs the function of the cochlea by converting sound energy to electricity and stimulating the auditory nerve in a tonotopic manner.
- *Conditions treated*
  - Sensorineural hearing loss due to cochlear dysfunction
  - Sensorineural hearing loss due to Auditory Neuropathy/Auditory Dys-synchrony assuming an auditory nerve is present.
- *Risks*
  - Loss of residual hearing.
  - Dizziness.
  - Facial nerve injury.
  - Meningitis.
  - Infection of the implant.
  - CSF leak.
  - Although not a surgical complication, device failure can occur.
- *Benefits*
  - At this time, cochlear implantation is the only medical treatment available to restore sensorineural hearing.
- *Additional notes*
  - The decision of when cochlear implantation may permit better auditory performance compared to hearing aids is important to make on an individual patient basis. However, cochlear implant technology continues to improve regularly, and the latest guidelines should be followed for optimal outcomes.

J.S. Oghalai, C.L.W. Driscoll, *Atlas of Neurotologic and Lateral Skull Base Surgery*,
DOI 10.1007/978-3-662-46694-0_10,

1. The cochlea. The traveling wave originates with vibrations of the stapes within the oval window (*OW*). It travels up the cochlear duct through scala vestibuli (*SV*). The sensory hair cells sit within scala media (*SM*). A cochlear implant electrode should be placed within scala tympani (*ST*), the portion of the cochlear duct in continuity with the round window (*RW*). The modiolus is the central core of the cochlea and is where the auditory nerve travels.

2. Cross section of the cochlear duct showing scala vestibuli (*SV*), scala media (*SM*), and scala tympani (*ST*). The organ of Corti contains one row of inner hair cells (*arrowhead*), three rows of outer hair cells (*arrow*), and the supporting cells (*SC*), all of which sit on top of the basilar membrane (*BM*). The basilar membrane is attached to the osseous spiral lamina (*OSL*) medially and the spiral ligament (*SL*) laterally. The tectorial membrane (*TM*) produces deflections of the hair cell stereocilia, resulting in sound transduction. The auditory nerve (*AN*) carries the electrical signals to the brain.

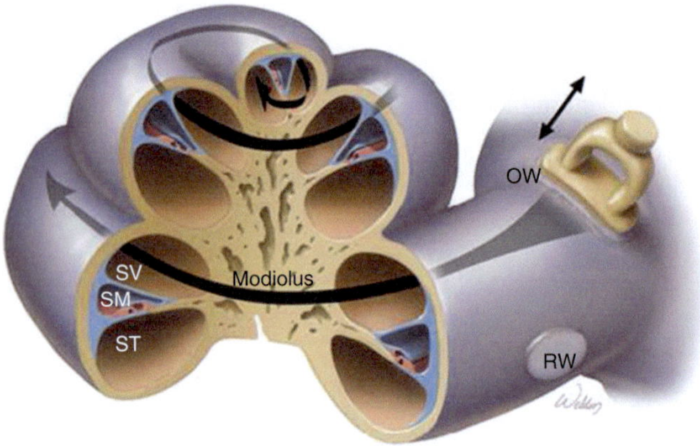

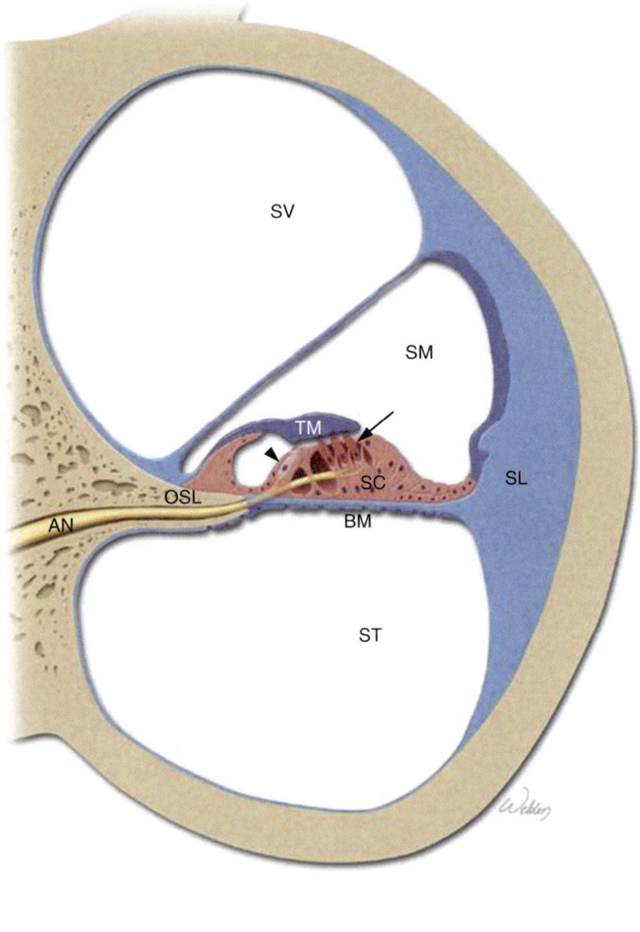

3. Schematic of the steps in cochlear implantation. Coronal view of a normal temporal bone.

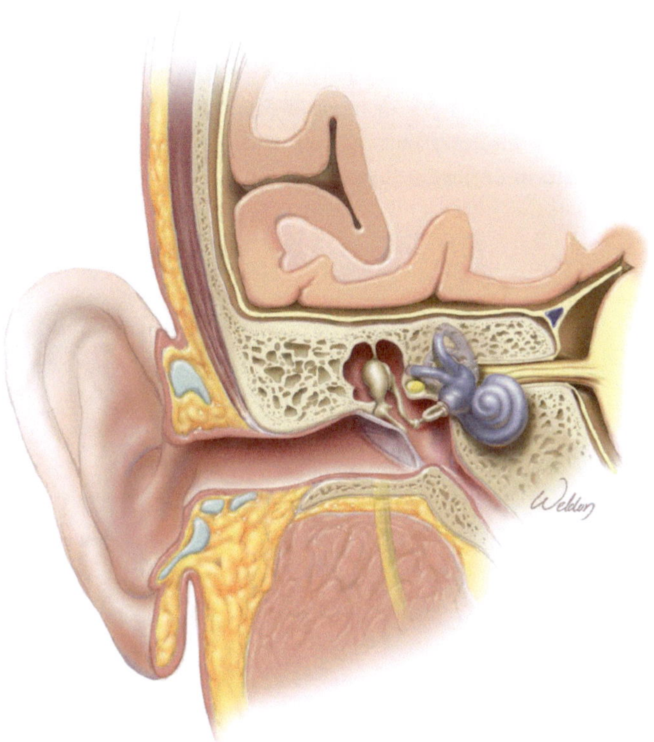

4. A simple mastoidectomy has been performed.

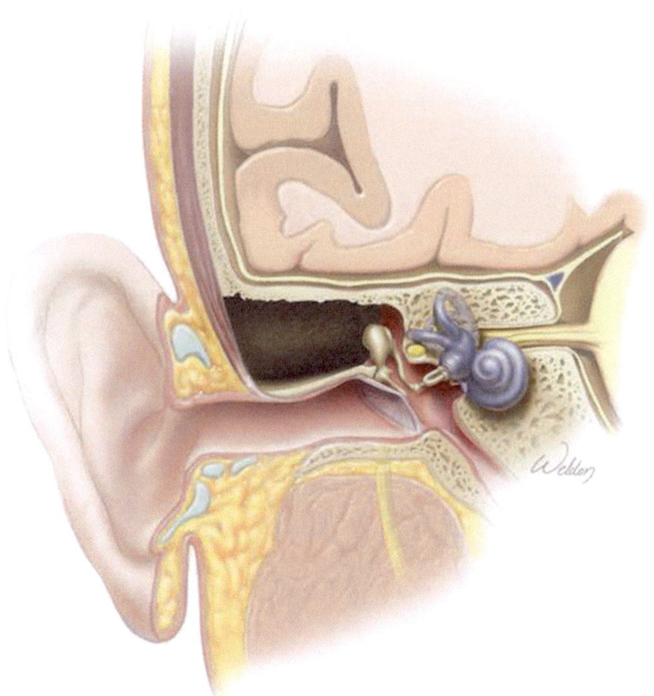

5. A facial recess approach has been performed.

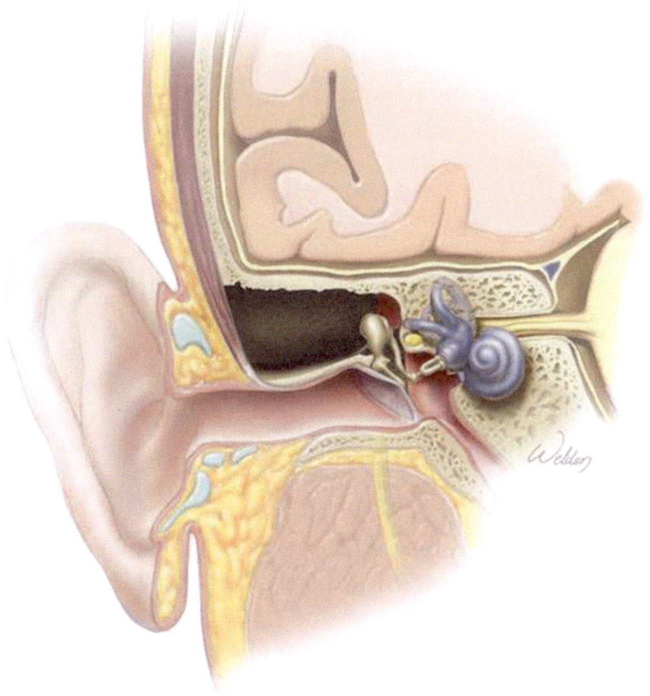

6. A cochlear implant has been placed. Note the electrode passing through the facial recess and entering the cochlea at the round window.

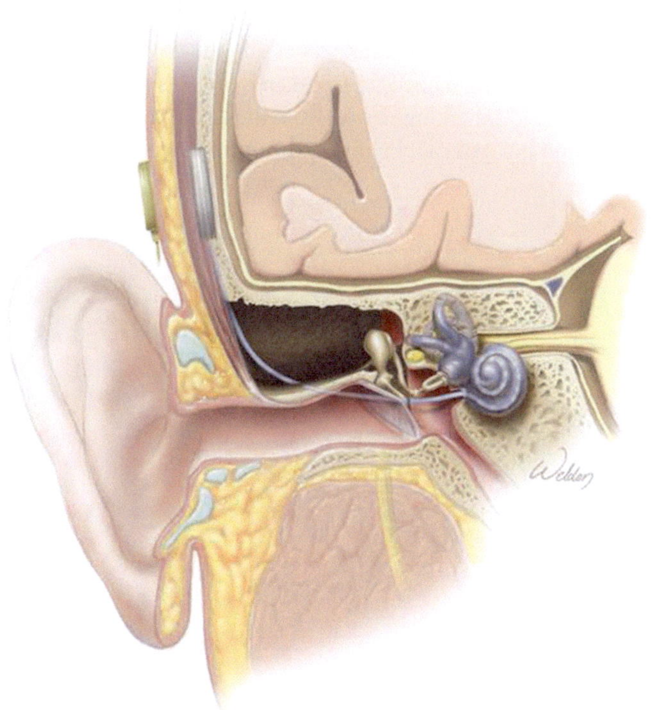

7. The surgical technique of cochlear implantation. An S-shaped postauricular incision is made. This type of incision has a lower risk of skin flap necrosis than the older C-shaped incision.

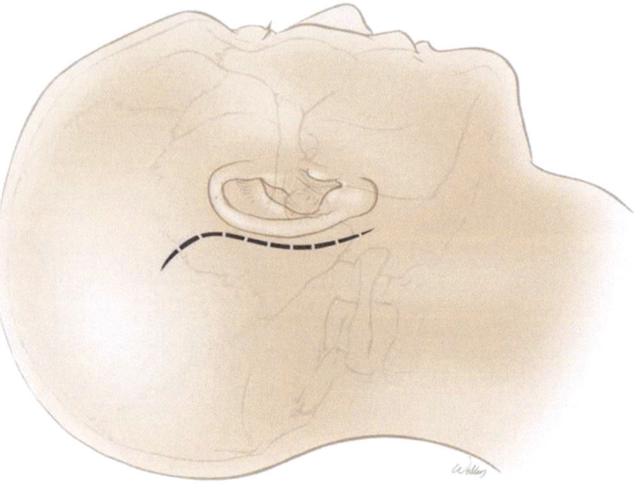

8. The incision can be carried straight down through the soft tissues to the skull. Alternatively, the incision through the subcutaneous tissues and the temporalis muscle can be staggered slightly from the skin incision to create flaps. While the theory is that the flaps will help reduce the risk of bacteria penetrating through the incision and colonizing the implant, we've not seen this be an issue in practice. In fact, the additional dead space created by the flaps may permit fluid accumulation and make it easier for bacteria to begin growing in the area of the implant.

   In young children with growing heads, an incision that extends into the hair-bearing region will tend to develop a wide scar and potentially significant area of alopecia. We try to make our incisions <5 cm long. Naturally, this does make recessing the device more difficult, and care needs to be taken to make sure the device is placed far enough away from the ear so that it does not bump the external behind-the-ear component.

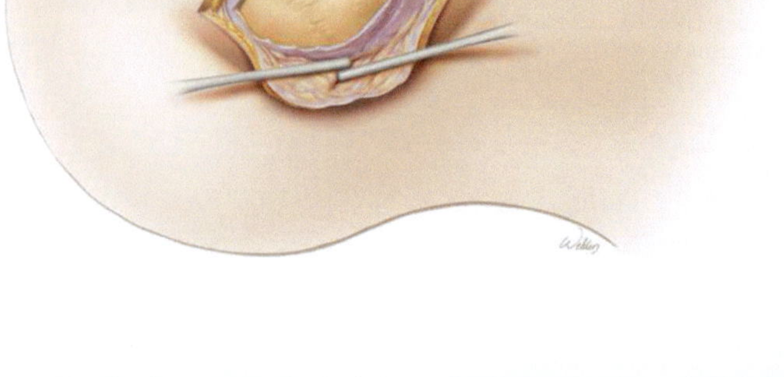

9. A simple mastoidectomy is then performed with identification of the sigmoid sinus, tegmen, and mastoid antrum. The short process of the incus should be identified, particularly where it attaches to the incudal buttress. Most importantly, the ear canal needs to be thinned. There should be no air cells left along its course because a thick ear canal will block the view of the round window through the facial recess. A larger cutting burr (5–6 mm) is used for most of the mastoidectomy, and a 4 mm diamond burr is used to thin the ear canal and begin to expose a few of the air cells within the facial recess.

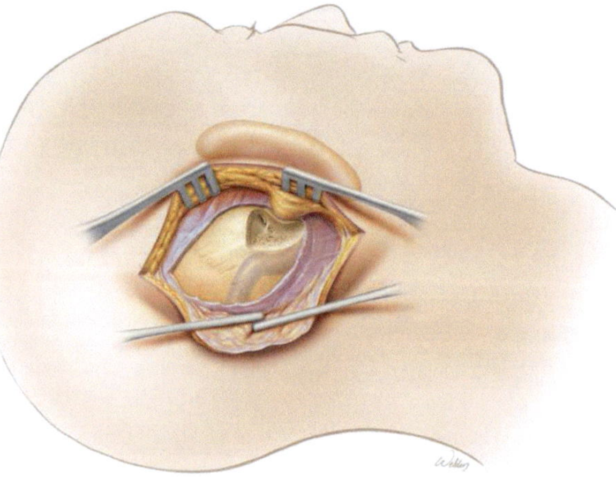

10. The facial recess approach is performed using a 2 mm diamond burr. A constant flow of water should be maintained to minimize heat transfer to the facial nerve. Note that this opening is in the shape of a triangle. The shaft of the drill should parallel the ear canal, and not be back over the sigmoid sinus. This allows the facial recess to follow the correct pathway and open into the middle ear space medial to the tympanic membrane. The boundaries are the facial nerve medially, the chorda tympani nerve and tympanic annulus laterally, and the incudal buttress superiorly. The incudal buttress should be left in place in order to maintain the ability of the ossicular chain to transmit sound vibrations to the cochlea. This is important if one desires to preserve as much acoustical hearing as possible.

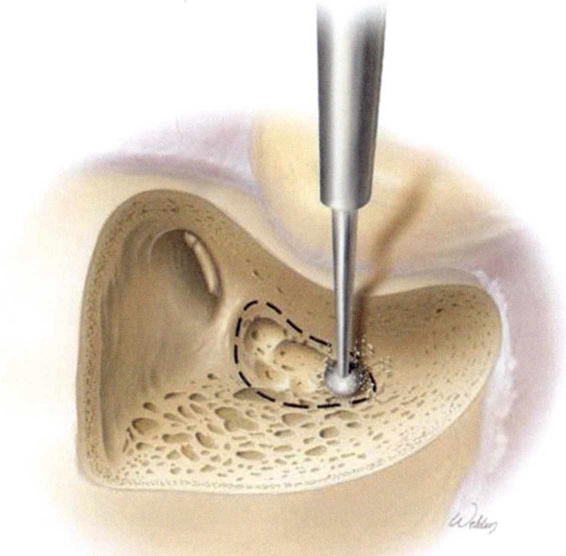

11. After the middle ear space has been entered through the facial recess, the 2 mm diamond bit can be brought through the facial recess and "back ended" on the bone in front of the facial nerve to enhance visualization. The drill speed should be slowed and the facial nerve monitored carefully during this procedure. This may well be the only time during otologic/neurotologic surgery where the interface between the drill burr and the bone is not visible.

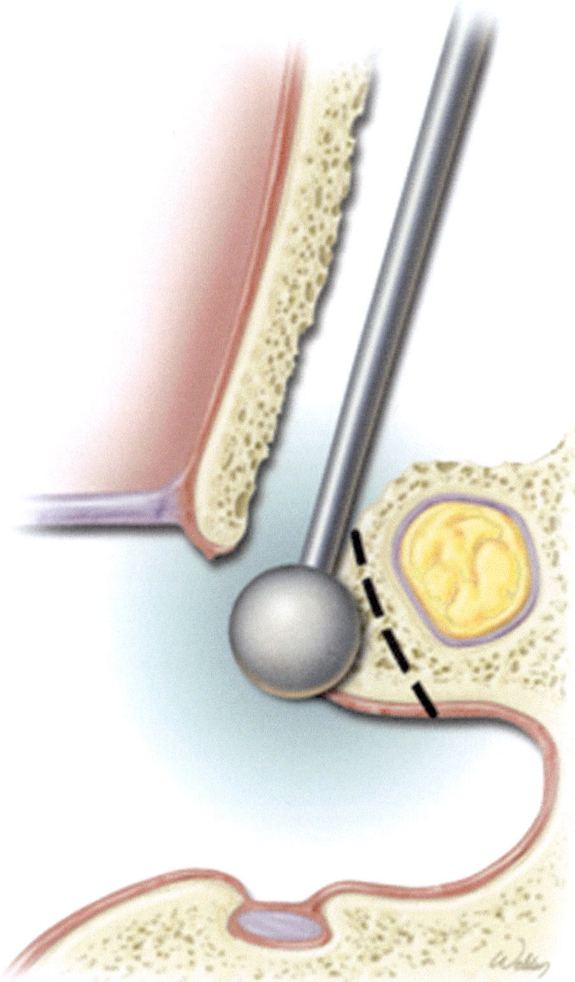

12. A completed facial recess. The microscope needs to be oriented so that the surgeon is looking down parallel to and just behind the ear canal. The incudal–stapedial joint, stapedial tendon, and the round window niche should be visible. If the undersurface of the tympanic membrane or the long process of the malleus is visible, the orientation angle of the microscope is too shallow. If the round window niche is not visible, it means that either the ear canal has not been thinned enough or that there is too much bone on top of the facial nerve.

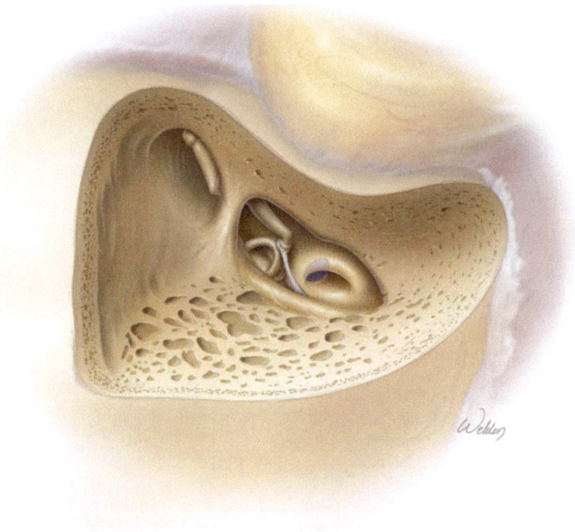

13. The templates for the device should be used to locate the appropriate location for the device and bone well if one is planned. A subperiosteal pocket the size of the implant should be developed. If a well is to be used, it can be drilled to the depth of the template if the skull is thick enough. Alternatively, for children with thin skulls, the well can be drilled down to the dura circumferentially using a bony "island" technique (shown in the illustration). The island of bone in the center should be thinned to the inner cortex of the skull. Over the next year, the well will reossify with a step depression. The use of the newer implants with thinner external devices has reduced the need to drill the well down to dura.

    The implant can be sutured down to holes made through the skull if desired, although we have largely abandoned this step. The thinner implants available today permit the option of not drilling a well, but we feel a trough should always be drilled to protect the electrode array. If no well is drilled, it is critical to create a tight periosteal pocket and insert the device sufficiently to limit the risk of anterior device migration.

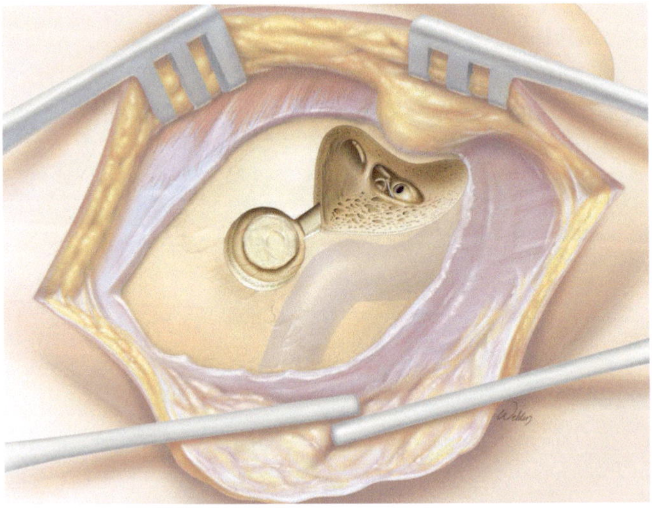

14. The lip of bone overhanging the round window membrane creates the round window niche. This lip should be removed so that the full circumference of the round window membrane can be seen. This is done using a 1 mm diamond burr at a slow speed. Care must be taken that the shaft of the drill does not contact the facial nerve. It is safest to begin bone removal posteriorly since this locates the drill further away from the membrane. When removing the bone more anteriorly, the membrane becomes increasingly at risk. An inadvertent opening along the superior part of the membrane is not catastrophic, but the electrode should not be inserted in this location because of the proximity of the basilar membrane.

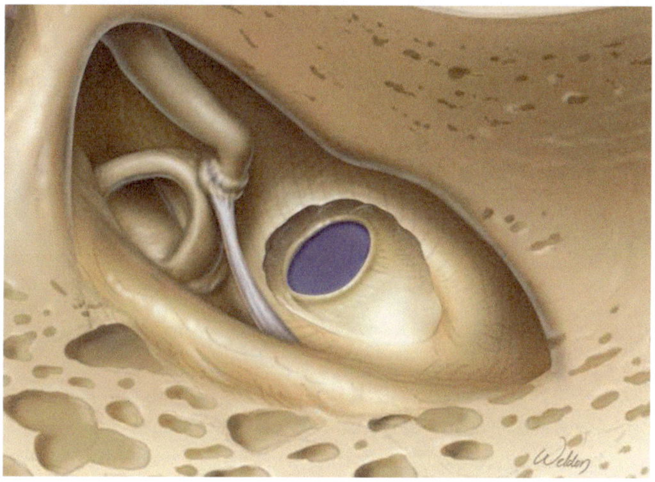

15. There are two ways of opening the cochlea. For a true round window insertion, a small angled pick or other sharp instrument (i.e., an angiocatheter needle or ophthalmologic knife) can be used to open the round window membrane directly. The instrument should not penetrate beyond the round window membrane to limit the risk of injuring the basilar membrane. Currently, we use this approach for the vast majority of cochlear implants because they are thin and flexible enough to allow full insertion through the round window.

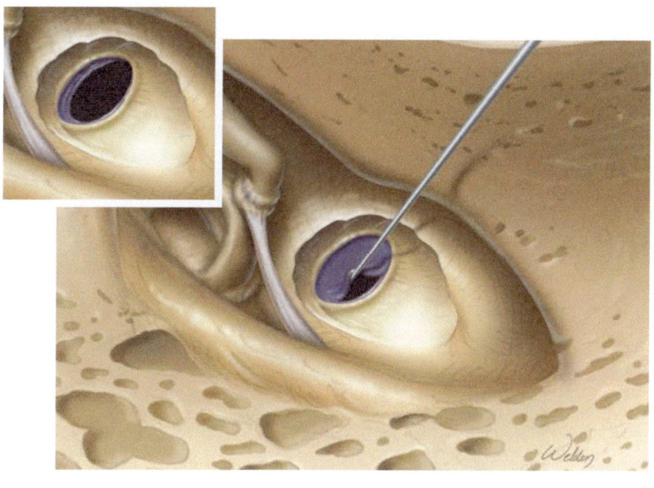

16. When using a cochlear implant with a larger and/or stiffer electrode, a cochleostomy is drilled to straighten out the electrode insertion angle and decrease the risk of trauma to the basilar membrane and modiolus. The cochleostomy is drilled tangential to the anterior–inferior aspect of the round window membrane using a 1 mm diamond burr. The round window membrane can also be opened to join the two openings. If the opening is made superiorly rather than inferiorly, the implant will go into scala vestibuli instead of scala tympani. Care must be taken not to aspirate the perilymph with the suction. As bone dust and blood clot collect in the area, a syringe of saline or low-viscosity hylauronic acid can be inserted into the round window niche and gently injected. This will push the bone dust out of the niche and allow it to be safely aspirated without aspirating the perilymph. Bone dust or blood clot that enters the cochlea makes electrode insertion difficult and will likely produce postoperative inflammation within the cochlea that may adversely affect outcomes.

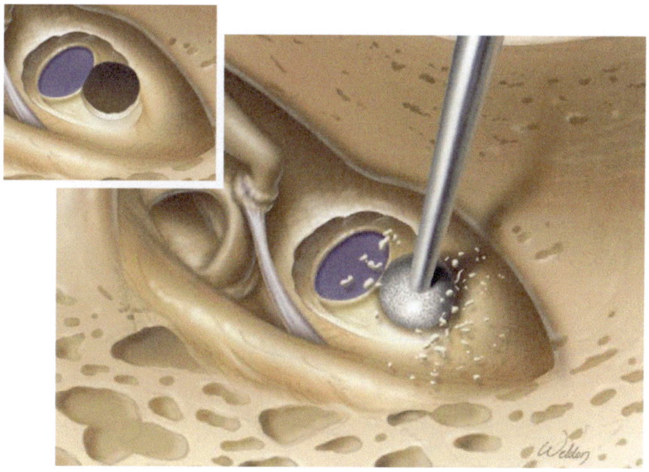

17. The electrode is held just behind the hub using the electrode forceps (the part number is listed in Chap. 2). This position is held throughout the insertion process. Alternatively, a nontoothed jeweler's forceps can be used. The tip of the electrode is then guided to the cochleostomy or opened round window. The electrode is inserted into the cochlea, aiming inferiorly and anteriorly. Slowly and steadily, the electrode is advanced into the cochlea to the hub. During this process, the tips of the forceps pass through the facial recess. The Y-fork is not desirable to use for cochlear implant insertion as its edge can damage the thin Silastic covering of the electrode array. A second forceps is then used to steady the electrode in the mastoid while the first set of forceps is carefully pulled back out of the facial recess.

    This picture shows the device body nearly fully exposed. Such a large incision is not our typical practice at this time.

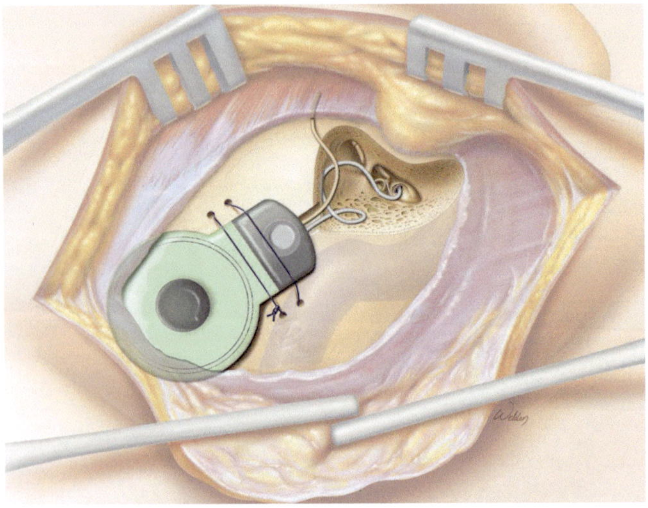

18. Case 1: In most cases, we use a 3–3.5 cm incision that drifts posteriorly at the superior end. Minimal shaving of hair is needed. The thicker the scalp, the longer the incision needs to be.

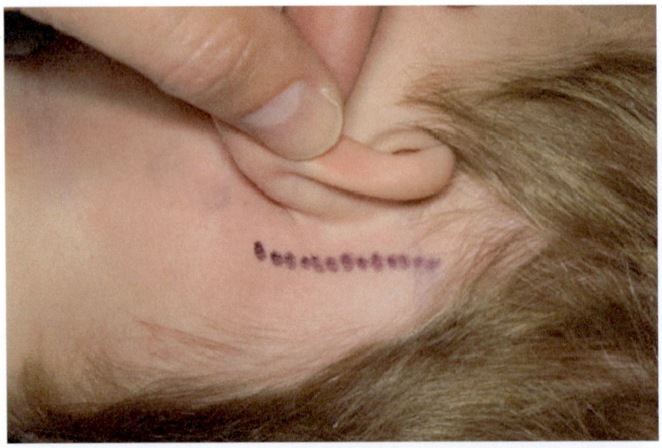

19. The side of the head is widely prepped so we can visualize the area where the coil will be located. This allows us to avoid drapes over the coil that can interfere with intraoperative testing of the device. Also, when performing bilateral implantation (sequential or simultaneous), we can accurately place the device so that it is symmetrical to the device on the contralateral side. The location is measured and marked prior to prepping and draping.

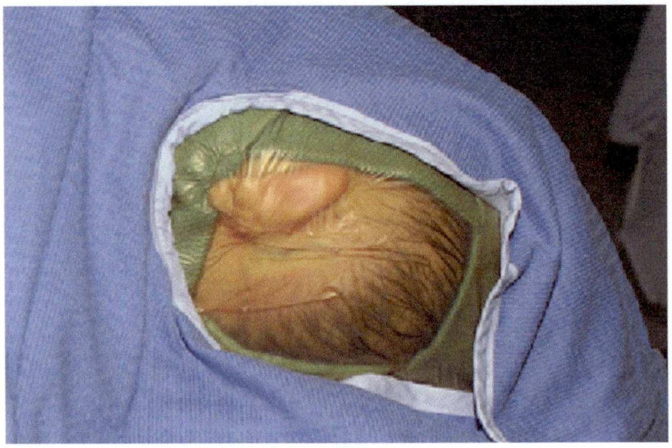

20. Using fish hooks to hold the ear and periosteal flap forward avoids having the posterior arm of a self-retaining retractor coming in conflict with the device once it is in place. A retractor can be added at the beginning of the case to help expose the mastoid and protect the skin from the drill shaft. The mastoid only needs to be large enough to gain access to the facial recess.

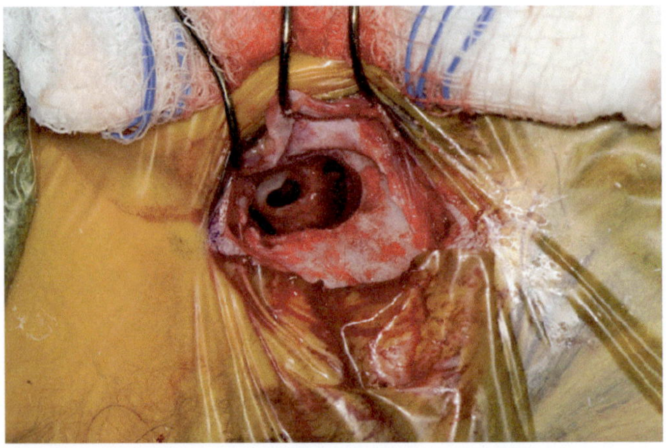

21. The electrode array is vulnerable as it traverses the skull and as it enters the mastoid cavity. It seems prudent to create a trough to protect this part of the device. While we continue to recess devices to some degree, others have had success without drilling any well. The benefits of recessing include improved cosmesis, less pressure on overlying skin, and less risk of device migration.

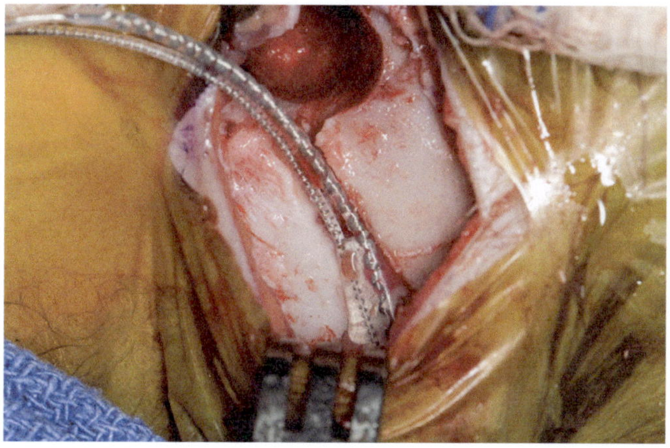

22. Case 2: It is important to coil the electrode into the mastoid in a manner that provides stable positioning. Keeping the walls of the mastoid cavity steep facilitates electrode retention. The short electrodes used in patients with residual low-frequency hearing have been effective in hearing preservation but may be more likely to migrate out of the cochlea if not secured. We have found that packing some muscle tightly into the facial recess results in better stabilization of these short electrodes.

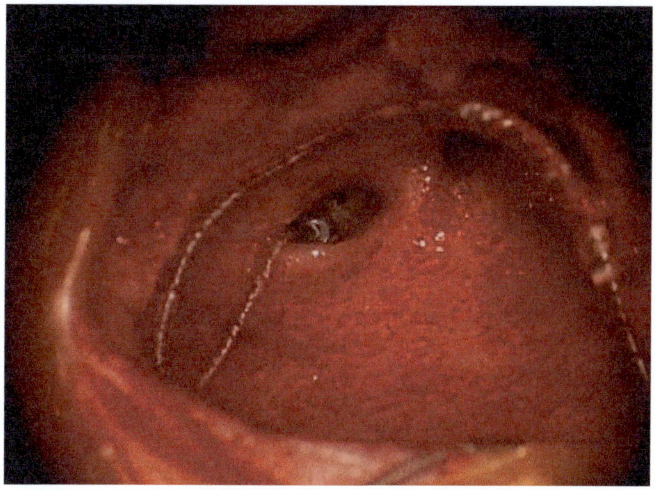

23. Case 3: Round window insertion (right ear). The view through the facial recess. The round window membrane is not visible because of the overhanging bone of the niche.

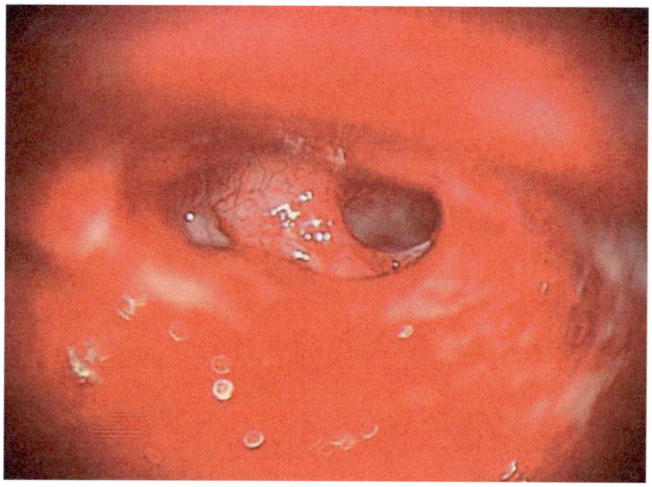

24. The overhanging bone of the round window niche was drilled away to expose the full circumference of the round window membrane.

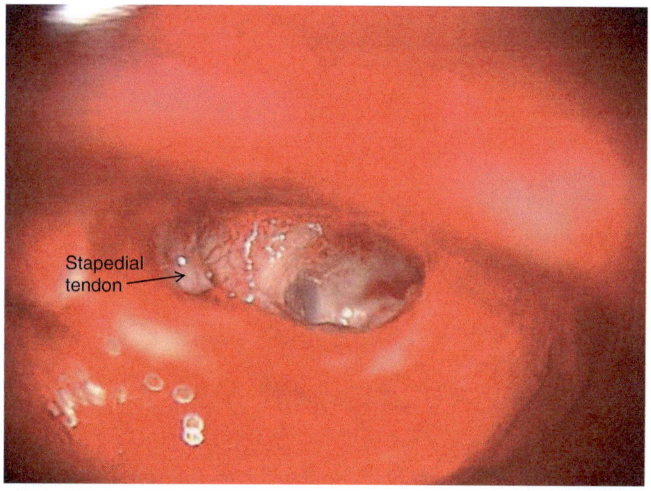

25. The round window membrane was teased open and the perilymph noted.

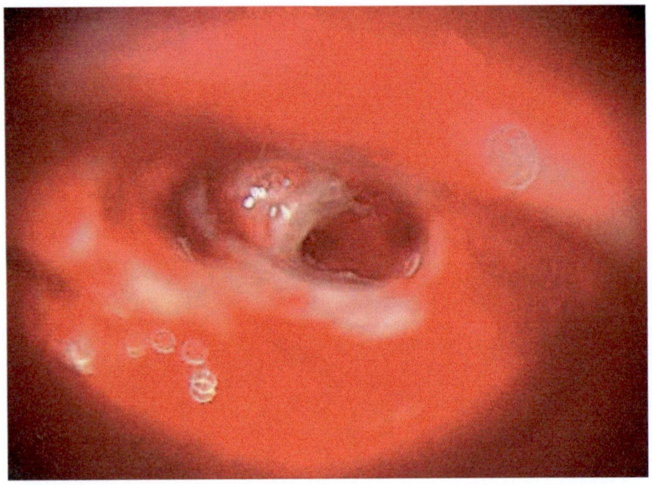

26. Full insertion of a Med-El electrode through the round window. The hub ring was seen at the round window, indicating that a full insertion was achieved.

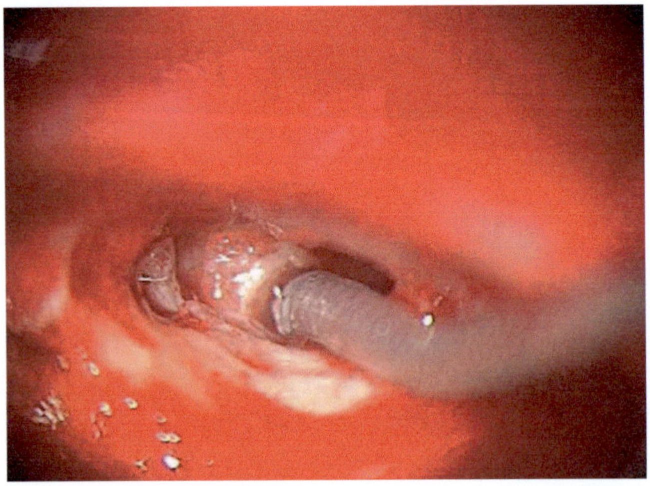

27. Case 4: Cochleostomy insertion (left ear). The view through the facial recess. A sliver of the round window membrane is visible.

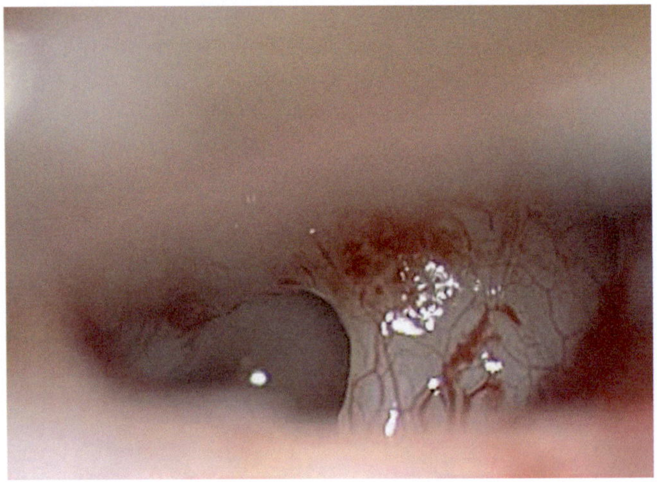

28. The overhanging bone of the round window niche was drilled away.

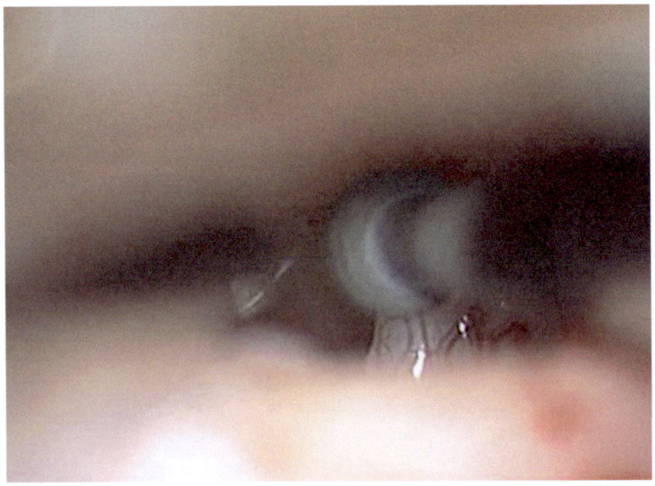

29. Partial view of the round window.

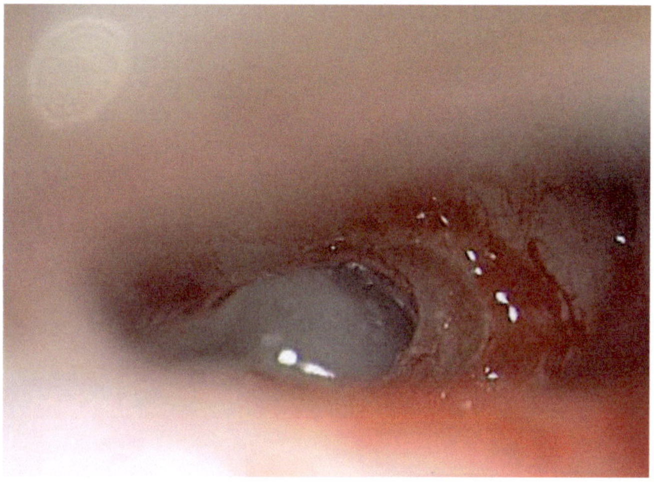

30. Complete view of the round window.

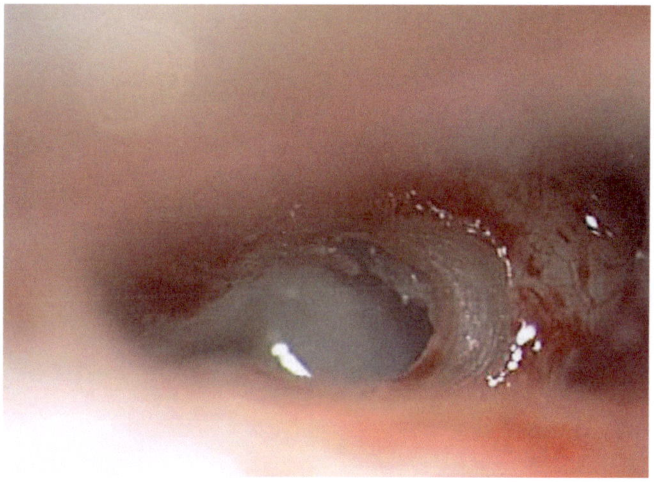

31. The round window was enlarged by drilling at its anterior–inferior aspect. The perilymph was not aspirated. Note the bone dust in the area which can be washed away by inserting a small blunt-tip needle through the cochleostomy and gently instilling saline or hyaluronic acid.

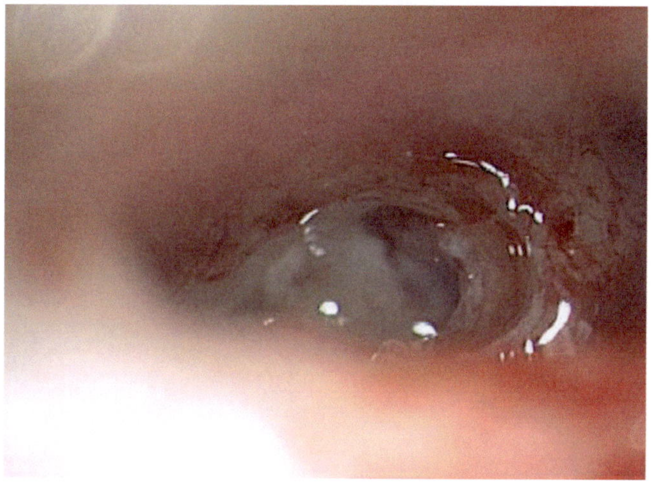

32. The tip of the Med-El electrode is entering the cochleostomy.

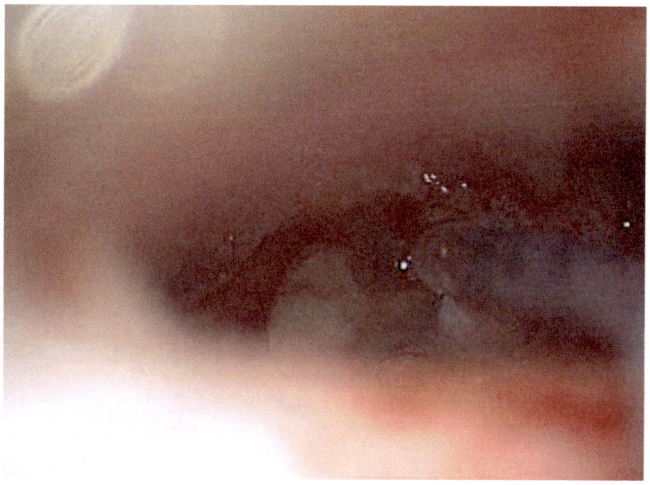

33. Lower power view after full insertion. The stapedial tendon (*ST*) and pyramidal eminence (*PE*) can be seen superior to the round window.

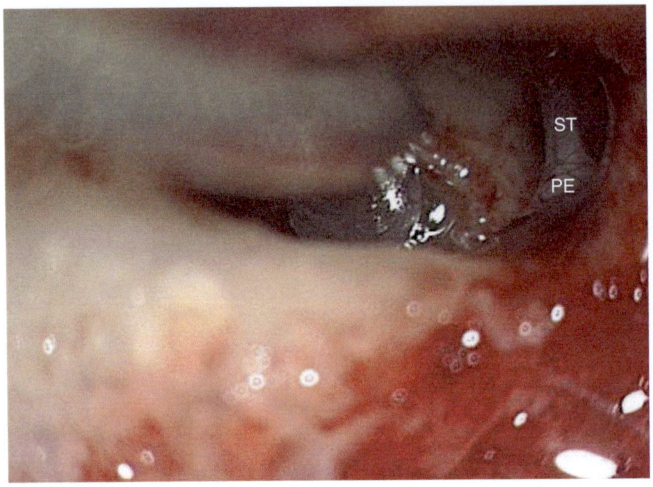

34. Case 5: Scala vestibuli insertion (right ear). The view through the facial recess. A cochleostomy was first made at the level of the round window, but the electrode could not be inserted due to ossification. The promontory and stapedial tendon (*ST*) are visible superior to the round window.

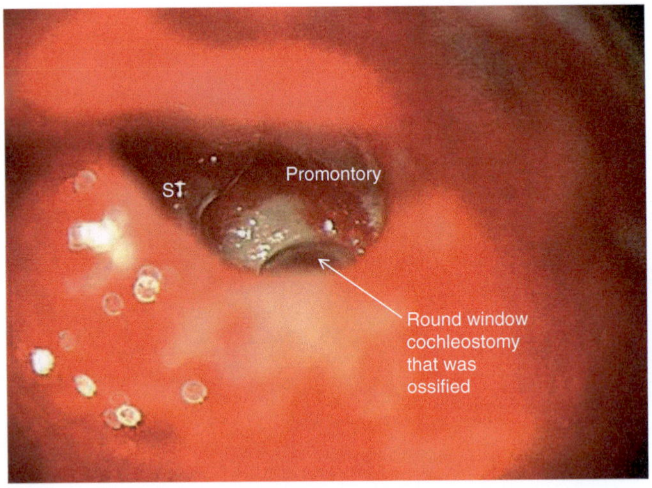

35. A second cochleostomy was then drilled into scala vestibuli by going between the stapes and the round window cochleostomy. The basilar membrane (*BM*) is the gray tissue bridging the gap between the two cochleostomies.

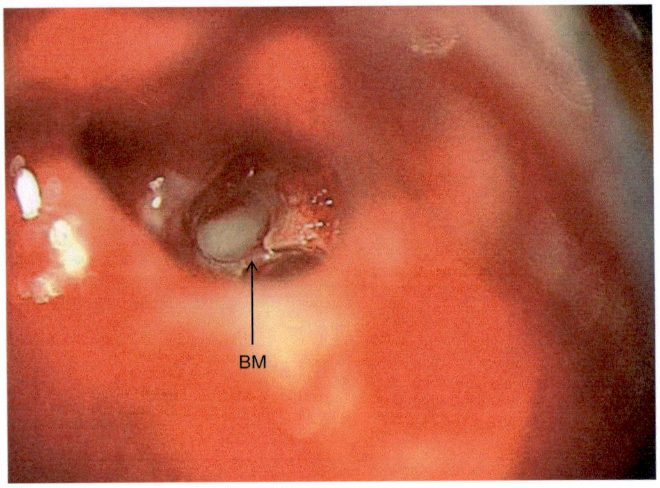

36. Complete insertion of a Med-El electrode into scala vestibuli.

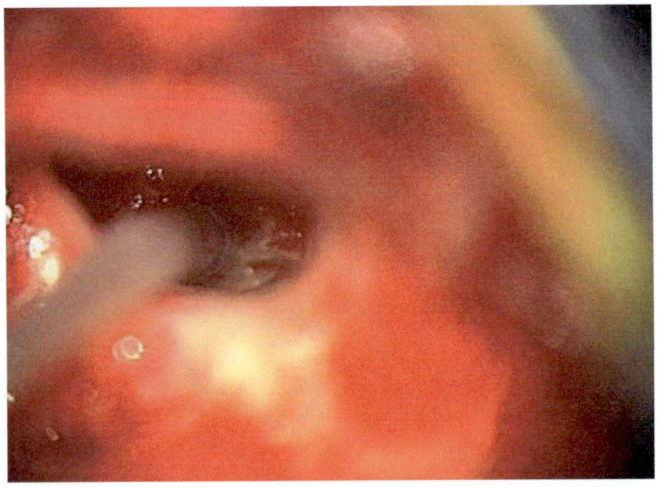

37. Case 6: Common cavity insertion of a custom Med-El electrode (right ear). Axial CT of a patient with a common cavity malformation.

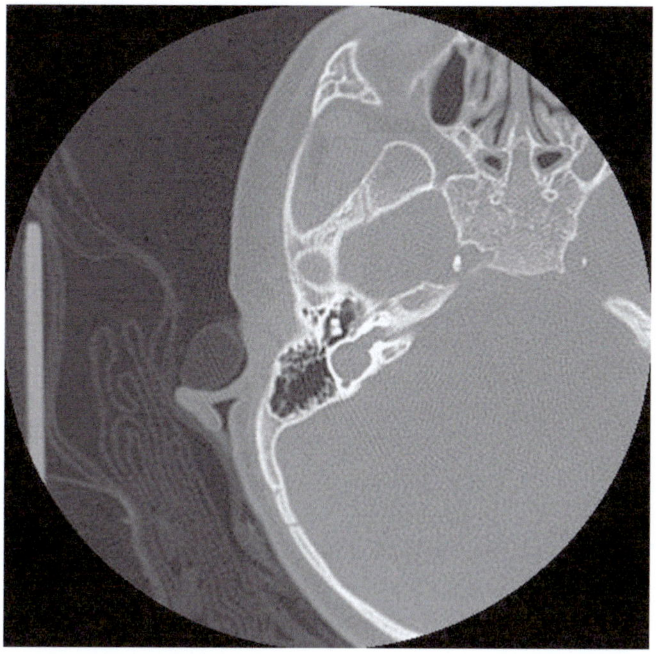

38. Axial MRI of the same patient. Particularly with a patient who has an inner ear malformation, it is important to verify that an eighth nerve complex (*arrows*) is visible prior to proceeding with cochlear implantation.

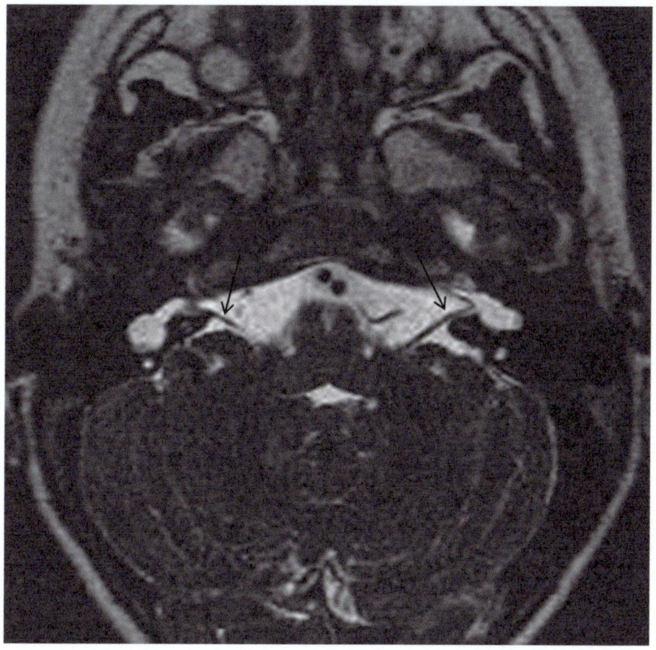

39. The custom electrode has additional length on the end distal to the electrical contacts. There is a small ball at the tip.

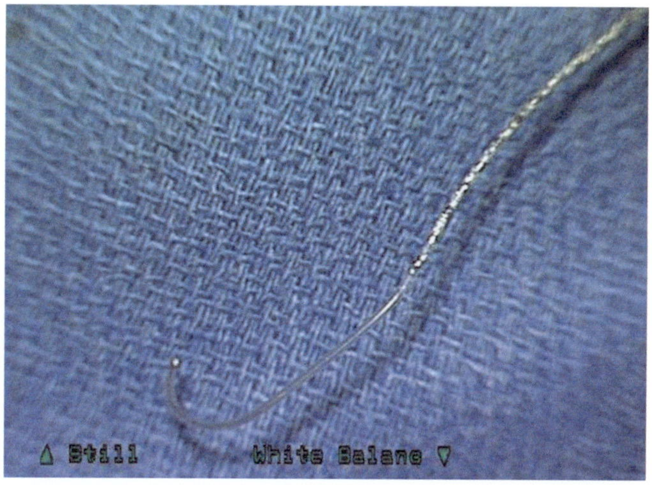

40. The common cavity is exposed in the mastoid antrum. Intraoperatively, this malformation typically looks like an enlarged lateral semicircular canal. The incudal buttress, the incus, and the head of the malleus are removed. Two cochleostomies are drilled on either end of the common cavity.

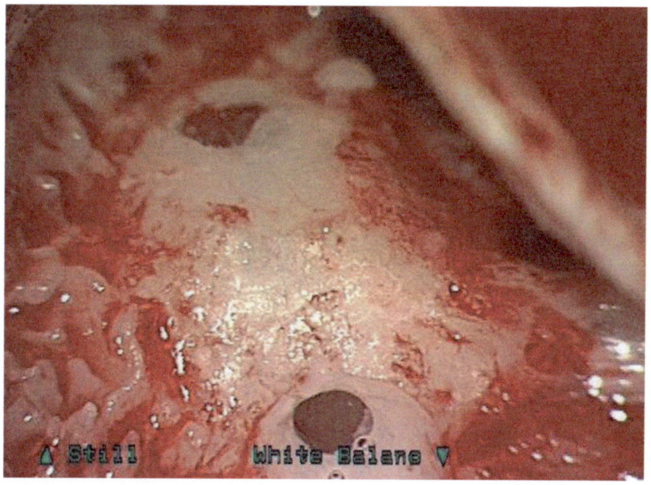

41. The electrode array is inserted in through the posterior cochleostomy, and the tip is guided through the common cavity until it comes out the anterior cochleostomy. It is then pulled through until the electrical contacts are visible at both cochleostomies.

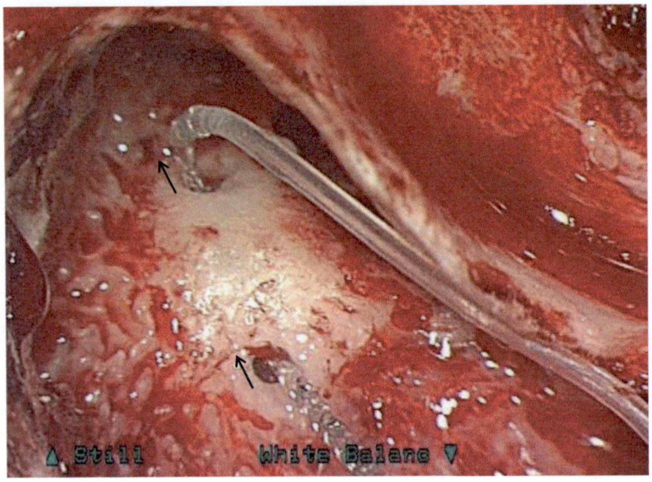

42. Both ends of the electrode are then gently pushed into the common cavity so as to position the electrical contacts along the deep wall of the cavity and be in close proximity to where the neural elements rest. The hub ring can be seen at the posterior cochleostomy.

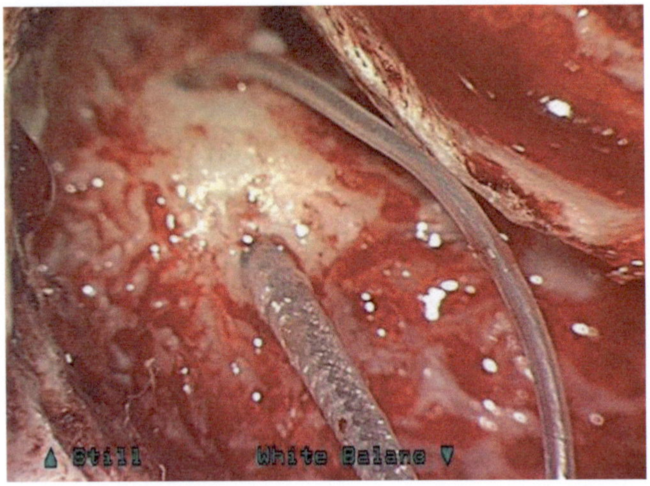

43. Temporalis fascia is then placed around both cochleostomies.

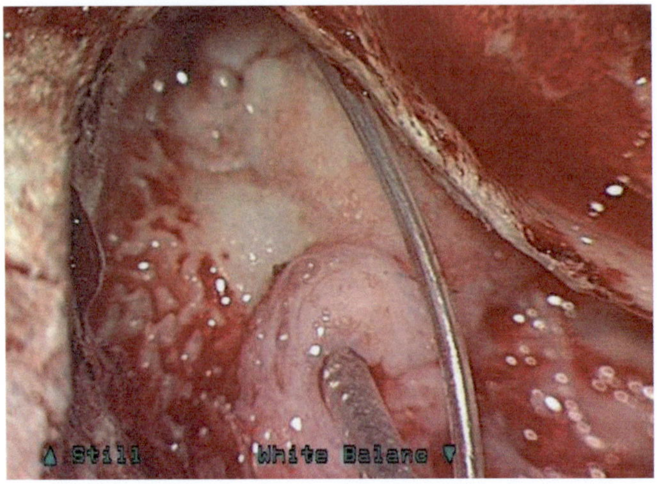

44. A post-op axial CT of the temporal bone can be performed to verify that the electrode contacts are in the proper position and that the electrode does not enter the internal auditory canal or cerebellopontine angle.

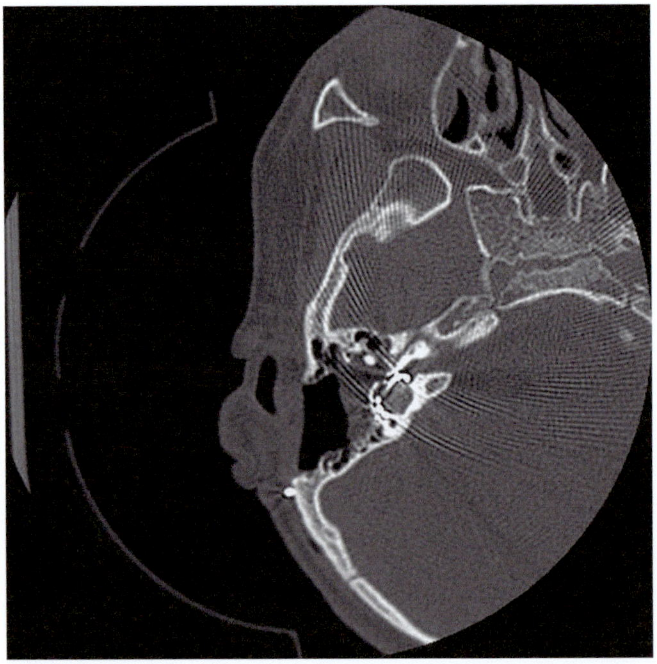

45. An axial cut at a slightly more inferior position. Note how the electrode coils around the interior of the common cavity. By counting the electrode channels on the postoperative CT scan, the surgeon can give the audiologist information regarding which channels are closest to the nerve and hence likely to provide the best stimulation.

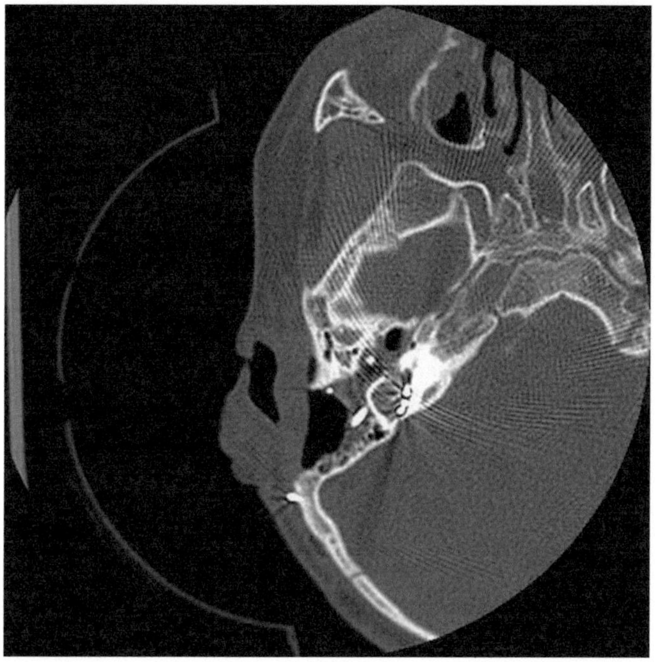

46. Case 7: Normal postoperative axial CT scan after cochlear implantation into a normal cochlea from inferior to superior. Image 1

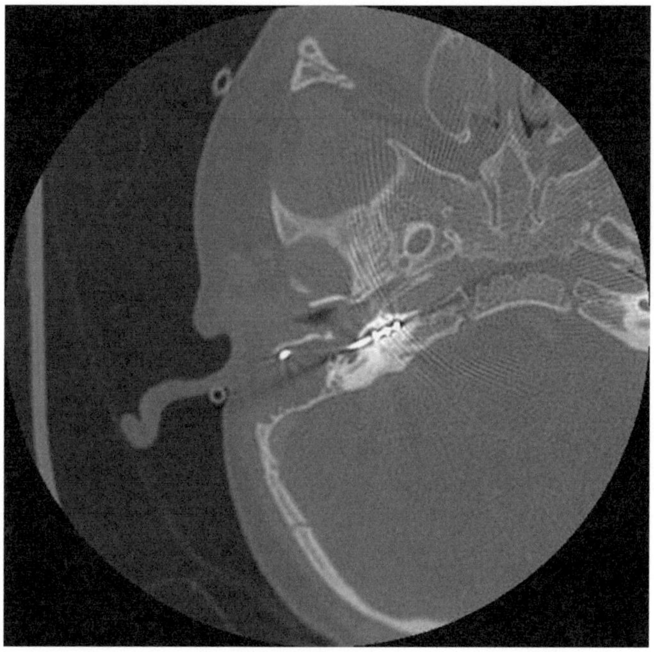

47. Image 2

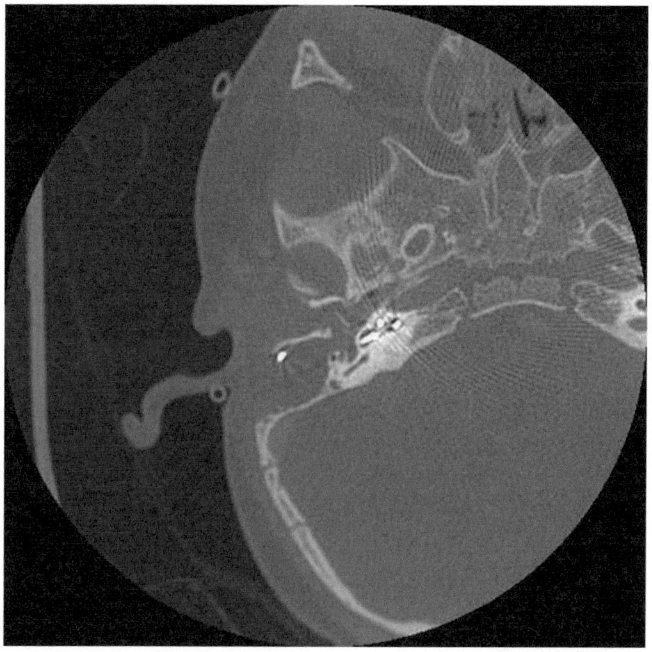

48. Image 3

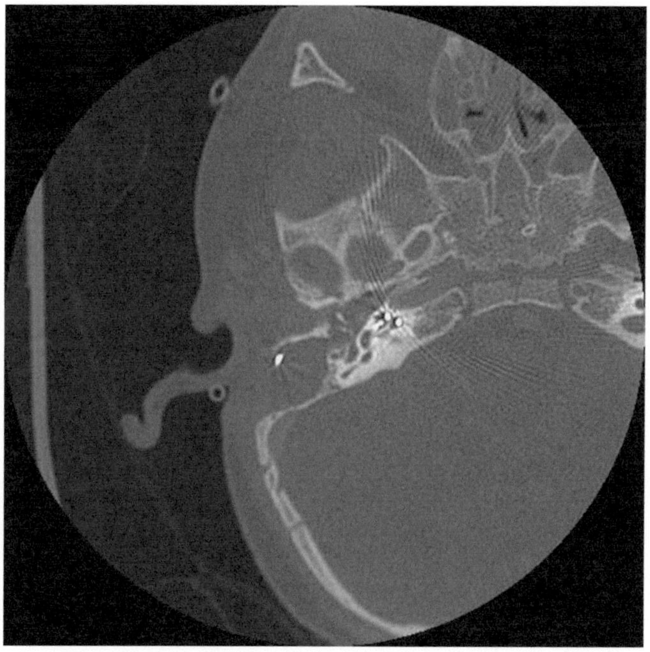

49. Image 4

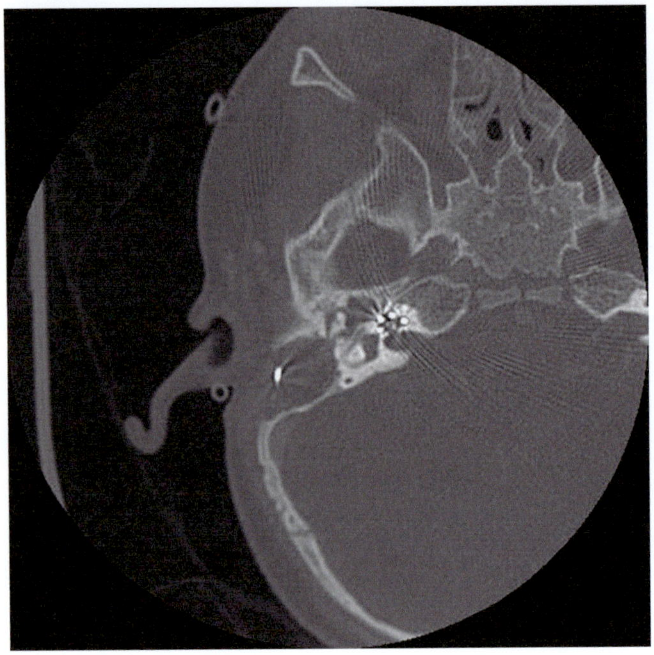

50. Case 8: Axial CT scan of a cochlear implant that was mistakenly inserted into the Eustachian tube.

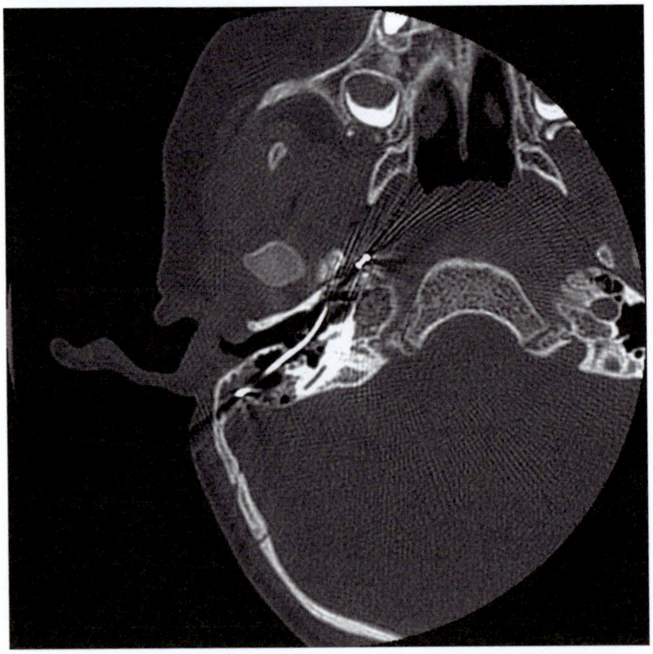

51. A slightly more inferior position shows the tip of the electrode array at the nasopharynx.

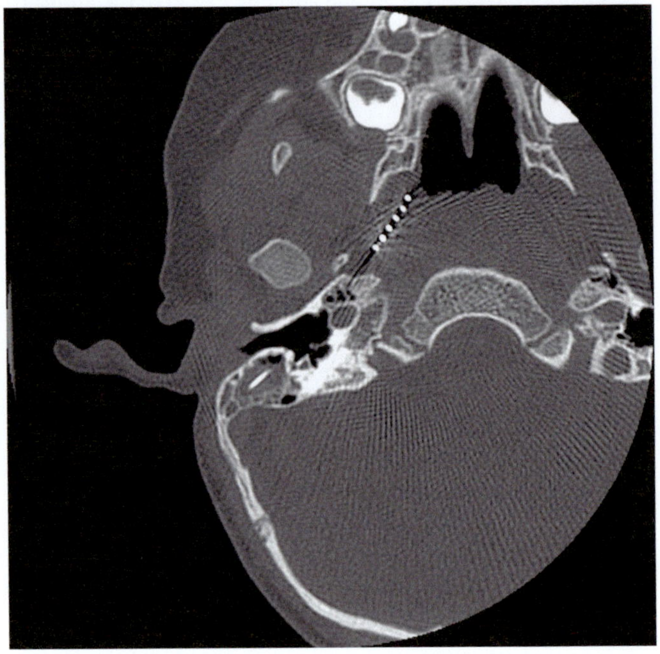

52. Case 9: CT scan of a cochlear implant that entered the jugular foramen and carotid canal. These types of insertion problems can occur when the mastoidectomy and facial recess are not large enough or the angle of visualization is inadequate. A straightforward way of preventing these types of problems is to clearly identify the round window membrane prior to performing the cochleostomy.

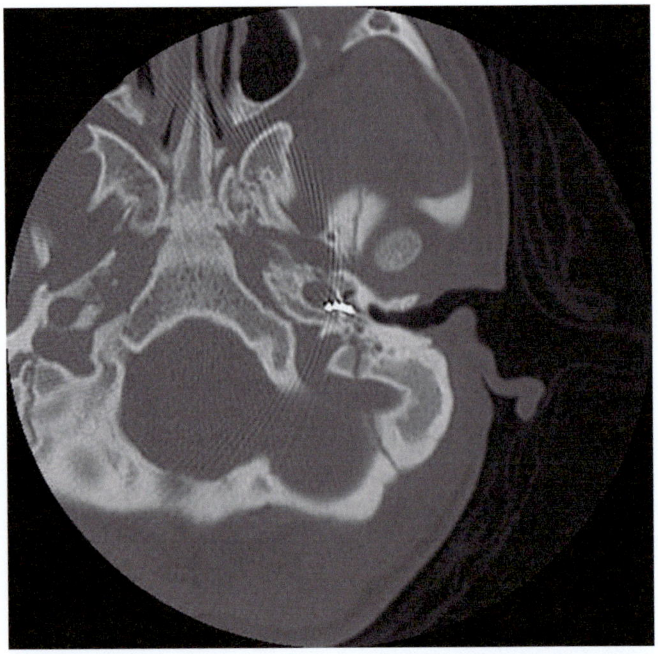

53. Case 10: Skin flap irritation. A patient with a cochlear implant that had mild skin breakdown due to an overly strong magnet. When mild like this, this problem can usually be treated conservatively. It is important to reduce the strength of the magnet, decrease implant usage for a few weeks, and use moleskin and/or duoderm to reduce skin irritation.

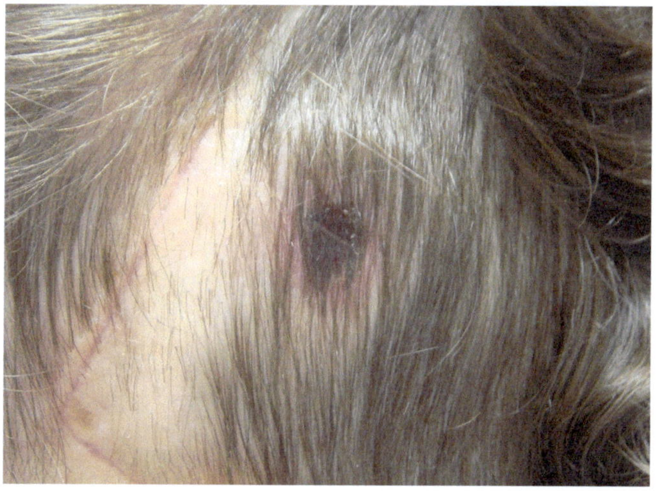

54. Skin flap necrosis: If a full thickness breakdown of the skin occurs (typically found with the older C-flap incision style), revision surgery may be necessary.

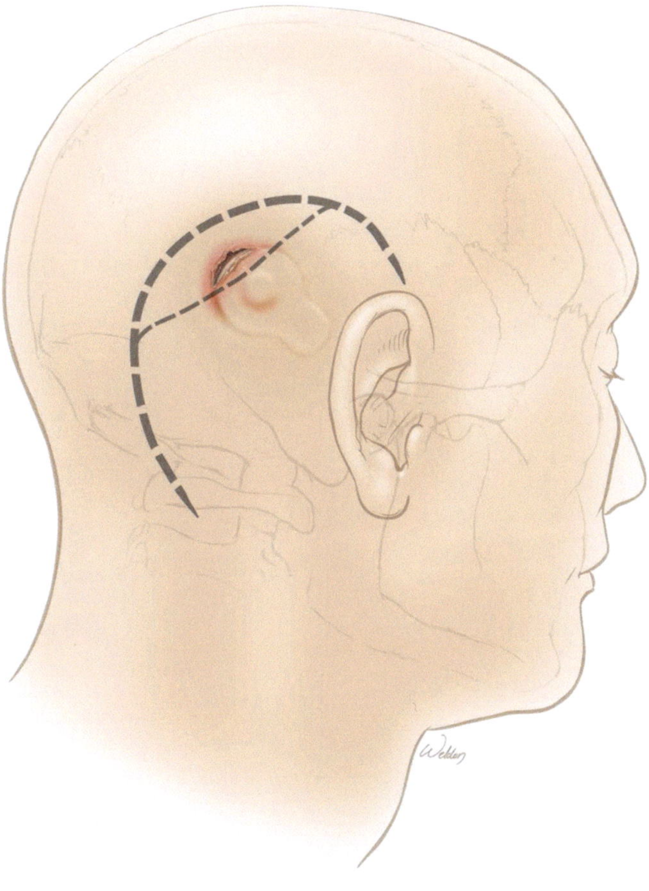

55. The previously used incision can be opened and the skin and subcutaneous tissues elevated off the deeper tissues that form the capsule around the implant.

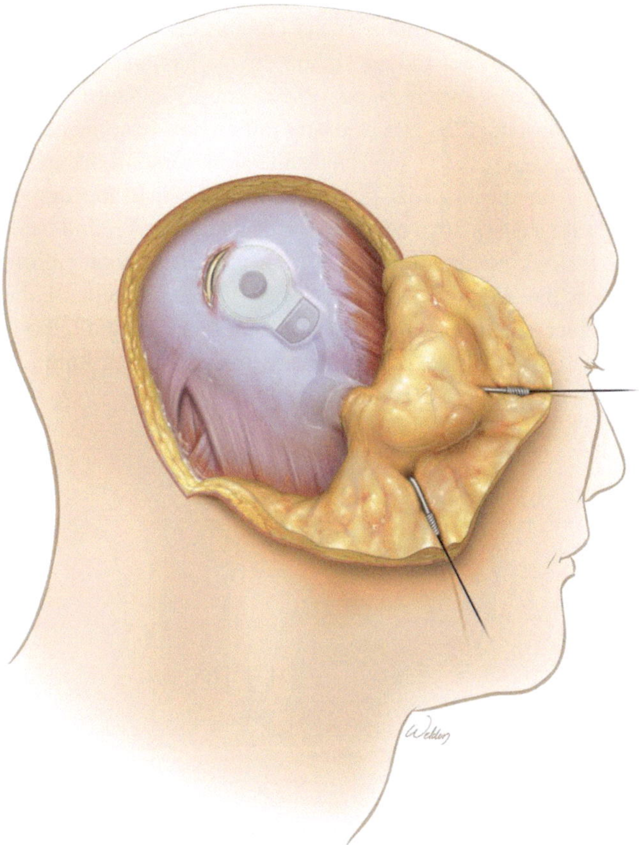

56. A separate flap is raised to expose the implant. A new well is drilled and the implant moved to its new position. Care must be taken not to tug on the electrode as it is easily pulled out of the cochlea. When we are repositioning implants, we obtain an intra-op x-ray before surgery begins and then at the conclusion to confirm the device has not moved. If the device has been partially withdrawn, it may be possible to simply advance it. The electrodes often can be easily pulled out. In some cases, we reopen the postauricular incision, remove the existing device from its pocket, and secure it to the drapes with a Steri-Strip before creating a new pocket and well. Delivering the device from the pocket without pulling on the electrode requires dissecting a segment of the electrode free from the scar tissue; this can be a tedious and difficult task putting the electrode at risk of injury. A backup device is always available.

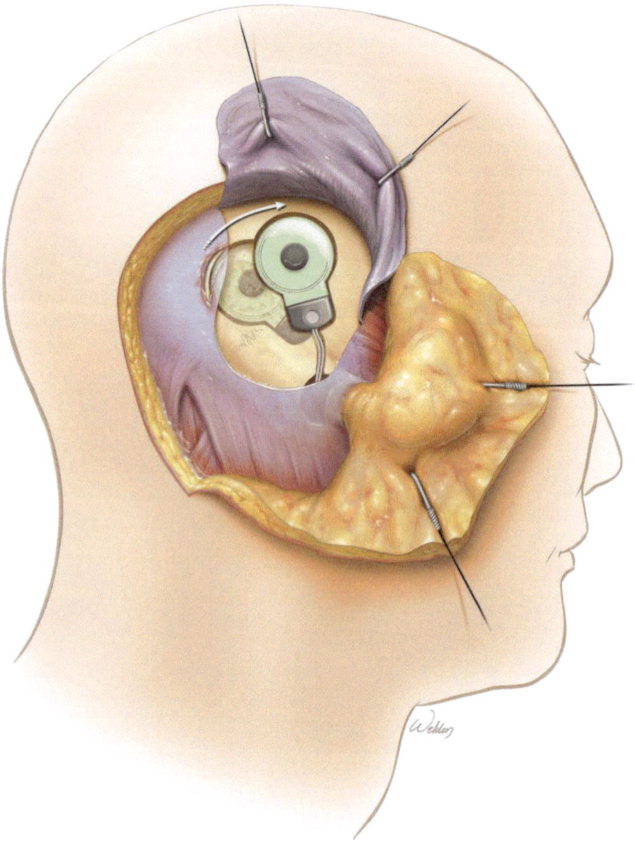

57. The staggered incisions are then closed. The wound should be given several weeks to heal before using the cochlear implant. Long-term antibiotics would be typically given as well. While it is reasonable to try and salvage a device that has become exposed, there is a significant chance of recurrent skin breakdown and infection due to biofilm on the device. Devices that have become exposed because of thin skin and breakdown or trauma are more likely to be salvaged as opposed to devices that have become infected and then begin to drain. These devices are rarely saved. We routinely remove these devices and proceed with reimplantation at a later date.

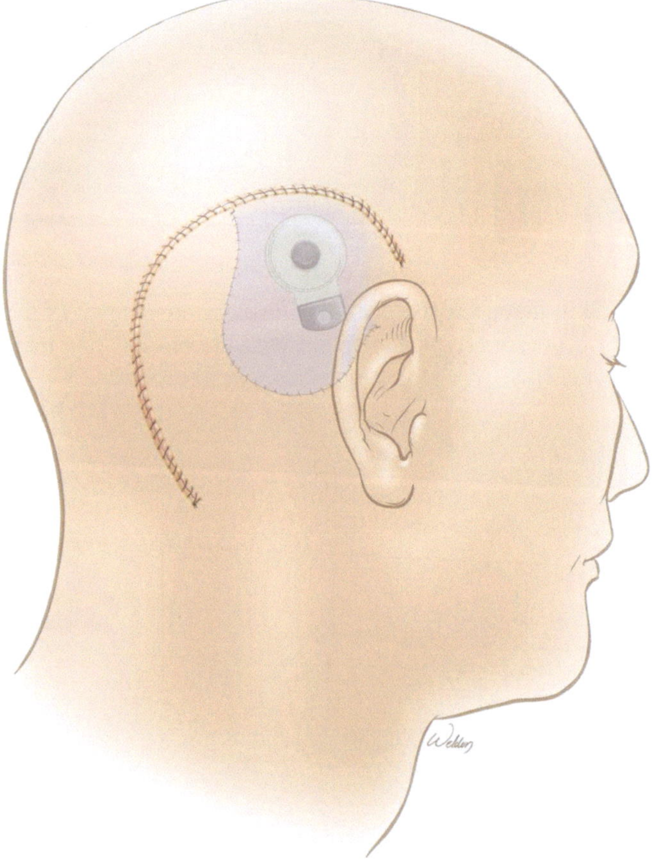

58. Case 11. An example of an extruding cochlear implant. When this much of the implant has become exposed, it cannot be saved. Replacement should be performed after excising the devitalized tissues and rotational flap coverage of the defect.

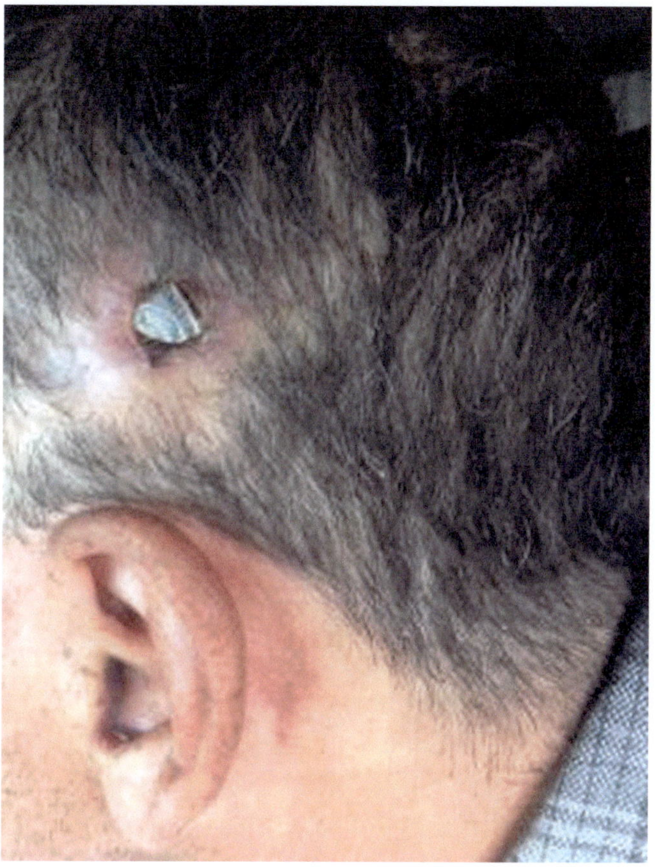

59. Cochlear implants can break, particularly those with the older-style ceramic casing. This implant stopped working after the child fell out of his/her high chair onto a tile floor. The CT scan was unremarkable, but we assumed the fall damaged the implant. Thus, we took him to surgery. Intraoperatively, upon opening the soft tissue capsule, the magnet inside leapt out through the fractured implant casing and stuck to the surgeon's dissecting hemostat. These are the pieces of the implant we removed from the child's head.

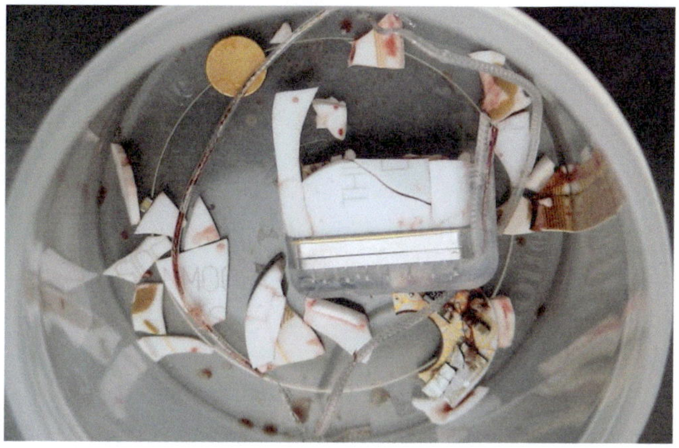

60. Case 12: Acute otitis media after cochlear implantation. Acute otitis media can occur in any child, but after having a mastoidectomy for cochlear implantation, it is not unusual for this to produce postauricular edema and induration indicative of acute mastoiditis. In this patient, the infection occurred 3 years after the implantation surgery. Note that the skin overlying the implant body was not swollen or red.

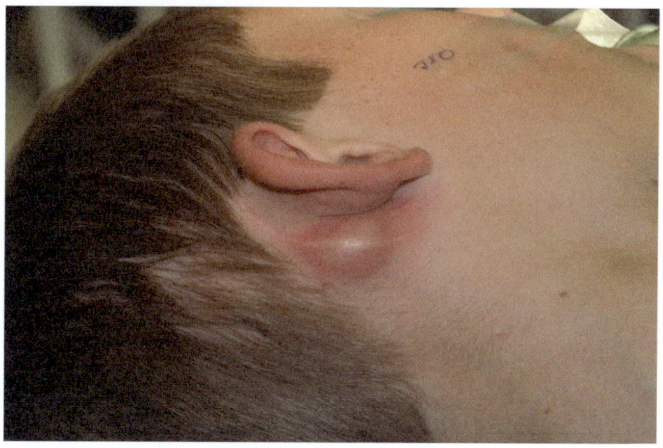

61. A CT scan of the temporal bones with contrast should be performed to verify that there are no intracranial complications. If not, a limited drainage procedure should be performed without exposing the cochlear implant or dislodging the electrode from the cochlea.

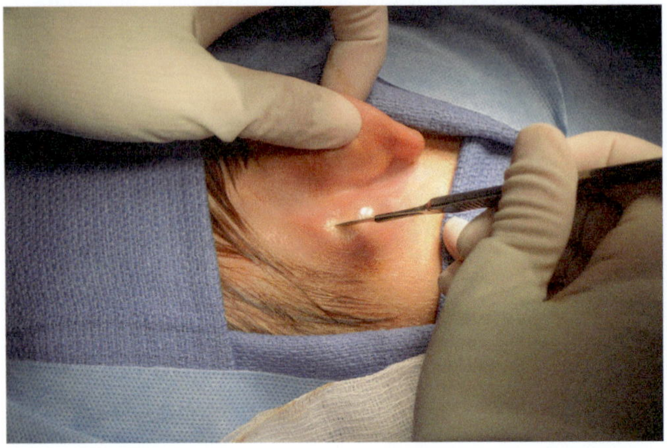

62. After making a small skin incision, the tissues were gently probed with a hemostat to drain out the pus.

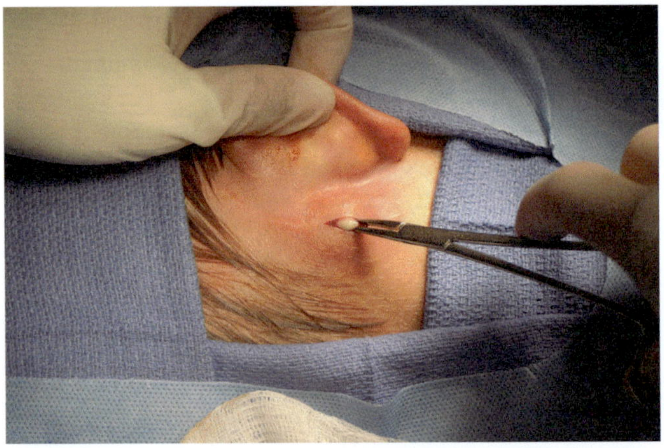

63. Cultures were taken to guide the choice of long-term antibiotics (typically 2–6 weeks). Despite the presence of extensive infection in the vicinity of the device, these infections almost always resolve without requiring device removal.

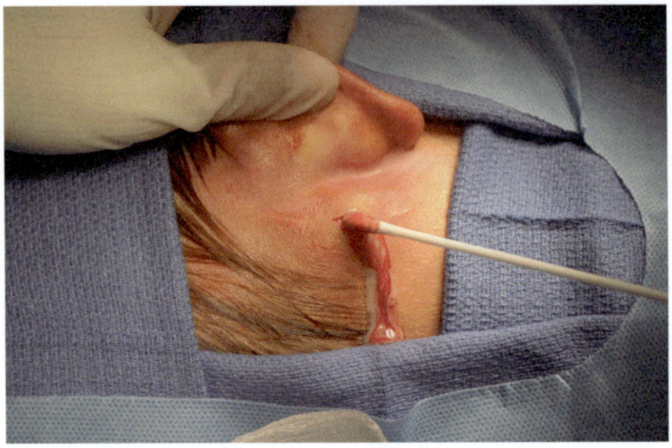

64. The mastoid cavity was irrigated out gently.

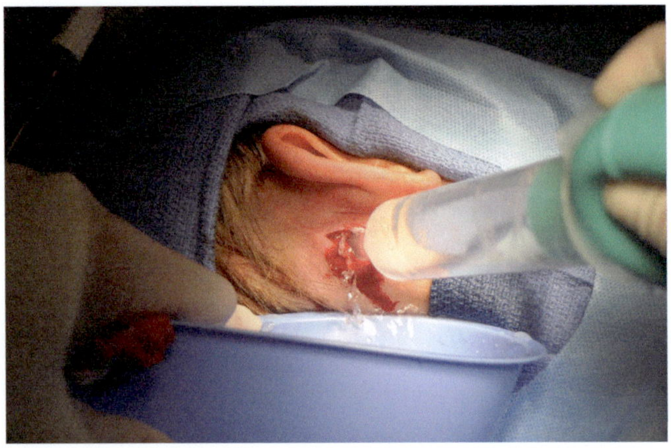

65. A PE tube was placed to aid drainage of the middle ear. The postauricular wound was closed without leaving a drain in place so as to reduce the risk of external bacteria entering the wound and seeding the implant.

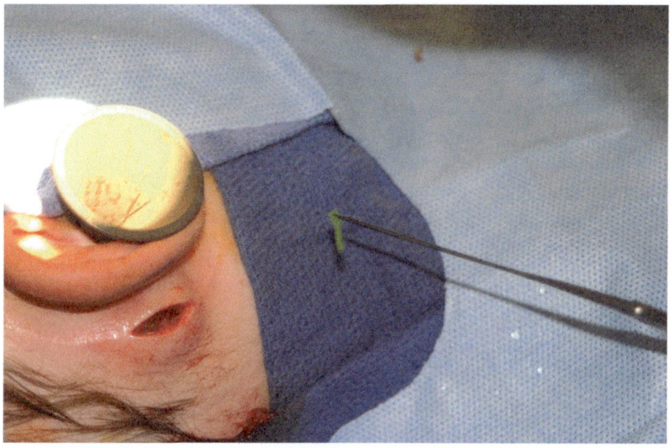

Surgery for Vertigo

11

Endolymphatic Shunt

- *Concept*
  - Endolymphatic hydrops is the most agreed-upon pathology associated with Meniere's disease. The postulated mechanism of this procedure is to stent open the endolymphatic sac to relieve the pressure buildup within the endolymphatic compartment. In reality, the mechanism by which this procedure can help patients is unknown and its efficacy is questioned. Nevertheless, it is a valuable procedure for the neurotologist to know how to perform as it has a low side-effect profile compared to other invasive treatments for recalcitrant Meniere's disease.
- *Conditions treated*
  - Meniere's disease refractory to medical management in patients with serviceable hearing or in whom there is desire to avoid a destructive labyrinthine procedure (e.g., bilateral disease, poor pre-existing balance)
- *Risks*
  - Hearing loss
  - Dizziness
  - Facial nerve injury
  - CSF leak
  - Disease recurrence (estimated at ~40–50 %)
- *Benefits*
  - This is a nondestructive outpatient surgical procedure that preserves hearing. If it doesn't work, other treatment strategies can be still used.
- *Additional notes*
  - Only the posterior fossa dura need be exposed. If the sigmoid sinus is small, bone can be left over it. If the sigmoid sinus is large, the bone can be egg-shelled to allow it to be compressed and aid exposure of the endolymphatic sac.

J.S. Oghalai, C.L.W. Driscoll, *Atlas of Neurotologic and Lateral Skull Base Surgery*,
DOI 10.1007/978-3-662-46694-0_11, © Springer-Verlag Berlin Heidelberg 2016

1. Approach to the endolymphatic sac. A right ear is shown. A simple mastoidectomy is first performed. The lateral semicircular canal (*LSCC*) is identified at the floor of the antrum. Donaldson's line (*dotted line*) is helpful in finding the posterior semicircular canal (*PSCC*). It travels posteriorly along the plane of the LSCC and bisects the PSCC. The dura inferior to the PSCC is then exposed to identify the endolymphatic sac (*ELS*). This involves careful delineation of the sigmoid sinus and the vertical portion of the facial nerve so as not to inadvertently damage them.

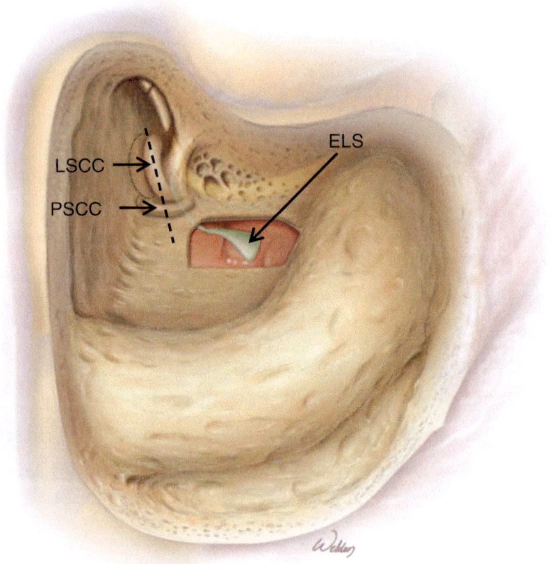

2. Case 1. Placement of a right endolymphatic shunt. A standard postauricular incision was used and a standard mastoidectomy performed. The mastoid antrum was opened, and the lateral semicircular canal (*LSCC*) can be seen. There were large retrofacial air cells that were opened. As a landmark, Donaldson's line (*dotted line*) is shown.

   There is some debate regarding how much bone removal should be performed. It is nice to widely decompress the sigmoid sinus and posterior fossa dura. The dura is then exposed from Donaldson's line inferiorly to the sigmoid sinus. Removal of bone this far superiorly makes it easier to identify the most lateral aspect of the sac. The demarcation between normal dura which is thinner and bluish can be differentiated from the thicker and whiter sac. Also, the region where the sac enters the temporal bone can be seen when the dura is dissected from the petrous bone superior to the sac. A large retrofacial air cell tract like in this picture facilitates decompression of the most medial part of the sac. The dura is often very thin medial to the sac and needs to be carefully decompressed and elevated from the bone to avoid a CSF leak. This is an area not easily repaired.

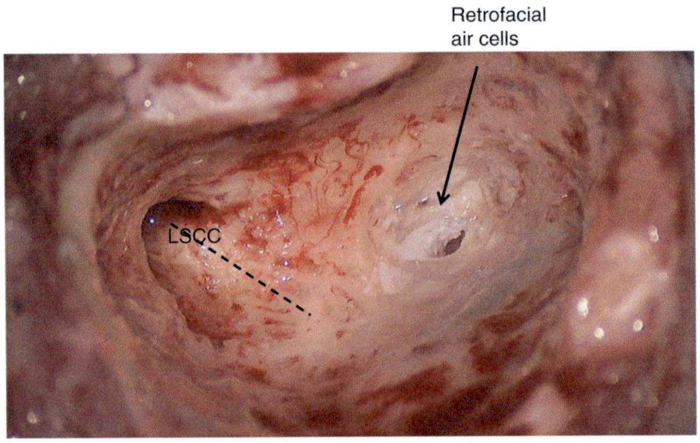

3. The presigmoid posterior fossa dura was identified and dissected free from the posterior temporal bone. Note how the dense otic capsule bone of the posterior semicircular canal is clearly delineated at the tip of the suction. Dura should not be exposed superior to this or the posterior canal may be inadvertently opened.

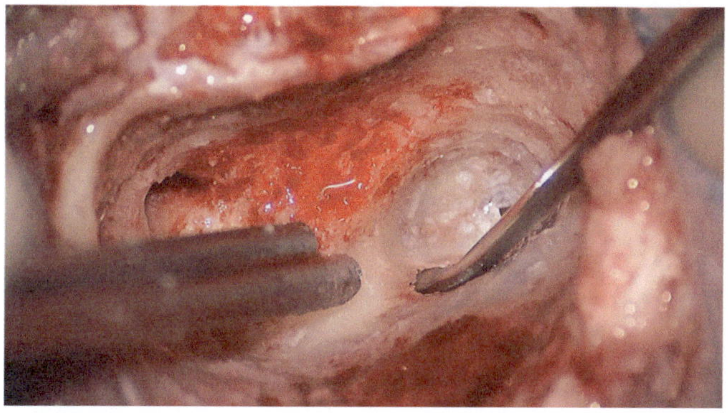

4. Drilling was continued deeper within the retrofacial air cells to fully expose the endolymphatic sac (*ELS*). The sac is simply a thickening of the dura in this region. It is often difficult to distinguish its margins, and so it is best to drill deep enough so that the endolymphatic duct can be identified coursing from the sac into the temporal bone. The lateral semicircular canal (*LSCC*) and posterior semicircular canal (*PSCC*) are shown.

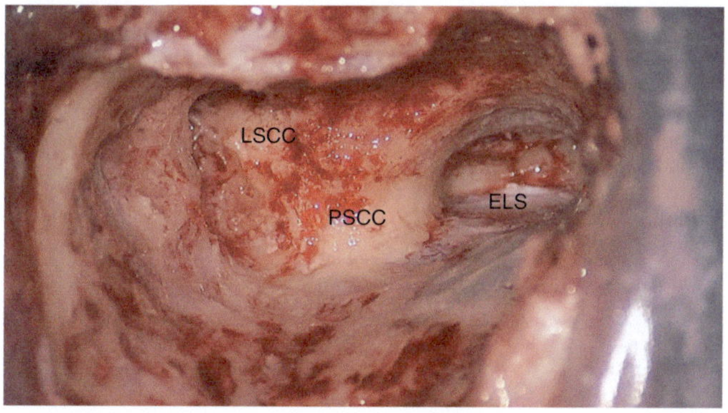

5. A small knife was used to incise the outer leaflet of the endolymphatic sac. A #5910 Beaver blade works well for this. It is possible to create a false lumen between the leaves of dura, but you can always find the true lumen which will have fluid and has a distinct shiny appearance. Care should be taken not to cut too deeply or a CSF leak will ensue.

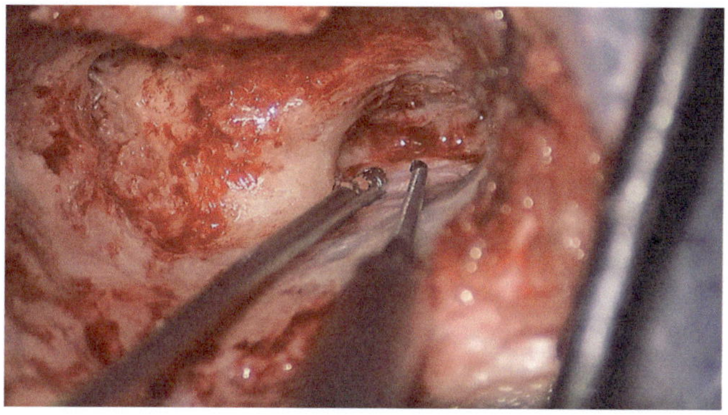

6. The endolymphatic sac can be probed to open it widely. Some surgeons will simply decompress the sac, others open the sac only, and still others insert a stent. Unfortunately, at this time, there is no good science to guide us in deciding which approach is best.

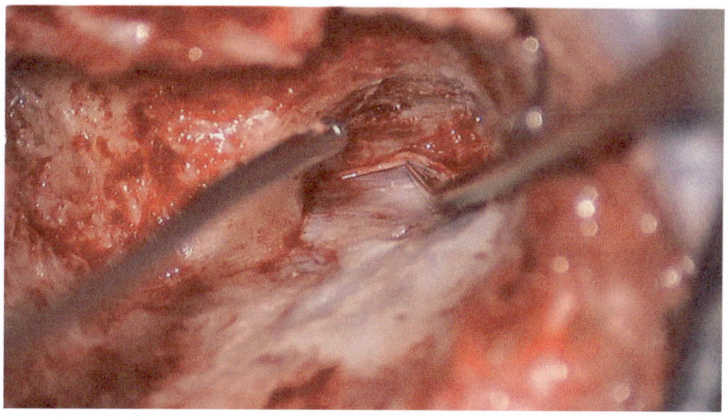

7. A thin piece of Silastic was inserted through the opening. We often cut it into the shape of an *arrow*.

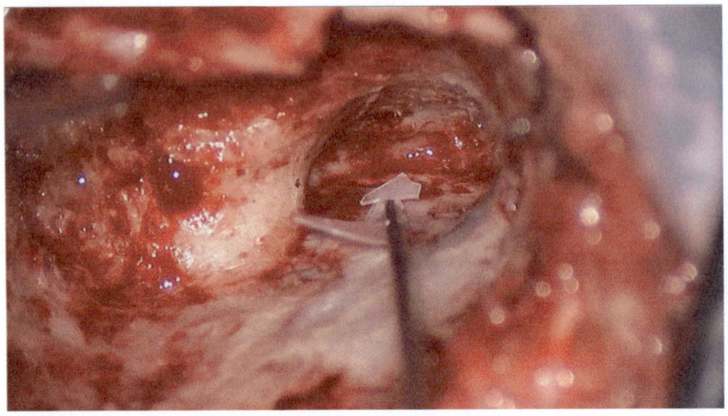

8. The *arrowhead* was inserted into the sac while the tail sat in the mastoid.

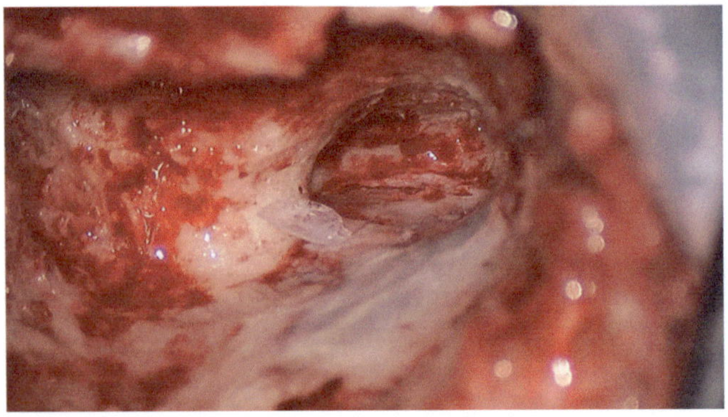

9. Gelfoam was placed around the area, and the mastoid incision is closed.

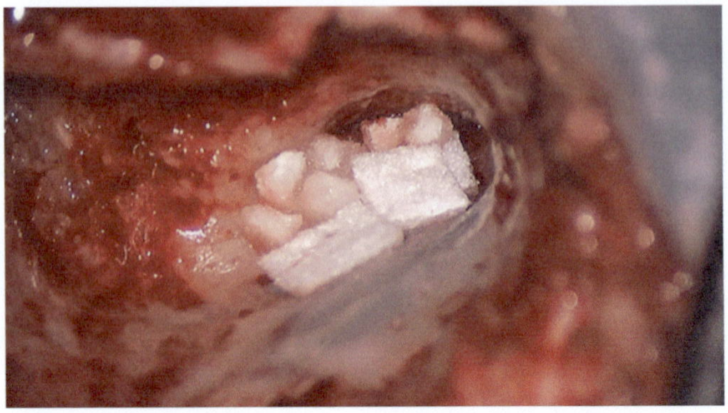

10. Post-op CT demonstrating the extent of bone removal after the procedure. Note that the drilling extended medial to the vertical segment of the facial nerve (*arrow*) to the area of the jugular bulb.

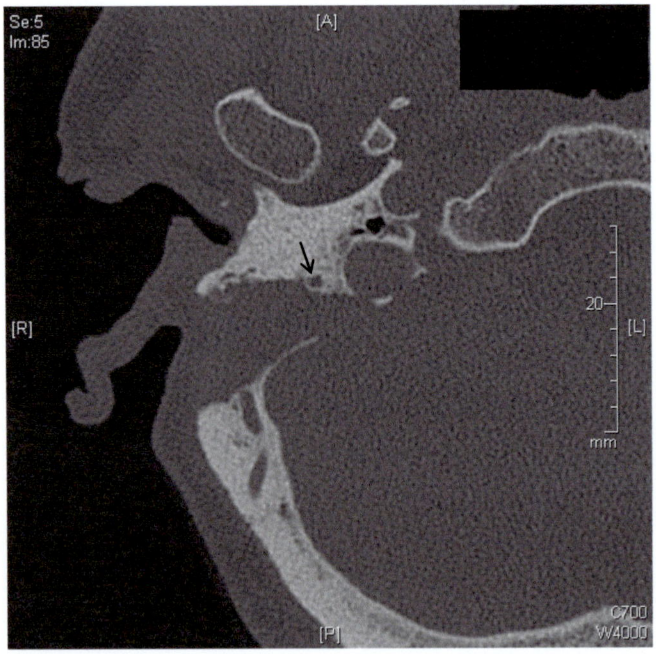

Vestibular Nerve Section

- *Concept*
  - A retrosigmoid craniotomy is performed to visualize CN VIII at the brainstem. The vestibular nerve is sectioned and the auditory nerve preserved.
- *Conditions treated*
  - Meniere's disease refractory to medical management in patients with serviceable hearing
- *Risks*
  - Hearing loss
  - Dizziness
  - Facial nerve injury
  - CSF leak
  - Stroke
  - Oscillopsia if there is also vestibular weakness on the contralateral side
- *Benefits*
  - This is an excellent way to prevent abnormal vestibular signals from being sensed by the brain and producing vertigo.
- *Additional notes*
  - This procedure is currently not as popular as in the past. This is largely because of the adoption of intratympanic gentamicin, which performs a similar function while not requiring a craniotomy and a postoperative stay in the hospital.
  - The surgical approach is the retrosigmoid approach. For details, please see Chap. 4.
  - Intraoperative ABR and facial nerve monitoring should be performed.

11. Retrosigmoid exposure of the cerebellopontine angle. Cranial nerves V, VII, VIII, IX, X, and XI can be seen. CN VII is deep to CN VIII.

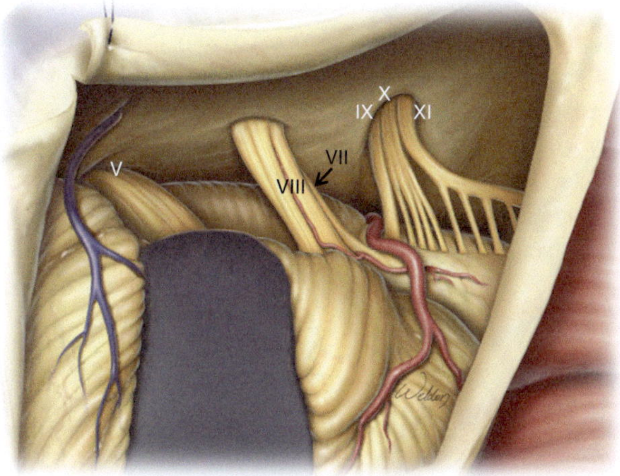

12. Separating the vestibular nerve from the auditory nerve using a straight Rhoton #2 dissector. A Rhoton #11 oblique pick also works nicely. There is typically a very small artery that defines this border. However, it is often difficult to find a specific plane. It is better to err on the side of not cutting all the vestibular nerve fibers rather than to include auditory nerve fibers in the resection. Deep to CN VIII, there is a slightly larger artery that separates CN VIII from CN VII at the brainstem. Care should be taken to minimize trauma to these arteries as one does not want to cauterize in this area. Bleeding can be controlled with Gelfoam and gentle pressure.

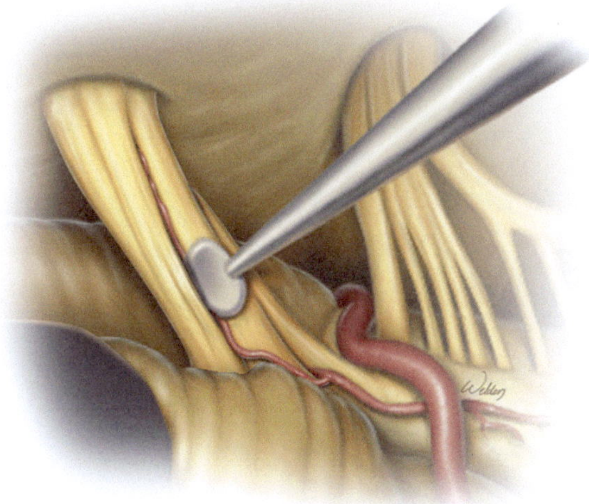

13. After separating the auditory nerve from the vestibular nerve, a microscissors is used to divide the vestibular nerve. In the operating room, it can be tough to remember which branch is the vestibular nerve and which is the auditory nerve. Remember that the vestibular nerve (which begins with the letter V) is closer to CN V (also the letter V). As the nerve is divided, it may become clear that there are additional vestibular nerve fibers that can be gently separated from the cochlear nerve fibers. Keep watching for subtle differences in color and small vessels. After sectioning the nerve and separating the ends or sometimes cutting out a segment, the craniotomy is closed in a standard watertight fashion.

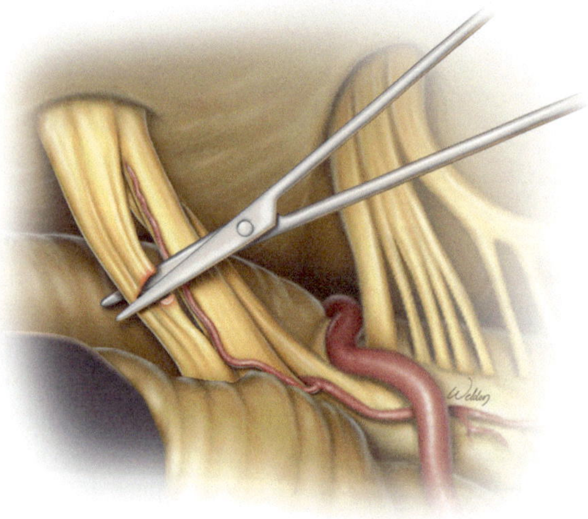

Labyrinthectomy

- *Concept*
  - The vestibular portion of the inner ear is physically drilled away and all neuroepithelial elements removed. Any residual hearing is sacrificed.
- *Conditions treated*
  - Meniere's disease refractory to medical management
- *Risks*
  - Facial nerve injury
  - Oscillopsia if the disease affects the contralateral side
- *Benefits*
  - This is the gold-standard treatment. All vestibular input to the brain from that ear is removed.
- *Additional notes*
  - If the patient is not vertiginous after surgery, he/she may be discharged the same day. However, postoperative care for 1–2 days to treat vertigo is common.
  - Surgical examples of the labyrinthectomy procedure can be found in the translabyrinthine approach section (Chap. 4) and in the temporal bone resection section (Chap. 8).

14. Overview of the bone to be removed (*gray*).

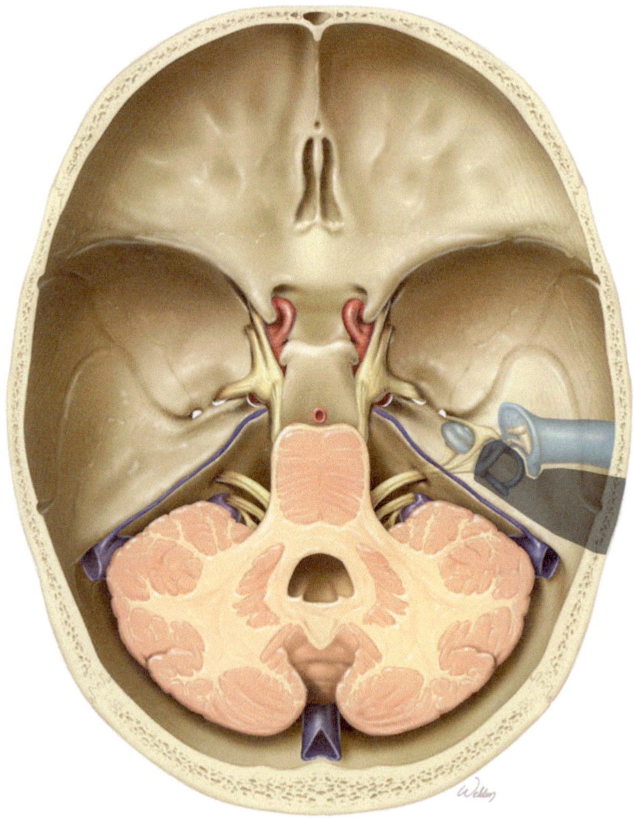

15. A mastoidectomy has been performed and the semicircular canals skeletonized. The labyrinthectomy is begun by opening the lateral canal and following this posteriorly to identify the posterior canal. The superior limb of the posterior canal can then be followed to identify the common crus and superior canal. This systematic approach helps keep the less experienced surgeon oriented.

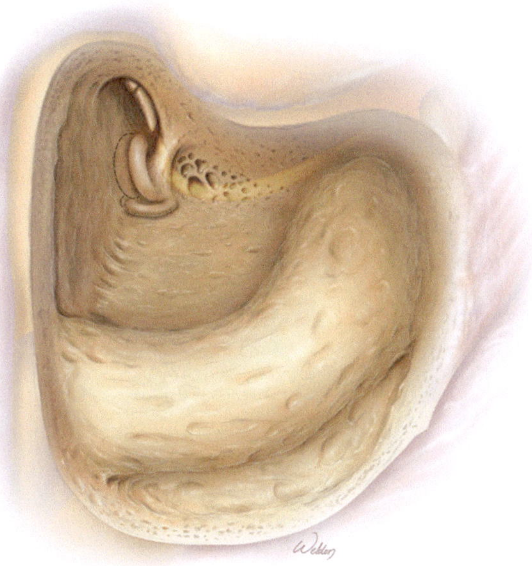

16. The labyrinth has been drilled away, the ampullae removed, and the vestibule opened. Maintaining the inferior aspect of the lateral canal will protect the facial nerve. Preservation of the superior aspect of the superior canal and the posterior aspect of the posterior canal will guard against injury of the dura. Drilling "within the labyrinth" will prevent injury to the bordering structures, the facial nerve and dura. The ampullated limb (inferior) of the posterior canal extends medial to the facial nerve, and it is possible to injure the nerve with the backside of the burr. The contents of the vestibule (the utricle and saccule) should be removed with a Crabtree dissector. Nothing needs to be placed in the mastoid cavity, and there should be no CSF leak. Closure of the skin can then be performed.

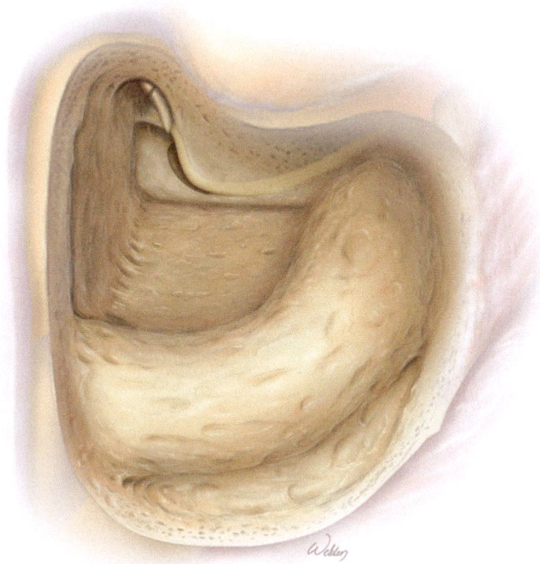

Complications and Additional Thoughts

12

Below are listed additional issues that we have experienced in the past. Hopefully, reading this list will help prevent them from happening to you. If not, perhaps the framework we give will help you in moments of stress.

- Teamwork. We believe in the team concept for skull base surgery, that is, the key combination of a neurotologist and a neurosurgeon. While many of the surgeries described in this book could be done by either type of surgeon solo, having a team provides several advantages. First, these can be long procedures, and it is beneficial to have a partner to trade-off with to rest and to get lunch. Second, discussing the nuances of the case with another person usually leads to better results. Two heads are better at rationally looking at a difficult tumor and deciding how to proceed. Third, having multiple surgeons helps to share the psychological burden of postoperative complications. It is also more fun to have a friend to share the victories.
- Differentiating pathology specimens from grafts. Make sure the scrub nurse knows that the bone flap, abdominal fat graft, etc. will be going back into the patient at the end of the procedure so he/she can label it appropriately. On long cases, as most skull base procedures are, OR staff often rotate in and out of the room. It is easy for them to forget to verbally pass along this information, and so a written label is preferable. One doesn't want the fat graft handed off the table and sent to pathology.
- Bone flap falls on the floor. If the bone flap falls on the floor, the person who dropped it already feels bad enough. Do not make it worse by complaining. If you are the person who dropped it, take a breath, and move on. This is not the end of the world. Some people say to flash sterilize the bone flap, but this is not necessary. Simply soak the bone flap in pure Betadine (the non-soapy version) for ~5 min. Then, rinse it profusely with saline. It can then be used safely. We have had this incident happen and have never had a postoperative wound infection.
- Operating on the wrong side. This is a mistake that cannot be fixed once it has happened. Thankfully, we've never made this mistake, yet we always worry about it. The "time-out" now commonly done in the OR is designed to prevent this issue. Nevertheless, we believe that sharing this responsibility with the family preoperatively is also very helpful. It is good for the attending surgeon to visit with the family in the preoperative holding area before any sedatives are given. The surgeon can verify and mark the operative site personally in full view of the patient and his/her family. The consent should also be double-checked for accuracy at this time. Although there are many "checks" to prevent this from occurring, the ultimate responsibility rests with the surgeon.
- Unexpected postoperative cranial neuropathies, CNS infarcts, deep vein thromboses, pulmonary issues, etc. These complications are very disconcerting to the patient, the family members, and the physician. It is important to maintain a good postoperative relationship with the patient and the family after such a complication. We follow several key steps:
  - Be as sure as possible preoperatively that the patient really needs surgery at this time in their life. Make sure the patient and his/her family know that you are always looking for ways not to operate if at all possible. Then, when surgery is indicated, postoperative complications will be understood to be a result of the disease and not the surgeon's desire to rush a patient to surgery.
  - Make sure the patient and their family members understand clearly why they need surgery.
  - Review the risks carefully and explicitly preoperatively with the patient. Do not minimize the risks.
  - We like to include family members in the preoperative discussion of risks, benefits, and alternatives to surgery. Because they had been involved in the decision-making process preoperatively, this minimizes their surprise if a poor outcome occurs.
  - Even if you have residents/fellows/PAs/NPs/etc., make rounds on your patient who has a complication every day and possibly twice a day when they are in the hospital. It is important to show concern and be there for them during this stressful time. Your attentiveness matters.

J.S. Oghalai, C.L.W. Driscoll, *Atlas of Neurotologic and Lateral Skull Base Surgery*,
DOI 10.1007/978-3-662-46694-0_12, © Springer-Verlag Berlin Heidelberg 2016

- The scrub nurse doesn't have the instrument you need, and you need it NOW. First, RELAX. Next, make a mental note to plan ahead next time and make sure all anticipated instruments and materials are ready at the beginning of the case. Remember coping strategies you were taught to use as a child when in a stressful situation: take a deep breath, count to 10, get up and stretch, don't say anything if you can't say anything nice, etc. Unfortunately, yelling at the nurse doesn't get the instrument into your hand any quicker. This has been tried before, and it doesn't work. While waiting, work on another part of the operation, or if there is nothing else to do, sit nicely and wait. Carry on a conversation with the nurse, your assistant, or the anesthesiologist about something completely unrelated to the surgery; this may take the pressure down a notch. The scrub tech and circulating nurse want the case to go smoothly as much as you do. They like to be well prepared, and it is your job to make sure they understand the procedures and help them anticipate our needs. Having a consistent well-trained team is important. You are responsible for educating and training them.
- Anesthesia issues during surgery such as the patient moving, becoming too hot or too cold, electrolyte imbalances, ventilation issues, etc. As with the missing instrument issue, complaining doesn't help. Respect the anesthesiologist's role, and be prepared to sit and wait. You and your patient will both do better in the long run. However, we do admit that these issues can be particularly frustrating when you have a full OR schedule that day and need to keep things moving. Communication is critical. Know their names; keep them informed about the progress of the case.
- Controlling bleeding from dural sinuses. This is low-pressure bleeding and can be controlled with the application of hemostatic agents (such as Surgicel, Gelfoam, and Flowseal). A cottonoid should then be placed on top of it and gentle pressure applied with a malleable retractor. You can continue the surgery, and after 5–10 min, the malleable can usually be safely removed. By the time surgery is done, the cottonoid can be removed while applying copious irrigation. The hemostatic agent is simply left in place to dissolve. As a general rule, it is safest to never have more than one area bleeding at a time. Arterial or venous bleeding from a single source can always be controlled, but multiple sites may result in loss of visualization and create an unsafe situation.
- Controlling bleeding from larger arteries. This is what you hope never happens, i.e., a tear in the basilar artery or internal carotid artery. Rapid application of Gelfoam wrapped in Surgicel followed by the application of pressure can be used to stop bleeding from small punctures.

  Larger tears or disruptions are more difficult. If arterial resection was not contemplated and planned for before surgery (by performing preoperative balloon occlusion testing with SPECT scanning), the goal should be to reestablish blood flow through the artery. One or more nonpermanent aneurysm clips can be applied to the vessel to stop the bleeding and give you time to decide what to do. Typically, treatment involves getting a vascular neurosurgeon involved to patch the artery or asking interventional neuroradiology to stent the artery. If arterial resection was planned for preoperatively, permanent aneurysm clips can be applied.
- Substantial blood loss. This can be nerve racking when it happens. However, dealing with it is part of being a skull base surgeon as we are often operating around major blood vessels and some tumors are extremely vascular. With current techniques, instrumentation, and experience, this rarely happens.
  - Communicate with your anesthesiologist. He/she can't keep up with continuing blood loss if they don't know about it. You don't want them to have to play "catch-up."
  - If you think a patient may need blood during surgery, remember to have several units typed and cross-matched ahead of time. If you think the patient may need a lot of blood during surgery, also get platelets and FFP ready ahead of time.
  - Repeatedly ask the anesthesiologist to check hemoglobin, PT/PTT, and ionized calcium levels during surgery if you are losing blood. It is critical to keep these levels as close to normal as possible to maintain hemodynamic stability and clotting ability.
  - If the labs get too abnormal or the patient becomes unstable, you may need to halt the procedure and plan for a second stage on another day. There is nothing wrong with this. Ultimately, the patient wants to remain alive and have the problem fixed. Following a philosophy of staged surgery is occasionally needed to accomplish both of these goals.
- High-speed drilling close to vital structures. This is a common technique used in skull base surgery. Supporting the elbow, wrist, or lateral surface of the hand on a rigid surface is helpful in maintaining stability. The irrigating suction can also be used between the drill and the vital structure as a "guard". Lastly, slowing down the drill speed can reduce the potential for the drill to skip out of position. Avoid drilling on edges. Beware of surgical or cottonoid threads that may get wrapped around the spinning drill shaft. An ultrasonic bone removal device can also be used when working in tight areas. Because it doesn't spin, control can be improved.
- Dissecting tumor from brain and cranial nerves. The most important tip is to find and dissect within the correct plane. There should not be very many blood vessels when the correct arachnoid plane is identified between brain

and tumor. Keeping the field free of active bleeding is also important. This allows for accurate visual definition of the plane.

When dissecting tumor off nerves, particularly the facial nerve within the internal auditory canal, finding the correct plane initially at the fundus is critical to being able to remove all of the tumor. Once you get out of the plane and start leaving a thin layer of tumor on the nerve, it is very difficult to find the right plane again. If this happens, you should go back to the fundus, figure out where you lost the plane within the internal auditory canal, and work to reestablish it.

- Approaches to the skull base continue to evolve. Our Rhinology and Head and Neck colleagues have become increasingly ingenious at accessing areas previously not possible. Thoughtful discussions should occur preoperatively to determine what each expert has to offer so risks and benefits of the various approaches can be considered. What are the goals of surgery? What needs to be resected and what is likely going to be left behind? How does the location and extent of residual tumor affect risk of recurrence and radiation options? These are just a few of many aspects to consider. There is often more than one reasonable strategy. Teamwork is essential.
- Debriefing the case. At the conclusion of a case, spend some time reflecting on how it went. Many institutions have instituted a team debriefing which we have found useful. Beyond this, you and your surgical colleagues can review the specific surgical decisions you made and the result. Was the exposure correct and not excessive or limiting? What was a struggle and what was easy? Why? Were you well prepared or did you encounter unanticipated difficulties? Could these have been predicted? Lessons learned?

1. Always identify landmarks prior to the skin incision. It is important to envision what is underneath the skin before you cut so that you don't burn any bridges when opening. For example, if you may need a temporalis flap, you should not cut through it down to the skull during the opening.

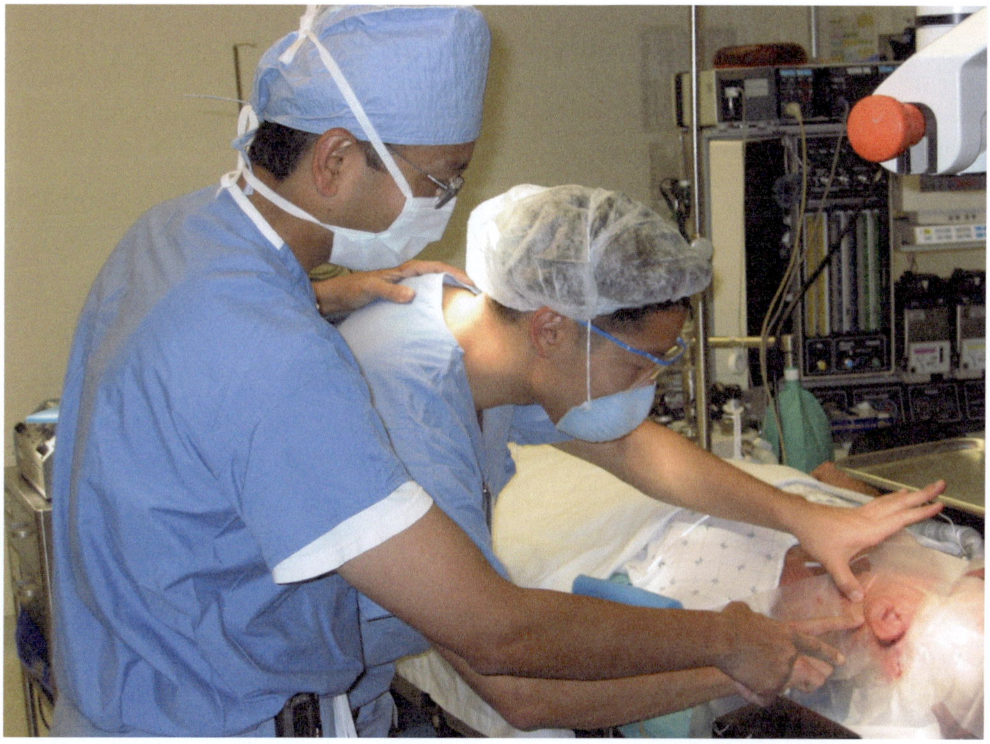

2. Case 1. Don't tie the mastoid dressing too tight. Erosion of the skin can occur and lead to long-term pigment change (*arrows*). Also, when hand-tying knots to hold the mastoid dressing, they should be placed more laterally so that they lie against the temporalis muscle rather than the forehead.

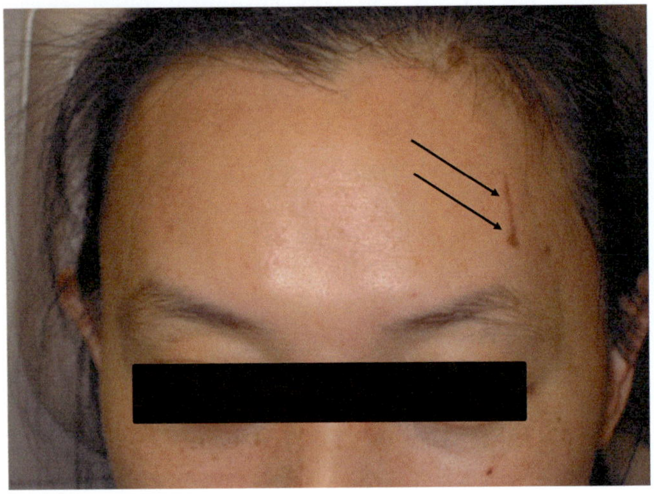

3. Case 2. Tension pneumocephalus after skull base surgery. This patient was blowing his nose shortly after having an orbitocraniozygomatic approach. Air can enter the intracranial cavity through the skull base defect. This typically causes altered mental status. If this happens, the patient should be placed on bed rest, 100 % oxygen, and observed. Surgery may be necessary if hemodynamic instability ensues.

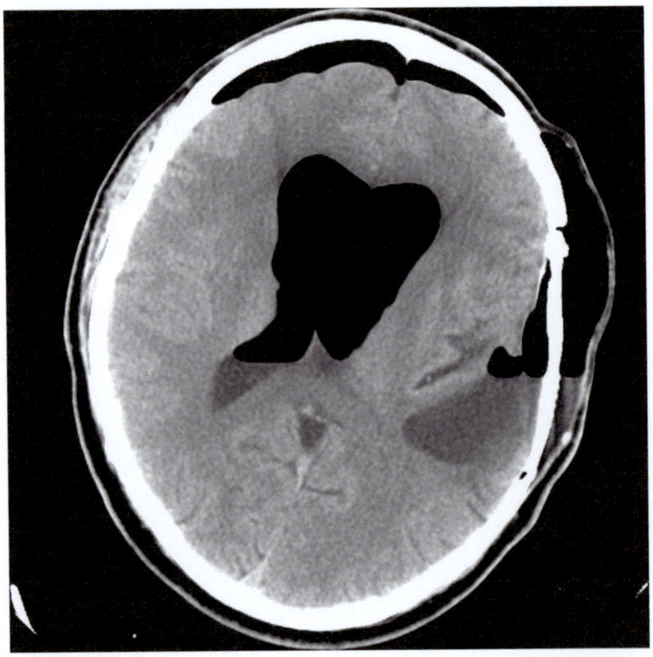

4. A lower cut in the same patient shows the large skull base defect.

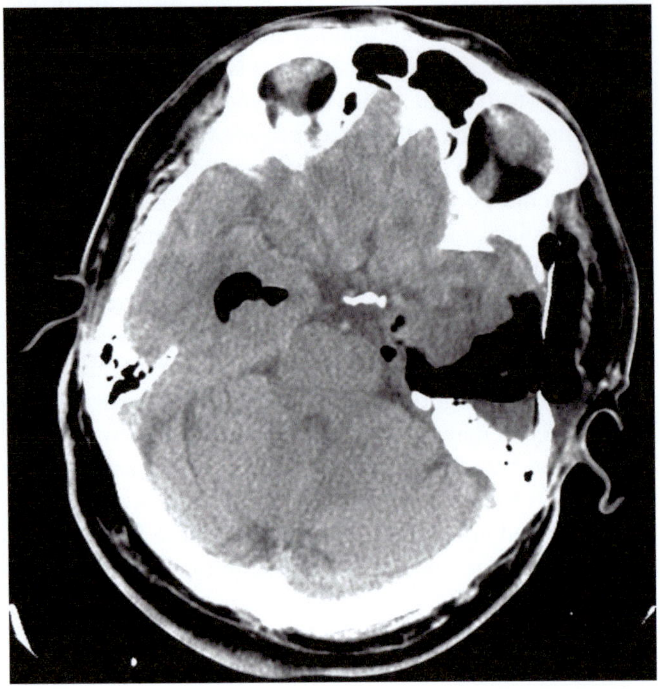

5. Case 3. Vein of Labbe infarct 12 h postoperatively. Acute blood products can be seen within the left temporal lobe.

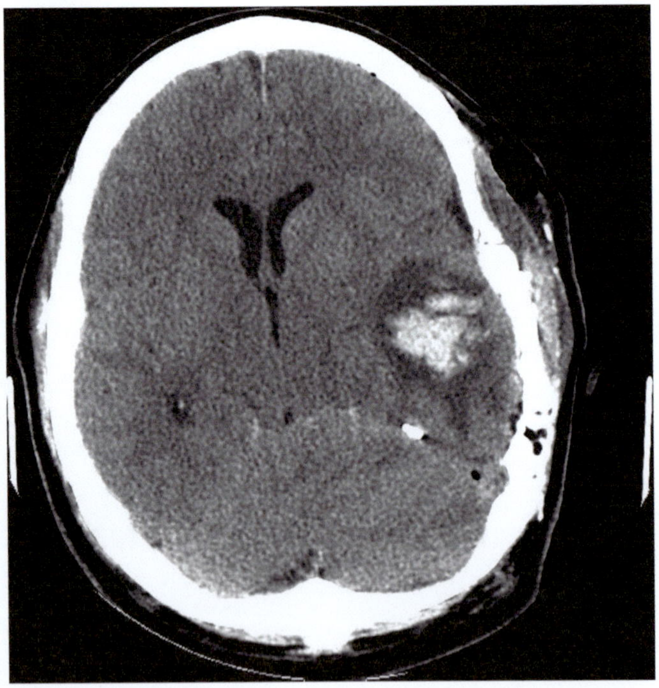

6. The same patient 36 h postoperatively. There was now loss of sulci and intracranial hypertension. The patient expired.

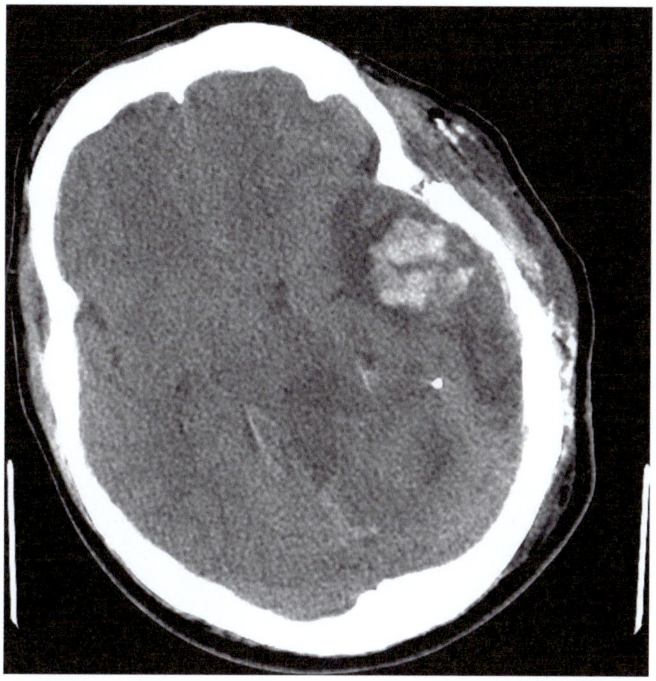

7. Case 4. T1 MRI of a vertebral artery pseudoaneuysm (*arrow*) 9 months after resection of a left vestibular schwannoma via a translabyrinthine approach. He was asymptomatic, and this was found on a routine follow-up MRI to assess for tumor recurrence. It was treated by interventional radiology.

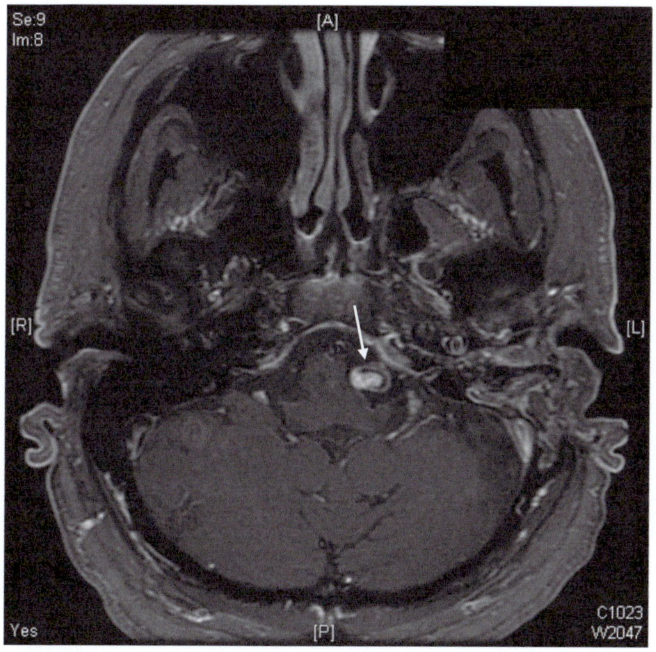

8. T2 MRI of the same patient.

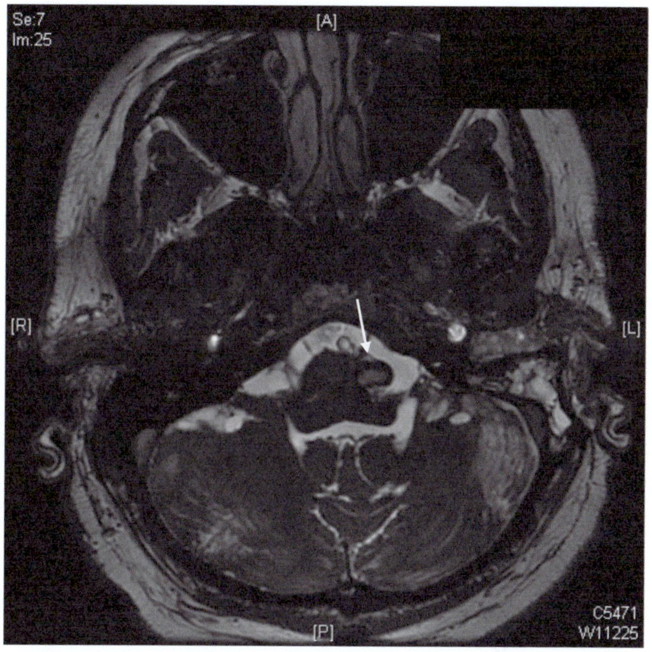

9. Case 5. An aberrant internal carotid artery (*arrow*) was found on axial CT after a white middle ear mass was noted on clinical exam.

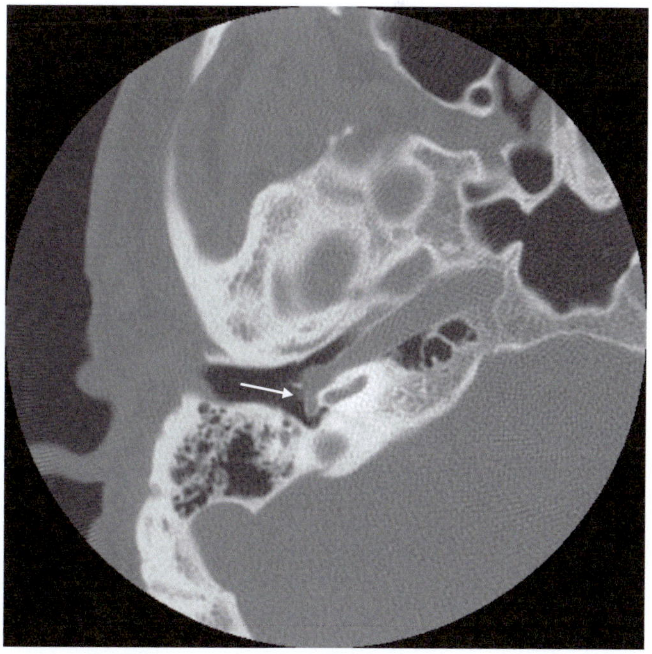

10. Coronal CT of the same patient.

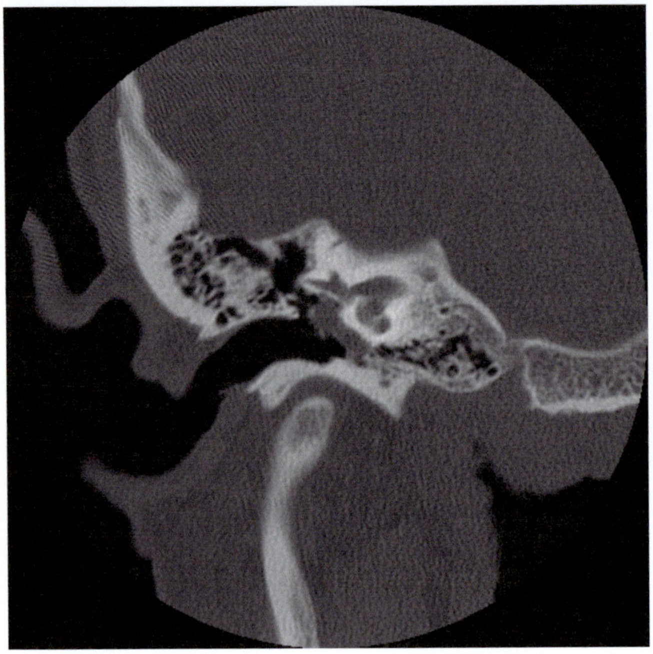

11. Case 6. Dehiscent jugular bulb (*arrow*). This was identified on clinical exam as a purple-colored mass in the hypotympanum.

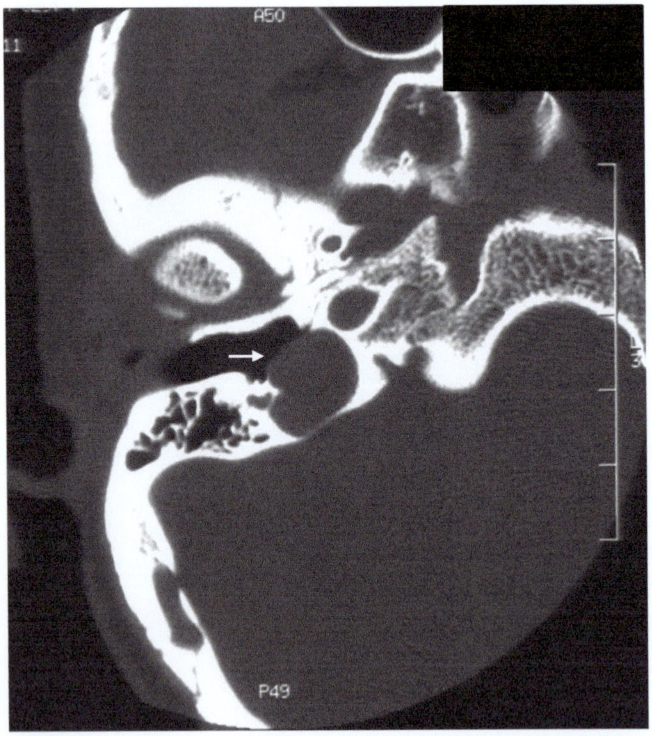

12. Case 7. Merocel in a dehiscent jugular bulb. This child had massive bleeding during routine placement of a pressure equalization tube. The incised dehiscent jugular bulb (*asterisk*) was packed with a Merocel sponge (*arrow*) to stop the bleeding before the patient was transferred to us for care. We removed the sponge the next day, and no bleeding occurred.

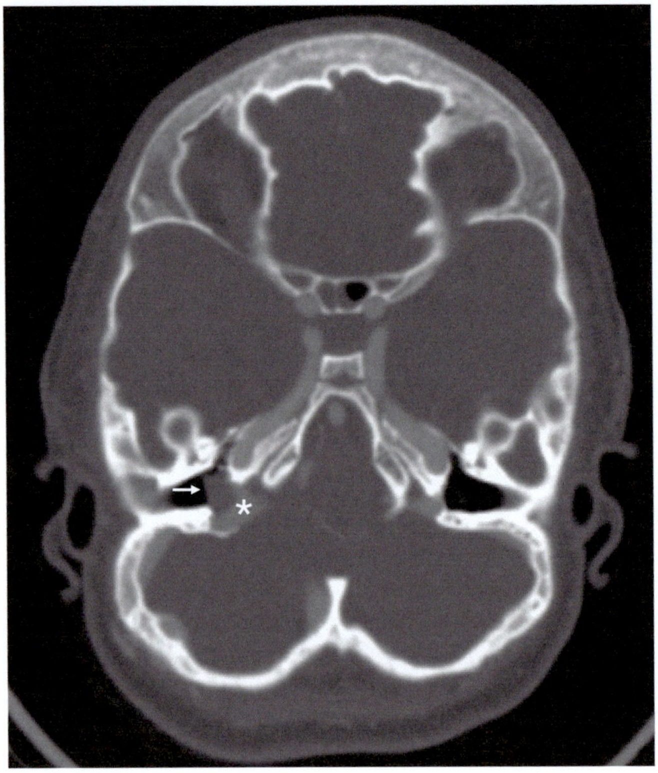

13. Case 8. Make sure your counts are correct at the end of the case! In this skull film taken after closing a large skull base procedure, a cottonoid was left on top of sigmoid sinus. We had to reopen the wound to remove it.

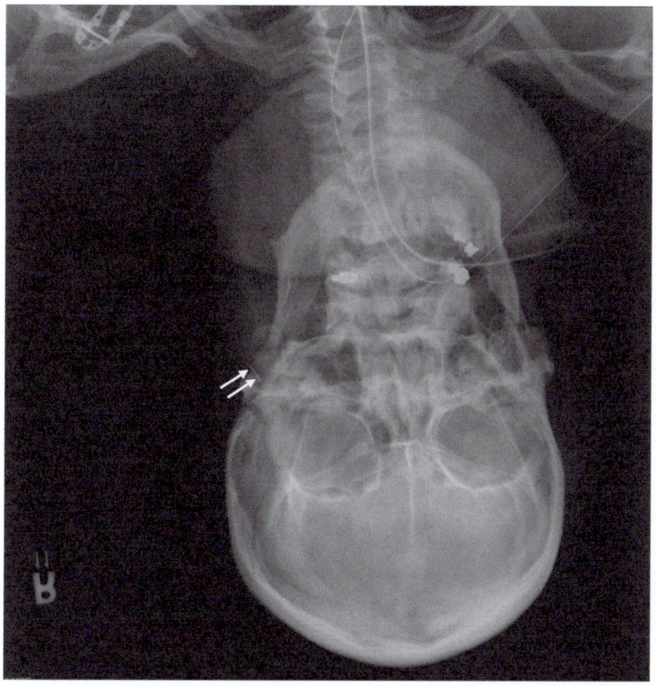

14. Case 9. Good anesthesiology colleagues to manage patient comorbidities. Here, a team of qualified anesthesiologists manage the airway of a patient with morbid obesity and obstructive sleep apnea with awake fiberoptic intubation. A team like this is worth their weight in gold!

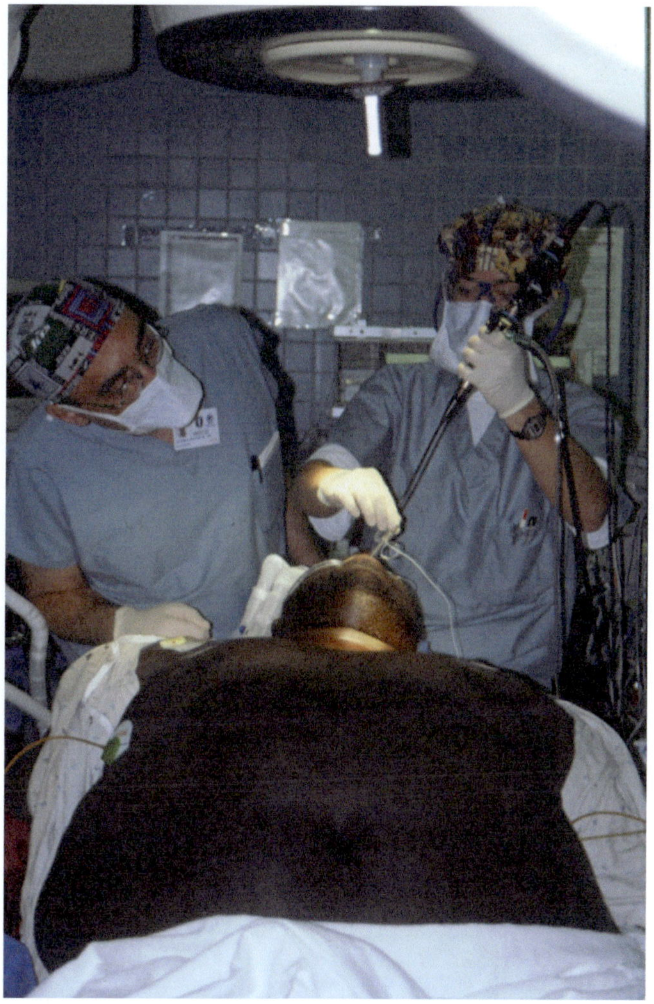

15. The training of residents and fellows is an important component of working in an academic center. Progressive responsibilities can be given to trainees as their skills and knowledge improve. To be a well-rounded skull base surgeon, trainees must be given the opportunity to learn from both the neurotologist and the neurosurgeon. Developing competence in both fields is important to having the best surgical outcomes.

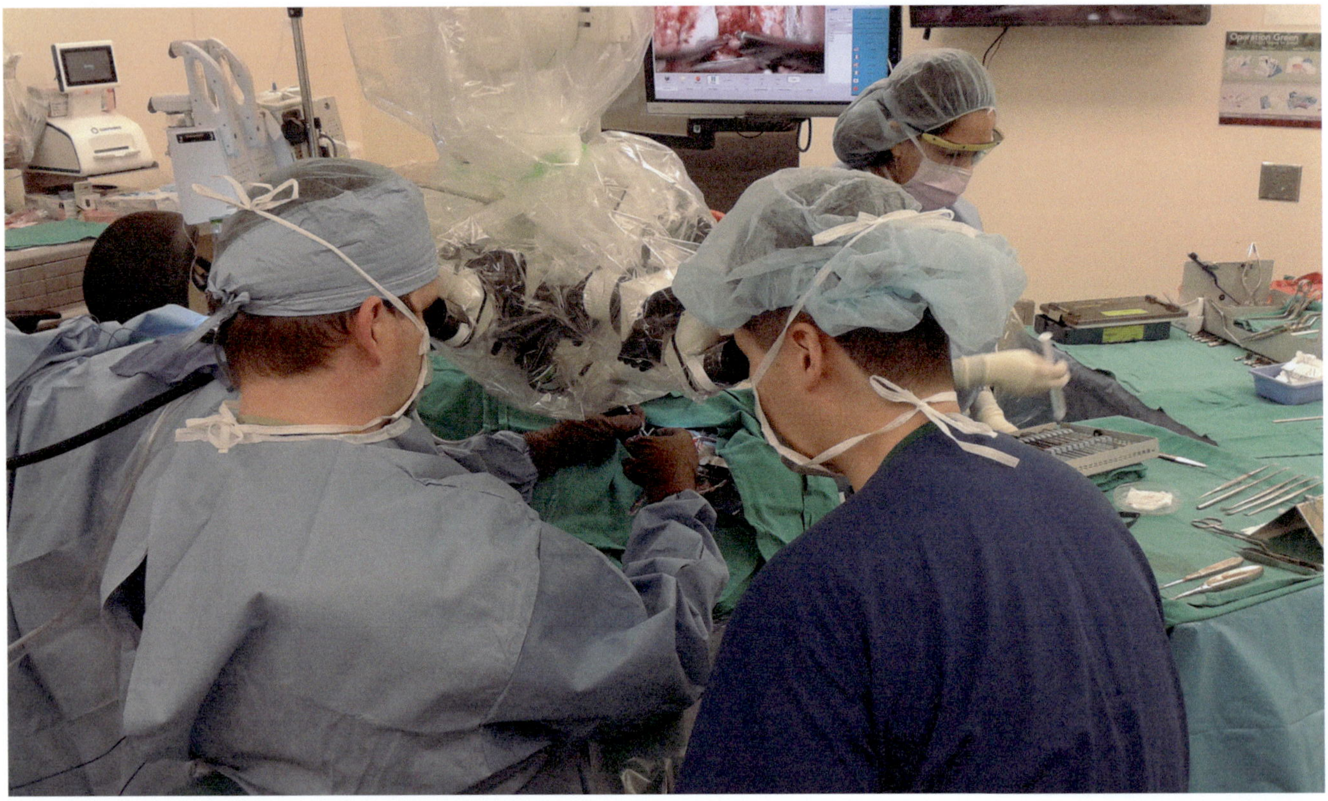

Index

A

Acute mastoiditis
- retrolabyrinthine craniotomy (*see* Retrolabyrinthine craniotomy, acute mastoiditis)
- simple mastoidectomy, 193–195

Adaptic strip use, 91
Auditory nerve (AN), 282

B

Basilar membrane (BM), 245, 282
Bilobed hypoglossal schwannoma, 108–111

C

Cerebrospinal fluid (CSF) management
- flow, 12–13
- lumbar subarachnoid drain (LSAD), 11
- rhinorrhea, 10

Cholesteatoma surgery, 104, 139, 254, 263
- anterior epitympanic region, 272
- canal wall up mastoidectomy, 272
- duckbill elevator, 273
- gadolinium, 272

Cholesterol granuloma (CG), 258
Clival chordoma, teenage boy, 154–160
Cochlear dysfunction, 281
Cochlear implantation, 285
- acute otitis media, 299
- auditory nerve, 282
- axial MRI, inner ear malformation, 293
- BM, 292
- bony island technique, 286
- cochleostomy, 287, 290–292
- concept, 281
- conditions, 281
- coronal CT, 256
- Eustachian tube, 296
- facial recess approach, 283, 284
- hearing loss, 281
- incision, 288
- mastoid, coil electrode, 289
- mastoidectomy, 283, 284
- nasopharynx, 296
- otologic/neurotologic surgery, 285
- PE tube, 301
- perilymph, 290
- periosteal flap, 288
- prepping and draping, 288
- promontory and ST, 292
- risks, 281
- RW insertion, 289–290
- S-shaped postauricular incision, 284
- sigmoid sinus, tegmen and mastoid antrum, 284
- skin flap, 297
- small skin incision, 300
- subcutaneous tissues and temporalis muscle, 284, 297
- SV insertion, 292
- trauma, 298

Cochleostomy insertion, 292. *See also* Cochlear implantation
- bone dust, 291
- round window niche, 290
- ST and PE, 292
- SV, 292

Common cavity insertion
- anterior and posterior cochleostomy, 294
- electrode coils, 295
- inner ear malformation, 293
- temporalis fascia, 294

Complications
- anesthesia issues, 312
- bleeding, 312
- bone flap, 311
- debriefing
  - anesthesiology, 317
  - coronal CT, 316
  - cottonoid, 317
  - dehiscent jugular bulb, 316
  - erosion of skin, 314
  - internal carotid artery, 315
  - intracranial hypertension, 315
  - skin incision, 313
  - skull base defect, 314
  - tension pneumocephalus, 314
  - vertebral artery pseudoaneuysm, 315
- dissecting tumor, 312–313
- drilling, 312
- grafts, pathology specimens, 311
- instrument, 312
- postoperative cranial neuropathies, 311
- teamwork, 311, 313

Computer-guided stereotactic navigation
- Mayfield head holder, 8
- Stealth system, 8

Cranial nerve monitoring
- earphone placement, 10
- hearing preservation middle fossa approach, 9
- orbicularis oculus and oris muscles, activation, 9

J.S. Oghalai, C.L.W. Driscoll, *Atlas of Neurotologic and Lateral Skull Base Surgery*,
DOI 10.1007/978-3-662-46694-0, © Springer-Verlag Berlin Heidelberg 2016

E

Ear canal closure, 241–242, 252–254
Endolymphatic sac tumor
  characteristic, 77
  coronal MRI, 77
  gadolinium-enhanced MRI, 77
  post-op T1 MRI, 78
  post-op T2 MRI, 78
  temporal bone, substantial erosion, 77
  transcochlear resection, 78
  translabyrinthine approach, 71
Endolymphatic shunt
  Beaver blade, 305
  Donaldson's line, 304
  drilling, 305
  endolymphatic hydrops, 303
  LSCC and PSCC, 304
  postauricular incision, 304
  presigmoid posterior fossa dura, 305
  risks and benefits, 303
  silastic piece, 306
  treatment, 303
Epidermoid posterior fossa, 102–104
Epidermoid, cerebellopontine angle
  basilar artery, 120
  CN IV and V, 125
  Duragen, 127
  Malleable retractors, 122
  mastoidectomy, 122
  middle fossa dura, 123, 124
  presigmoid posterior fossa dura, 123
  residual disease, 126
  residual epidermoid, 126
  superior petrosal sinus, 123, 124
  Tegaderms, 121
  Telfa strips, 127
  temporalis fascia, 127
  tentorium, 124
  yellow fishhook retractors, 121
  zygomatic arch, 122
Extracranial hypoglossal schwannoma, 185, 188–189

F

Facial nerve decompression
  anterior horizontal segment, 269
  canal wall up mastoidectomy, 272
  GSPN, 268
  intracranial procedure, 269
  labyrinthine segment (LS), 269
  middle fossa craniotomy, 267
  standard canal wall up mastoidectomy, 266
  stylomastoid foramen, 266
  temporal lobe dura, 267
  transmastoid approach, 269
Facial nerve surgery
  auricular nerve graft harvest, 274, 275, 277
  Bell's palsy, 263
  cholesteatoma, 272–273
  cortical mastoidectomy, 264
  decompression, 265–269
  ENoG testing, 265
  geniculate hemangiomas, 271
  hearing loss, 263
  hearing/non hearing preservation, 265
  House–Brackmann grade function, 263
  interpositional graft, 270
  mastoid cortex, 264
  mucoepidermoid carcinoma, 274
  nerve decompression, 263
  pes anserinus, 277
  primary nerve repair/interpositional nerve grafting, 263
  stapes and round window, 273
  sternocleidomastoid muscle, 277
  sural nerve graft harvest, 274–276
  sural nerve interposition graft, 274
  XII-VII jump graft anastomosis, 276, 277
Far lateral approach
  bilobed hypoglossal schwannoma, 108–111
  bones for removal, 116
  cervical spinal cord dura dissection, 106
  concept, 104
  decompression, 104
  dural opening, 107
  hypoglossal nerve schwannoma, 104, 107
  incision, 105
  left posterior fossa meningioma, 111–114
  malleable retractor, 106
  mastoidectomy, 106
  meningiomas, 104
  retrosigmoid craniotomy, 105
  risks, 104
  rongeur, 106
  soft tissues and periosteum dissection, 105
  Telfa strip, 107
  visualization, 104
Fossa tumor (small right posterior), retrosigmoid approach, 89–98

G

Geniculate hemangiomas
  facial paralysis, 271
  subtotal resection, 271
Gigantic tumor, head and neck, 190–192
Glomus jugulare tumor (aural polyp), 161
Greater superficial petrosal nerve (GSPN), 29, 268

H

Hypoglossal nerve tumors, 113, 183
Hypoglossal schwannoma
  extracranial, 185, 188–189
  left bilobed, 186–188

I

Incudostapedial joint, 235
Inferior petrosal sinus (IPS), 34
Instrumentation
  cochlear implant instruments, 18
  craniotomy set, 16–17
  fat graft set, 18
  House-Urban and Fisch retractors, 15
  neurotology set, 17–18
  skull base surgery, 14
Internal auditory canal approach
  ABR, changes in, 27
  anterior-inferior exposure, 21
  arcuate eminence (AE), 23
  auditory nerve (cochlear nerve, C), 27
  burr hole (BH), 22
  cerebrospinal fluid, 34
  craniotome, 22
  decompression, 25
  evaluation, headaches, 32

facial nerve, 26
FIESTA T2-weighted sequence, 29
GSPN, dissection, 23, 29
hearing preservation, 19
incision choice, 22
labyrinthine course, 19
layout of nerves, 25
Mayfield head holder, 23
middle fossa dura, elevation of, 20
middle meningeal artery (MMA), 23
MRI techniques, 28, 31
petrous apex bone, 32
petrous bone drilling, 28, 30
posterior fossa dura, 24, 25, 31
proximal vestibular nerve (V), 27
retractors, 23–24
risks, 19
superior petrosal sinus (SPS), 23
temporal bone, coronal view, 20
temporal lobe dura, 29
Internal carotid artery (ICA), 255, 256, 258
Intracochlear schwannoma
asymmetric sensorineural hearing loss, 78
fallopian bridge, 79
fat piece, 80
FIESTA T2 MRI, 79
internal auditory canal, 79
post-op T2 MRI, 80
transcochlear approach, 79
Invasive fungal sinusitis, 166–171

J
Jugular bulb (JB), 255, 256, 258

K
Kawase's triangle approach, 217
cholesterol granuloma, 35
fat graft, 35
petrous apex bone, 33, 36
posterior fossa approaches, 33
posterior fossa dura, 34
posterior fossa meningioma, 36
retrosigmoid craniotomy, 36
risks, 33

L
Labyrinthectomy
gold-standard treatment, 308
labyrinth, 309
mastoidectomy, 309
risks, 308
vestibular portion, 308
Lateral semicircular canal (LSCC), 304
Left posterior fossa meningioma, 111–114
Left posterior fossa schwannoma, 139–141
Left vestibular schwannoma with nonserviceable hearing, 62, 70
Luc's abscess, 211

M
Mastoidectomy, 54, 62, 66
erosion of mastoid cortex, 195
myringotomy and placement of pressure equalization, 193
periosteum, elevation, 194
risks, 193
simple mastoidectomy, 194
subperiosteal abscess, 194, 195
Mayfield head holder
Budde Halo system, 4
Greenberg retractor system, 4
head and neck positioning, 7
pinning, 4–6
Medium-sized right vestibular schwannoma, 65–70
Middle and posterior fossa
cerebellopontine angle, 120–128
Circle of Willis, 115, 121
CSF, 119
labyrinthine injury, 115
mastoid and petrous apex, 130
mastoidectomy, 118, 122
petroclival junction, 120
petroclival meningioma, 128–130
retrofacial/retrolabyrinthine exposure, 118
sigmoid sinus curves, 119
superficial tissues, 117
superior petrosal sinus, 115, 123
Telfa strips, 119
temporal lobe dura, 118
tentorium, 119
translabyrinthine approach, 118
trigeminal nerve schwannoma, 118
vein of Labbé, 115
Middle fossa approaches
internal auditory canal, 19–32
Kawase's triangle approach, 33–36
orbitocraniozygomatic approach, 37–50
Middle meningeal artery (MMA), 23
Multicystic vestibular schwannoma, 64

N
Neoplasia. *See* Superior semicircular canal dehiscence

O
Orbitocraniozygomatic approach, 314
artificial dura (DuraGen), 48
benefits, 37
bicoronal incision, 46
bone flap, removal of, 38, 42
burr holes, 38, 42
cavernous sinus meningioma, 48
clinoid process, 39
clivus, erosion, 46
CSF rhinorrhea, 49
debulking, 47
deep temporal fascia, 41
extracranial vascular feeding vessels, embolization, 41
extradural drilling, 43
incision, 37
inflammatory changes, 44
lateral rhinotomy incision, 45
residual tumor, 50
risks, 37
skull base procedures, 41, 47
temporalis muscle (T), 38, 46
transfacial approach, 43
tumor resection, 44, 47
tumor, intracranial extension, 40
zygoma, removal of, 38
Osseous spiral lamina (OSL), 245, 282

Osteomyelitis, skull base. *See* Petrosectomy, subtotal (circumferential)
Otolaryngology residency training, 132
Oval window (OW), 282

P

Petroclival meningioma
 axial T1 MRI, 129
 cerebellopontine angle, 128
 coronal T1 MRI, 129
 internal auditory canal, 128
 jugular bulb, 129
 mastoid and petrous apex, 130
 ventral pons, 128
Petrosectomy, subtotal (circumferential)
 CN VI palsy, 218
 craniotomy bone flap, 217
 facial nerve, 216
 incision, 215
 Kawase's triangle approach, 217
 long-term IV antibiotics, 220
 middle fossa dura, 217
 petrous apex disease, 218–220
 preservation, 214
 risks, 214
 skull base osteomyelitis, 219
 temporalis muscle, 216
 translabyrinthine approach, 216
Petrositis, acute. *See* Petrosectomy, subtotal (circumferential)
Petrous apex lesions
 cholesterol granulomas, 254, 260
 cochlea and jugular bulb, 258
 cyst, 254, 257, 259, 260
 fat suppression techniques, 257, 261
 gadolinium, 257
 hearing preservation, 254
 inferior ear canal bone, 255, 258
 inferior tympanic annulus, 258
 infracochlear approach, 255, 258
 left bilobed cholesterol granuloma, 260
 mild brainstem compression, 260
 outpatient procedure, 254
 pituitary gland, 233
 retrofacial and retrolabyrinthine dissection, 254
 risks, 254
 silastic, 259
 soft tissues, 255
 temporalis fascia, 259
 treatment, 254
 tympanic membrane, 259
 tympanoplasty, 256
Plexiform neurofibroma, 179–181
Postauricular approach
 and preauricular approach, 181
 brain, venous outflow, 132
 canal wall up procedure, 132–134
 cholesteatoma, 139
 clival chordoma, teenage boy, 154–160
 congenital variants, sigmoid sinus, 132
 dissection, 131
 extracranial hypoglossal schwannoma, 181, 185, 188–189
 facial nerve, 131, 132, 184
 fallopian bridge technique, 131
 fossa schwannoma, left posterior, 139–141
 gigantic tumor, head and neck, 190–192
 glomus jugulare tumor (aural polyp), 131, 161
 hypoglossal nerve tumors, 183
 hypoglossal schwannoma, left bilobed, 186–188
 incision, 183
 infratemporal fossa approach, 131, 181
 internal carotid artery, 131
 jugular bulb, exposed, 130
 jugular foramen schwannoma/meningioma, 131
 lateral skull base, 131
 mastoidectomy, 132
 nerves, 182
 otolaryngology residency training, 132
 parapharyngeal space, 162
 recurrent neuroblastoma, child with, 148–153
 risks, 131, 162
 SCM, 132, 184
 skull base meningioma, 141–147
 stylohyoid muscle, 185
 Surgicel, extraluminal packing, 133
 Telfa strips, 145
 transjugular craniotomy, 134
 traverses, mastoid, 131
 vascular supply to head, 182
Posterior fossa approaches
 far lateral, 104–114
 retrosigmoid (*see* Retrosigmoid approach)
 transcochlear, 72–82
 translabyrinthine (*see* Translabyrinthine approach)
Posterior Semicircular canal (PSCC), 304
Preauricular approach. *See also* Postauricular approach
 cavernous sinus tumors, 162
 CN VI palsy, 177–178
 incision, 162
 infratemporal fossa and parapharyngeal space, 162
 invasive fungal sinusitis, 166–171
 juvenile nasopharyngeal angiofibroma, 162
 mandible-splitting approach, 162
 middle ear/jugular bulb, 162
 plexiform neurofibroma, 179–181
 recurrent nasopharyngeal carcinoma, 162
 risks, 162
 styloid process, 163
 temporomandibular joint capsule, 164
 teratoma, upper jugular region, 172–177
 transcervical approach, 162

R

Recurrent glomus jugulare tumor
 Fisch type A approach, 80
 Onyx, 81
 post-op CT, 81, 82
 post-op MRI, 82
 postoperative pseudomeningocele, 82
 T2 MRI, 80
Recurrent meningitis
 and profound left sensorineural hearing loss, 73
 bony defects, well-circumscribed, 75
 canal wall, mastoidectomy, 75
 cochlea removal, 75
 coronal T2 MRI, 74
 facial nerve, 75
 fallopian bridge, 76
 jugular foramen, 74
 labyrinthectomy, 75
 post-op axial CT, 76
 post-op coronal CT, 76

post-op T2 MRI, 76
unusual cystic erosion, 73
Recurrent neuroblastoma, child with, 148–153
Retractors, 52
Retrolabyrinthine craniotomy, acute mastoiditis
abscess/clot/granulation tissue, curettage, 199
axial CT, 200, 206–207
axial MRI, 207
bone removal, 208, 210
cerebral ischemia, 206
clots, 204
cortex of mastoid, 209
cortical mastoidectomy, 224
cottonoid pledget, 205
CSF leak, 200
epidural abscess, 199, 202, 203, 211
erosion of bony cortex, 208
Fogarty catheter, 204
intracranial abscess, 196
intravenous antibiotic therapy, 200
Joseph/Freer elevator, 197
Luc's abscess, 211
malleable retractors, 198
MRI with gadolinium, 201
MRV, 208
otitic hydrocephalus, 206
postauricular incision, 196
posterior cranial fossa subdural abscess, 199
posterior fossa dura, 202, 211
retrosigmoid dura, 197
risks, 196
sigmoid sinus thrombosis, 198, 203, 209–210
simple mastoidectomy, 197
SPECT, 206
subdural abscess, 213
subperiosteal abscess, 208
thrombosis, 201
venous occlusion, 213
Retrosigmoid approach
and transverse sinus (TS), 85, 86
arachnoid mater, 92
bleeding, sigmoid and transverse sinuses, 86
bone removal, 84
bone wax application, 96
debulking, 87, 94
decompression, 86
diamond burrs, 95
epidermoid posterior fossa, 102–104
fossa tumor, small right posterior, 89–98
Gelfoam, 95
hearing preservation approach, 83
incision, 85
internal auditory canal, 86–88
intraparenchymal abscess, 83
jugular foramen schwanommas, 83
malleable, 86
mastoid, 89, 90
meningiomas and posterior fossa tumors, 83
posterior cranial fossa subdural, 83
retrosigmoid dura exposed., 90
Rhoton dissector, 93
risks, 83
sigmoid sinus (SS), 85
skull, 83
Surgicel layer, 97
translabyrinthine approach, 83
vestibular schwannomas, 83, 89, 98–100
watertight closure, 97
Y-shaped dural opening, 91
Yingling stimulator probe, 93
Room layout, 3
Round window (RW) insertion. *See also* Cochlear implantation
facial recess, 289
overhanging bone, 289
perilymph, 290

S

Scala media (SM), 282
Scala tympani (ST), 282
Scala vestibuli (SV) insertion. *See also* Cochlear implantation
cochleostomy, 292
tissue bridging, 292
Skull base meningioma, 141–146
Skull base surgery, 1
Spiral ligament (SL), 282
Stapedial tendon, 235
Stereotactic radiotherapy, 1
Sternocleidomastoid muscle (SCM), 132, 184
Subtotal (circumferential) petrosectomy, 214–220
Superior petrosal sinus (SPS), 23, 34
Superior semicircular canal dehiscence
arcuate eminence, 237
canal plugging, 235
dehiscence, 237
direct view, 235
dura, 236
erosion, bone, 235
fistulas, 235
hydroxyapatite bone paste, 238
incision, 236
malleable retractors, 237
patient with symptomatic, 236
posterior limb, 237
risks, 235
Rosen needle, 237
tegmen, 237
temporalis muscle, 236
transmastoid approach, 235
treatement, 235
Sural nerve graft harvest
direct XII-VII anastomosis, 276
hypoglossal–facial nerve anastomosis, 276
intact and Botox, 275
trigeminal–facial nerve anastamosis, 275
zygomatic branch, 275
Sural nerve interposition graft
multiple interrupted sutures, 274
stylomastoid foramen, 274
Surgical decision-making, 1
Surgicel (S)
and Gelfoam use, 55
postauricular approach, 133
retrosigmoid approach, 97

T

Tectorial membrane (TM), 282
Telfa strips, 119, 127
and cottonoids removal, 61, 67
far lateral approach, 107
postauricular approach, 145

Temporal bone resection
after completion of dural patch, 2
Allis clamp, 345
artificial dural graft, 247
axial CT, extensive bone erosion, 242
BCCA of left pinna, 249
bone wax, 252, 253
bony ear canal, 262
chronic left otorrhea refractory, 242
cochlea, 346
CSF rhinorrhea, 242
dura, 249
ear canal with temporalis muscle, 264
Eustachian tube, 241, 252, 257
exophytic SCCA, 253
extended facial recess approach, 264, 344
external ear canal, 241
facial nerve, 254
fallopian canal bridge, post-op coronal CT, 356
free-flap reconstruction, 253
gadolinium, 222, 224
incus, 264
large venous infarct, 3
lateral temporal bone resection, 229
left small encephalocele, 228
left temporal lobe encephalocele, 230
mastoid and temporalis muscle, 243
mastoid cavity, 230
meatus of ear canal, 243
middle cranial fossa, 241
middle fossa dura, 246
otic antimicrobial drops, 342
parotid gland, 244
patient with mastoid bowl, 228
pedicled trapezius myocutaneous flap, 251
Penfield 4 elevator, 246
periosteum, 252
permits complete resection, 228
pinna, 240
post-op axial CT, 249
postoperative XRT, 228
right temporal lobe encephalocele, 228
risks, 228
SCCA of ear, 242
sigmoid-transverse sinus junction, 250
skin and soft tissues, 249
sleeve resection, 229
specimen, bone erosion, 250
standard canal wall up mastoidectomy, 240, 244
sternocleidomastoid and occipital musculature, 248
subcutaneous tissues, 242
Telfa strip, 248
temporal bone resection with facial nerve, 262
temporalis muscle, 245, 247
tisseal, 247
total temporal bone resection, 365
tragal and conchal cartilages, 253
transcochlear approach, 245
treatement, 228
tumor eroded the tegmen, 243
tumor invasion, inner ear, 244
tympanic membrane, 228
vein of Labbé, 250, 251
vertical segment, 253
Temporal bone surgery
acute mastoiditis
retrolabyrinthine craniotomy (*see* Retrolabyrinthine craniotomy, acute mastoiditis)
simple mastoidectomy, 193–195
acute petrositis/skull base osteomyelitis, 214–220
Temporal lobe encephalocele
after insetting, 231
after removal, 234, 235
asterisk, 224
bipolar cautery, 225
bone graft, 229
brain herniation, 221
canal wall up procedure, 226
cartilage graft, 221
chronic CSF leak, 221
CPAP, 221
craniotomy site, 225
CSF leak, 221, 223
direct and wide exposure, 221
divided and facial ridge lowered, 228
Duragen, 225
dural defect, 227
elevated and bone graft, 230
extradural dissection, 224
Gelfoam, 234
herniated brain, 231
iatrogenic injury, 221
identification and resection, 231
inadvertent injury, 223
incision, 223
intradural patch, 225
malleable retractor in extradural fashion, 229
mastoid antrum, 232
mastoid process, 223
mastoidectomy, 222
meticulous hemostasis, 226
microdissected out of middle ear, 233
middle fossa approach, 235
middle fossa craniotomy, 224, 227
normal coronal view, 221
post-op CSF leak, risk, 226
posterior half, 229
posterior-superior ear canal, 222
reduced and dura closed, 229
removal of, 234
risks, 221
Rosen needle, 245
routine otologic techniques, 228
sagittal T1 MRI, pituitary gland, 241
spontaneous CSF leaks, 221
sternocleidomastoid muscle, 223
superior semicircular canal dehiscence, 233
tegmen, 222
temporalis muscle, 227
titanium plate, 231
tympanic membrane, 227
vascularized muscle flap, 221, 231
Temporomandibular joint (TMJ), 164, 241
Teratoma, upper jugular region, 172–176
Transcochlear approach
bone amount removed, 73
endolymphatic sac tumors, 72, 77–79
fallopian canal, 72

intracochlear schwannoma, 80–83
malignant tumors, 72
parotid gland carcinomas, 72
posterior fossa, 72
recurrent glomus jugulare tumor, 80–82
recurrent meningitis, 73–76
risks, 72
translabyrinthine approach, 72
unusual temporal bone lesions, 72
ventral brainstem and central skull base, 72
Transjugular craniotomy, 134
Translabyrinthine approach, 216, 315
endolymphatic sac tumor, 71
facial nerve, 51
mastoid and semicircular canals, 51
retrosigmoid approach, 51
risks, 51
vestibular schwannoma, 51 (*see also* Vestibular schwannoma)
Trigeminal schwannomas, 115, 118
Tympani tendon (TT), 241
Tympanic membrane (TM), 258

V
Vertigo
endolymphatic shunt, 303–309
nerve section (*see* Vestibular nerve section)
Vestibular nerve section
abnormal vestibular signals, 307
auditory nerve, 307
retrosigmoid craniotomy, 307
Rhoton dissector, 307
risks, 307
treatment, 307
Vestibular schwannoma
capsule dissection, 68
cerebrospinal fluid, release of, 59
coronal view, 65
distal internal auditory canal, 65
endolymphatic duct, 56, 66
facial nerve, 60, 63, 67, 69
fat graft placement, 69
fat saturation, 64
internal auditory canal (IAC), 60, 67, 68
jugular bulb (JB) identification, 58, 66
labyrinthectomy, 57
lateral semicircular canal (LSSC), 66
left, with nonserviceable hearing, 61, 70
mastoid cortex, 53
mastoid emissary vein, 54
medium-sized right, 65–69
moist Telfa pledget, 59
multicystic, 65
porus acusticus (PA) identification, 58
retrosigmoid approach, 89, 98–102
retrosigmoid dura identification, 54
sternocleidomastoid muscle (SCM), 53
subtotal resection, 65, 69, 70
Surgicel and Gelfoam use, 55
T1 MRI without fat saturation, 64
Telfa strips and cottonoids removal, 61, 67
temporal bone drilling, 57
tentorium, 65
tumor capsule, 59
tumor size and location, 53
ultrasonic aspirator, 60

MIX
Papier aus verantwortungsvollen Quellen
Paper from responsible sources
FSC® C105338

If you have any concerns about our products,
you can contact us on
ProductSafety@springernature.com

In case Publisher is established outside the EU,
the EU authorized representative is:
Springer Nature Customer Service Center GmbH
Europaplatz 3, 69115 Heidelberg, Germany

Printed by Libri Plureos GmbH
in Hamburg, Germany